A Clinician's Guide to Pulmonary Fibrosis

A Clinician's Guide to Pulmonary Fibrosis

Edited by Kimberly Dawson

hayle medical

New York

Hayle Medical,
750 Third Avenue, 9th Floor,
New York, NY 10017, USA

Visit us on the World Wide Web at:
www.haylemedical.com

ISBN: 978-1-64647-516-2

Cataloging-in-Publication Data

A clinician's guide to pulmonary fibrosis / edited by Kimberly Dawson.
p. cm.
Includes bibliographical references and index.
ISBN 978-1-64647-516-2
1. Pulmonary fibrosis. 2. Pulmonary fibrosis--Diagnosis. 3. Pulmonary fibrosis--Treatment.
4. Lungs--Diseases. I. Dawson, Kimberly.
RC776 .F5 P85 2023
616.24--dc23

Table of Contents

Preface

Fibrosis is refers to the excessive matrix deposition that results in the impairment of organ function and tissue destruction. It is the end result of chronic inflammatory responses brought on by a variety of stimuli such as autoimmune responses, tissue damage, persistent infections, allergic reactions and radiation. The fibrosis of lung tissue is known as pulmonary fibrosis. Some of its prominent symptoms are fatigue, shortness of breath, aches in joints and muscles, and clubbed toes or fingers. It can lead to a variety of medical complications such as respiratory failure, pulmonary hypertension, lung cancer, and other lung complications. There are various tests which can be used to diagnose pulmonary fibrosis. These include pulse oximetry, echocardiogram, chest X-ray, and pulmonary function testing. This book is compiled in such a manner, that it will provide in-depth knowledge about pulmonary fibrosis. It aims to shed light on some of the unexplored aspects of this disease. A number of latest researches have been included to keep the readers up-to-date with the global concepts in this medical condition.

All of the data presented henceforth, was collaborated in the wake of recent advancements in the field. The aim of this book is to present the diversified developments from across the globe in a comprehensible manner. The opinions expressed in each chapter belong solely to the contributing authors. Their interpretations of the topics are the integral part of this book, which I have carefully compiled for a better understanding of the readers.

At the end, I would like to thank all those who dedicated their time and efforts for the successful completion of this book. I also wish to convey my gratitude towards my friends and family who supported me at every step.

Editor

1

Myeloid Fbxw7 Prevents Pulmonary Fibrosis by Suppressing TGF-β Production

Jia He[1,2†], Yue Du[1,2†], Gaopeng Li[1,2†], Peng Xiao[1,2], Xingzheng Sun[1,2], Wenjun Song[1,2], Lihua Lai[1,2], Meng Xia[1,2], Jianhua Zhang[3] and Qingqing Wang[1,2*]*

[1] *Institute of Immunology, Zhejiang University School of Medicine, Hangzhou, China,* [2] *The Key Laboratory for Immunity and Inflammatory Diseases of Zhejiang Province, Hangzhou, China,* [3] *Department of Medical Laboratory, School of Medicine, Shaoxing University, Shaoxing, China*

***Correspondence:**
Qingqing Wang
wqq@zju.edu.cn
Jianhua Zhang
sxzjh1018@126.com

†*These authors have contributed equally to this work and share first authorship*

Idiopathic pulmonary fibrosis (IPF) is a group of chronic interstitial pulmonary diseases characterized by an inexorable decline in lung function with limited treatment options. The abnormal expression of transforming growth factor-β (TGF-β) in profibrotic macrophages is linked to severe pulmonary fibrosis, but the regulation mechanisms of TGF-β expression are incompletely understood. We found that decreased expression of E3 ubiquitin ligase *Fbxw7* in peripheral blood mononuclear cells (PBMCs) was significantly related to the severity of pulmonary fibrosis in IPF patients. Fbxw7 is identified to be a crucial suppressing factor for pulmonary fibrosis development and progression in a mouse model induced by intratracheal bleomycin treatment. Myeloid cell-specific *Fbxw7* deletion increases pulmonary monocyte-macrophages accumulation in lung tissue, and eventually promotes bleomycin-induced collagen deposition and progressive pulmonary fibrosis. Notably, the expression of TGF-β in profibrotic macrophages was significantly upregulated in myeloid cell-specific *Fbxw7* deletion mice after bleomycin treatment. C-Jun has long been regarded as a critical transcription factor of *Tgfb1*, we clarified that Fbxw7 inhibits the expression of TGF-β in profibrotic macrophages by interacting with c-Jun and mediating its K48-linked ubiquitination and degradation. These findings provide insight into the role of Fbxw7 in the regulation of macrophages during the pathogenesis of pulmonary fibrosis.

Keywords: IPF – idiopathic pulmonary fibrosis, TGF-β, Fbxw7, macrophage, c-Jun

INTRODUCTION

Idiopathic pulmonary fibrosis (IPF) is a lung disease characterized by fibroblast hyperproliferation and extracellular matrix (ECM) deposition (1), which can cause pulmonary fibrosis and eventually lead to respiratory failure. However, the etiology of IPF remains unclear. Transforming growth factor-β (TGF-β) is one of the best-characterized pro-fibrotic factors (2). In mammals, there are three isoforms of TGF-β (TGF-β1, TGF-β2, and TGF-β3), of which TGF-β1 most closely related to the development of IPF (2). Disturbances of the pulmonary microenvironment induced by TGF-β are critical to promote the recruitment of circulating fibrocytes and bone marrow–derived progenitor cells to the lung (3), and enhance the pro-fibrotic capacities of these cells or induce their differentiation into activated myofibroblasts (4), eventually leading to the typical IPF symptoms like ECM deposition and abnormal collagen accumulation (5). Moreover, TGF-β1 induces macrophage recruitment and stimulates the expression of several pro-inflammatory and profibrogenic cytokines in macrophages, such as TNF-α and IL-1β (5). IPF patients have much higher TGF-β1 mRNA expression in profibrotic macrophages compared to normal volunteers (6, 7). Previous studies have reported that TGF-β1 expression can be induced by cytokines, such as IL-1β, TNF-α (8), IL-13 (9, 10) and IL-24 (11), the increased generation of ROS also induces TGF-β1 production (12). Moreover, the activation of TGF-β1 in fibrotic disorders can be induced by multiple factors, such as matrix metalloproteinases (MMP) 3 and MMP9 (13), thrombospodin-1 (14) and integrins $\alpha_V\beta_6$ (15). TGF-β1 signaling pathways and their downstream signal transduction mechanisms have been extensively studied, but there are few reports involved in the regulation mechanism of TGF-β1 expression.

Pulmonary macrophages derived from blood monocytes and classified into $CD64^+SiglecF^+$ alveolar macrophages (AMs) and $CD11b^+CD206^+$ interstitial macrophages (IMs) based on the different anatomical locations (16), both of those macrophage subsets derived from blood monocytes have been known to play a crucial role in IPF pathogenesis. Pulmonary macrophages polarized into alternatively activated anti-inflammatory phenotypes to promote tissue repair and fibrosis after lung injury (17). Aberrant immune function of anti-inflammatory macrophages present profibrogenic phenotypes, which induce the dysfunction of wound repair and accumulate in fibrotic lung, further support fibrogenesis of lung by generating reactive oxygen species (ROS) (6), contributing to collagen synthesis and ECM remodeling. Increased accumulation of profibrotic AMs have been detected in lung of IPF patients (6). During lung fibrogenesis, profibrotic macrophages release soluble factors to create and sustain the profibrotic lung microenvironment (18–20), such as TGF-β1, CCL8 (21), IGF-I (22), PDGF (23), and arginase 1 (24). In contrast, loss of profibrotic macrophages promotes the resolution of established pulmonary fibrosis (25) and the reduction of lung collagen deposition (26). Importantly, in rodents with bleomycin-induced lung fibrosis, pulmonary macrophages have been demonstrated to be the predominant source of profibrogenic mediator TGF-β (27). However, the specific mechanism of TGF-β1 secreted by macrophages in the pathogenesis of IPF is remain poorly understood.

F-box and WD repeat domain–containing 7 (Fbxw7) is a member of the F-box protein family, which is a component of the SKP1-cullin-F-box-protein (SCF) ubiquitin ligase complex. Many studies have shown that Fbxw7 is a tumor suppressor by targeting c-Myc, Notch, MCL1 and c-Jun (28). Fbxw7 mutation was detected in squamous cell carcinoma developed on IPF (29). Fbxw7 also participates in the regulation of Parkinson's disease (30) and circadian rhythm (31). Moreover, Fbxw7 controls neural stem cell differentiation (32) and myelination (33). Fbxw7 has immunoregulatory capacities, it controls effector T cell polyfunctionality and survival in tumor environment by inhibiting Notch activation (34). Our previous studies have shown that Fbxw7 enhances antiviral innate immune response (35) and aggravate intestinal inflammation (36). These observations implicate that Fbxw7 may act as a transducer of tissue microenvironment, regulating the plastic function of macrophages. In this work, we further investigated the function of Fbxw7 in pulmonary macrophages during the pathogenesis of IPF. Our findings demonstrate that *Fbxw7* expression decreased significantly in peripheral blood mononuclear cells (PBMCs) of IPF patients and lung tissues of the mice model of bleomycin-induced fibrosis. *Fbxw7* deletion in myeloid cells increased the release of fibrogenic factors and the recruitment of monocytes into lung tissues. In terms of the mechanism, the *Fbxw7* deletion promoted the TGF-β expression in macrophages through reducing c-Jun ubiquitination, thereby aggravating the severity of pulmonary fibrosis.

MATERIALS AND METHODS

Mice Information

$Fbxw7^{fl/fl}$ mice (C57BL/6J background) were obtained from Jackson Laboratories. *LysM-Cre* mice C57BL/6J were kindly provided by Dr. Ximei Wu (Zhejiang University School of Medicine, Hangzhou, China). $LysM^+Fbxw7^{fl/fl}$ mice were generated by crossing $Fbxw7^{f/f}$ mice with *LysM-Cre* transgenic mice as previously described (36). All mice were bred at the laboratory animal center of Zhejiang University under specific pathogen-free conditions. In all experiments, age-matched (8-12 week) mice were randomized into the experimental or control groups. All animal experiments were performed according to the protocol approved by the Animal Ethics Committee of Zhejiang University and were in compliance with institutional guidelines.

Cell Culture and DNA Transfection

Bone marrow cells were isolated by flushing femurs and tibias of 6- to 8-week-old mice with PBS and differentiated into BMDMs in RPMI-1640 medium with 10% (vol/vol) FCS and 10 ng/ml recombinant mouse M-CSF (R&D, 416-ML). To induce M2 macrophages, BMDMs were stimulated by adding the recombinant mouse IL-4 (30 ng/ml, PeproTech, 214-14). Proteasome inhibitors MG132 (M8699), protein synthesis inhibitor CHX (C4859), and JNK inhibitor SP600125 (420119) were from Sigma-Aldrich. TGF-β neutralizing antibody (MAB1835) and mouse IgG1 isotype control (MAB002) were from R&D systems.

Mouse embryonic fibroblast cell line (MEF) was obtained from American Type Culture Collection (ATCC) and maintained in Dulbecco's modified Eagle medium (DMEM) with 10% fetal bovine serum (FBS; BI). Murine macrophage-like RAW264.7 cells were cultured in RPMI 1640 medium with 10% fetal bovine serum (FBS; BI), 100 U/ml penicillin and 100 mg/ml streptomycin in an atmosphere of humidified 5% CO_2 at 37°C.

Recombinant vectors encoding mouse c-Jun (NM_010591) were cloned into pcDNA3.1-c-Myc eukaryotic expression vector. The RAW264.7 cells (3×10^5 cells/well, in 24-well plate) were incubated with NATE^{TM} (*In vivo*gen, lyec-nate) for 30 min to enhance the transfection efficiency and transient expression of target plasmid. Then RAW264.7 cells were transfected with c-Jun plasmid (Roche, FuGENE HD Reagent) and treated with IL-4 for the indicated time.

Co-Culture Experiments

MEF cells (2×10^5) were cultured in the lower chamber and macrophages (5×10^5) were added to the upper chamber of a 12-well transwell apparatus (0.4 mm pore size, Costar, Cambridge, MA). The MEF were subjected to the further analysis at 48 h after co-culturing.

Induction of Pulmonary Fibrosis

An experimental pulmonary fibrosis model was established using the direct endotracheal injection of bleomycin (37). Briefly, 6- to 8-week-old C57BL/6 mice were anesthetized with pentobarbital by intraperitoneal injections. Neck area of mice was sterilized using povidone-iodine swabs after depilation of hairs, and 1 cm midline incision was made with sterile scissors. Intratracheal administration of 3.5 mg/kg bleomycin hydrochloride (Hisun-Pfizer Pharmaceuticals, Taizhou, China) in sterile PBS, an equal volume of sterile PBS for controls by using 1 ml syringe fitted with a 26 G needle (carefully insert the needle into the visualized trachea and rapidly inject the bleomycin solution during a single inspiration). The incision was closed with surgical sutures after withdrawing the needle. The mice were placed on warmer pads and monitored until fully awake. Mouse lung tissues were sacrificed at 14 days and 21 days post-bleomycin injection for subsequent experiments.

LPS induced pulmonary injury model (38, 39) were established using the direct endotracheal injection of 5 mg/kg LPS (Sigma-Aldrich, St. Louis, Missouri, USA). Mouse lung tissues were sacrificed at 10 days post-LPS injection for subsequent experiments.

Flow Cytometry

Cells were stained with fluorochrome-labeled mAbs and analyzed with an LSRII flow cytometer (BD). Flow cytometric analysis was performed using FlowJo software. The following fluorochrome-labeled mAbs were purchased from Biolegend, Inc. and used according to the manufacturers' protocols: anti-CD11b-FITC (101205, RRID: AB_312788), anti-CD206-APC (141707, RRID: AB_10896057), anti-Ly6C-APC-Cy7 (128026, RRID: AB_10640120), anti-Ly6G-PE (127608, RRID: AB_1186099), anti-F4/80-Brilliant Violet 421 (123132, RRID: AB_11203717), anti-CD64-PE (139303, RRID: AB_10613467), and anti-Siglec-F-APC (155507, RRID: AB_2750236).

Immunoprecipitation and Immunoblot Analysis

Immunoprecipitation, SDS-PAGE and immunoblot analysis were performed according to a standard protocol as described previously (35). The following antibodies were used according to the manufacturers' protocols: anti-Fbxw7 (Abcam, ab12292, RRID: AB_442966), anti-Lys48-specific linked polyubiquitin (MilliporeSigma, 05-1307, RRID: AB_1587578), anti-c-Jun (CST, #9165S, RRID: AB_2130165), anti-p65 (CST, #8242, RRID: AB_10859369), anti-p-p65 (CST, #3036, RRID: AB_331281), Collagen-I(Abcam, ab34710, RRID: AB_731684), Collagen-III (Abcam, ab7778, RRID: AB_306066), EGR-1 (CST, #4154S, RRID: AB_2097035). The PVDF membranes were incubated with corresponding primary antibodies followed by horseradish peroxidase-linked secondary antibodies. The images were developed and captured using Chemiluminescence imaging system (ChemiScope 3000 Mini, Clinx Science Instruments Co., Ltd). Relative quantities of target protein were determined comparing to β-actin expression using densitometric analysis (ImageJ 1.52v). The standard deviation was calculated for biological duplicates.

Lung Histology

Lungs from bleomycin-treated or control mice were dissected, fixed in 10% phosphate-buffered formalin, and embedded into paraffin. Tissue sections were stained with H&E for morphological analysis and with Masson's trichrome for the detection of collagen fibers according to the manufacturers' instructions (Nanjing Jiancheng, Nanjing, China). The Szapiel's score was used to evaluate the severity of fibrosis using the following criteria (40): none (0), no evidence of fibrosis; mild (1), <20% of the lung affected; moderate (2), 20%–50% affected; severe (3), >50% affected.

Hydroxyproline Assay

To assess collagen synthesis in the lung, pulmonic hydroxyproline levels were determined using a hydroxyproline assay kit obtained from Jiancheng Bioengineering Institute (Nanjing, China), according to manufacturer's instructions. Hydroxyproline content was expressed as μg/mg lung wet weight.

Quantitative RT-PCR

Total RNA was extracted from tissues or cells using RNAiso Plus (TakaRa), and then reversely transcribed to cDNA using the PrimeScript RT reagent kit (TaKaRa) with random primers according to the manufacturer's instructions. Quantitative PCR was performed using KAPA SYBR Green (SYBR Green Fast qPCR Master Mix) on CFX96 Touch^{TM} Real-Time PCR Detection System (BioRad). Expression data were normalized to the mRNA levels of the β-actin gene and calculated using the $2^{-\Delta\Delta Ct}$ method (41). The sequences for primers were listed in **Supplementary Table 1**.

ELISA

The levels of mouse TGF-β in bronchoalveolar lavage fluid (BALF) or culture supernatants were measured with ELISA kits (Invitrogen, 88-8350-88) according to the manufacturer's instructions.

Statistical Analysis

Statistical analysis was performed with GraphPad Prism 7.0. All data are shown as mean ± SD. The comparisons of two experimental groups were determined using an unpaired, 2-tailed student's t-test. Multiple comparisons were assessed by one-way ANOVA with Tukey's multiple comparisons test. P-values less than 0.05 were considered significant.

RESULTS

Decreased Expression of *Fbxw7* Is Related to IPF

We first investigated whether Fbxw7 was related to the development of IPF, the expression level of *Fbxw7* from IPF patients was analyzed in the data from Gene Expression Omnibus (GEO) database (GSE70867) (42). The result showed that *Fbxw7* mRNA expression in bronchoalveolar lavage (BAL) cells of IPF patients was significantly lower than that in healthy controls (**Figure 1A**). In another database of microarray expression profiling of PBMCs from IPF patients in the training cohort (GSE132607) (43), *Fbxw7* mRNA expression level in 12-months IPF patients was significantly lower than that in baseline, 4-months, and 8-months IPF patients (**Figure 1B**). We then used the bleomycin-induced mouse model of pulmonary fibrosis to observe the expression of *Fbxw7* in lung tissues (**Figure 1C**) and peripheral blood monocytes (**Figure 1D**). qRT-PCR results showed that the expression level of *Fbxw7* was significantly reduced after 21 days of intratracheal bleomycin administration compared to the PBS controls. Moreover, the expression of *Fbxw7* in the macrophages in mice pulmonary fibrosis tissue was markedly decreased compared with those in healthy control subjects detected by immunofluorescence staining (**Figure 1E**). These results suggest that the decreased expression of Fbxw7 is associated with the formation of pulmonary fibrosis.

Myeloid Deficiency of *Fbxw7* Aggravates Bleomycin-Induced Collagen Deposition in Lung Tissue

Augmented collagen deposition within the interstitium (44, 45) and the remodeling of ECM (46) are recognized as one of the primordial pathophysiological events of IPF. To investigate the role of Fbxw7 in macrophages in the pathogenesis of IPF, we generated LysM-Cre$^+$Fbxw7$^{fl/fl}$ (*LysM$^+$Fbxw7$^{fl/fl}$*) mice (**Supplementary Figure 1A**) and confirmed that myeloid

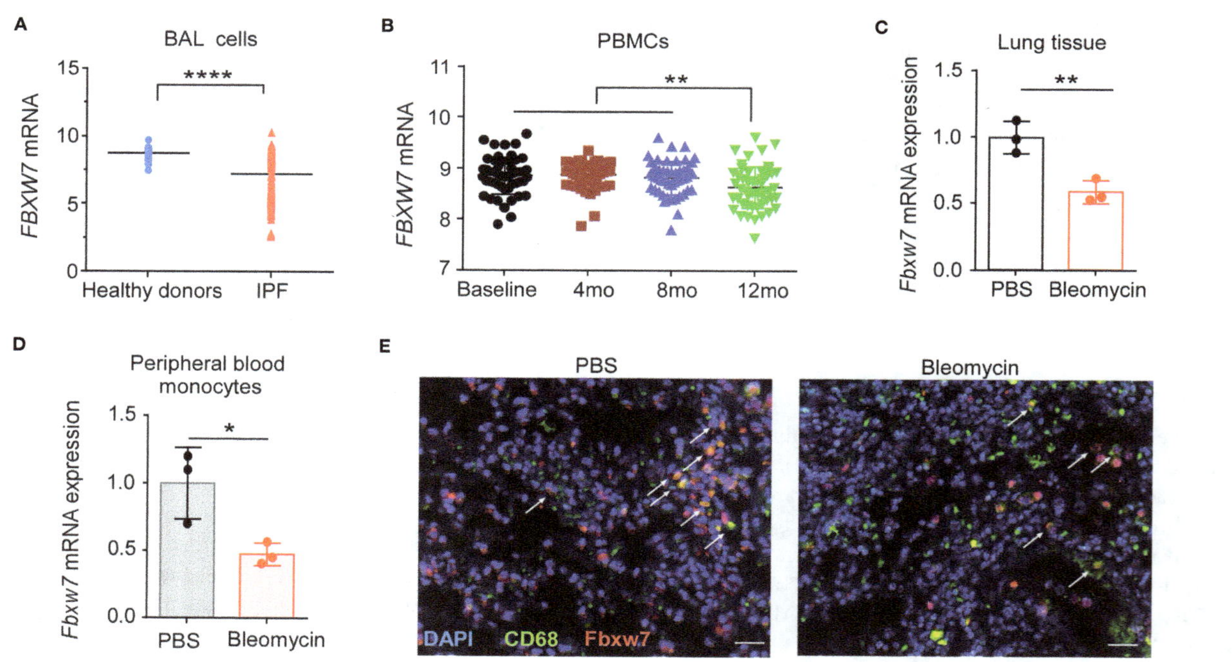

FIGURE 1 | Decreased Fbxw7 expression is related to pulmonary fibrosis. **(A)** Fbxw7 mRNA expression in bronchoalveolar lavage (BAL) cells from healthy donors (n=48) and from IPF patients (n=176), the data were collected from GEO database (GSE70867), P value was obtained using two-tailed Student's t test, ****P < 0.0001. **(B)** *Fbxw7* mRNA expression in PBMCs from baseline (n=74), 4 months (4 mo, n=74), 8 months (8 mo, n=68) and 12 months (12 mo, n=60) IPF patients, the data were collected from the GEO database (GSE132607). Statistical significance was assessed by one-way ANOVA with Tukey's multiple comparisons test, **P < 0.01. qRT-PCR analysis of lung tissues **(C)** and peripheral blood monocytes **(D)** obtained from mice after 21 days of bleomycin-induced lung injury and healthy controls. Data are expressed as mean ± SD of biological duplicates (n=3) and are representative of three independent experiments. P value was obtained using two-tailed Student's t test, *P < 0.05, **P < 0.01. **(E)** Immunofluorescence staining for FBXW7 (red), CD68 (green), and DAPI for nuclei (blue) in lung tissues obtained from mice after 21 days of bleomycin-induced lung injury and healthy control mice. Scale bars: 20 μm. Data shown are the representative of three independent experiments.

specific deletion of *Fbxw7* does not affect the differentiation and development of myeloid cells (**Supplementary Figures 1B-F**).

LysM$^+$*Fbxw7*$^{fl/fl}$ mice and their *Fbxw7*$^{fl/fl}$ littermates were subjected to establish experimental pulmonary fibrosis model. Masson staining of lung tissues showed that collagen deposition was significantly increased in *LysM*$^+$*Fbxw7*$^{fl/fl}$ mice 14 days after bleomycin administration, compared with *Fbxw7*$^{fl/fl}$ *mice* (**Supplemental Figure 2A**), and further increased after 21 days (**Figure 2A**). Szapiel scores also showed that Fbxw7 knockout exacerbated the degree of fibrosis (**Supplemental Figure 2B** and **Figure 2B**). The expression of collagen III and α-SMA observed by immune-histochemical staining was also significantly higher in the fibrotic lung tissue of *LysM*$^+$*Fbxw7*$^{fl/fl}$ mice compared with *Fbxw7*$^{fl/fl}$ littermates (**Figure 2C**). Furthermore, *LysM*$^+$*Fbxw7*$^{fl/fl}$ mice had significantly higher levels of hydroxyproline in lung tissues compared with *Fbxw7*$^{fl/fl}$ mice (**Figure 2D**).

Moreover, we examined the mRNA expression levels of collagen-related genes in the lung tissues after bleomycin administration. Fibronectin 1 (Fn1), a pro-fibrotic marker, is an important member of the fibronectin family (47). Col1α1 and

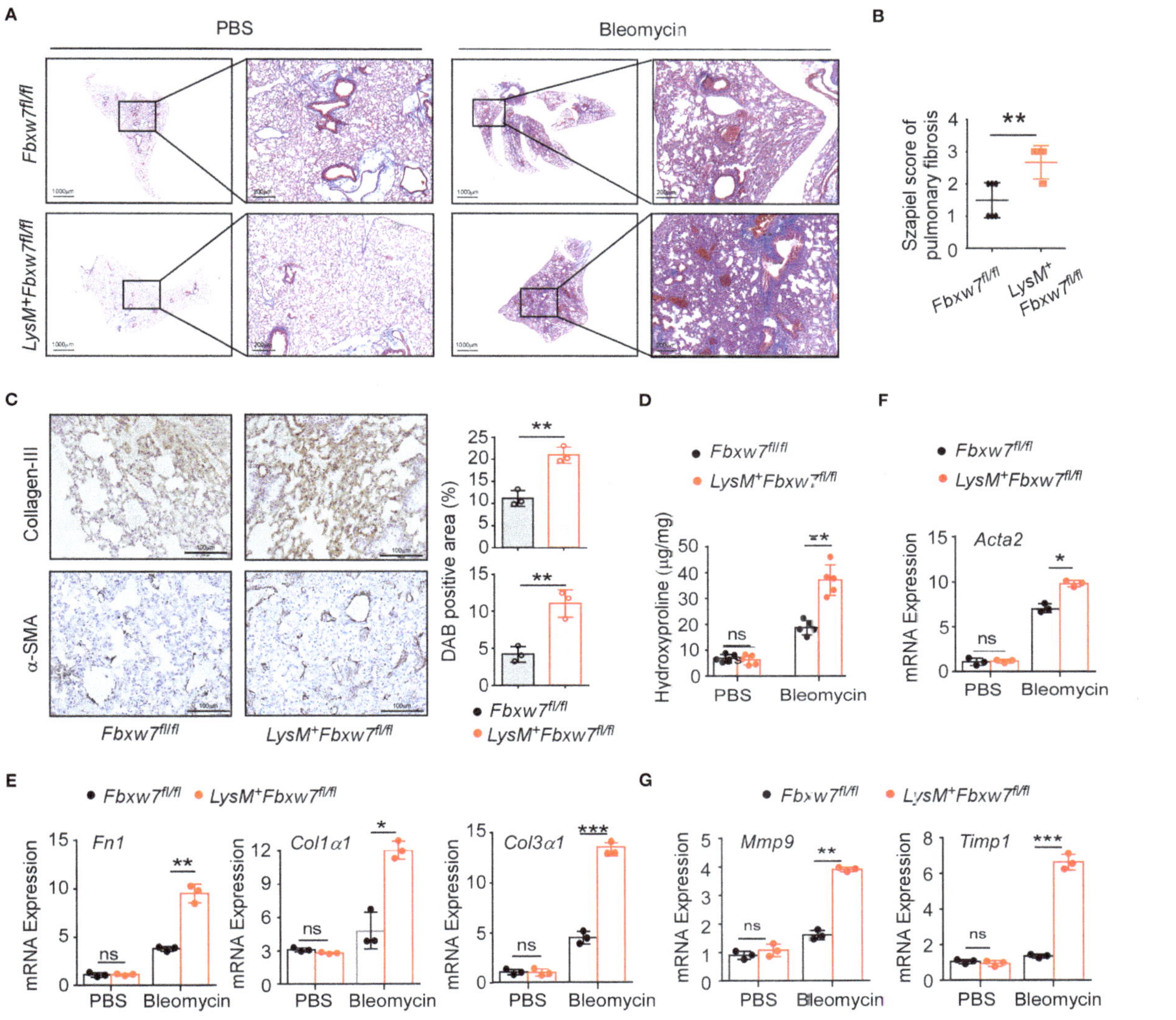

FIGURE 2 | *LysM*$^+$*Fbxw7*$^{fl/fl}$ mice show aggravated pulmonary fibrosis. *Fbxw7*$^{fl/fl}$ and *LysM*$^+$*Fbxw7*$^{fl/fl}$ mice were administered bleomycin by direct endotracheal injection to induce pulmonary fibrosis. Three weeks later, lung tissues were isolated for Masson staining and RT-PCR analysis. **(A)** Masson staining of collagen fiber, scale bars 1000 μm (whole pulmonary section), and 200 μm (detail) and sapiel score of pulmonary tissue **(B)** obtained from *Fbxw7*$^{fl/fl}$ and *LysM*$^+$*Fbxw7*$^{fl/fl}$ mice. **(C)** Representative collagen III and α-SMA immunohistochemical staining of lung tissues obtained from *Fbxw7*$^{fl/fl}$ and *LysM*$^+$*Fbxw7*$^{fl/fl}$ mice after 21 days of bleomycin-induced lung injury, scale bars 100 μm. Comparison of DAB staining intensity (Image J) among the groups is shown. Quantification of hydroxyproline contents **(D)** and relative mRNA expression of collagen genes **(E)**, Acta2 gene (α-SMA) **(F)**, and matrix metalloproteinases **(G)** in the lungs from *Fbxw7*$^{fl/fl}$ and *LysM*$^+$*Fbxw7*$^{fl/fl}$ mice after bleomycin treatment for 21 days. Data are expressed as mean ± SD of biological duplicates (n≥3) and are the representative of three independent experiments. P values were obtained using two-tailed Student's *t* test. $^*P < 0.05$, $^{**}P < 0.01$, $^{***}P < 0.001$, ns, not significant.

Col3α1 is component of the ECM in IPF. qRT-PCR results showed that the expression of *Fn1* and *Col3α1* increased significantly in *LysM⁺Fbxw7^fl/fl^* mice (**Supplemental Figure 2C** and **Figure 2E**). Furthermore, as a surface molecular marker of myofibroblasts, the mRNA expression of α-smooth muscle actin (*α-SMA* or *Acta2*) was also significantly increased in *LysM⁺Fbxw7^fl/fl^* mice (**Supplemental Figure 2D** and **Figure 2F**). Matrix metalloproteinases (MMPs) and their specific inhibitors (tissue inhibitors of metalloproteinases, TIMPs) participate in the formation and degradation of ECM, and the imbalance between MMPs and TIMPs plays a pivotal role in pulmonary fibrosis pathogenesis. qRT-PCR results demonstrated that *Fbxw7* deletion significantly increased the expression of *Mmp9* and *Timp1* (**Figure 2G**). These results suggest that the myeloid cell specific *Fbxw7* knockout mice have increased collagen deposition in their lung tissue that may aggravate the degree of fibrosis induced by bleomycin.

Myeloid Deficiency of *Fbxw7* Aggravates Bleomycin-Induced Lung Injury and Monocytes Recruitment

Tissue damage and inflammation are important triggers for pulmonary fibrosis (48). To determine whether *Fbxw7* deletion in myeloid cells aggravates lung injury and inflammation, we evaluated the morphological characteristics in mouse lung tissues. The H & E staining results showed that the lung tissues of *Lysm⁺Fbxw7^fl/fl^* mice were more severely damaged 14 days (**Supplemental Figure 3A**) and 21 days (**Figure 3A**) after bleomycin administration. Lung tissues of *LysM⁺Fbxw7^fl/fl^* mice appeared to be denser, congestion and edema, as well as loss of alveolar structures compared with *Fbxw7^fl/fl^* mice. Moreover, we examined the mRNA expression of surfactant protein-D (*Sftpd*) and qRT-PCR results showed that myeloid deficiency of *Fbxw7* resulted in higher levels of *Sftpd* in fibrotic lung tissues (**Supplemental Figure 3B** and **Figure 3B**).

Furthermore, *LysM⁺Fbxw7^fl/fl^* mice had higher degree of inflammatory cell infiltration in the alveolar space observed by H & E staining (**Figure 3A**). Flow cytometric analysis was used to investigate the changes in mononuclear phagocyte subpopulations in bronchoalveolar lavage fluid (BALF) and lung tissue during pulmonary fibrosis development. After 21 days of bleomycin-induced pulmonary fibrosis in mice, *Fbxw7* knockout did not increase $CD64^+SiglecF^+$ AMs accumulation (**Supplemental Figure 3C**), but significantly increased $CD11b^+Ly6C^+$ monocytes recruitment (**Figure 3C**) in BALF. Moreover, a single-cell suspension was prepared by digesting lung tissues and analyzed by flow cytometry. Compared with the PBS group, the percentages of $CD11b^+CD206^+$ IMs (**Figure 3D**) and $CD11b^+Ly6C^+$ monocytes (**Figure 3E**) in lung tissues of mice treated with bleomycin were increased. Importantly, *LysM⁺Fbxw7^fl/fl^* mice showed an obviously increased accumulation of IM and monocyte cell populations compared with *Fbxw7^fl/fl^* littermates (**Figures 3D, E**). These results suggest that the deletion of *Fbxw7* exacerbates injury-induced lung fibrosis by promoting the recruitment and accumulation of mononuclear phagocytes.

Fbxw7 Deficiency Upregulates TGF-β Expression in Macrophages

Macrophages are the major source of multiple profibrotic mediators in pulmonary fibrosis (49). We next investigated whether myeloid *Fbxw7* deletion altered the cytokine profile in fibrotic lung tissues. The qRT-PCR results showed that the mRNA expressions of *Tnf-α*, and *Il1β* in lung tissues of *LysM⁺Fbxw7^fl/fl^* mice was significantly higher than that of *Fbxw7^fl/fl^* mice 14 days after bleomycin administration, but the expression of *Il6* and *Il10* was not significantly different (**Supplemental Figure 4A**). In contrast, *LysM⁺Fbxw7^fl/fl^* mice had significantly higher levels of *Il6* and *Il1β*, but not *Tnf-α* and *Il10*, compared with *Fbxw7^fl/fl^* mice 21 days after administration of bleomycin (**Supplemental Figure 4B**). Furthermore, we evaluated cytokines expression in alveolar macrophages and found that the mRNA expressions of *Il1β*, *Tnf-α*, *Il6* and *Il10* were significantly increased after bleomycin administration, however, there were no significant differences in the expression level between *LysM⁺Fbxw7^fl/fl^* mice and *Fbxw7^fl/fl^* littermates (**Figure 4A**). Interestingly, mRNA expression of *Tgfb1*, the macrophage-derived fibrogenic cytokine, was significantly increased in lung tissues and alveolar macrophages in *LysM⁺Fbxw7^fl/fl^* mice compared to *Fbxw7^fl/fl^* littermates (**Figure 4B**). ELISA further confirmed that the concentration of TGF-β protein in BALF from *LysM⁺Fbxw7^fl/fl^* mice was significantly higher than that from *Fbxw7^fl/fl^* littermates (**Figure 4C**). In lung injury model established by LPS, more severe lung injury, fibrosis associated collagen deposition as well as higher expression of *Tgfb1* were found in lung tissue and BAL cells from *LysM⁺Fbxw7^fl/fl^* mice compared to *Fbxw7^fl/fl^* littermates (**Supplemental Figures 4C, D** and **Figure 4D**). The significantly elevated concentration of TGF-β protein in BALF and serum from *LysM⁺Fbxw7^fl/fl^* mice was observed by ELISA compared with that from *Fbxw7^fl/fl^* littermates (**Figure 4E**). These data suggest that deficiency of *Fbxw7* in macrophages exacerbates pulmonary fibrosis, which may be related to the up-regulation of TGF-β expression.

IL-4, as a Th2 cytokine, was reported to induce TGF-β expression in profibrotic macrophage to activate fibroblasts and promotes extensive tissue fibrosis (50, 51). qRT-PCR confirmed that the expression of *Il4* was abundant in fibrotic lung tissues, but the level of *Il4* was similar between *LysM⁺Fbxw7^fl/fl^* mice and their *Fbxw7^fl/fl^* littermates (**Supplemental Figure 4E**). Next, we performed a Transwell co-culture assay to evaluate the profibrogenic capability of macrophages from *LysM⁺Fbxw7^fl/fl^* mice and *Fbxw7^fl/fl^* littermates after IL-4 treatment *in vitro* (**Figure 4F**), the results consistently showed that myeloid *Fbxw7* deficiency resulted in higher secretion levels of TGF-β in co-cultured macrophages after IL-4 treatment (**Figure 4G**), *Fbxw7* deficient macrophages treated with IL-4 mediates a higher activation of co-cultured fibroblasts by the examination of the expression levels of collagen-I and collagen-III through western blot (**Figure 4H**). To further confirm that the enhanced profibrogenic capability of macrophages from *LysM⁺Fbxw7 ^fl/fl^* mice is TGF-β-dependent, transwell co-culture assay was performed after IL-4 treatment with or without TGF-β neutralizing antibody. Neutralization of TGF-β abrogated the

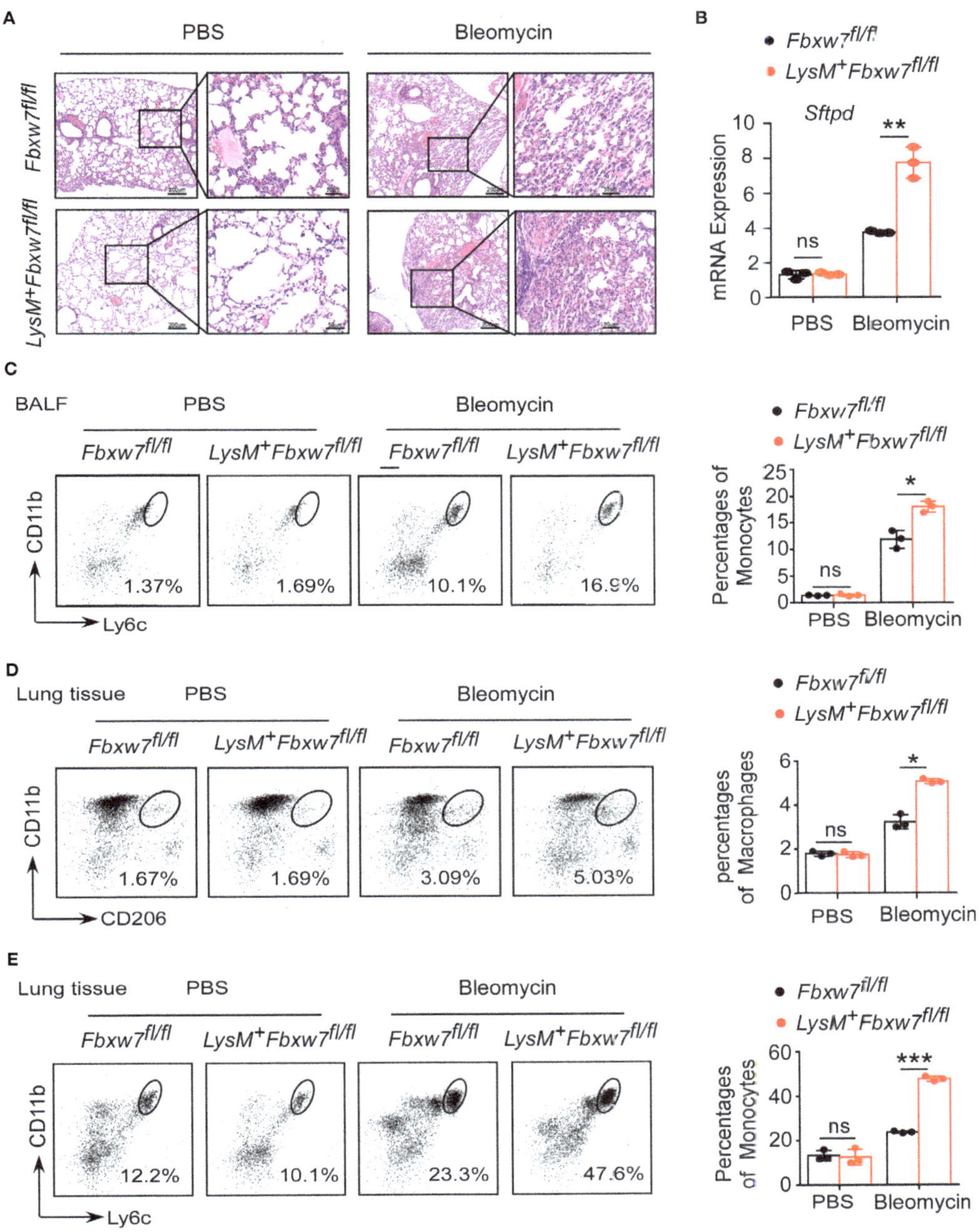

FIGURE 3 | *Fbxw7* deficiency increases recruitment of monocytes and macrophages after bleomycin-induced lung injury. *Fbxw7*$^{fl/fl}$ and *LysM*$^{+}$*Fbxw7*$^{fl/fl}$ mice were administered PBS or bleomycin for 21 days to induce pulmonary fibrosis. **(A)** H&E staining of lung sections, scale bars 200 μm (whole pulmonary section), and 50 μm (detail). **(B)** qRT-PCR analysis of relative expression of *Sftpd* in lung tissue. Flow cytometry and statistical analysis of the percentage of CD11b^{+}Ly6C^{+} monocytes in bronchoalveolar lavage fluid (BALF) **(C)**, CD11b^{+}CD206^{+} IMs **(D)** and CD11b^{+}Ly6C^{+} monocytes **(E)** in lung tissues, data are expressed as mean ± SD of biological duplicates (n=3) and are the representative of three independent experiments. P values were obtained using two-tailed Student's *t* test. $^{*}P < 0.05$, $^{**}P < 0.01$, $^{***}P < 0.001$, ns, not significant.

difference of profibrogenic ability between *LysM*$^{+}$*Fbxw7*$^{fl/fl}$ macrophages and *Fbxw7*$^{fl/fl}$ macrophages (**Figure 4I**). Collectively, these data further support that *Fbxw7* deletion in myeloid cells can exacerbate bleomycin-induced production of TGF-β and promote the development of pulmonary fibrosis.

Fbxw7 Regulates TGF-β Expression by Mediating the Ubiquitination and Degradation of c-Jun

Transcription factors including early growth response protein 1 (EGR-1) (52, 53) and NF-κB (54) have been reported to be

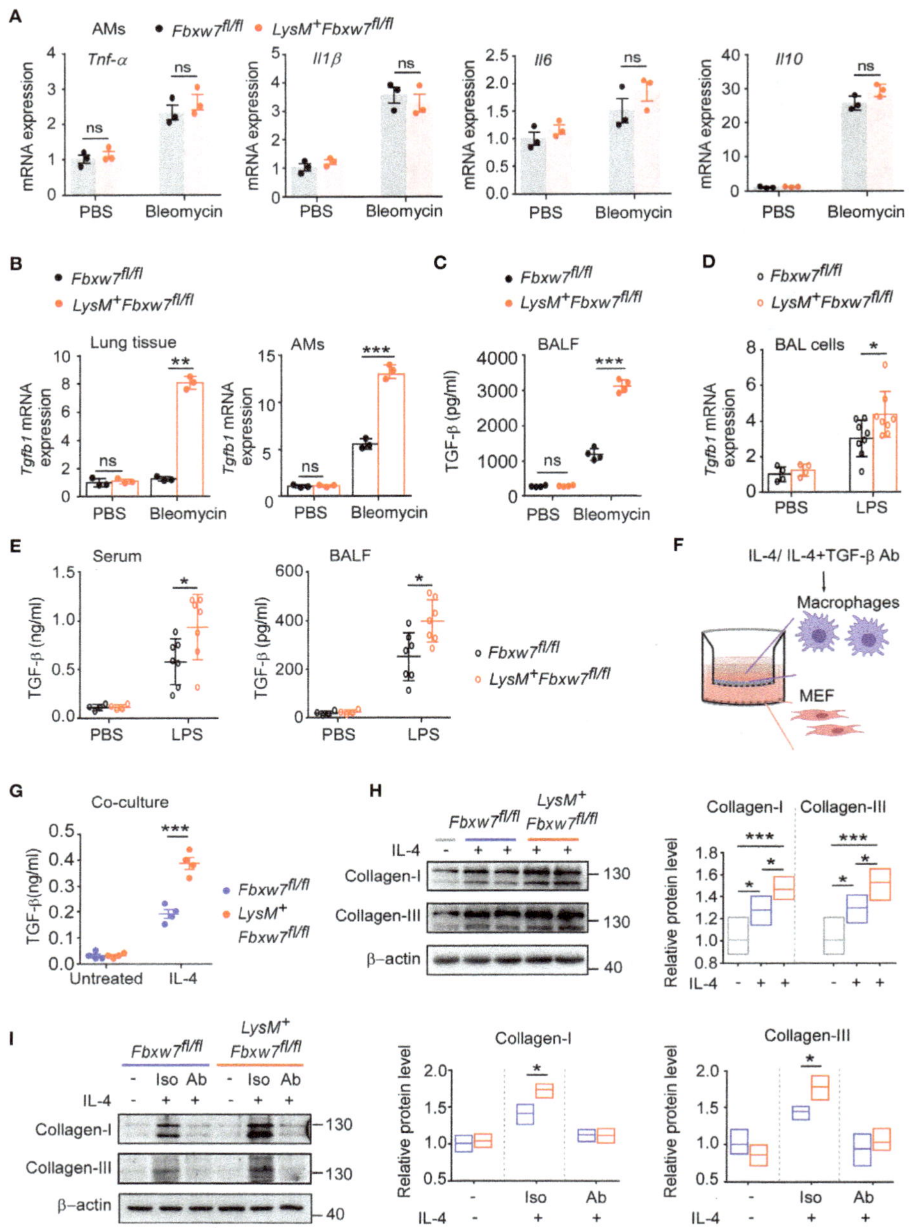

FIGURE 4 | *Fbxw7* deletion upregulates TGF-β expression in lung fibrosis model induced by bleomycin. qRT-PCR analysis of *Tnf-α*, *Il1β*, *Il6*, and *Il10* relative mRNA expression of AMs **(A)** after *Fbxw7*$^{fl/fl}$ and *LysM*$^{+}$*Fbxw7*$^{fl/fl}$ mice were administered PBS or bleomycin for 21 days to induce pulmonary fibrosis. After a 21d period of bleomycin-induced lung injure, qRT-PCR analysis of *Tgfb1* relative mRNA expression in lung tissue and AMs **(B)**, TGF-β content in BALF was detected by ELISA **(C)**. *Tgfb1* relative mRNA expression in BAL cells was analyzed by qRT-PCR **(D)**, TGF-β content in serum and BALF was detected by ELISA **(E)** after 10 days of LPS-induced lung injury. Macrophages from *Fbxw7*$^{fl/fl}$ and *LysM*$^{+}$*Fbxw7*$^{fl/fl}$ mice were stimulated with IL-4 (30 ng/ml) and treated with or without TGF-β neutralizing antibody for 12 h, then co-cultured with MEF for another 48 h. **(F)** The schematics of the approach. **(G)** TGF-β in the media of the macrophage co-culture system. Data are expressed as mean ± SD of biological duplicates (n≥3) and are the representative of three independent experiments. P values were obtained using two-tailed Student's *t* test, $^{*}P < 0.05$, $^{**}P < 0.01$, $^{***}P < 0.001$, ns, not significant. **(H)** Representative images of western blot analysis of collagen-I and collagen-III in co-cultured MEF after IL-4 treatment. Densitometric fold change of target proteins based on IL-4 untreated group was calculated. **(I)** Representative images of western blot analysis of collagen-I and collagen-III in co-cultured MEF after IL-4 with TGF-β neutralizing antibody (Ab) treatment (3 μg/ml). Iso: Isotype. Relative protein levels were presented by densitometric fold change quantified by ImageJ based on *Fbxw7*$^{fl/f}$ untreated group, the floating bars indicate the min, mean and max value of biological duplicates (n=3), which are the representative of three independent experiments. P values were obtained using One-way ANOVA with Tukey's Multiple Comparison test **(H)** or two-tailed Student's *t* test **(I)**. $^{*}P < 0.05$, $^{**}P < 0.01$, $^{***}P < 0.001$.

involved in the pathogenesis of fibrosis *via* enhancing TGF-β dependent signaling. To further elucidate the mechanisms how Fbxw7 regulates TGF-β production in profibrotic macrophages, we investigated the effect of *Fbxw7* deletion on the protein levels of EGR-1 and NF-κB by western blot. The protein levels of EGR1 and NF-κB in alveolar macrophages after bleomycin stimulation were not significantly changed between *Fbxw7*$^{fl/fl}$ and *LysM*$^{+}$*Fbxw7*$^{fl/fl}$ mice, but the level of c-Jun was significantly higher in *LysM*$^{+}$*Fbxw7*$^{fl/fl}$ mice than that in *Fbxw7*$^{fl/fl}$ mice (**Figure 5A**). Subsequently, we found significantly higher protein expression of c-Jun in IL-4-stimulated BMDMs after *Fbxw7* deletion (**Figure 5B**). We then overexpressed c-Jun in RAW264.7 cells (**Supplemental Figure 5A**) and analyzed the expression of TGF-β by qRT-PCR and ELISA, the results showed that the expression level of TGF-β was significantly increased after c-Jun overexpression (**Supplemental Figure 5B**), indicating

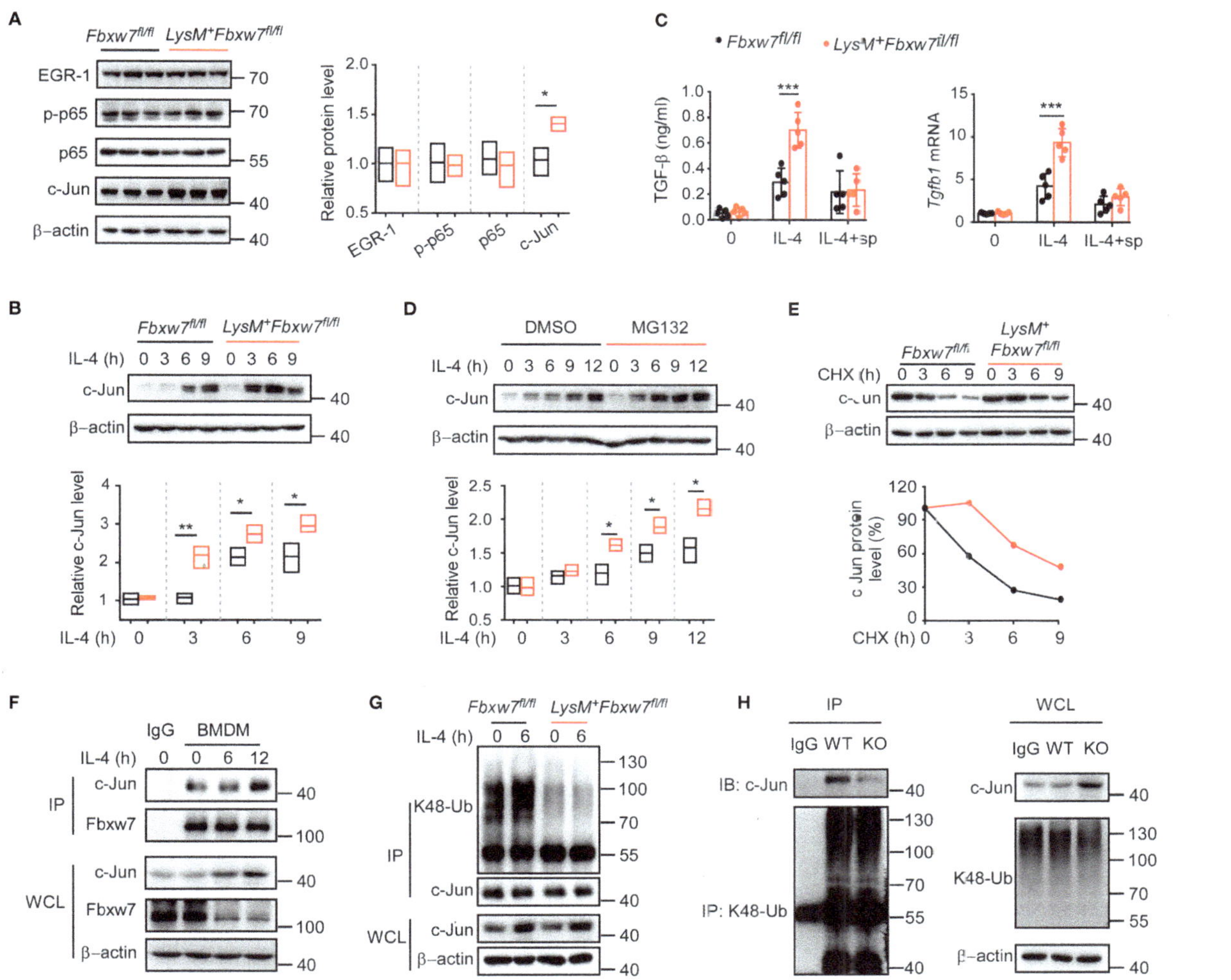

FIGURE 5 | Fbxw7 regulates TGF-β expression *via* mediating the ubiquitination of c-Jun. **(A)** Immunoblot analysis of phosphorylated and/or total proteins in lysates of lung tissues obtained from bleomycin-treated *Fbxw7*$^{fl/fl}$ and *LysM*$^{+}$*Fbxw7*$^{fl/fl}$ mice. Densitometric fold change of target proteins based on *Fbxw7*$^{fl/fl}$ group was calculated. **(B)** Immunoblot analysis of c-Jun protein levels in lysates of IL-4 (30 ng/ml) stimulated BMDMs from *Fbxw7*$^{fl/fl}$ and *LysM*$^{+}$*Fbxw7*$^{fl/fl}$ mice. Densitometric fold change for the relative c-Jun level based on *Fbxw7*$^{fl/fl}$ untreated group was calculated. **(C)** *Fbxw7*$^{fl/fl}$ and *LysM*$^{+}$ *Fbxw7*$^{fl/fl}$ BMDMs stimulated with IL-4 and treated or not with SP600125 (15 μM), qRT-PCR analysis for *Tgfb1* relative mRNA expression and ELISA for TGF-β protein expression. Data are expressed as mean ± SD of biological duplicates (n=5) and are the representative of three independent experiments. P values were obtained using two-tailed Student's *t* test, $^{***}P <$ 0.001. **(D)** Immunoblot analysis of c-Jun expression in BMDMs treated or not with MG132 (20 μM) for 8 hours and stimulated with IL-4 for the indicated durations. Densitometric fold change of c-Jun based on IL-4, MG132 untreated group was calculated. **(E)** Immunoblot analysis and relative protein levels of c-Jun in lysates of *Fbxw7*$^{fl/fl}$ and *LysM*$^{+}$*Fbxw7*$^{fl/fl}$ BMDMs treated with CHX (40 μg/ml) for indicated hours after stimulation with IL-4 for 6 h. **(F)** Coimmunoprecipitation and immunoblot of BMDMs stimulated with IL-4 for indicated hours. **(G)** Immunoblot analysis of the K48 ubiquitination of c-Jun in *Fbxw7*$^{fl/fl}$ and *LysM*$^{+}$*Fbxw7*$^{fl/fl}$ BMDMs stimulated with IL-4 for 6 h. **(H)** Peritoneal macrophages from *LysM*$^{+}$*Fbxw7*$^{fl/fl}$ (WT) and *Fbxw7*$^{fl/fl}$ (KO) mice were stimulated with IL-4 for 6 h, coimmunoprecipitation was performed with K48-Ub to pull-down ubiquitylated proteins, followed by IB with c-Jun. Relative protein levels were presented by densitometric fold change quantified by ImageJ, the floating bars indicate the min, mean and max value of biological duplicates and are the representative of three independent experiments. P values were obtained using two-tailed Student's *t* test. $^{*}P < 0.05$, $^{**}P < 0.01$, $^{***}P < 0.001$.

that c-Jun expression is sufficient for TGF-β in macrophages. SP600125 is a specific JNK inhibitor that competes with ATP to inhibit the phosphorylation of c-Jun (55). qRT-PCR analysis and ELISA results showed that the mRNA and protein expression of TGF-β increased significantly after the deletion of *Fbxw7* (**Figures 4C, D**), but this effect was abrogated after inhibition of c-Jun phosphorylation by SP600125 (**Figure 5C**). The MEF cells, co-cultured with peritoneal macrophage from $LysM^{+}Fbxw7^{fl/fl}$ mice or $Fbxw7^{fl/fl}$ littermates after inhibiting the phosphorylation of c-Jun, showed similar protein levels of collagen-I and collagen-III, which were detected by western blot (**Supplemental Figures 5C, D**). Taken together, *Fbxw7* deletion leads to the upregulation of TGF-β expression and severity of pulmonary fibrosis through the regulation of c-Jun.

It has been demonstrated that the transcription factor c-Jun can be degraded by the ubiquitin-proteasome system as a substrate for Fbxw7 (56). As expected, western blot analysis showed that the degradation of c-Jun protein could be inhibited by protease inhibitor MG132 (**Figure 5D**). A cycloheximide chase assay showed that *Fbxw7* deletion extended the half-life of endogenous c-Jun protein in BMDMs (**Figure 5E**). Immunoprecipitation assay results showed that Fbxw7 can physically bind to c-Jun protein (**Figure 5F**) and induce K48-linked polyubiquitination of c-Jun (**Figure 5G**). Moreover, immunoprecipitation assay was performed by using K48-Ub to pull-down c-Jun and the peritoneal macrophages from $LysM^{+}Fbxw7^{f/f}$ mice showed weaker ability of mediating c-Jun ubiquitination and proteasomal degradation compared with cells from $Fbxw7^{f/f}$ littermates (**Figure 5H**). This result further revealed that the myeloid *Fbxw7* deficiency leads to a significantly accumulation of c-Jun by abolishing its K48 ubiquitination. Collectively, these data confirmed that Fbxw7 promotes TGF-β expression by inducing K48-linked polyubiquitination and proteasome degradation of c-Jun in macrophages.

DISCUSSION

The E3 ubiquitin ligase Fbxw7 has been well characterized as a critical tumor suppressor that can mediate the degradation of various oncoproteins by the ubiquitin-proteasome system (57). Our studies and others have presented compelling evidence that Fbxw7 plays a crucial role in inflammation and antivirus immune response through regulating the function of macrophages (35, 36, 58). In this study, we demonstrated that the deletion of *Fbxw7* in the myeloid lineages aggravates bleomycin-induced lung injury, collagen deposition, and monocyte recruitment, and eventually leads to the exacerbation of pulmonary fibrosis in mice. We revealed its underlying mechanism that *Fbxw7* deletion will upregulate TGF-β expression by inhibiting the degradation of c-Jun in macrophages. These findings will be beneficial for understanding the role of innate immune response in the pathogenesis of IPF.

Macrophages are the most abundant immune cell population in the lung environment and are involved in tissue repair and lung fibrosis progression, it has also been recognized to play a significant role in driving the fibrogenesis and matrix remodeling. Given the high plasticity of lung macrophages, the relative roles of tissue-resident alveolar macrophages, interstitial macrophages and monocyte-derived infiltrating macrophages in pulmonary fibrosis is complicated (59). High numbers of both interstitial and alveolar macrophages were detected in pulmonary fibrosis (24), the depletion of macrophages, including alveolar and infiltrating macrophage, reduces fibrogenesis (25, 60). Experimental fibrosis leads to the recruitment of bone marrow-derived AMs that are more profibrogenic than their disrupted resident counterparts (61). Selectively targeting alveolar macrophage differentiation without affecting global monocytes or tissue-resident alveolar macrophage may ameliorate fibrosis depletion, while the depletion of tissue-resident AMs cannot alter fibrosis severity (61). In addition, IMs are also thought to arise from monocytes, and highly expression of monocyte-related genes, such as *Cd14*, *Cd163*, and *Csfr1* (62), activated IMs have been reported to induce myofibroblastic activation and ECM production (24). Furthermore, those more profibrogenic macrophages which play a vital role in airway remodeling in pulmonary fibrosis biases alternatively activated macrophages, so we used IL-4-stimulated BMDMs for *in vitro* experiments to mimic profibrogenic macrophages *in vivo*. Our data showed that more monocytes are recruited into the lung tissues and BALF of *Fbxw7*-KO mice, these monocytes further differentiate into profibrogenic macrophages and then participate in the development of pulmonary fibrosis.

The abundant expression of *Fbxw7* mRNA and protein can be detected in most human and mice tissues. The decreased level of *Fbxw7* mRNA in IPF may be regulated by many factors, including DNA or RNA silencing. The expression of microRNA-155 (miR-155) has been reported to be correlated to the damage degree of IPF (63), and miR-155 reduces the levels of *Fbxw7* mRNA (64). The *Fbxw7* promoter can be regulated through epigenetic mechanism during lung fibrosis, including histone modifications. Aberrant elevation of DNA methyltransferase 1 (Dnmt1) can mediate the hypermethylation of *Fbxw7* promoter and result in decreased gene level of *Fbxw7* (65), subsequently contributes significantly to the development of pulmonary fibrosis (66). Moreover, the expression of enhancer of zeste homolog 2 (Ezh2) is increased in IPF patients, increased Ezh2 recruitment and hypermethylated H3K27 at the promoter of fibrotic related genes have been demonstrated, such as *Cox-2* (67) and *Cxcl10* (68). We speculate the function of Ezh2 in inducing the increase of H3K27me3 at *Fbxw7* promotor and silencing of *Fbxw7* gene (34) might also be involved in regulating pulmonary fibrosis. IL-4 has been shown to induce TGF-β expression in profibrotic macrophage to activate fibroblasts and promotes extensive tissue fibrosis (50). In our study, we found IL-4 was highly expressed in lung fibrosis tissue of bleomycin-induced mice, and the expression of Fbxw7 was significantly decreased in bleomycin-induced mice lung issue and in BMDMs after IL-4 stimulation as shown in **Figures 1**, **S4B** and **5G**. These findings suggest that IL-4 in the profibrotic microenvironment might downregulate Fbxw7 expression and block c-Jun degradation.

TGF-β can be produced by a wide variety of cell types, including lung macrophages, alveolar epithelial cells, endothelial cells, fibroblasts and myofibroblasts. However, lung macrophages are revealed to be the main source of TGF-β (6, 69). In bleomycin induced pulmonary fibrosis, macrophages induce fibroblast differentiation and proliferation by producing TGF-β, thereby exacerbating pulmonary fibrosis (70, 71). The widespread accumulation of collagen in lungs, which was observed in WT mice, disappeared in the myeloid *TGF-β* deficient mice, which showed similar lung architecture to saline controls (6). Several factors have previously been implicated in the transcriptional induction of *Tgfb1*, bacterial induction of *Tgfb1* mRNA expression in human intestinal epithelial cells is butyrate and SP1-dependent (72). P38/MAPK signal, MEK-1 and JNK are involved in *Tgfb1* transcription (73). The higher mRNA expression of *Tgfb1* was detected in *Egr-1* overexpressed mesangial cell compared with control cells (74). Moreover, p65 and c-Jun were recruited to the promoter of *Tgfb1* in A549 cells upon IL-1β stimulation, this result suggesting the role of NF-κB and AP-1 in regulating *Tgfb1* expression (75).

C-Jun protein is a component of the dimeric transcription factor activator protein 1 (AP-1) (76), it has been shown to play essential roles in most fibrotic conditions, which can activate multiple signaling pathways, resulting in the expression of many fibrogenesis-associated genes (77). C-Jun N-terminal kinase JNK1 has been reported to promote fibrosis in the lung (78), inhibition of c-Jun phosphorylation *in vivo* reduced fibrosis and mRNA levels of *Tgfb1* in the unilateral ischemia reperfusion injury model (79). C-Jun expression in non-parenchymal liver cells (NPLCs) promotes the fibrogenesis and was particularly correlated with liver fibrosis during non-alcoholic steatohepatitis (80). Moreover, studies have shown that c-Jun can be degraded by the ubiquitin-proteasome system as the substrate of Fbxw7 (81, 82), which was also confirmed by our study. Our data show that deletion of *Fbxw7* in macrophages does not affect the levels of P65, EGR-1 and their phosphorylation, but significantly increases the level of AP-1 transcription factor subunit c-Jun.

Notably, the published data from Wang et al. (83) showed that FBXW7 deficiency prevents fibrogenesis by increasing telomere capping, which is contrary to the conclusion of our finding. Several potential possibilities exist for this discrepancy. Wang et al. used a mouse model of Fbw7 conditional knockout in pulmonary alveolar epithelial type 2 (AEC2) stem cells, while we used a model of *Fbxw7* conditional knockout in myeloid cells. Those reverse effects of Fbxw7 in AEC2 stem cells and myeloid cells in regulating lung fibrosis indicated that the pathogenesis of IPF is complicated, it involves the abnormal repair of lung tissue injury by alveolar epithelial cells, the disordered differentiation and proliferation of fibroblasts, or the hyperactivated recruitment and activation of innate immune cells. The dysfunction in any cell type can lead to different outcomes of IPF. Moreover, subtle genetic background differences in the strains of the mice used and microbiome differences between the mouse colonies may also contribute to these discrepancies.

In conclusion, our study revealed that Fbxw7 plays a crucial role in regulating pulmonary fibrosis progression. Myeloid-specific deletion of *Fbxw7* exacerbates pulmonary fibrosis by inhibiting c-Jun degradation and upregulating TGF-β expression in macrophages.

AUTHOR CONTRIBUTIONS

QW, JZ, and JH designed the research. JH, YD, GL, XS, WS, LL, and MX performed experiments and acquired and analyzed data. JZ, JH, and PX drafted the manuscript. QW revised the manuscript. All authors read and approved the submitted version.

ACKNOWLEDGMENTS

We would like to thank Prof. Ximei Wu for providing the Lysm-Cre mice. We thank the Core Facilities, Zhejiang University School of Medicine for technical support.

REFERENCES

Wolters PJ, Blackwell TS, Eickelberg O, Loyd JE, Kaminski N, Jenkins G, et al. Time for a Change: Is Idiopathic Pulmonary Fibrosis Still Idiopathic and Only Fibrotic? *Lancet Respir Med* (2018) 2:154–60. doi: 10.1016/s2213-2600(18) 30007-9

Xaubet A, Marin-Arguedas A, Lario S, Ancochea J, Morell F, Ruiz-Manzano J, et al. Transforming Growth Factor-Beta1 Gene Polymorphisms Are Associated With Disease Progression in Idiopathic Pulmonary Fibrosis. *Am J Respir Crit Care Med* (2003) 4:431–5. doi: 10.1164/rccm.200210-1165OC

Mura M, Porretta MA, Bargagli E, Sergiacomi G, Zompatori M, Sverzellati N, et al. Predicting Survival in Newly Diagnosed Idiopathic Pulmonary Fibrosis: A 3-Year Prospective Study. *Eur Respir J* (2012) 1:101–9. doi: 10.1183/09031936.00106011

King TEJr., Tooze JA, Schwarz MI, Brown KR, Cherniack RM. Predicting Survival in Idiopathic Pulmonary Fibrosis: Scoring System and Survival Model. *Am J Respir Crit Care Med* (2001) 7:1171–81. doi: 10.1164/ ajrccm.164.7.2003140

Fernandez IE, Eickelberg O. The Impact of Tgf-Beta on Lung Fibrosis: From Targeting to Biomarkers. *Proc Am Thorac Soc* (2012) 3:111–6. doi: 10.1513/pats.201203-023AW

Larson-Casey JL, Deshane JS, Ryan AJ, Thannickal VJ, Carter AB. Macrophage Akt1 Kinase-Mediated Mitophagy Modulates Apoptosis Resistance and Pulmonary Fibrosis. *Immunity* (2016) 3:582–96. doi: 10.1016/j.immuni.2016.01.001

Yu X, Buttgereit A, Lelios I, Utz SG, Cansever D, Becher B, et al. The Cytokine Tgf- Beta Promotes the Development and Homeostasis of Alveolar Macrophages. *Immunity* (2017) 5:903–12 e4. doi: 10.1016/j.immuni.2017.10.007

Phillips AO, Topley N, Steadman R, Morrisey K, Williams JD. Induction of Tgf-Beta 1 Synthesis in D-Glucose Primed Human Proximal Tubular Cells by Il-1 Beta and Tnf Alpha. *Kidney Int* (1996) 5:1546–54. doi: 10.1038/ ki.1996.470

Zhu Z, Homer RJ, Wang Z, Chen Q, Geba GP, Wang J, et al. Pulmonary Expression of Interleukin-13 Causes Inflammation, Mucus Hypersecretion, Subepithelial Fibrosis, Physiologic Abnormalities, and Eotaxin Production. *J Clin Invest* (1999) 6:779–88. doi: 10.1172/JCI5909

Lee CG, Homer RJ, Zhu Z, Lanone S, Wang X, Koteliansky V, et al. Interleukin-13 Induces Tissue Fibrosis by Selectively Stimulating and Activating Transforming Growth Factor Beta(1). *J Exp Med* (2001) 6:809– 21. doi: 10.1084/jem.194.6.809

Rao LZ, Wang Y, Zhang L, Wu G, Zhang L, Wang FX, et al. Il-24 Deficiency Protects Mice Against Bleomycin-Induced Pulmonary Fibrosis by Repressing Il-4-Induced M2 Program in Macrophages. *Cell Death Differ* (2021) 4:1270– 83. doi: 10.1038/s41418-020-00650-6

Sunaga H, Matsui H, Ueno M, Maeno T, Iso T, Syamsunarno MR, et al. Deranged Fatty Acid Composition Causes Pulmonary Fibrosis in Elovl6-Deficient Mice. *Nat Commun* (2013) 4:2563. doi: 10.1038/ncomms3563

Mahalanobish S, Saha S, Dutta S, Sil PC. Matrix Metalloproteinase: An Upcoming Therapeutic Approach for Idiopathic Pulmonary Fibrosis

Pharmacol Res (2020) 152:104591. doi: 10.1016/j.phrs.2019.104591

Murphy-Ullrich JE, Suto MJ. Thrombospondin-1 Regulation of Latent Tgf- Beta Activation: A Therapeutic Target for Fibrotic Disease. *Matrix Biol* (2018) 68-69:28–43. doi: 10.1016/j.matbio.2017.12.009

Dong X, Zhao B, Iacob RE, Zhu J, Koksal AC, Lu C, et al. Force Interacts With Macromolecular Structure in Activation of Tgf-Beta. *Nature* (2017) 7639:55– 9. doi: 10.1038/nature21035

Byrne AJ, Maher TM, Lloyd CM. Pulmonary Macrophages: A New Therapeutic Pathway in Fibrosing Lung Disease? *Trends Mol Med* (2016) 4:303–16. doi: 10.1016/j.molmed.2016.02.004

Laskin DL, Malaviya R, Laskin JD. Role of Macrophages in Acute Lung Injury and Chronic Fibrosis Induced by Pulmonary Toxicants. *Toxicol Sci* (2019) 2:287–301. doi: 10.1093/toxsci/kfy309

Gibbons MA, MacKinnon AC, Ramachandran P, Dhaliwal K, Duffin R, Phythian-Adams AT, et al. Ly6chi Monocytes Direct Alternatively Activated Profibrotic Macrophage Regulation of Lung Fibrosis. *Am J Respir Crit Care Med* (2011) 5:569–81. doi: 10.1164/rccm.201010-1719OC

Fernandez IE, Eickelberg O. New Cellular and Molecular Mechanisms of Lung Injury and Fibrosis in Idiopathic Pulmonary Fibrosis. *Lancet* (2012) 9842:680–8. doi: 10.1016/S0140-6736(12)61144-1

Zhang L, Wang Y, Wu G, Xiong W, Gu W, Wang CY. Macrophages: Friend or Foe in Idiopathic Pulmonary Fibrosis? *Respir Res* (2018) 1:170. doi: 10.1186/ s12931-018-0864-2

Prasse A, Pechkovsky DV, Toews GB, Jungraithmayr W, Kollert F, Goldmann T, et al. A Vicious Circle of Alveolar Macrophages and Fibroblasts Perpetuates Pulmonary Fibrosis *via* Ccl18. *Am J Respir Crit Care Med* (2006) 7:781–92. doi: 10.1164/ rccm.200509-1518OC

Wynes MW, Frankel SK, Riches DW. Il-4-Induced Macrophage-Derived Igf-I Protects Myofibroblasts From Apoptosis Following Growth Factor Withdrawal. *J Leukoc Biol* (2004) 5:1019–27. doi: 10.1189/jlb.0504288

Nagaoka I, Trapnell BC, Crystal RG. Upregulation of Platelet-Derived Growth Factor-A and -B Gene Expression in Alveolar Macrophages of Individuals With Idiopathic Pulmonary Fibrosis. *J Clin Invest* (1990) 6:2023–7. doi: 10.1172/JCI114669

Meziani L, Mondini M, Petit B, Boissonnas A, Thomas de Montpreville V, Mercier O, et al. Csf1r Inhibition Prevents Radiation Pulmonary Fibrosis by Depletion of Interstitial Macrophages. *Eur Respir J* (2018) 3:1702120. doi: 10.1183/13993003.02120-2017

Redente EF, Keith RC, Janssen W, Henson PM, Ortiz LA, Downey GP, et al. Tumor Necrosis Factor-Alpha Accelerates the Resolution of Established Pulmonary Fibrosis in Mice by Targeting Profibrotic Lung Macrophages. *Am J Respir Cell Mol Biol* (2014) 4:825–37. doi: 10.1165/ rcmb.2013-0386OC

Murray LA, Chen Q, Kramer MS, Hesson DP, Argentieri RL, Peng X, et al. Tgf-Beta Driven Lung Fibrosis Is Macrophage Dependent and Blocked by Serum Amyloid P. *Int J Biochem Cell Biol* (2011) 1:154–62. doi: 10.1016/ j.biocel.2010.10.013

Khalil N, Bereznay O, Sporn M, Greenberg AH. Macrophage Production of Transforming Growth Factor Beta and Fibroblast Collagen Synthesis in Chronic Pulmonary Inflammation. *J Exp Med* (1989) 3:727–37. doi: 10.1084/jem.170.3.727

Sailo BL, Banik K, Girisa S, Bordoloi D, Fan L, Halim CE, et al. Fbxw7 in Cancer: What Has Been Unraveled Thus Far? *Cancers (Basel)* (2019) 2:246. doi: 10.3390/ cancers11020246

Guyard A, Danel C, Theou-Anton N, Debray MP, Gibault L, Mordant P, et al. Morphologic and Molecular Study of Lung Cancers Associated With Idiopathic Pulmonary Fibrosis and Other Pulmonary Fibroses. *Respir Res* (2017) 1:120. doi: 10.1186/s12931-017-0605-y

Ekholm-Reed S, Goldberg MS, Schlossmacher MG, Reed SI. Parkin-Dependent Degradation of the F-Box Protein Fbw7beta Promotes Neuronal Survival in Response to Oxidative Stress by Stabilizing Mcl-1. *Mol Cell Biol* (2013) 18:3627–43. doi: 10.1128/MCB.00535-13

Zhao X, Hirota T, Han X, Cho H, Chong LW, Lamia K, et al. Circadian Amplitude Regulation *via* Fbxw7-Targeted Rev-Erbalpha Degradation. *Cell* (2016) 7:1644–57. doi: 10.1016/j.cell.2016.05.012

Hoeck JD, Jandke A, Blake SM, Nye E, Spencer-Dene B, Brandner S, et al. Fbw7 Controls Neural Stem Cell Differentiation and Progenitor Apoptosis *via* Notch and C-Jun. *Nat Neurosci* (2010) 11:1365–72. doi: 10.1038/nn.2644

Kearns CA, Ravanelli AM, Cooper K, Appel B. Fbxw7 Limits Myelination by Inhibiting Mtor Signaling. *J Neurosci* (2015) 44:14861–71. doi: 10.1523/ JNEUROSCI.4968-14.2015

Zhao E, Maj T, Kryczek I, Li W, Wu K, Zhao L, et al. Cancer Mediates Effector T Cell Dysfunction by Targeting Micrornas and Ezh2 *via* Glycolysis Restriction. *Nat Immunol* (2016) 1:95–103. doi: 10.1038/ni.3313

Song Y, Lai L, Chong Z, He J, Zhang Y, Xue Y, et al. E3 Ligase Fbxw7 Is Critical for Rig-I Stabilization During Antiviral Responses. *Nat Commun* (2017) 8:14654. doi: 10.1038/ncomms14654

He J, Song Y, Li G, Xiao P, Liu Y, Xue Y, et al. Fbxw7 Increases Ccl2/7 in Cx3cr1hi Macrophages to Promote Intestinal Inflammation. *J Clin Invest* (2019) 129:3877–93. doi: 10.1172/JCI123374

Liu T, De Los Santos FG, Phan SH. The Bleomycin Model of Pulmonary Fibrosis. *Methods Mol Biol* (2017) 1627:27–42. doi: 10.1007/978-1-4939-7113-8_2

Li Y, Li H, Liu S, Pan P, Su X, Tan H, et al. Pirfenidone Ameliorates Lipopolysaccharide-Induced Pulmonary Inflammation and Fibrosis by Blocking Nlrp3 Inflammasome Activation. *Mol Immunol* (2018) 99:134–44. doi: 10.1016/j.molimm.2018.05.003

Liu YY, Shi Y, Liu Y, Pan XH, Zhang KX. Telomere Shortening Activates Tgf- Beta/ Smads Signaling in Lungs and Enhances Both Lipopolysaccharide and Bleomycin-Induced Pulmonary Fibrosis. *Acta Pharmacol Sin* (2018) 11:1735– 45. doi: 10.1038/s41401-018-0007-9

Szapiel SV, Elson NA, Fulmer JD, Hunninghake GW, Crystal RG. Bleomycin- Induced Interstitial Pulmonary Disease in the Nude, Athymic Mouse. *Am Rev Respir Dis* (1979) 4:893–9. doi: 10.1164/arrd.1979.120.4.893

Schmittgen TD, Livak KJ. Analyzing Real-Time Pcr Data by the Comparative C(T) Method. *Nat Protoc* (2008) 6:1101–8. doi: 10.1038/nprot.2008.73

Prasse A, Binder H, Schupp JC, Kayser G, Bargagli E, Jaeger B, et al. Data From: BAL Cell Gene Expression is Predictive of Mortality in Idiopathic Pulmonary Fibrosis and Enriched for Genes of Airway Basal Cells. *Gene Expression Omnibus* (2018), GSE70867.

Huang Y, Oldham JM, Ma S, Martinez FJ, Noth I. Data From: Longitudinal Blood Transcriptomic Changes Predict Lung Function Decline in Idiopathic Pulmonary Fibrosis. *Gene Expression Omnibus* (2019), GSE132607.

Desogere P, Tapias LF, Hariri LP, Rotile NJ, Rietz TA, Probst CK, et al. Type I Collagen-Targeted Pet Probe for Pulmonary Fibrosis Detection and Staging in Preclinical Models. *Sci Transl Med* (2017) 384:eaaf4696. doi: 10.1126/ scitranslmed.aaf4696

Tsukui T, Sun KH, Wetter JB, Wilson-Kanamori JR, Hazelwood LA, Henderson NC, et al. Collagen-Producing Lung Cell Atlas Identifies Multiple Subsets With Distinct Localization and Relevance to Fibrosis. *Nat Commun* (2020) 1:1920. doi: 10.1038/s41467-020-15647-5

Tschumperlin DJ. Matrix, Mesenchyme, and Mechanotransduction. *Ann Am Thorac Soc* (2015) 12:S24–9. doi: 10.1513/AnnalsATS.201407-320MG

Ryu C, Sun H, Gulati M, Herazo-Maya JD, Chen Y, Osafo-Addo A, et al. Extracellular Mitochondrial DNA Is Generated by Fibroblasts and Predicts Death in Idiopathic Pulmonary Fibrosis. *Am J Respir Crit Care Med* (2017) 12:1571–81. doi: 10.1164/rccm.201612-2480OC

Dong J, Ma Q. Type 2 Immune Mechanisms in Carbon Nanotube-Induced Lung Fibrosis. *Front Immunol* (2018) 9:1120. doi: 10.3389/fimmu.2018.01120

He C, Murthy S, McCormick ML, Spitz DR, Ryan AJ, Carter AB. Mitochondrial Cu,Zn-Superoxide Dismutase Mediates Pulmonary Fibrosis by Augmenting H2o2 Generation. *J Biol Chem* (2011) 17:15597–607. doi: 10.1074/jbc.M110.187377

Su S, Zhao Q, He C, Huang D, Liu J, Chen F, et al. Mir-142-5p and Mir-130a- 3p Are Regulated by Il-4 and Il-13 and Control Profibrogenic Macrophage Program. *Nat Commun* (2015) 6:8523. doi: 10.1038/ncomms9523

Zhu L, Fu X, Chen X, Han X, Dong P. M2 Macrophages Induce Emt Through the Tgf-Beta/Smad2 Signaling Pathway. *Cell Biol Int* (2017) 9:960–68. doi: 10.1002/cbin.10788

Lee CG, Cho SJ, Kang MJ, Chapoval SP, Lee PJ, Noble PW, et al. Early Growth Response Gene 1-Mediated Apoptosis Is Essential for Transforming Growth Factor Beta1-Induced Pulmonary Fibrosis. *J Exp Med* (2004) 3:377–89. doi: 10.1084/ jem.20040104

Ghosh AK, Bhattacharyya S, Lafyatis R, Farina G, Yu J, Thimmapaya B, et al. P300 Is Elevated in Systemic Sclerosis and Its Expression Is Positively Regulated by Tgf-Beta: Epigenetic Feed-Forward Amplification of Fibrosis. *J Invest Dermatol* (2013) 5:1302–10. doi: 10.1038/jid.2012.479

Freudlsperger C, Bian Y, Contag Wise S, Burnett J, Coupar J, Yang X, et al. Tgf-Beta and Nf-Kappab Signal Pathway Cross-Talk Is Mediated Through Tak1 and Smad7 in a Subset of Head and Neck Cancers. *Oncogene* (2013) 12:1549–59. doi: 10.1038/onc.2012.171

Zhang S, Che D, Yang F, Chi C, Meng H, Shen J, et al. Tumor-Associated Macrophages Promote Tumor Metastasis *via* the Tgf-Beta/Sox9 Axis in Non-Small Cell Lung Cancer. *Oncotarget* (2017) 59:99801–15. doi: 10.18632/ oncotarget.21068

Babaei-Jadidi R, Li N, Saadeddin A, Spencer-Dene B, Jandke A, Muhammad B, et al. Fbxw7 Influences Murine Intestinal Homeostasis and Cancer, Targeting

Notch, Jun, and Dek for Degradation. *J Exp Med* (2011) 2:295– 312. doi: 10.1084/jem.20100830

Yeh CH, Bellon M, Nicot C. Fbxw7: A Critical Tumor Suppressor of Human Cancers. *Mol Cancer* (2018) 1:115. doi: 10.1186/s12943-018-0857-2

Zhang C, Chen F, Feng L, Shan Q, Zheng GH, Wang YJ, et al. Fbxw7 Suppresses Hmgb1-Mediated Innate Immune Signaling to Attenuate Hepatic Inflammation and Insulin Resistance in a Mouse Model of Nonalcoholic Fatty Liver Disease. *Mol Med* (2019) 1:29. doi: 10.1186/s10020-019-0099-9

Guilliams M, Scott CL. Does Niche Competition Determine the Origin of Tissue-Resident Macrophages? *Nat Rev Immunol* (2017) 7:451–60. doi: 10.1038/nri.2017.42

Osterholzer JJ, Olszewski MA, Murdock BJ, Chen GH, Erb-Downward JR, Subbotina N, et al. Implicating Exudate Macrophages and Ly-6c(High) Monocytes in Ccr2-Dependent Lung Fibrosis Following Gene-Targeted Alveolar Injury. *J Immunol* (2013) 7:3447–57. doi: 10.4049/jimmunol.1200604

Misharin AV, Morales-Nebreda L, Reyfman PA, Cuda CM, Walter JM, McQuattie-Pimentel AC, et al. Monocyte-Derived Alveolar Macrophages Drive Lung Fibrosis and Persist in the Lung Over the Life Span. *J Exp Med* (2017) 8:2387–404. doi: 10.1084/jem.20162152

Gibbings SL, Thomas SM, Atif SM, McCubbrey AL, Desch AN, Danhorn T, et al. Three Unique Interstitial Macrophages in the Murine Lung at Steady State. *Am J Respir Cell Mol Biol* (2017) 1:66–76. doi: 10.1165/rcmb.2016- 0361OC

Li P, Zhao GQ, Chen TF, Chang JX, Wang HQ, Chen SS, et al. Serum Mir-21 and Mir-155 Expression in Idiopathic Pulmonary Fibrosis. *J Asthma* (2013) 9:960–4. doi: 10.3109/02770903.2013.822080

Cao S, Wang Y, Li J, Lv M, Niu H, Tian Y. Tumor-Suppressive Function of Long Noncoding Rna Malat1 in Glioma Cells by Suppressing Mir-155 Expression and Activating Fbxw7 Function. *Am J Cancer Res* (2016) 11:2561–74.

Kitade S, Onoyama I, Kobayashi H, Yagi H, Yoshida S, Kato M, et al. Fbxw7 Is Involved in the Acquisition of the Malignant Phenotype in Epithelial Ovarian Tumors. *Cancer Sci* (2016) 10:1399–405. doi: 10.1111/cas.13026

Wei A, Gao Q, Chen F, Zhu X, Chen X, Zhang L, et al. Inhibition of DNA Methylation Derepresses Ppargamma and Attenuates Pulmonary Fibrosis. *Br J Pharmacol* (2021). doi: 10.1111/bph.15655

Coward WR, Feghali-Bostwick CA, Jenkins G, Knox AJ, Pang L. A Central Role for G9a and Ezh2 in the Epigenetic Silencing of Cyclooxygenase-2 in Idiopathic Pulmonary Fibrosis. *FASEB J* (2014) 7:3183–96. doi: 10.1096/fj.13- 241760

Coward WR, Brand OJ, Pasini A, Jenkins G, Knox AJ, Pang L. Interplay Between Ezh2 and G9a Regulates Cxcl10 Gene Repression in Idiopathic Pulmonary Fibrosis. *Am J Respir Cell Mol Biol* (2018) 4:449 60. doi: 10.1165/ rcmb.2017-0286OC

Broekelmann TJ, Limper AH, Colby TV, McDonald JA. Transforming Growth Factor Beta 1 Is Present at Sites of Extracellular Matrix Gene Expression in Human Pulmonary Fibrosis. *Proc Natl Acad Sci USA* (1991) 15:6642–6. doi: 10.1073/pnas.88.15.6642

Toossi Z, Hirsch CS, Hamilton BD, Knuth CK, Friedlander MA, Rich EA. Decreased Production of Tgf-Beta 1 by Human Alveolar Macrophages Compared With Blood Monocytes. *J Immunol* (1996) 9:3461–8.

Young LR, Gulleman PM, Short CW, Tanjore H, Sherrill T, Qi A, et al. Epithelial-Macrophage Interactions Determine Pulmonary Fibrosis Susceptibility in Hermansky-Pudlak Syndrome. *JCI Insight* (2016) 17: e88947. doi: 10.1172/jci.insight.88947

Martin-Gallausiaux C, Beguet-Crespel F, Marinelli L, Jamet A, Ledue F, Blottiere HM, et al. Butyrate Produced by Gut Commensal Bacteria Activates Tgf-Beta1 Expression Through the Transcription Factor Sp1 in Human Intestinal Epithelial Cells. *Sci Rep* (2018) 1:9742. doi: 10.1038/s41598-018-28048-y

Xiao Y, Freire-de-Lima C, Schiemann W, Bratton D, Vandivier R, Henson P, et al. Transcriptional and Translational Regulation of Tgf-Beta Production in Response to Apoptotic Cells. *J Immunol* (2008) 5:3575–85. doi: 10.4049/ jimmunol.181.5.3575

Peng W, Huang S, Shen L, Tang Y, Li H, Shi Y. Long Noncoding Rna Nonhsag053901 Promotes Diabetic Nephropathy *via* Stimulating Egr-1/Tgf-Beta-Mediated Renal Inflammation. *J Cell Physiol* (2019) 10:18492–503. doi: 10.1002/jcp.28485

Lee KY, Ito K, Hayashi R, Jazrawi EP, Barnes PJ, Adcock IM. Nf-Kappab and Activator Protein 1 Response Elements and the Role of Histone Modifications in Il-1beta-Induced Tgf-Beta1 Gene Transcription. *J Immunol* (2006) 1:603– 15. doi: 10.4049/jimmunol.176.1.603

Eferl R, Wagner EF. Ap-1: A Double-Edged Sword in Tumorigenesis. *Nat Rev Cancer* (2003) 11:859–68. doi: 10.1038/nrc1209

Wernig G, Chen SY, Cui L, Van Neste C, Tsai JM, Kambham N, et al. Unifying Mechanism for Different Fibrotic Diseases. *Proc Natl Acad Sci USA* (2017) 18:4757–62. doi: 10.1073/pnas.1621375114

Velden JL, Alcorn JF, Guala AS, Badura EC. And Janssen-Heininger Y M. C-Jun N-Terminal Kinase 1 Promotes Transforming Growth Factor-Beta1- Induced Epithelial-To-Mesenchymal Transition *via* Control of Linker Phosphorylation and Transcriptional Activity of Smad3. *Am J Respir Cell Mol Biol* (2011) 4:571–81. doi: 10.1165/rcmb.2009-0282OC

Yang L, Besschetnova TY, Brooks CR, Shah JV. Bonventre JV. Epithelial Cell Cycle Arrest in G2/M Mediates Kidney Fibrosis After Injury. *Nat Med* (2010) 5:535–43. doi: 10.1038/nm.2144

Schulien I, Hockenjos B, Schmitt-Graeff A, Perdekamp MG, Follo M, Thimme R, et al. The Transcription Factor C-Jun/Ap-1 Promotes Liver Fibrosis During Non-Alcoholic Steatohepatitis by Regulating Osteopontin Expression. *Cell Death Differ* (2019) 9:1688–99. doi: 10.1038/s41418-018- 0239-8

Nateri AS, Riera-Sans L, Da Costa C, Behrens A. The Ubiquitin Ligase Scffbw7 Antagonizes Apoptotic Jnk Signaling. *Science* (2004) 5662:1374–8. doi: 10.1126/science.1092880

Kravchick DO, Karpova A, Hrdinka M, Lopez-Rojas J, Iacobas S, Carbonell AU, et al. Synaptonuclear Messenger Prr7 Inhibits C-Jun Ubiquitination and Regulates Nmda-Mediated Excitotoxicity. *EMBO J* (2016) 17:1923–34. doi: 10.15252/ embj.201593070

Wang L, Chen R, Li G, Wang Z, Liu J, Liang Y, et al. Fbw7 Mediates Senescence and Pulmonary Fibrosis Through Telomere Uncapping. *Cell Metab* (2020) 5:860–77e9. doi: 10.1016/j.cmet.2020.10.004

2

Protective Effect of Remdesivir against Pulmonary Fibrosis in Mice

Xiaohe Li[1,2†], Rui Liu[1,2†], Yunyao Cui[1,2†], Jingjing Liang[1,2†], Zhun Bi[1†], Shimeng Li[1,2], Yang Miao[1], Liang Zhang[3], Xiaoping Li[3], Honggang Zhou[1,2] and Cheng Yang[1,2]*

[1]State Key Laboratory of Medicinal Chemical Biology, College of Pharmacy and Tianjin Key Laboratory of Molecular Drug Research, Nankai University, Tianjin, China, [2]Tianjin Key Laboratory of Molecular Drug Research, Tianjin International Joint Academy of Biomedicine, Tianjin, China, [3]Department of Thoracic Surgery, Tian Jin First Central Hospital, Tianjin, China

***Correspondence:**
Honggang Zhou
honggang.zhou@nankai.edu.cn

[†]These authors have contributed equally to this work

Pulmonary fibrosis is a known sequela of severe or persistent lung damage. Existing clinical, imaging and autopsy studies have shown that the lungs exhibit a pathological pulmonary fibrosis phenotype after infection with coronaviruses, including severe acute respiratory syndrome coronavirus 2 (SARS-CoV-2). Pulmonary fibrosis may be one of the most serious sequelae associated with coronavirus disease 2019 (COVID-19). In this study, we aimed to examine the preventative effects of the antiviral drug remdesivir on pulmonary fibrosis. We used a mouse model of bleomycin-induced pulmonary fibrosis to evaluate the effects of remdesivir on pulmonary fibrosis *in vivo* and further explored the potential pharmacological mechanisms of remdesivir in lung fibroblasts and alveolar epithelial cells *in vitro*. The preventive remdesivir treatment was started on the day of bleomycin installation, and the results showed that remdesivir significantly alleviated bleomycin-induced collagen deposition and improved pulmonary function. *In vitro* experiments showed that remdesivir dose-dependently suppressed TGF-β1-induced lung fibroblast activation and improved TGF-β1-induced alveolar epithelial to mesenchymal transition. Our results indicate that remdesivir can preventatively alleviate the severity of pulmonary fibrosis and provide some reference for the prevention of pulmonary fibrosis in patients with COVID-19.

Keywords: remdesivir (RDV), COVID-19, pulmonary fibrosis, bleomycin, TGF-β1

INTRODUCTION

The novel coronavirus severe acute respiratory syndrome coronavirus 2 (SARS-CoV-2) causes coronavirus disease 2019 (COVID-19), was identified in December 2019 and has triggered an outbreak and spread rapidly across the world (Wang et al., 2020). As of January 7, 2021, SARS-COV-2 is still prevalent, with a total of 87.7 million confirmed cases worldwide (WHO, 2020), but there are still no effective treatments. SARS-CoV-2 is the sixth international public health emergency after the emergence of H1N1, poliovirus, Ebola virus, and Zika virus (Lai et al., 2020). The SARS-CoV-2 pandemic not only brings physical and psychological burdens to patients but also had a major impact on the development of all aspects of society.

Most COVID-19 patients have common respiratory and gastrointestinal symptoms, such as fever, dry cough and diarrhea, and some patients may progress to severe manifestations, including acute respiratory distress syndrome (ARDS), respiratory failure, multiorgan failure, and even death (Bajwah et al., 2020; Wang et al., 2020). According to former reports, many patients survive the acute phase of ARDS but die as a result of subsequent progressive pulmonary fibrosis (Meduri et al.,

1995). A large amount of clinical evidence also confirms that coronavirus infection in the respiratory system can cause lung damage and develop into irreversible pulmonary fibrosis (George et al., 2020). For example, Xie et al. showed that 45% of patients infected with SARS-CoV develop the appearance of "ground glass" (a sign of fibrosis) in the lungs (Xie et al., 2005). Up to 33% of patients infected with Middle East respiratory syndrome (MERS)-CoV have pulmonary fibrosis sequelae (Das et al., 2017). SARS-CoV-2 has similar gene sequences as SARS-CoV and MERS-CoV, with consistencies of 79 and 50%, respectively (Jiang et al., 2020; Lu et al., 2020). Therefore, pulmonary fibrosis may also be the main sequelae in SARS-CoV-2 patients during the recovery period. Recently, a clinical study showed the formation of fibrosis during the rehabilitation of patients with COVID-19 (Xu et al., 2020). Other studies also showed that 17.5–33.9% of COVID-19 patients had fibrotic changes on chest CT scans (Pan et al., 2020; Zhou et al., 2020). Hence, although long-term follow-up studies are needed to determine the exact proportion of post-COVID-19 fibrosis, antifibrotic therapy should be a key concern for COVID-19 survivors.

Remdesivir is a nucleoside analog drug that inhibits viral RNA-dependent RNA polymerase (RdRP) through triphosphate metabolites, which can stop the transcription of viral RNA and prevent viral replication (Warren et al., 2016; Tchesnokov et al., 2019). In 2015, the FDA approved remdesivir for the treatment of Ebola virus (Mulangu et al., 2019); while remdesivir did not show significant efficacy in the treatment of Ebola virus but did show significant antiviral activity against coronaviruses such as SARS-CoV and MERS-CoV (Brown et al., 2019; de Wit et al., 2020). Recently, a series of *in vitro* and *in vivo* studies showed that remdesivir also has a strong inhibitory effect on SARS-CoV-2 (Sheahan et al., 2020). Some clinical trials and case reports also support remdesivir as a potentially effective drug for the treatment of COVID-19 (Beigel et al., 2020; Goldman et al., 2020; Spinner et al., 2020). At present, remdesivir has been approved by the FDA and EMA for the treatment of COVID-19 (Agency, 2020; Diseases, 2020). However, the effect of remdesivir on subsequently occurring pulmonary fibrosis in patients with COVID-19 has not been reported.

Since our laboratory is not qualified for viral testing, we used a bleomycin (BLM)-induced pulmonary fibrosis mouse model to evaluate the preventative effect of remdesivir on pulmonary fibrosis and further explored the potential pharmacological mechanisms, which may provide a reference for the clinical prevention of pulmonary fibrosis in COVID-19 patients.

MATERIALS AND METHODS

Materials

Recombinant human transforming growth factor-β1 (TGF-β1) was purchased from Peprotech (United States). Antibodies against collagen I, fibronectin, P-Smad3/Smad3, P-Akt/Akt, P-ERK/ERK, P-JNK/JNK, P-P38/P38, GAPDH, E-cadherin, vimentin, and N-cadherin were purchased from Cell Signaling Technology (United States). The β-tubulin antibody was obtained from Proteintech (China) The α-SMA antibody was obtained from Santa Cruz Biotechnology (China). Goat pAbs against Rb IgG (HRP) and Rb pAbs against Ms IgG were obtained from ImmunoWay (China). TRIzol reagent was acquired from Ambion Life Technology (China). DEPC-treated H_2O and RNase Away H_2O were purchased from Life Technologies. Fastking gDNA Dispelling RT SuperMix was purchased from Tiangen (Beijing, China). UNICON® qPCR SYBR Green Master Mix and liposomal transfection reagents were purchased from Yevsen (Shanghai, China) The Masson's trichrome staining kit was obtained from Solarbio (China). Recombinant Mouse Platelet-derived Growth Factor-BB were purchased from MedChemExpress (China).

Cell Culture

Human pulmonary epithelial cells (A549, ATCC) were maintained in RPMI-1640 (KeyGEN BioTECH, China) with 10% fetal bovine serum (FBS, ExCell Bio, China). Mouse embryonic fibroblasts (NIH-3T3, ATCC) were maintained in DMEM (KeyGEN BioTECH, China) with 10% FBS. NIH-3T3 cells were stably transfected with the $(CAGA)_{12}$-Lux reporter to generate CAGA-NIH-3T3 reporter cells. All cells were incubated with 5% CO_2 at 37°C.

Animals

Male C57BL/6 mice (6–8 weeks old, 20–25 g) were purchased from the Weitong Lihua Experimental Animal Technology Co. Ltd. (Beijing, China). The animal experimental protocol was performed in accordance with the Health Guide for Care from the National Institutes (NIH Publications No. 85–23, revised 1996). All animal care and experimental procedures complied with guidelines approved by the Institutional Animal Care and Use Committee (IACUC) of Nankai University (Permit No. SYXK 2019-0001).

BLM Administration

A mouse pulmonary fibrosis model was established by intratracheal BLM administration as described previously (Guo et al., 2019). Briefly, mice were intratracheally administered BLM (2 U/ Kg) dissolved in physiological saline (0.9% NaCl). Forty mice were randomly divided into five groups: the NaCl group, the BLM group, the positive control group (BLM + nintedanib, 100 mg kg^{-1}), the low-dose remdesivir group (BLM + remdesivir, 10 mg kg^{-1}) and the high-dose remdesivir group (BLM + remdesivir, 20 mg kg^{-1}). The mice in the remdesivir groups were intraperitoneally injected daily with 10 mg kg^{-1} or 20 mg kg^{-1} remdesivir, which was suspended in 5% DMSO, 10% PEG and 2.5% polyoxyl 40-hydrogenated castor oil, while mice in the control and BLM groups received equal volumes of vehicle. Mice in the positive control group were intragastrically administered 100 mg kg^{-1} nintedanib daily. The mice were sacrificed on the 14th day after BLM administration for subsequent analysis, including hydroxyproline content determination.

Isolation of Primary Pulmonary Fibroblasts

Primary pulmonary fibroblasts (PPF) were isolated from C57BL/6 J mice. Briefly, the lungs were lavaged three times with 1 ml of PBS, digested with 2.5 mg/ ml dispase II (Roche, United States), and 2.5 mg/ ml Collagenase Type 4 (Worthington, United States) for 30 min at 37°C and then centrifuged. The cell pellet was resuspended in DMEM containing 10% FBS and cultured in 5% CO_2 at 37°C in a humidified atmosphere. PPF cells at passages two to five were used for various assays.

Hydroxyproline Assay

Hydroxyproline was analyzed according to previously described methods (Li et al., 2019).

Histological Examination

The left lung was fixed in 10% formalin, dehydrated and embedded in paraffin. Tissue sections with a thickness of 4 μm were incubated for 4 h at 60°C and stained with hematoxylin and eosin (H and E) and Masson's trichrome. Quantification of pulmonary fibrosis was performed as described previously (Jiang et al., 2004). In brief, Masson staining slides were examined under low power and the whole lung images were captured. Images were analyzed by Image-Pro Plus version 6.0 to demarcate the entire lung area and automatically calculate the total pixel Pw of the region and then calculate the total pixel Pf of the fibrotic region (fibrosis ratio = fibrotic area total pixel Pf/total lung total pixel Pw).

Pulmonary Function Testing

After the mice were anesthetized, the trachea was exposed, and a tracheal cannula was placed and fixed. The mice were transferred to a plethysmography chamber for pulmonary function analysis using an Anires2005 system according to the manufacturer's instructions (Beijing Biolab, Beijing, China).

Cell Viability Analysis

Cell viability was measured using 3-(4,5-dimethylthiazol-2-yl)-2,5-diphenyltetrazolium bromide (MTT) as previously described (Li et al., 2019).

Luciferase Assay

Luciferase reporter assays were performed as previously described (Guo et al., 2019).

Wound Healing Assay

Wound healing assays were performed as previously described (Li et al., 2019).

Transwell Migration Assays

The influence of Remdesivir to NIH-3T3 cells migration was evaluated with a Transwell system. (Corning Costar, 3,422, United States) Briefly, serum-starved cells were trypsin-harvested in DMEM with 0.1% FBS. Next, 600 μL of medium containing 20% FBS was added to the lower chambers, while 200 μL NIH-3T3 cells (1×10^5) were plated in the upper chambers. At the same time, NIH-3T3 cells were treated with/ without PDGF-bb (10 ng/ ml) and remdesivir (12.5, 25, and 50 μM). After 24 h incubation, the cells on the bottom of the transwell membrane were fixed with 4% paraformaldehyde at 37 °C for 20 min and stained with 1% crystal violet at 37°C for 15 min, the nonmigrating cells in the upper chamber were removed with blunt-end swabs. The membranes were washed three times with PBS and photographed under a microscope.

Quantitative Real-Time PCR

The mRNA expression level of genes was determined by qRT-PCR using primers according to a previously described protocol (Li et al., 2020). Primer pairs of target genes used were as follows:

Mouse β-actin (NM_007393.3), 5′-AGGCCAACCGTGAAA AGATG-3′ and 5′-AGAGCA TAGCCCTCGTAGATGG-3′; Human GAPDH (NM_001256799), 5′-GGAGCGAGATCC CTCCAAAAT-3′ and 5′-GGCTGTTGTCATACTTCTCAT GG-3′; Mouse α-SMA (NM_001297715.1), 5′-TGGGTGAACTCCATCGCTGTA-3′and 5′-GTCGAA TGCAACAAGGAAGCC-3′; Mouse Collagen I (NM_000088.4), 5′-AAGCCGGAGGACAACCTTTTA-3′and 5′-GCGAAGAGAATGACCAGATCC-3′; Mouse Fibronectin (NM_001306132.1), 5′-GTGCCCGGAATACGCATGTA-3′and 5′-CTGGTGGACGGGATCATCCT-3′; Human E-cadherin (NM_0,01317185.2), 5′-A TTTTTCCCTCGACACCCGA T-3′and 5′- TCCCAGGCGTAGACCAAGA-3′; Human Vimentin (NM_003380.5), 5′-AGTCCACTGAGTACCGGA GAC-3′ and 5′-CA TTTCACGCA TCTGGCGTTC-3′; Human N-cadherin (NM_001792.5), 5′-TTTGA TGGAGGTCTCCT AACACC-3′ and 5′- ACGTTTAACACGTTGGAAA TGTG-3′; Mouse P16 (NM_058197), 5′-GGCAGGTTCTTGGTCACT GT-3′ and 5′-TGTTCACGAAAGCCAGAGCG-3′; Mouse P21 (NM_001111099), 5′-CCTGGTGATGTCCGACCTG-3′ and 5′-CCATGAGCGCATCGCAATC-3′.

Western Blot Analysis

All proteins were collected from cells or lung tissues as reported previously (Ning et al., 2004). The monoclonal antibodies used in this study were: α-SMA (Affinity, BF9212), Collagen I (Affinity, AF7001), Fibronectin (Affinity, AF5335), β-tubulin (Affinity, T0023), GAPDH (Affinity, AF7021), Phospho-Smad3 (Affinity, AF3362), Smad3 (Affinity AF6323), Smad2 (Affinity, AF6449), Phospho-Smad2 (Affinity, AF3450 Phospho-p38 (Affinity, AF4001), p38 (Affinity, BF8015), Phospho-JNK (Affinity, AF3318), JNK (Affinity, AF6318), Phospho-ERK (Affinity, AF1015), ERK (Affinity, AF0155), Phospho-AKT (Affinity, AF0832), AKT (Affinity, AF6212), Cleaved PARP (Affinity, AF7023), E-cadherin (Cell Signaling Technology, 14472S), N-cadherin (Cell Signaling Technology, 13,116), Vimentin (Cell Signaling Technology, 5,741). The monoclonal antibodies are diluted 1:1,000 with skimmed milk powder.

Immunofluorescence Analysis

NIH-3T3 or A549 cells were seeded in a 24-well chamber. At the end of the treatment, the cells were fixed with a 4% fixative solution for 15 min (Solarbio), permeabilized with 0.2% Triton X-100 for 20 min, and incubated in 5% BSA for 30 min. NIH-3T3 cells were cultured overnight with α-SMA primary antibodies (Affinity, BF9212), and A549 cells were probed with E-cadherin (Cell Signaling Technology, 14472S) and vimentin antibodies (Cell Signaling Technology, 5,741) diluted in 5% BSA, the monoclonal antibodies are diluted 1:200 with skimmed milk powder. Then, the cells were incubated with TRITC-conjugated or FITC-conjugated secondary antibodies. The cells were washed with PBST, and DAPI (Beyotime Biotechnology) was used to stain the nuclei. The fluorescence was examined with a confocal microscope (Nikon, Japan).

Immunohistochemical Staining

Paraffin-embedded lung tissue was dewaxed with xylene, and the sections were heated in a microwave oven with antigen-fixing solution (0.01 M citrate buffer) for 20 min. After the sections were cooled to room temperature and blocked with an immunohistochemistry kit, the primary antibody was added and incubated at 4 °C overnight. The primary antibodies were as follows: mouse anti-α-SMA (1:200 dilution, Affinity, BF9212), mouse anti-fibronectin (1:200 dilution, Affinity, AF5335). After being washed with TBST three times, the tissue sections were incubated with the secondary antibody at room temperature for 1 h. Subsequently, the tissue sections were rehydrated through a series of ethanol solutions and were stained with hematoxylin to observe histological changes and target gene expression under an optical microscope.

Cell Cycle

NIH-3T3 cells were seeded in 6-well plates at a density of 1×10^6cells/well and cultured at 37°C in a humidified 5% CO_2 atmosphere until the cell confluency reached 60–70%. After treated with remdesivir at the desired concentrations (12.5, 25, and 50 μM), NIH-3T3 cells were washed with precooled phosphate buffered saline (PBS) twice and then fixed in 70% ethanol overnight at 4°C. The fixed cells which were washed twice with pre-cooled PBS after fixation were then stained with Propidium (PI)/Rnase A and incubated at 37°C in the dark for 30 min. The DNA content of NIH-3T3 cells were assessed by using a flow cytometer (Thermo Fisher Scientific). FlowJo software (Version 7.6.1) was used to analyze the data.

Statistical Analysis

The data are presented as the means ± SD and were analyzed using Prism version 7.0 software. Differences between the experimental and control groups were assessed by Student's t tests. Significant differences among multiple groups were analyzed by one-way ANOVA. A value of $p < 0.05$ was considered statistically significant.

RESULTS

Remdesivir Attenuates BLM-Induced Pulmonary Fibrosis in Mice

To determine the role of remdesivir in pulmonary fibrosis *in vivo*, C57BL/6 J mice were administered BLM (2 U), and then different doses of remdesivir (10 and 20 mg kg^{-1}) were administered for 14 days (day 1-day 14) (**Figure 1A**). Nintedanib (100 mg kg^{-1}) was used as a positive control. We found that the weight ratio, hydroxyproline level and percentage of fibrotic areas were significantly decreased in the remdesivir-treated group and that the inhibitory effect of remdesivir was better than that of nintedanib, while the survival rate of remdesivir was comparable to nintedanib (**Figures 1B–E**). Moreover, H and E and Masson's trichrome staining were performed to assess the degree of pulmonary fibrosis. As shown in **Figure 1F**, BLM-induced collagen deposition was markedly reduced by remdesivir treatment. Lung function is a decisive factor in the diagnosis and treatment of pulmonary fibrosis in clinical trials. As shown in **Figure 2**, remdesivir significantly improved lung function in BLM-induced fibrotic mice, as seen by the increases in forced vital capacity (FVC) and dynamic compliance (Cdyn) and decreases in inspiratory resistance (Ri) and expiratory resistance (Re), and the effects were superior to those of the positive control drug nintedanib. These data revealed that remdesivir could ameliorate BLM-induced pulmonary fibrosis in mice.

Remdesivir Suppresses TGF-β1-Induced Proliferation and Migration of Lung Fibroblasts

The proliferation and migration of activated fibroblasts contribute to the development of lung fibrosis (Coward et al., 2010). First, we examined whether remdesivir affected the proliferation of normal fibroblasts using the MTT assay. We found that remdesivir had no obvious toxicity on normal fibroblasts, and the IC_{50} value of remdesivir in NIH-3T3 cells was 60.32 μM (**Figure 3A**). We also examined the effect of remdesivir on the cell cycle and senescence of normal fibroblasts in absence of TGF-β1 stimulation and the results showed that after treated with different doses of remdesevir, the fibroblasts didn't arrest and becoming senescent (**Supplementary Figure S1**). To further investigate the effect of remdesivir on cell proliferation of active fibroblasts, we co-treated NIH3T3 cells with TGF-β1 (5 ng ml^{-1}) and remdesivir (12.5, 25, and 50 μM), then used immunofluorescence and western blot to detect the expression of cell proliferation marker Ki67 and cell apoptosis maker cleaved PARP. As shown in **Figures 3B–D**, remdesivir could dose-dependently inhibit the proliferation and apoptosis of TGF-β1-activated fibroblasts.

Then, we used wound healing assay and transwell assay to test the effects of remdesivir on the migration of activated fibroblasts. NIH-3T3 cells were co-treated with remdesivir (12.5, 25, and 50 μM) and TGF-β1 (5 ng ml^{-1}) for 6, 12, 24, and 48 h. As shown in **Figures 4A–C**, remdesivir dose-dependently inhibited the migration of TGF-β1-activated fibroblasts. The transwell assay also indicated that remdesivir could dose-dependently inhibit PDGF-induced migration of fibroblasts (**Figure 4D**).

Remdesivir Attenuates TGF-β1-Induced Activation of Lung Fibroblasts

To further examine whether remdesivir could inhibit the activation of TGF-β1-induced fibroblasts, we treated NIH-3T3 cells and PPF cell with TGF-β1 (5 ng ml^{-1}) and remdesivir (12.5, 25, and 50 μM) to assess the gene expression levels of the typical

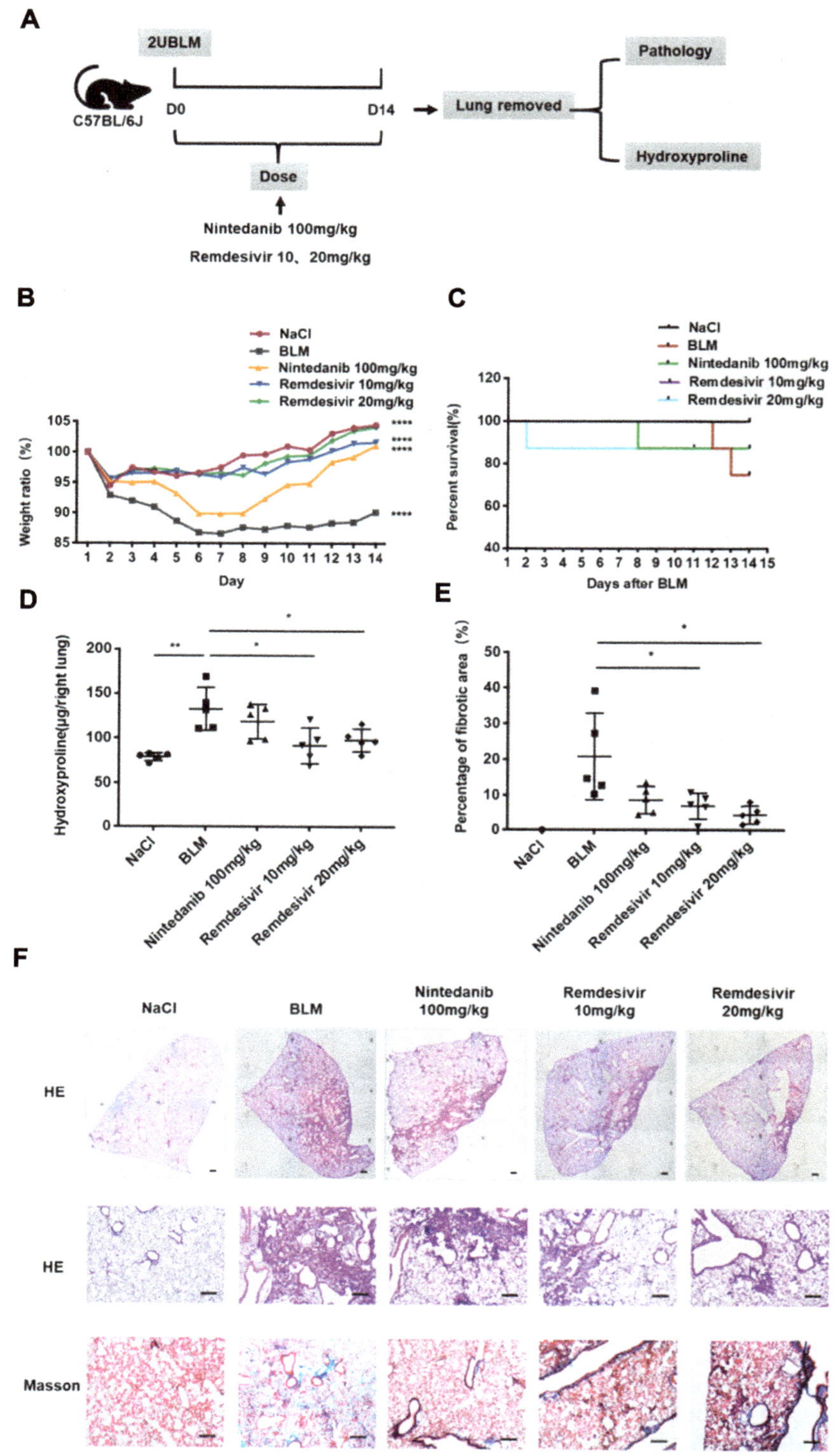

FIGURE 1 | Remdesivir ameliorates BLM-induced pulmonary fibrosis in mice. **(A)** Dosing regimen in BLM-induced pulmonary fibrosis model. **(B)** Changes in body weight relative to initial body weight during administration. **(C)** Percentages of surviving mice were plotted from day 1–14 after BLM treatment. **(D)** Hydroxyproline contents of lung tissues in mice. **(E)** Statistics of lung fibrosis area among groups. **(F)** Lung tissue sections were stained with hematoxylin-eosin (H and E) and Masson Trichrome staining. Scale bar = 50 μm. Data was noted as the means ± SD, $n = 5$. * $p < 0.05$, ** $p < 0.01$, **** $p < 0.0001$.

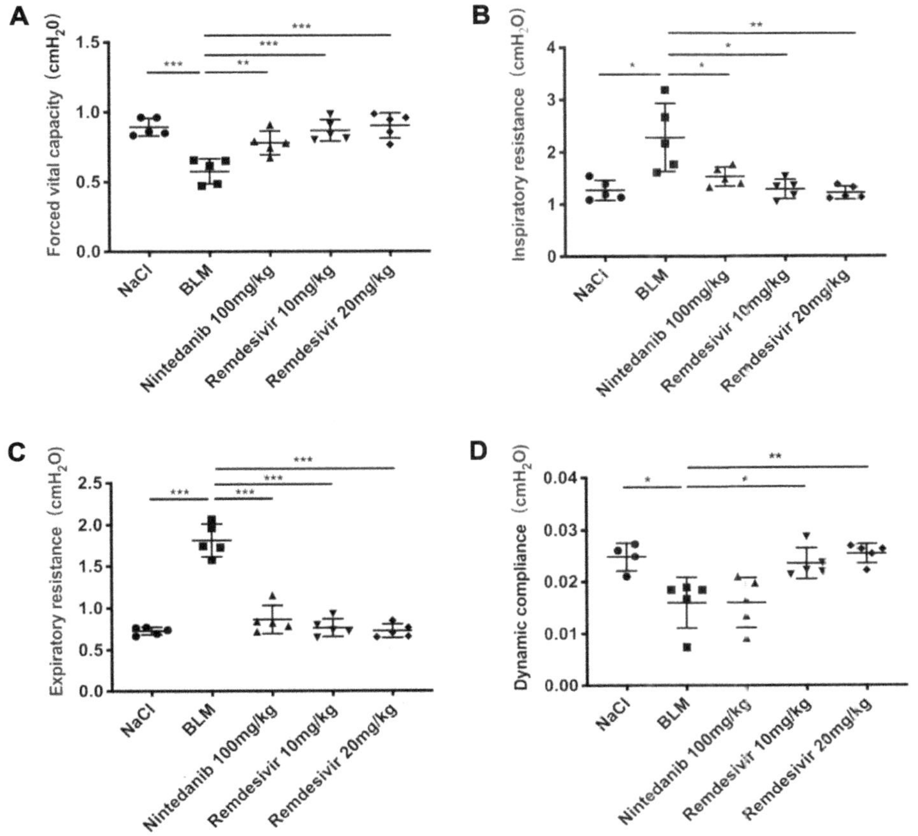

FIGURE 2 | Remdesivir improves pulmonary function in BLM-treated mice. **(A)** Forced vital capacity of mice. **(B)** Inspiratory resistance of mice. **(C)** Expiratory resistance of mice. **(D)** Dynamic compliance of mice. Data was noted as the means ± SD, $n = 5$. * $p < 0.05$, ** $p < 0.01$, *** $p < 0.001$, **** $p < 0.0001$.

fibroblast activation marker α-SMA and the extracellular matrix (ECM) proteins collagen I and fibronectin. As shown in **Figure 5A**, remdesivir dose-dependently decreased TGF-β1-induced expression of the α-SMA, collagen I and fibronectin genes. Similarly, remdesivir treatment reduced the protein expression levels of α-SMA, and fibronectin in TGF-β1-stimulated fibroblasts, including NIH3T3 cell and PPF cell (**Figures 5B,C**). Immunofluorescence assays were used to evaluate α-SMA expression in NIH-3T3 cells, and the results were consistent (**Figures 5D,E**). Accordingly, these results indicated that remdesivir suppressed TGF-β1-induced myofibroblast differentiation and reduced ECM production in myofibroblasts.

Remdesivir Inhibits TGF-β1-Induced Activation of Smad and Non-smad Signaling Pathways in Lung Fibroblasts

The TGF-β1 signaling pathway is critical in regulating the proliferation and activation of fibroblasts in pulmonary fibrosis (Aschner and Downey, 2016). Therefore, we examined whether remdesivir could regulate TGF-β1/Smad and non-Smad signaling in active pulmonary fibroblasts. We stably transfected the $(CAGA)_{12}$-luciferase reporter, which contain repeated canonical Smad3-binding element (SBE) 5′-CAGA-3′ in NIH-3T3 fibroblasts. CAGA-NIH-3T3 cells were used to examine the inhibitory effects of compounds on the TGF-β/Smad3 signaling pathway. After the administration of $5\ \text{ng ml}^{-1}$ TGF-β1, the fluorescence value was obviously increased in CAGA-NIH-3T3 cells, while remdesivir inhibited fluorescence in a dose-dependent manner (**Figure 6A**). Next we used the western blot assay to detect the effect of remdesivir on the activation of TGF-β1/Smad and non-Smad signaling in fibroblasts. We first examined the effect of TGF-β1 on the protein phosphorylation level of Smad and non-Smad under the time gradient, and the results revealed that the phosphorylation level of the protein was positively correlated with the time of adding TGF-β1 and the phosphorylation levels were more significant after 1 h of TGF-β stimulation (**Supplementary Figure S2**). Then we assessed the effect of remdesivir on the activation of Smad3 signaling in NIH-3T3 cells and PPF cells after 1 h treatment of TGF-β1. As shown in **Figures 6B,C**, remdesivir significantly reduced the phosphorylation level of Smad3 and had no significant effect on the protein levels of total Smad3. Moreover, the levels of phosphorylated P38, JNK, ERK and Akt were examined in NIH-3T3 cells by western blotting. The results revealed that remdesivir restrained the activation of TGF-β1/Smad and non-Smad signaling (**Figure 6D**).

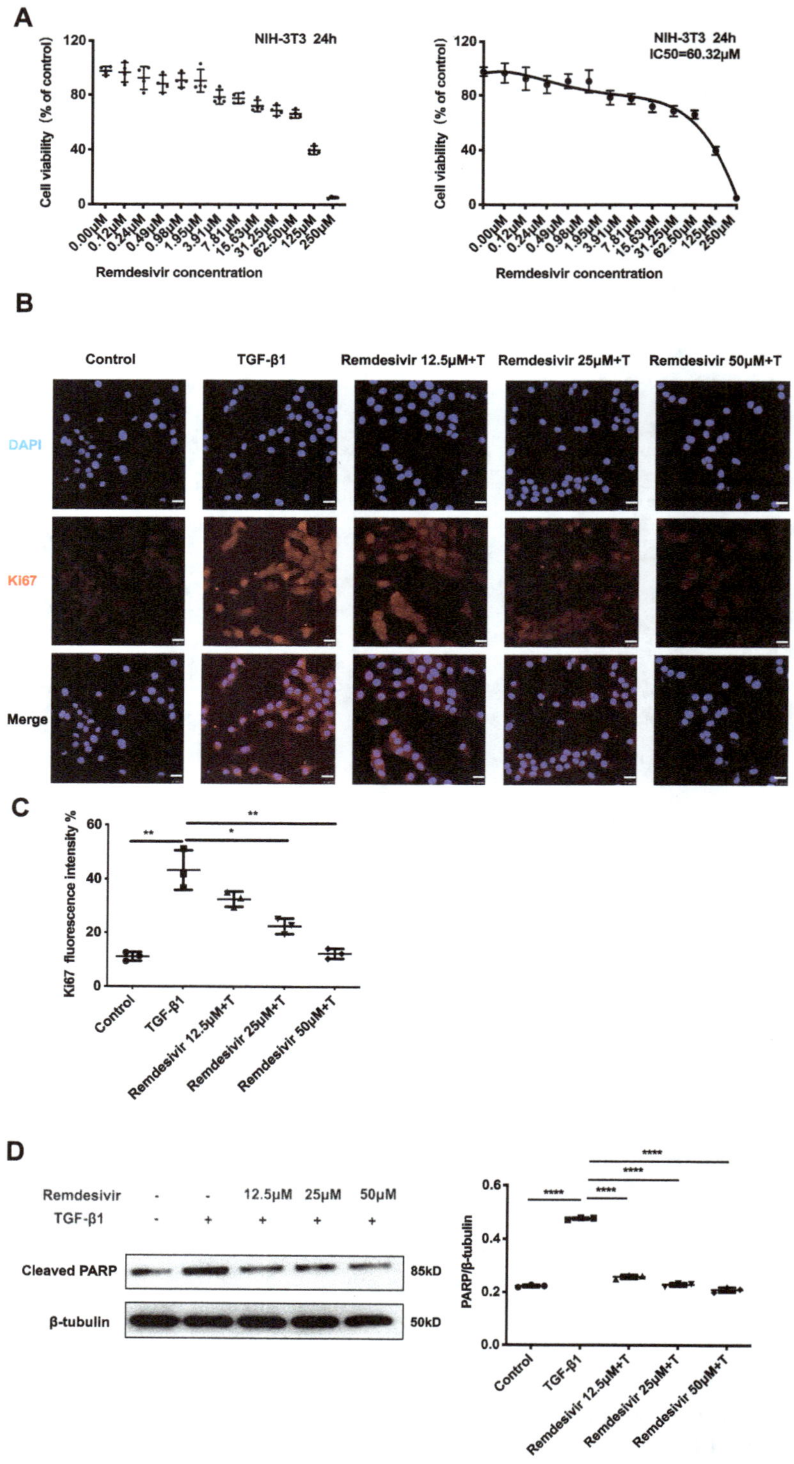

FIGURE 3 | Remdesivir suppresses TGF-β1-induced proliferation of lung fibroblasts. **(A)** MTT assays of NIH-3T3 cells. Cells were exposed to the indicated doses of Remdesivir (0–250 μM) for 24 h, IC_{50} = 60.32 μM (n = 4 per group). **(B–C)** NIH-3T3 cells were co-treated with TGF-β1 (5 ng ml^{-1}) and Remdesivir (12.5, 25, 50 μM) for 24 h to detect the Ki67 expression levels by immunofluorescence. The analyses of mean gray value were shown below. Scale bar = 60 μm (n = 3 per group). **(D)** NIH-3T3 cells were co-treated with TGF-β1 (5 ng ml^{-1}) and Remdesivir (12.5, 25, 50 μM) for 24 h. Cleaved PARP were assessed using western blot. GAPDH was used as the internal control, *n* = 3. Data was presented as the means ± SD. $^{*}p < 0.05$, $^{**}p < 0.01$, $^{***}p < 0.001$, $^{****}p < 0.0001$.

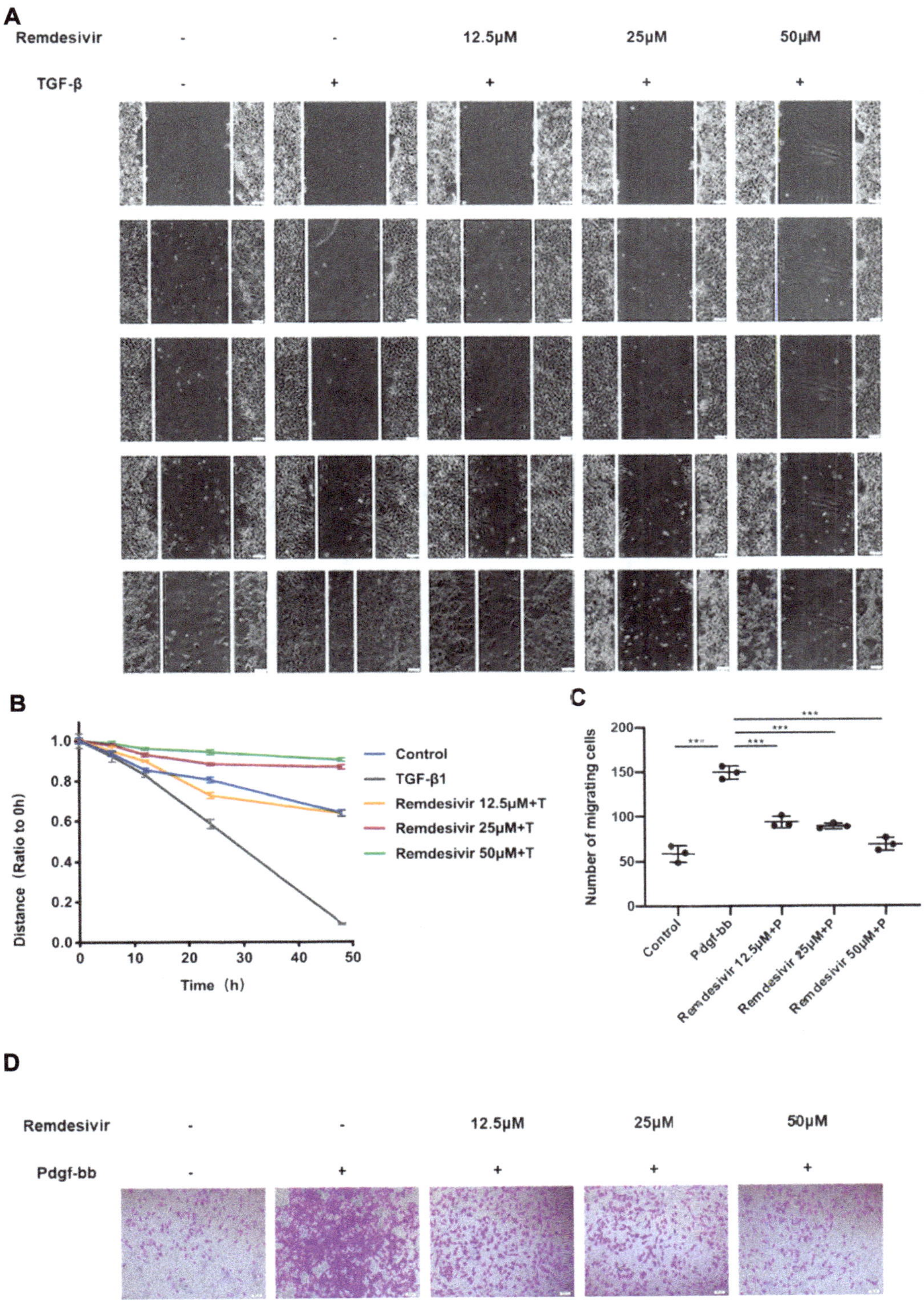

FIGURE 4 | Remdesivir suppresses TGF-β1-induced migration of lung fibroblasts. **(A–B)** Wound healing assays of NIH3T3 co-cultured with TGF-β1 (5 ng ml^{-1}) and Remdesivir (12.5, 25, 50 μM). The wound closure was photographed at 0, 6, 12, 24, and 48 h post-scratching **(C–D)** NIH-3T3 cells treated with/without Remdesivir (12.5, 25, 50 μM) and/or Pdgf-bb (5 ng ml^{-1}). Scale bar = 60 μm. Data was presented as the means ± SD, n = 3. * $p < 0.05$, ** $p < 0.01$, *** $p < 0.001$, **** $p < 0.0001$.

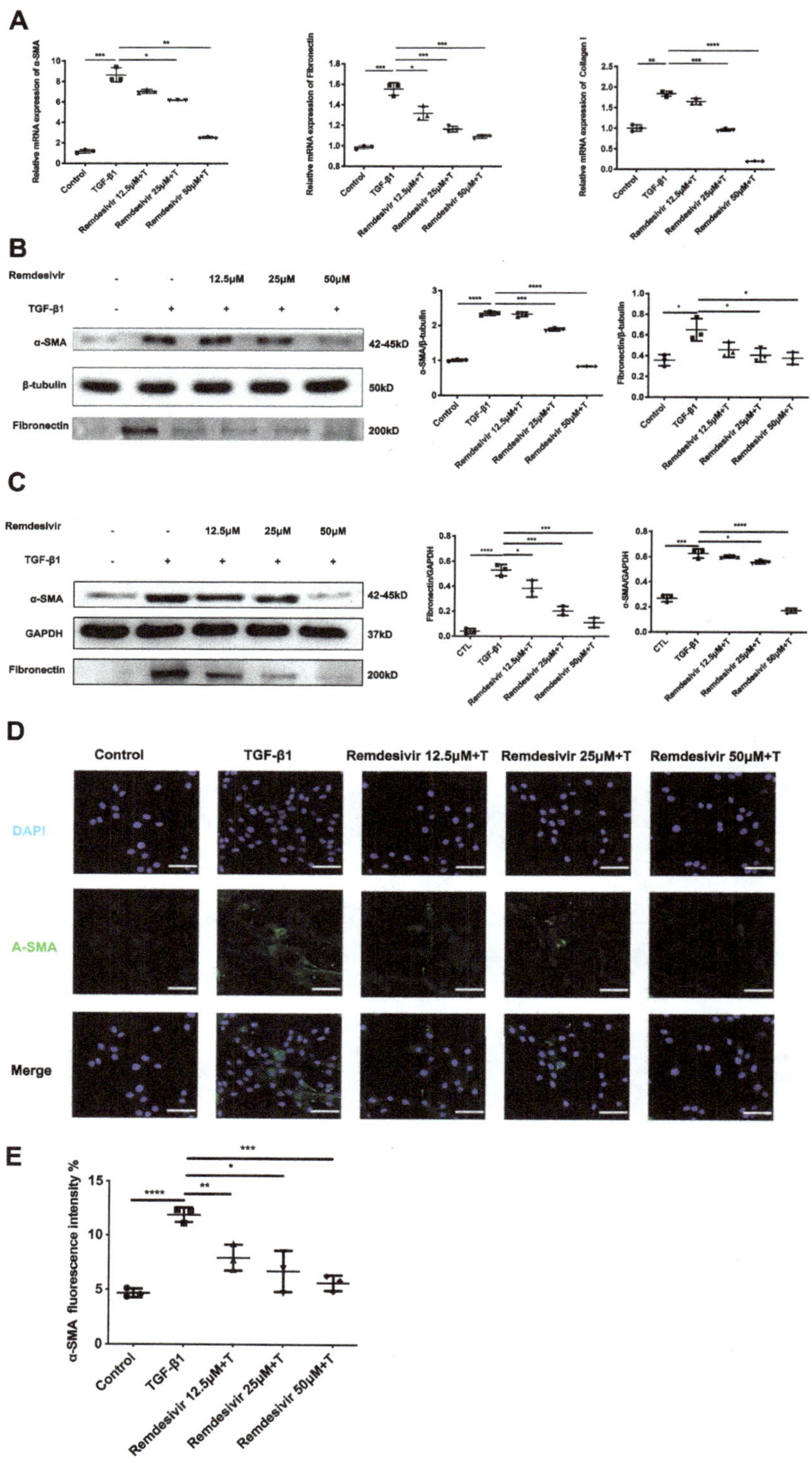

FIGURE 5 | Remdesivir attenuates TGF-β1-induced activation of lung fibroblasts. **(A)** NIH-3T3 cells were co-treated with TGF-β1 (5 ng ml^{-1}) and Remdesivir (12.5, 25, 50 μM) for 24 h. mRNA levels of α-SMA, Fibronectin and Collagen I were tested by RT-PCR in NIH-3T3 cells **(B)** NIH-3T3 cells were co-treated with TGF-β1 (5 ng ml^{-1}) and Remdesivir (12.5, 25, 50 μM) for 24 h. α-SMA and Fibronectin were assessed using western blot, GAPDH was used as the internal control **(C)** PPF cells were co-treated with TGF-β1 (5 ng ml^{-1}) and Remdesivir (12.5, 25, 50 μM) for 24 h. α-SMA and Fibronectin were assessed using western blot, β-tubulin was used as the internal control **(D)** Immunofluorescence staining of α-SMA were performed on NIH-3T3 cells treated with/without TGF-β1 (5 ng ml^{-1}) and/or Remdesivir (12.5, 25, 50 μM) for 24 h. Data was noted as the means ± SD, $n = 3$. $^{*}p < 0.05$, $^{**}p < 0.01$, $^{***}p < 0.001$, $^{****}p < 0.0001$.

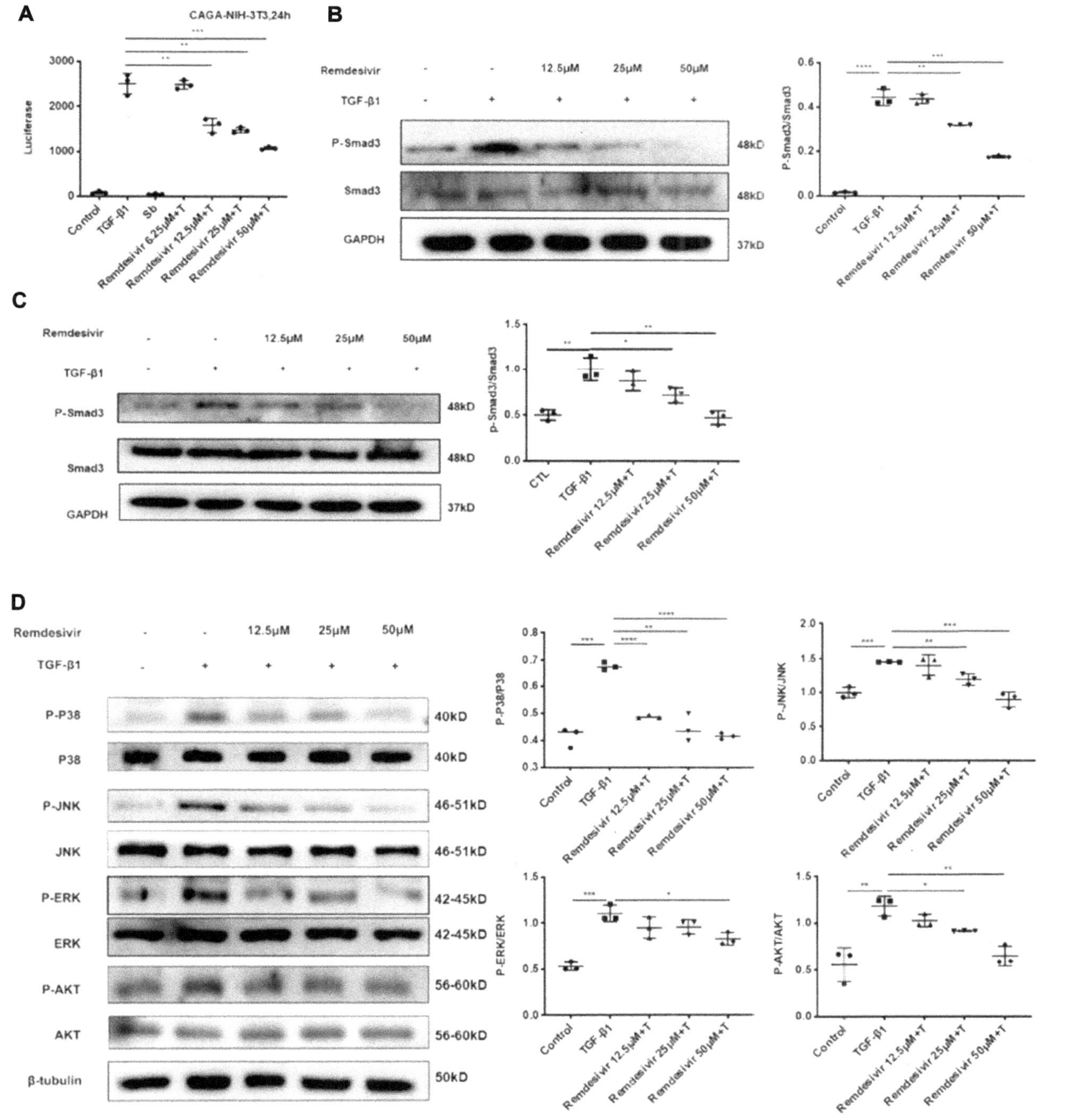

FIGURE 6 | Remdesivir inhibits TGF-β1-induced activation of Smad and non-Smad signaling pathway in lung fibroblasts **(A)** Luciferase assays of CAGA-NIH3T3 cells. Cells were pretreated with Remdesivir (0–50 μM) for 30 min and then incubated with TGF-β1 (5 ng ml^{-1}) for 24 h, then analyzed with luciferase assay. SB431542 is a TGF-β1/Smad pathway inhibitor and serves as a positive control **(B)** NIH-3T3 cells were co-treated with TGF-β1 (5 ng ml^{-1}) and Remdesivir (12.5, 25, 50 μM) for 1 h. P-Smad3 and Smad3 were assessed using western blot. GAPDH was used as the internal control **(C)** PPF cells were co-treated with TGF-β1 (5 ng ml^{-1}) and Remdesivir (12.5, 25, 50 μM) for 1 h. P-Smad3 and Smad3 were assessed using western blot. GAPDH was used as the internal control (D) NIH-3T3 cells were co-treated with TGF-β1 (5 ng ml^{-1}) and Remdesivir (12.5, 25, 50 μM) for 1 h and the phosphorylation levels of P-38, JNK, ERK and Akt were analyzed by Western blot. β-tubulin was used as a loading control in grayscale analysis. Scale bar = 60 μm. Data was presented as the means ± SD, $n = 3$. *$p < 0.05$, **$p < 0.01$, ***$p < 0.001$, ****$p < 0.0001$.

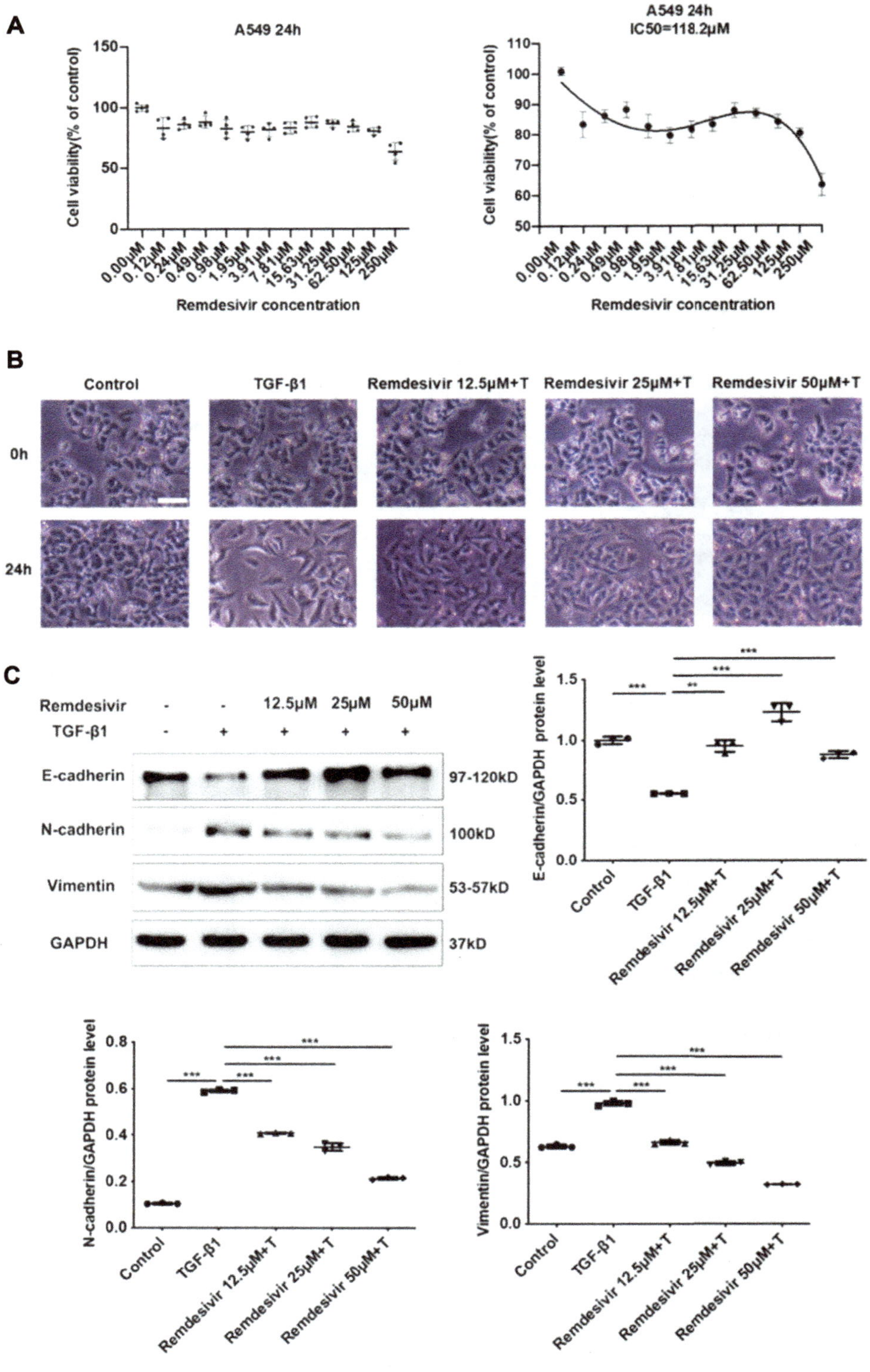

FIGURE 7 | Remdesivir inhibits TGF-β1-induced epithelial to mesenchymal transition in alveolar epithelial cells **(A)** MTT assays of A549 cells. Cells were exposed to the indicated doses of Remdesivir (0–250 μM) for 24 h, IC_{50} = 118.2 μM (n = 4 per group) **(B–C)** A549 cells were co-treated with Remdesivir (12.5, 25, 50 μM) and TGF-β1 (5 ng ml^{-1}) for 24 h **(B)** Morphological changes of A549 cells. **(C)** Protein expression levels of E-cadherin, Vimentin and N-cadherin were assessed by Western blot in A549 cells. GAPDH was used as a loading control. Data was presented as the means ± SD, n = 3. * p < 0.05, ** p < 0.01, *** p < 0.001, **** p < 0.0001.

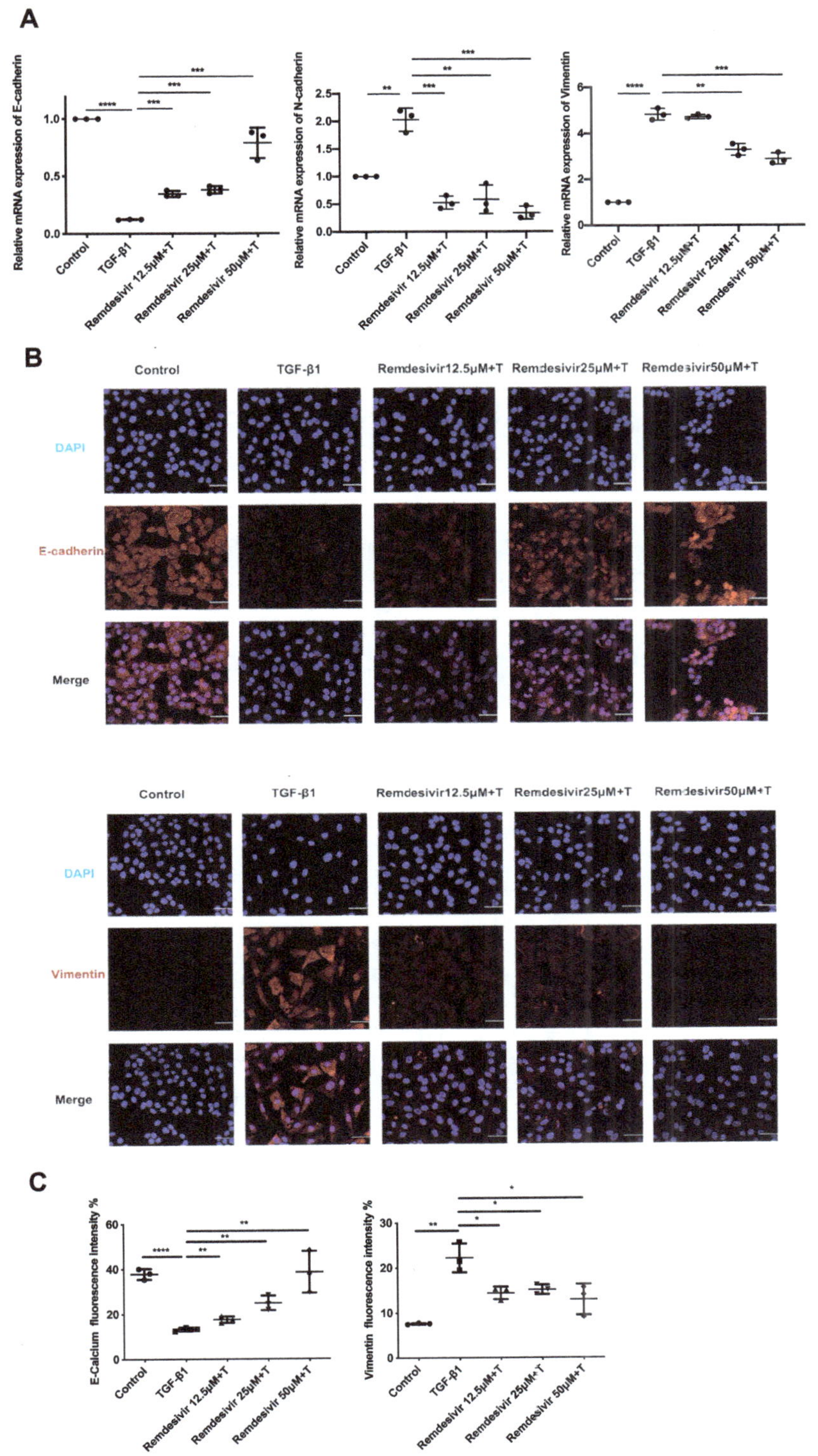

FIGURE 8 | Remdesivir inhibits TGF-β1-induced epithelial to mesenchymal transition in alveolar epithelial cells. A549 cells were co-treated with Remdesivir (12.5, 25, 50 μM) and TGF-β1 (5 ng ml^{-1}) for 24 h **(A)** mRNA levels of E-cadherin, N-cadherin and Vimentin were tested by RT-PCR in A549 cells. **(B–C)** Immunofluorescence analysis of E-cadherin and Vimentin in A549 cells. Scale bar = 50 μm. Data was presented as the means ± SD, n = 3. * $p < 0.05$, ** $p < 0.01$, *** $p < 0.001$.

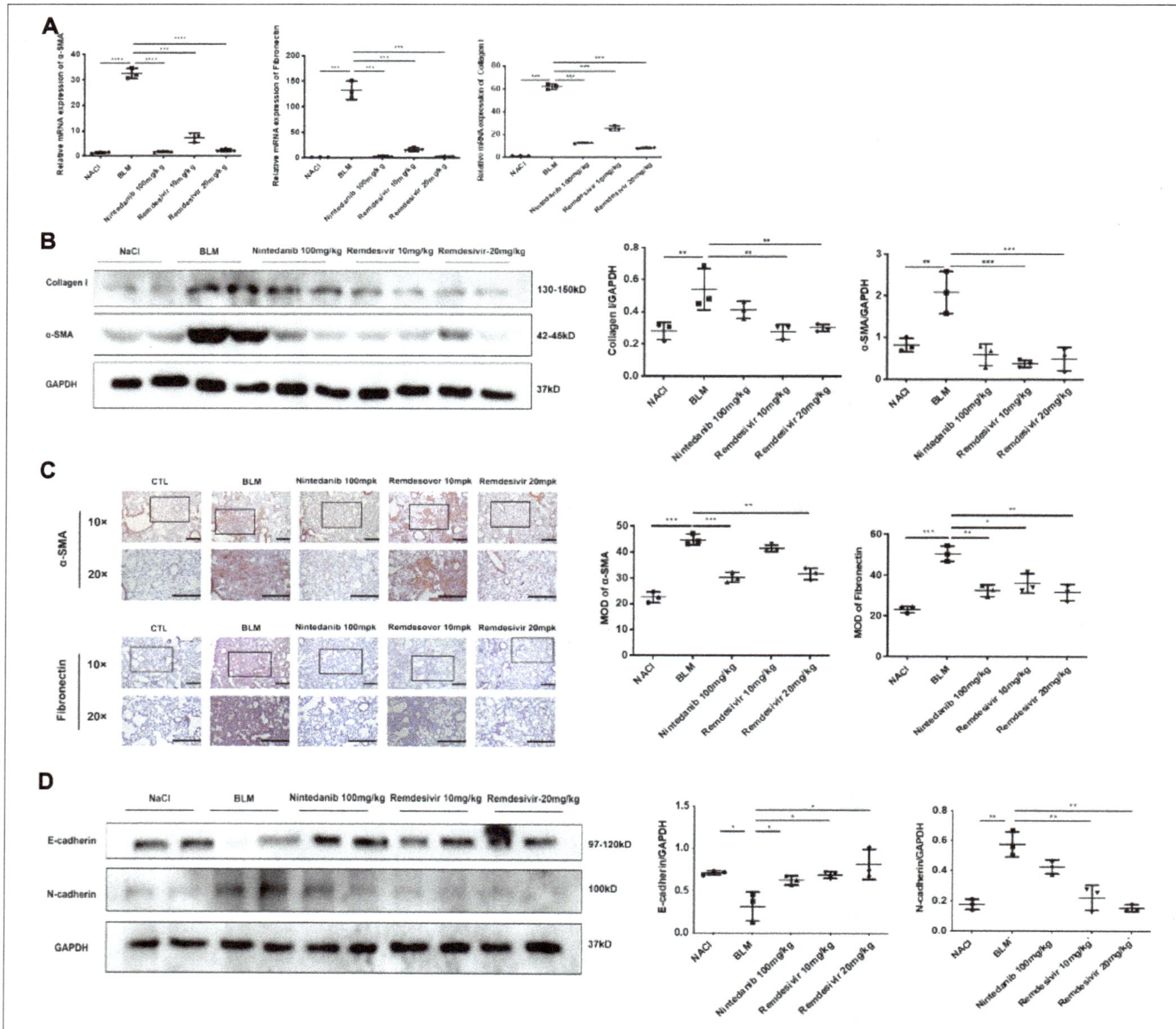

FIGURE 9 | Remdesivir attenuates BLM-induced fibroblast activation and epithelial injury *in vivo* **(A)** RT-PCR was performed to detect mRNA levels of α-SMA, Fibronectin and Collagen I in lung tissues. **(B)** Protein levels of α-SMA and Collagen I were verified by Western blot in lung tissues. GAPDH was used as an internal reference in densitometric analysis **(C)** Immunohistochemical staining analysis of α-SMA and Fibronectin in lung tissues. **(D)** Protein expression levels of E-cadherin and N-cadherin were assessed by Western blot in lung tissues. GAPDH was used as a loading control. Data was presented as the means ± SD, $n = 3$. * $p < 0.05$, ** $p < 0.01$, *** $p < 0.001$.

Remdesivir Inhibits TGF-β1-Induced Phenotypic Transition in Alveolar Epithelial Cells

Evidence suggests that lung fibrosis is a dysregulated epithelial-mesenchymal disorder in which epithelial injury is an initiating event (Selman and Pardo, 2002). The hallmark features of injured epithelial cells are the decreased expression of epithelial markers, including E-cadherin, and the increased expression of mesenchymal markers, such as N-cadherin and vimentin (King et al., 2011; Kage and Borok, 2012). First, we examined whether remdesivir affected the proliferation of A549 cells using the MTT assay. We found that remdesivir had no obvious toxicity on A549 cell, and the IC_{50} value of remdesivir in A549 cells was 118.2 μM (**Figure 7A**). To explore whether remdesivir exerted antifibrotic effects by protecting against epithelial to mesenchymal transition, we used stimulated human pulmonary epithelial cells (A549 cells) with TGF-β1 and then treated the cells with remdesivir (12.5, 25, and 500 μM). After 24 h, the morphological changes and expression of epithelial/mesenchymal phenotypic markers in A549 cells were examined. The results indicated that remdesivir could effectively reverse the

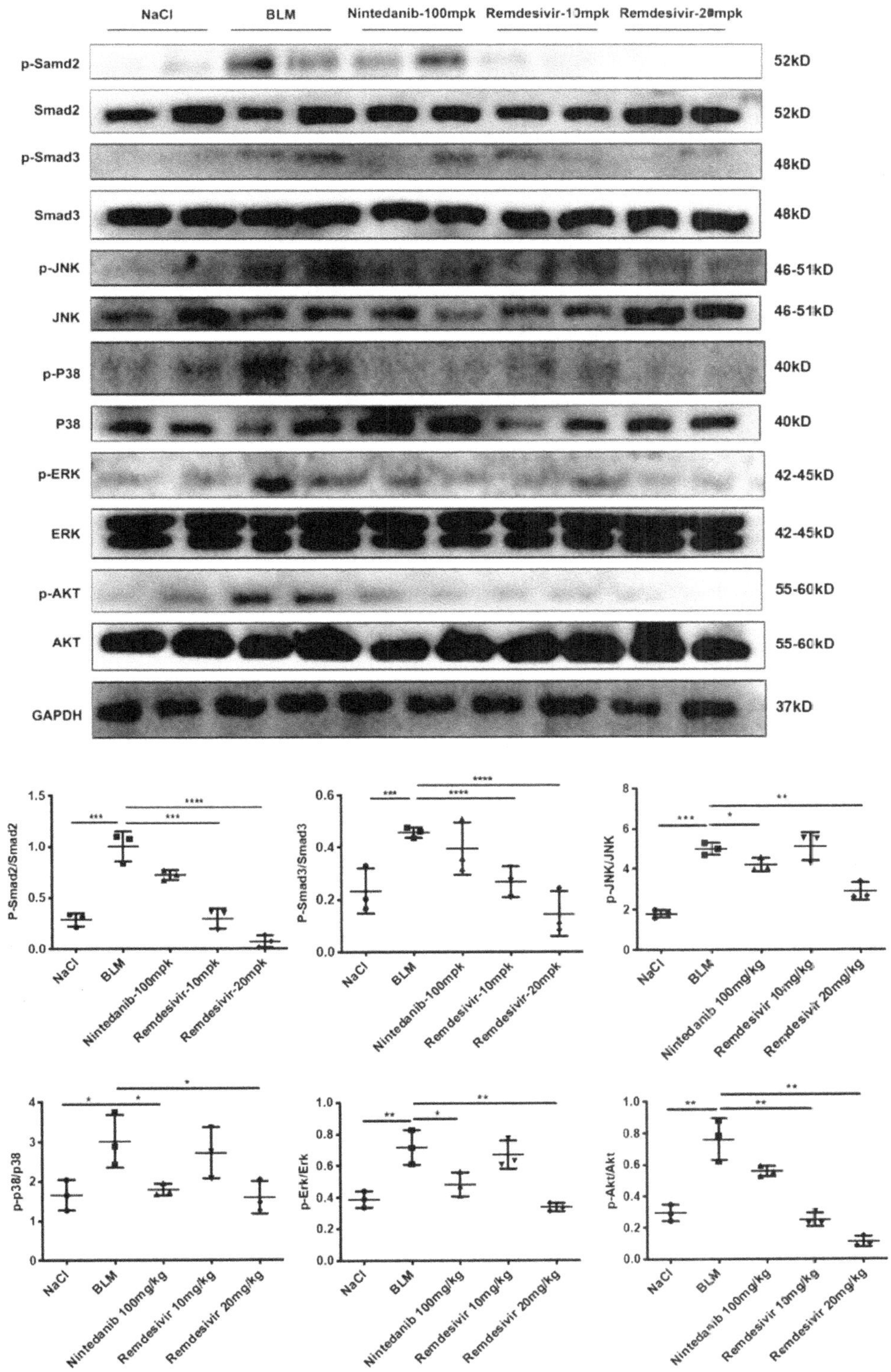

FIGURE 10 | Remdesivir suppress BLM-induced pulmonary fibrosis in mice via inhibiting TGF-β1-Smad and non-Smad signaling pathway *in vivo*. Protein levels of p-Smad2, Smad2, p-Smad3, Smad3, p-P38, P38, p-JNK, JNK, p-ERK, ERK, p-AKT, and AKT were verified by Western blot in lung tissues. GAPDH was used as an internal reference in densitometric analysis. Data was presented as the means ± SD, $n = 3$. ** $p < 0.01$, *** $p < 0.001$.

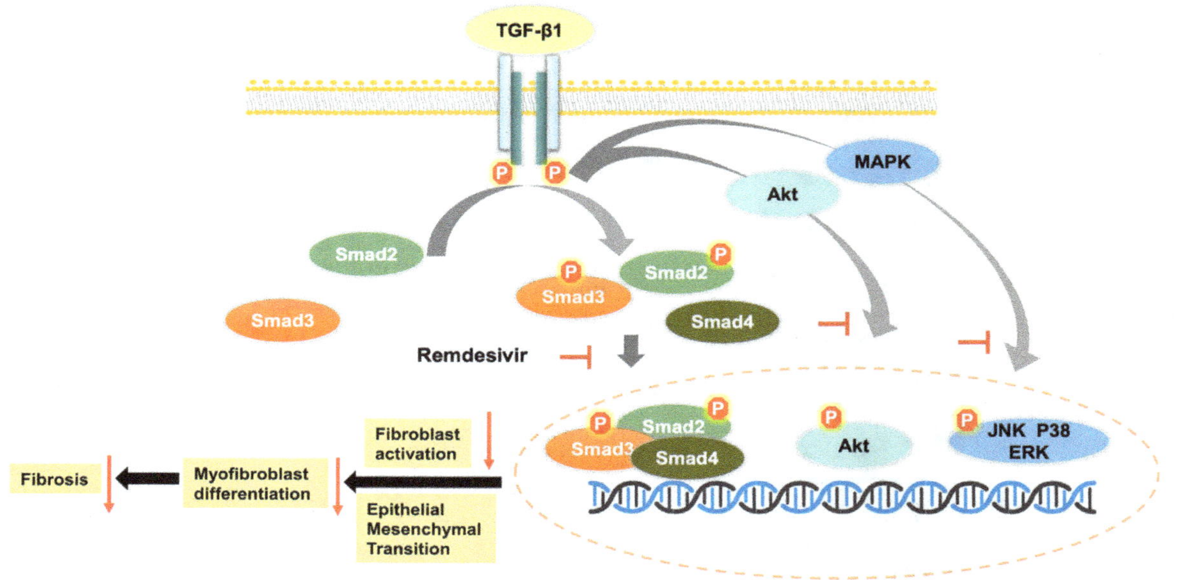

FIGURE 11 | Mechanism for the anti-pulmonary fibrosis effect of remdesivir.

morphological changes in TGF-β1-induced A549 cells (**Figure 7B**). The qRT-PCR and western blot results indicated that remdesivir could significantly increase the expression of the epithelial marker E-cadherin and decrease the expression of the mesenchymal markers N-cadherin and vimentin in A549 cells (**Figure 7C**; **Figure 8A**). Moreover, the immunofluorescence staining results were consistent with the above results (**Figures 8B,C**). Collectively, these data indicate that remdesivir inhibits TGF-β1-induced phenotypic transition in alveolar epithelial cells.

Remdesivir Attenuates BLM-Induced Fibroblast Activation and Epithelial to Mesenchymal Transition *in vivo*

To further verify whether remdesivir could reduce the activation of lung fibroblasts *in vivo*, we extracted protein and RNA from lung tissues and analyzed them by western blotting and qRT-PCR. The results confirmed that the protein and RNA expression levels of α-SMA and collagen I in the lung tissues of the remdesivir group were significantly lower than those in the BLM model group and better than those of the positive control group (**Figures 9A,B**). We also performed immunohistochemical analysis of lung tissue sections, and the expression levels of α-SMA and fibronectin in the lung tissues of remdesivir-treated mice were lower than those in the BLM model group (**Figure 9C**). Epithelial-mesenchymal transition markers were evaluated, and similar to our *in vitro* results, western blotting showed that E-cadherin expression was increased and N-cadherin expression was decreased by remdesivir treatment (**Figure 9D**). Then we further verified whether remdesivir could influence TGF-β1 signaling pathway *in vivo*, the western blotting results indicated that remdesivir significantly reduced the activation of Smad2/3 and MAPK signaling in the lung tissues of bleomycin-injured mice (**Figure 10**). In conclusion, remdesivir attenuated BLM-induced fibroblast activation and epithelial to mesenchymal transition *in vivo*.

DISCUSSION

In this study, we first reported that remdesivir could attenuate BLM-induced pulmonary fibrosis by suppressing the proliferation, migration and activation of lung fibroblasts and improving alveolar epithelial to mesenchymal transition. We confirmed that TGF-β1 signaling is the key pathway in the antifibrotic pharmacological mechanism of remdesivir. Thus, we propose that remdesivir may be a potential drug candidate for preventing pulmonary fibrosis.

In the past year, SARS-CoV-2 has spread around the globe, infecting millions and claiming far too many lives. According to a case report, 25.9% of COVID-19 patients were seriously ill, and 17.2–31% of COVID-19 patients suffered from viral-induced ARDS (Lai et al., 2020). A considerable proportion of ARDS patients will suffer from long-term damage to lung function, and CT follow-up of these patients also showed evidence of pulmonary fibrosis (Herridge et al., 2011; Masclans et al., 2011). The pathology of severe COVID-19-related lung damage also indicated the existence of pulmonary fibrosis, which was shown as hyperplastic and metaplastic changes in pneumocytes and interstitial collagen fiber deposits (Kommoss et al., 2020). In recent decades, a single tracheal instillation of BLM in rodents has been a widely used model for studying the occurrence of pulmonary fibrosis and evaluating the effects of antifibrotic treatments (Jenkins et al., 2017). BLM induces a significant fibrotic reaction in the lungs, and the pathological manifestations are similar to clinical manifestations, including destruction of alveolar structure, abnormal fibroblast proliferation and differentiation, and excessive deposition of ECM proteins (Kolb et al., 2020). The initiation of BLM-induced injury is also an acute inflammatory response, including the infiltration of inflammatory cells and the upregulation of acute inflammatory factors such as interleukins, and the disease will then progress to pulmonary fibrosis (Chaudhary et al., 2006). In our study, we used a BLM-induced model to mimic post-COVID-19 fibrosis and evaluated the effect of remdesivir on pulmonary fibrosis. The results indicated that remdesivir could attenuate BLM-induced collagen deposition, improve lung function *in vivo*, and inhibit myofibroblast activation and epithelial injury both *in vivo* and *in vitro*.

TGF-β is a widely expressed multifunctional cytokine that plays a key role in the tissue repair process after injury. TGF-β1 is the core regulatory factor in the pathological repair process associated with pulmonary fibrosis (Aschner and Downey, 2016). In the pathological process of pulmonary fibrosis, TGF-β1 activates Smad and non-Smad transcription factors via the serine-threonine kinase transduction pathway and then promotes the transcription of genes involved in ECM formation, stimulates fibroblast migration and proliferation, induces the deposition of collagen and fibronectin, and promotes alveolar epithelial cell injury (Fernandez and Eickelberg, 2012). Here, we first demonstrated that remdesivir attenuated pulmonary fibrosis by inhibiting the TGF-β signaling pathway. The *in vitro* data indicated that remdesivir suppressed TGF-β1-induced proliferation, migration, and activation of lung fibroblasts and improved TGF-β1-induced alveolar epithelial cell injury by inhibiting the TGF-β1/Smad and TGF-β1/non-Smad signaling pathways (**Figure 11**). These data indicate that in addition to antiviral targets, remdesivir may interfere with the TGF-β1 pathway through other targets, and these specific targets will be further studied.

AUTHOR CONTRIBUTIONS

HZ and CY designed the study. XHL, RL and YC performed the *in vivo* experiments. JL and ZB performed the *in vitro* experiments. SL and YM analyzed the experimental data. LZ and XPL wrote the manuscript with input from all co-authors.

REFERENCES

Agency, E. (2020). First COVID-19 Treatment Authorised for Use in the EU. Available from: https://www.ema.europa.eu/en/human-regulatory/overview/public-health-threats/coronavirus-disease-covid-19/treatments-vaccines-covid-19#remdesivir-section.

Aschner, Y., and Downey, G. P. (2016). Transforming Growth Factor-β: Master Regulator of the Respiratory System in Health and Disease. *Am. J. Respir. Cel Mol Biol* 54, 647–655. doi:10.1165/rcmb.2015-0391TR

Bajwah, S., Wilcock, A., Towers, R., Costantini, M., Bausewein, C., Simon, S. T., et al. (2020). Managing the Supportive Care Needs of Those Affected by COVID-19. *Eur. Respir. J.* 55. doi:10.1183/13993003.00815-2020

Beigel, J. H., Tomashek, K. M., Dodd, L. E., Mehta, A. K., Zingman, B. S., Kalil, A. C., et al. (2020). Remdesivir for the Treatment of Covid-19 - Final Report. *N. Engl. J. Med.* 383, 1813–1826. doi:10.1056/NEJMoa2007764

Brown, A. J., Won, J. J., Graham, R. L., Dinnon, K. H., 3rd, Sims, A. C., Feng, J. Y., et al. (2019). Broad Spectrum Antiviral Remdesivir Inhibits Human Endemic and Zoonotic Deltacoronaviruses with a Highly Divergent RNA Dependent RNA Polymerase. *Antivir. Res* 169, 104541. doi:10.1016/j.antiviral.2019.104541

Chaudhary, N. I., Schnapp, A., and Park, J. E. (2006). Pharmacologic Differentiation of Inflammation and Fibrosis in the Rat Bleomycin Model. *Am. J. Respir. Crit. Care Med.* 173, 769–776. doi:10.1164/rccm.200505-717OC

Coward, W. R., Saini, G., and Jenkins, G. (2010). The Pathogenesis of Idiopathic Pulmonary Fibrosis. *Ther. Adv. Respir. Dis.* 4, 367–388. doi:10.1177/1753465810379801

Das, K. M., Lee, E. Y., Singh, R., Enani, M. A., Al Dossari, K., Van Gorkom, K., et al. (2017). Follow-up Chest Radiographic Findings in Patients with MERS-CoV after Recovery. *Indian J. Radiol. Imaging* 27, 342–349. doi:10.4103/ijri.IJRI_469_16

de Wit, E., Feldmann, F., Cronin, J., Jordan, R., Okumura, A., Thomas, T., et al. (2020). Prophylactic and Therapeutic Remdesivir (GS-5734) Treatment in the Rhesus Macaque Model of MERS-CoV Infection. *Proc. Natl. Acad. Sci. U S A.* 117, 6771–6776. doi:10.1073/pnas.1922083117

Diseases, N. (2020). NIH Clinical Trial Shows Remdesivir Accelerates Recovery from Advanced COVID-19. Available from: www.nih.gov/news-events/news-releases/nih-clinical-trial-shows-remdesivir-accelerates-recovery-advanced-covid-19.

Fernandez, I. E., and Eickelberg, O. (2012). The Impact of TGF-β on Lung Fibrosis: from Targeting to Biomarkers. *Proc. Am. Thorac. Soc.* 9, 111–116. doi:10.1513/pats.201203-023AW

George, P. M., Wells, A. U., and Jenkins, R. G. (2020). Pulmonary Fibrosis and COVID-19: the Potential Role for Antifibrotic Therapy. *Lancet Respir. Med.* 8, 807–815. doi:10.1016/S2213-2600(20)30225-3

Goldman, J. D., Lye, D. C. B., Hui, D. S., Marks, K. M., Bruno, R., Montejano, R., et al. (2020). Remdesivir for 5 or 10 Days in Patients with Severe Covid-19. *N. Engl. J. Med.* 383, 1827–1837. doi:10.1056/NEJMoa2015301

Guo, J., Fang, Y., Jiang, F., Li, L., Zhou, H., Xu, X., et al. (2019). Neohesperidin Inhibits TGF-β1/Smad3 Signaling and Alleviates Bleomycin-Induced Pulmonary Fibrosis in Mice. *Eur. J. Pharmacol.* 864, 172712. doi:10.1016/j.ejphar.2019.172712

Herridge, M. S., Tansey, C. M., Matté, A., Tomlinson, G., Diaz-Granados, N., Cooper, A., et al. (2011). Functional Disability 5 Years after Acute Respiratory Distress Syndrome. *N. Engl. J. Med.* 364, 1293–1304. doi:10.1056/NEJMoa1011802

Jenkins, R. G., Moore, B. B., Chambers, R. C., Eickelberg, O., Königshoff, M., Kolb, M., et al. (2017). An Official American Thoracic Society Workshop Report: Use of Animal Models for the Preclinical Assessment of Potential Therapies for Pulmonary Fibrosis. *Am. J. Respir. Cel Mol Biol* 56, 667–679. doi:10.1165/rcmb.2017-0096ST

Jiang, D., Liang, J., Hodge, J., Lu, B., Zhu, Z., Yu, S., et al. (2004). Regulation of Pulmonary Fibrosis by Chemokine Receptor CXCR3. *J. Clin. Invest.* 114, 291–299. doi:10.1172/JCI16861

Jiang, S., Du, L., and Shi, Z. (2020). An Emerging Coronavirus Causing Pneumonia Outbreak in Wuhan, China: Calling for Developing Therapeutic and Prophylactic Strategies. *Emerg. Microbes Infect.* 9, 275–277. doi:10.1080/22221751.2020.1723441

Kage, H., and Borok, Z. (2012). EMT and Interstitial Lung Disease: a Mysterious Relationship. *Curr. Opin. Pulm. Med.* 18, 517–523. doi:10.1097/MCP.0b013e3283566721

King, T. E., Jr., Pardo, A., and Selman, M. (2011). Idiopathic Pulmonary Fibrosis. *Lancet* 378, 1949–1961. doi:10.1016/S0140-6736(11)60052-4

Kolb, P., Upagupta, C., Vierhout, M., Ayaub, E., Bellaye, P. S., Gauldie, J., et al. (2020). The Importance of Interventional Timing in the Bleomycin Model of Pulmonary Fibrosis. *Eur. Respir. J.* 55. doi:10.1183/13993003.01105-2019

Kommoss, F. K. F., Schwab, C. Tavernar, L., Schreck, J., Wagner, W. L., Merle, U., et al. (2020). The Pathology of Severe COVID-19-Related Lung Damage. *Dtsch Arztebl Int.* 117, 500–506. doi:10.3238/arztebl.2020.0500

Lai, C. C., Shih, T. P., Ko, W. C., Tang, H. J., and Hsueh, P. R. (2020). Severe Acute Respiratory Syndrome Coronavirus 2 (SARS-CoV-2) and Coronavirus Disease-2019 (COVID-19): The Epidemic and the Challenges. *Int. J. Antimicrob. Agents* 55, 105924. doi:10.1016/j.ijantimicag.2020.105924

Jiang, D., Liang, J., Hodge, J., Lu, B., Zhu, Z., Yu, S., et al. (2004). Regulation of Pulmonary Fibrosis by Chemokine Receptor CXCR3. *J. Clin. Invest.* 114, 291–299. doi:10.1172/JCI16861

Jiang, S., Du, L., and Shi, Z. (2020). An Emerging Coronavirus Causing Pneumonia Outbreak in Wuhan, China: Calling for Developing Therapeutic and Prophylactic Strategies. *Emerg. Microbes Infect.* 9, 275–277. doi:10.1080/22221751.2020.1723441

Kage, H., and Borok, Z. (2012). EMT and Interstitial Lung Disease: a Mysterious Relationship. *Curr. Opin. Pulm. Med.* 18, 517–523. doi:10.1097/MCP.0b013e3283566721

King, T. E., Jr., Pardo, A., and Selman, M. (2011). Idiopathic Pulmonary Fibrosis. *Lancet* 378, 1949–1961. doi:10.1016/S0140-6736(11)60052-4

Kolb, P., Upagupta, C., Vierhout, M., Ayaub, E., Bellaye, P. S., Gauldie, J., et al. (2020). The Importance of Interventional Timing in the Bleomycin Model of Pulmonary Fibrosis. *Eur. Respir. J.* 55. doi:10.1183/13993003.01105-2019

Kommoss, F. K. F., Schwab, C., Tavernar, L., Schreck, J., Wagner, W. L., Merle, U., et al. (2020). The Pathology of Severe COVID-19-Related Lung Damage. *Dtsch Arztebl Int.* 117, 500–506. doi:10.3238/arztebl.2020.0500

Lai, C. C., Shih, T. P., Ko, W. C., Tang, H. J., and Hsueh, P. R. (2020). Severe Acute Respiratory Syndrome Coronavirus 2 (SARS-CoV-2) and Coronavirus Disease-2019 (COVID-19): The Epidemic and the Challenges. *Int. J. Antimicrob. Agents* 55, 105924. doi:10.1016/j.ijantimicag.2020.105924

Disease Therapeutics. *N. Engl. J. Med.* 381, 2293–2303. doi:10.1056/NEJMoa1910993

Ning, W., Li, C. J., Kaminski, N., Feghali-Bostwick, C. A., Alber, S. M., Di, Y. P., et al. (2004). Comprehensive Gene Expression Profiles Reveal Pathways Related to the Pathogenesis of Chronic Obstructive Pulmonary Disease. *Proc. Natl. Acad. Sci. U S A.* 101, 14895–14900. doi:10.1073/pnas.0401168101

Pan, Y., Guan, H., Zhou, S., Wang, Y., Li, Q., Zhu, T., et al. (2020). Initial CT Findings and Temporal Changes in Patients with the Novel Coronavirus Pneumonia (2019-nCoV): a Study of 63 Patients in Wuhan, China. *Eur. Radiol.* 30, 3306–3309. doi:10.1007/s00330-020-06731-x

Selman, M., and Pardo, A. (2002). Idiopathic Pulmonary Fibrosis: an Epithelial/fibroblastic Cross-Talk Disorder. *Respir. Res.* 3, 3. doi:10.1186/rr175

Sheahan, T. P., Sims, A. C., Zhou, S., Graham, R. L., Pruijssers, A. J., Agostini, M. L., et al. (2020). An Orally Bioavailable Broad-Spectrum Antiviral Inhibits SARS-CoV-2 in Human Airway Epithelial Cell Cultures and Multiple Coronaviruses in Mice. *Sci. Transl Med.* 12. doi:10.1126/scitranslmed.abb5883

Spinner, C. D., Gottlieb, R. L., Criner, G. J., Arribas López, J. R., Cattelan, A. M., Soriano Viladomiu, A., et al. (2020). Effect of Remdesivir vs Standard Care on Clinical Status at 11 Days in Patients with Moderate COVID-19: A Randomized Clinical Trial. *JAMA* 324, 1048–1057. doi:10.1001/jama.2020.16349

Tchesnokov, E. P., Feng, J. Y., Porter, D. P., and Götte, M. (2019). Mechanism of Inhibition of Ebola Virus RNA-dependent RNA Polymerase by Remdesivir. *Viruses* 11, 11. doi:10.3390/v11040326

Wang, D., Hu, B., Hu, C., Zhu, F., Liu, X., Zhang, J., et al. (2020). Clinical Characteristics of 138 Hospitalized Patients with 2019 Novel Coronavirus-Infected Pneumonia in Wuhan, China. *JAMA* 323, 1061–1069. doi:10.1001/jama.2020.1585

Warren, T. K., Jordan, R., Lo, M. K., Ray, A. S., Mackman, R. L., Soloveva, V., et al. (2016). Therapeutic Efficacy of the Small Molecule GS-5734 against Ebola Virus in Rhesus Monkeys. *Nature* 531, 381–385. doi:10.1038/nature17180

Who (2020). Novel Coronavirus (2019-nCoV) Situation Reports. Available from: http://www.who.int/emergencies/diseases/novel-coronavirus-2019/situation-reports/.

Xie, L., Liu, Y., Xiao, Y., Tian, Q., Fan, B., Zhao, H., et al. (2005). Follow-up Study on Pulmonary Function and Lung Radiographic Changes in Rehabilitating Severe Acute Respiratory Syndrome Patients after Discharge. *Chest* 127, 2119–2124. doi:10.1378/chest.127.6.2119

Xu, Y. H., Dong, J. H., An, W. M., Lv, X. Y., Yin, X. P., Zhang, J. Z., et al. (2020). Clinical and Computed Tomographic Imaging Features of Novel Coronavirus Pneumonia Caused by SARS-CoV-2. *J. Infect.* 80, 394–400. doi:10.1016/j.jinf.2020.02.017

Zhou, S., Wang, Y., Zhu, T., and Xia, L. (2020). CT Features of Coronavirus Disease 2019 (COVID-19) Pneumonia in 62 Patients in Wuhan, China. *AJR Am. J. Roentgenol* 214, 1287–1294. doi:10.2214/AJR.20.22975

3

Study on the Mechanism of Astragalus Polysaccharide in Treating Pulmonary Fibrosis Based on "Drug-Target-Pathway" Network

Pingping Bing, Wenhu Zhou and Songwen Tan**

Academician Workstation, Changsha Medical University, Changsha, China

***Correspondence:**
Wenhu Zhou
zhouwenhuyaoji@163.com
Songwen Tan
tansongwening@gmail.com

Pulmonary fibrosis is a chronic, progressive and irreversible heterogeneous disease of pulmonary interstitial tissue. Its incidence is increasing year by year in the world, and it will be further increased due to the pandemic of COVID-19. However, at present, there is no safe and effective treatment for this disease, so it is very meaningful to find drugs with high efficiency and less adverse reactions. The natural astragalus polysaccharide has the pharmacological effect of anti-pulmonary fibrosis with little toxic and side effects. At present, the mechanism of anti-pulmonary fibrosis of astragalus polysaccharide is not clear. Based on the network pharmacology and molecular docking method, this study analyzes the mechanism of Astragalus polysaccharides in treating pulmonary fibrosis, which provides a theoretical basis for its further clinical application. The active components of Astragalus polysaccharides were screened out by Swisstarget database, and the related targets of pulmonary fibrosis were screened out by GeneCards database. Protein-protein interaction network analysis and molecular docking were carried out to verify the docking affinity of active ingredients. At present, through screening, we have obtained 92 potential targets of Astragalus polysaccharides for treating pulmonary fibrosis, including 11 core targets. Astragalus polysaccharides has the characteristics of multi-targets and multi-pathways, and its mechanism of action may be through regulating the expression of VCAM1, RELA, CDK2, JUN, CDK1, HSP90AA1, NOS2, SOD1, CASP3, AHSA1, PTGER3 and other genes during the development of pulmonary fibrosis.

Keywords: Astragalus polysaccharides, pulmonary fibrosis, network pharmacology, molecular docking, mechanism

INTRODUCTION

Pulmonary fibrosis is caused by many causes, and it is a chronic, progressive and irreversible heterogeneous disease of pulmonary interstitial tissue (Raghu et al., 2011). Including pulmonary fibrosis caused by secondary factors and idiopathic pulmonary fibrosis. The pathological features of pulmonary fibrosis are mainly the proliferation of lung fibroblasts and excessive deposition of extracellular matrix, which leads to the destruction of lung tissue structure and eventually leads to chronic respiratory failure (Datta et al., 2011; King et al., 2011). There are many factors leading to pulmonary fibrosis, mainly including smoking and environmental exposure, genetic factors, virus infection and complications (Renzoni et al., 2014; Zaman and Lee, 2018). The data show that the incidence of pulmonary fibrosis is increasing year by year in the world and is similar to that of liver cancer, gastric cancer and cervical cancer (Hutchinson et al., 2015). At present, with the global spread of Coronavirus Disease 2019 (COVID-19), there may be more patients with pulmonary fibrosis. COVID-19 can cause severe lung injury and may lead to pulmonary fibrosis. Previous data of coronavirus infection (SARS-CoV or MERS-CoV) and new data of COVID-19 pandemic indicate that severe fibrosis may occur after SARS-CoV-2 infection (George et al., 2020). Early diagnosis of pulmonary fibrosis is difficult and incurable, and the prognosis is very poor. The median survival time after diagnosis is 2–3 years, The 5-year survival rate is less than 30% (Vancheri and du Bois, 2013; Wuyts et al., 2020). At present, the main treatments for pulmonary fibrosis are drug therapy and lung transplantation. Lung transplantation is the most effective treatment at present, but it is limited by the supply of donor organs, economic situation and patients' situation (Kistler et al., 2014). As for drug therapy, so far only Pirfenidone and Nidanib have been approved by FDA for the treatment of pulmonary fibrosis worldwide (Mora et al., 2017; Lederer and Martinez, 2018). These two anti-fibrosis drugs can improve patients' lung function, but they still can't cure pulmonary fibrosis and have obvious side effects, such as diarrhea and drug-induced liver injury, anorexia, vomiting and photosensitive rash, etc. (Richeldi et al., 2014; King et al., 2014). At present, the pathogenesis of pulmonary fibrosis is not clear, but the incidence of pulmonary fibrosis is on the rise, especially with the pandemic of COVID-19, the incidence of pulmonary fibrosis secondary to COVID-19 will further increase, and seriously affect the health of patients. Although many treatments have been used to treat pulmonary fibrosis, there is still no safe and effective treatment. Therefore, it is of great significance to find drugs with high efficiency and less adverse reactions to improve the quality of life and survival rate of patients with pulmonary fibrosis. A large number of clinical and experimental studies show that traditional Chinese medicine can obviously improve many pathological links of pulmonary fibrosis, and the toxicity of traditional Chinese medicine is relatively small, which can improve the quality of life of patients and reduce the mortality rate, and has a good application prospect (Zhao et al., 2017). Among them, Astragalus membranaceus plays an important role in treating fibrosis (Ma et al., 2020). Astragalus membranaceus has been used in Chinese medicine for nearly 2000 years and is one of the most popular Chinese medicines in the world (Shahrajabian et al., 2019). As one of the traditional Chinese medicines commonly used in clinic, Astragalus membranaceus can improve and treat various diseases, and has many pharmacological effects, such as antioxidation (Shahzad et al., 2016), immunomodulation (Block and Mead, 2003), antifibrosis (Zhou et al., 2016), antitumor (Zhou et al., 2018) and analgesia (Di Cesare Mannelli et al., 2017). The main bioactive components in Astragalus membranaceus include polysaccharides, saponins, flavonoids and alkaloids (Shahrajabian et al., 2019). Among them, Astragalus polysaccharide is the most abundant component in Astragalus membranaceus, which has a variety of pharmacological activities (Zheng et al., 2020). The main components of Astragalus polysaccharides include dextran, heteropolysaccharide, acidic polysaccharide, and neutral polysaccharide. The monosaccharide components of Astragalus polysaccharide include glucose, glucuronic acid, arabinose, rhamnose, fructose, mannose, galactose, galacturonic acid, fucose, etc (Wang et al., 2019). Studies have shown that Astragalus polysaccharide has anti-fibrosis pharmacological activity, and the main active ingredient of Astragalus membranaceus in anti-pulmonary fibrosis may be Astragalus polysaccharide. However, due to the complex components of Astragalus polysaccharide, the research on the anti-pulmonary fibrosis mechanism of Astragalus polysaccharide is relatively lacking at present, and the anti-pulmonary fibrosis mechanism of Astragalus polysaccharide is still unclear (Li et al., 2011).

Network pharmacology is a new discipline of multi-target drug molecular design by network construction and selecting specific signal Nodes. Emphasis is placed on the multi-channel regulation of signal pathway, improving the therapeutic effect of drugs and reducing the toxic and side effects, thus opening up new ways for drug development and utilization and saving the research and development cost of drugs (Zhang et al., 2019). Molecular docking is a computer simulation of the recognition process between two or more molecules, which involves spatial matching and energy matching between molecules. Molecular docking methods are widely used in drug design, screening and other fields (Morris and Lim-Wilby, 2008). Based on network pharmacology and molecular docking technology, this study preliminarily explored the mechanism of Astragalus polysaccharides in anti-pulmonary fibrosis, provided possible therapeutic drugs for the treatment of pulmonary fibrosis, and laid a theoretical foundation for the clinical application of Astragalus polysaccharides in anti-pulmonary fibrosis.

METHODS

Screening of Key Active Components and Targets in Astragalus Polysaccharides

HERB (http://herb.ac.cn/) is a platform for pharmacology of Chinese herbal medicines. The database mainly includes the chemical substances, targets and drug target networks of Chinese herbal medicines (Ru et al., 2014). We searched the HERB database for related chemical components with "Astragalus membranaceus" as the key word, and finally screened the components of Astragalus membranaceus polysaccharides from the above-mentioned searched compounds by combining with references. Pubchem database (https://pubchem.ncbi.nlm.nih.gov/) is a biological activity database of small organic molecules supported by the National Institutes of Health and maintained by the National Biotechnology Information Center (Li et al., 2010). We get the SMILES numbers of the compound components through Pubchem database. SwissTargetPrediction database (www.swisstargetprediction.ch/) is a database for target prediction of more than 3,000 kinds of protein and more than 370,000 kinds of known active substances of different species (Zoete et al., 2016). We import the SMILES of the obtained compounds into Swiss Target Prediction database to predict the target of Astragalus polysaccharide.

Screening of Disease Targets

Enter the keyword "Pulmonary fibrosis" in the human gene database GeneCards (//www.genecards.org), and collect the disease targets related to pulmonary fibrosis (Safran et al., 2002). Then, with the help of jvenn (http://www.bioinformatics.com.cn/static/others/jvenn/example.html), the active ingredient targets of Astragalus polysaccharides screened out are intersected with the targets related to pulmonary fibrosis, and finally, the potential targets of Astragalus polysaccharides for treating pulmonary fibrosis are determined.

Network Construction

Through the software Cytoscape (v3.7.1), the screened active ingredients and the potential targets are visualized by constructing the network between the active ingredients and the potential targets (Lopes et al., 2010). And further construct the target topology network by using BisoGenet. STRING database is a database for searching protein-protein interactions, which contains a large number of PPI data verified by experiments and predicted by bioinformatics methods. In order to analyze the interaction between the potential target genes and proteins of Astragalus polysaccharide in anti-pulmonary fibrosis, a PPI(protein-protein interaction) network was built by STRING database (https://cn.string-db.org/), which was set as *Homo sapiens* and high confidence of 0.700, and the key targets were screened by visualization and network topology heterogeneity analysis in Cytoscape software.

KEGG and GO Enrichment Analysis

In order to describe and annotate the functions of target genes and explore the signal pathways of their functions, we input the selected core targets into the DAVID database (//www.genecards.org) (Huang et al., 2009). The species is limited to human, and the enrichment analysis of GO and KEGG is carried out with $p < 0.05$ as the screening condition. The enrichment analysis of GO includes the enrichment analysis of biological process, BP), cellular component, CC) and molecular function (MF). Through enrichment analysis, the biological processes and potential signal pathways involved in the treatment of pulmonary fibrosis by Astragalus polysaccharides were screened out. In addition, the pathway enrichment analysis of core targets is carried out by ClueGO.

Molecular Docking

Generally, we judge the binding degree of ligand and receptor by the level of energy. When the conformation of compound molecule and receptor is stable, the lower the energy, the greater the possibility of action. We use molecular docking technology to study the binding ability of the selected target protein to active compounds. We obtained the 3D structure of the target protein obtained by the above screening through PDB database. With the active ingredient of Astragalus polysaccharide as the ligand, the processed ligand was molecularly docked with the target protein in Autodock Vina 1.1.2 software (Trott and Olson, 2010). Finally, the docking results are visualized by PyMOL 2.3.4 software.

RESULT

Screening of Key Active Components and Targets in Astragalus Polysaccharides

We searched the HERB database for the keyword "huang qi" to obtain the active ingredient chemistry of Astragalus membranaceus. Finally, we determined the ingredients of Astragalus membranaceus polysaccharide from these ingredients screened from Astragalus membranaceus. We obtained 10 kinds of polysaccharide ingredients, namely D-Galacturonic acid, Alpha-L-Rhamnose, D-ascorbicacid, Vitamin C, L-Rhamnose, DL-Glucuronic acid, L-(-)-Fucose, DL-Xylose, glucose, arabinose. Search the HERB database for related targets of Astragalus polysaccharides, and predict the targets of some polysaccharide components through Swiss Target Prediction database, and finally get 142 targets of Astragalus polysaccharides (**Figure 1**).

Screening of Disease Targets

With "pulmonary fibrosis" as the key word, 5,783 genes were preliminarily screened out from Genecards database, and the potential targets of Astragalus polysaccharides for treating pulmonary fibrosis were obtained by intersecting the selected targets with disease targets by using jvenn (http://www.bioinformatics.com.cn/static/others/jvenn/example.html). As shown in **Figure 1A**, 142 related targets of Astragalus polysaccharides were screened, among which there were 92 potential targets for treating pulmonary fibrosis. We introduced ten compounds and corresponding targets in Astragalus polysaccharide into Cytoscape to construct a polysaccharide component-target network. As shown in **Figure 1B**, it can be seen from the network diagram that compounds act on multiple targets, and some targets also correspond to multiple compounds. Among them, the sub-network degree value of Vitamin C and related targets is high, and most targets are potential targets for treating pulmonary fibrosis, suggesting that Vitamin C may play an important role in the treatment of pulmonary fibrosis by Astragalus polysaccharides.

KEGG and GO Enrichment Analysis

DAVID database was used for GO and KEGG enrichment analysis of Astragalus polysaccharide in treating pulmonary fibrosis. The results of KEGG pathway enrichment analysis are shown in **Figure 2A**, mainly including Pathways in cancer, Malaria, TNF signaling pathway, NF-kappa B signaling pathway, Rheumatoid arthritis, Non-alcoholic fatty liver disease (NAFLD), Leishmaniasis, Pertussis, Inflammatory bowel disease (IBD), PPAR signaling pathway, Tuberculosis, Chagas disease (American trypanosomiasis), Amoebiasis, Herpes simplex infection, Hepatitis B, Amyotrophic lateral sclerosis (ALS), Small cell lung cancer, NOD-like receptor signaling pathway, MAPK signaling pathway etc.

GO enrichment analysis results show that it mainly involves response to hypoxia, response to drug, response to ethanol, aging, positive regulation of cell division, response to antibiotic, inflammatory response, negative regulation of apoptotic

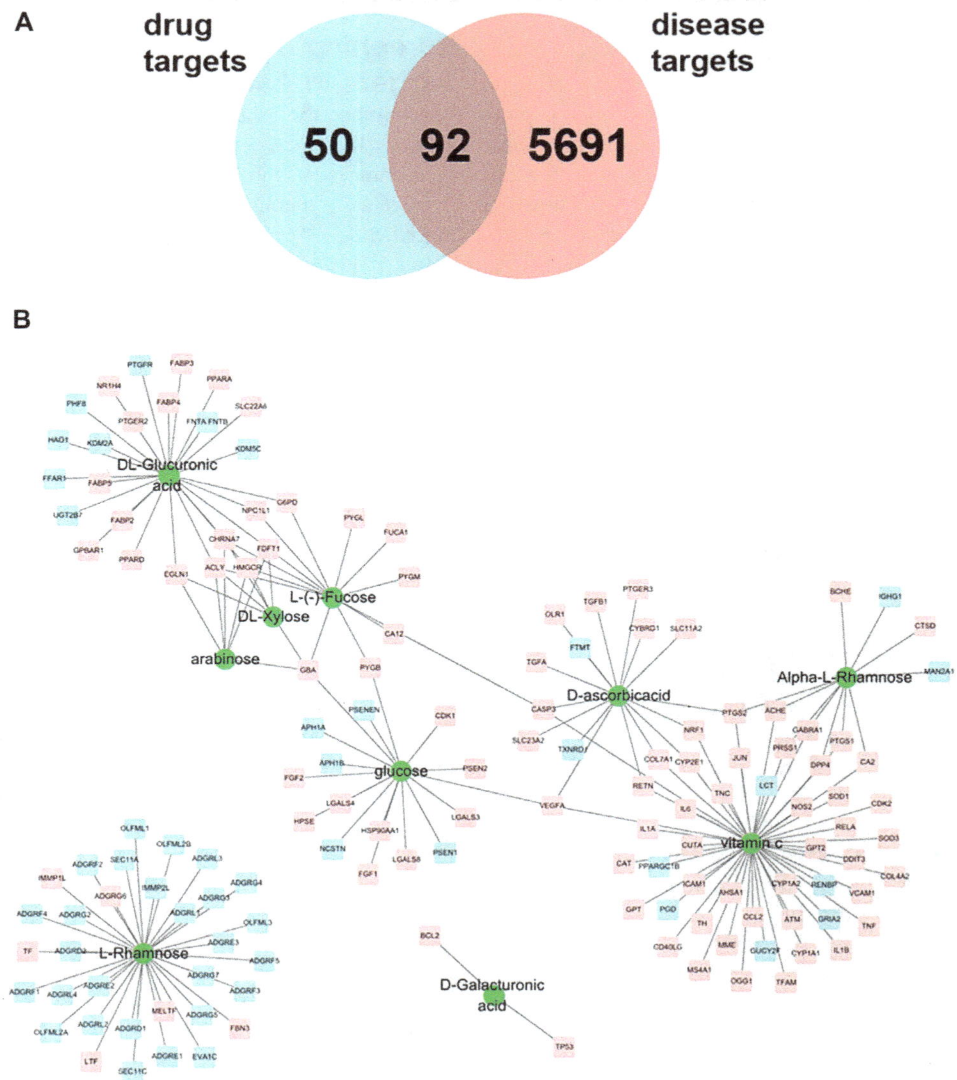

FIGURE 1 | (A) Venn maps of components and disease targets have 92 common targets. **(B)** Components-Target network of astragalus polysaccharide. The green circle indicated the component, and the square was the action target of polysaccharide component, and the pink square was the potential treatment target of pulmonary fibrosis.

process, positive regulation of ERK1 and ERK2 cascade, positive regulation of NF-kappaB transcription factor activity, extracellular space, extracellular exosome, cell surface, extracellular matrix, extracellular region, protein homodimerization activity, enzyme binding, cytokine activity, glycogen phosphorylase activity, heme binding etc. (**Figure 2B**).

Network Construction and Screening of Core Targets

The protein interaction network of potential targets of Astragalus polysaccharide in treating pulmonary fibrosis was obtained by using the BisoGenet plug-in in Cytoscape. As shown in **Figure 3**, there are 4,411 node in network a and 159,341 target interaction relationships. In order to screen out the core targets of the network more accurately, network b was extracted with the median values of the three evaluation indexes of Betweenness, Degree and Closeness as the boundaries, and there were 1770 nodes and 80,027 kinds of target interactions in network b. We continued to extract the targets of the top 500 indexes in network b to build interactive network c, which had 226 nodes and 6,281 kinds of target interactions. In the core network c, we found 11 direct targets, VCAM1, RELA, CDK2, JUN, CDK1, HSP90AA1, NOS2, SOD1, CASP3, AHSA1, PTGER3, which had the greatest

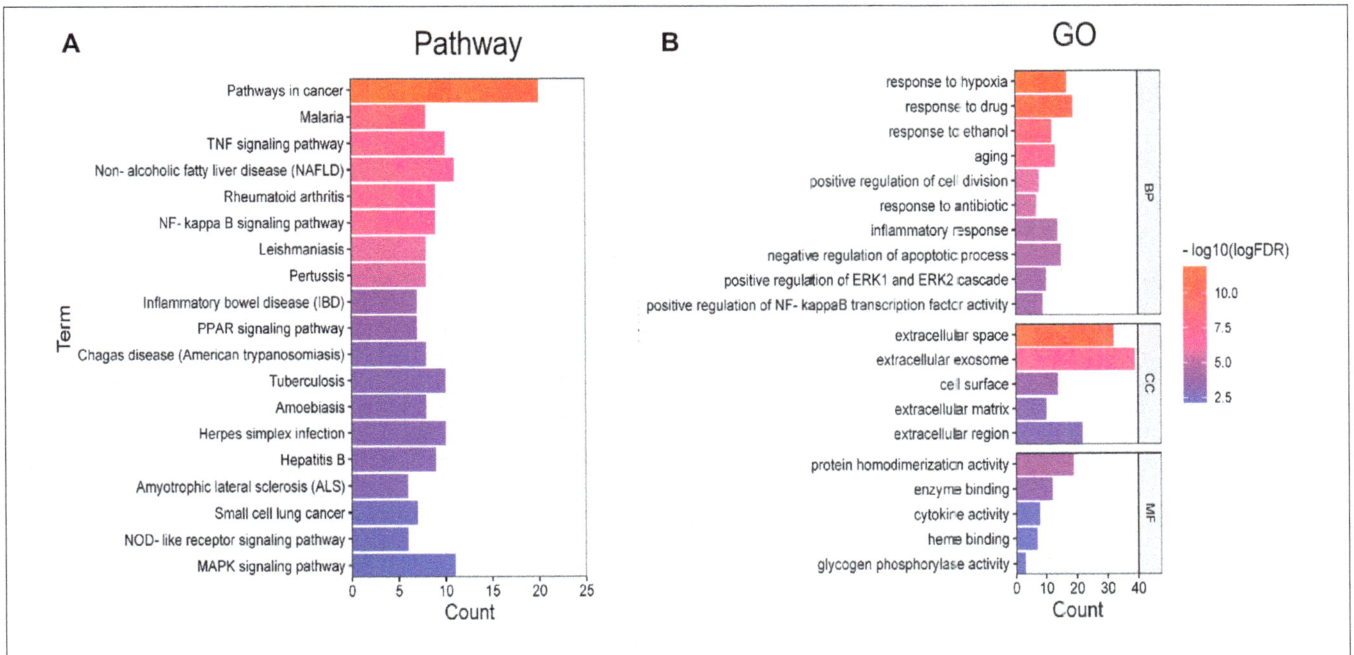

FIGURE 2 | Enrichment analysis of KEGG and GO. **(A)** Pathway enrichment analysis. **(B)** GO enrichment analysis.

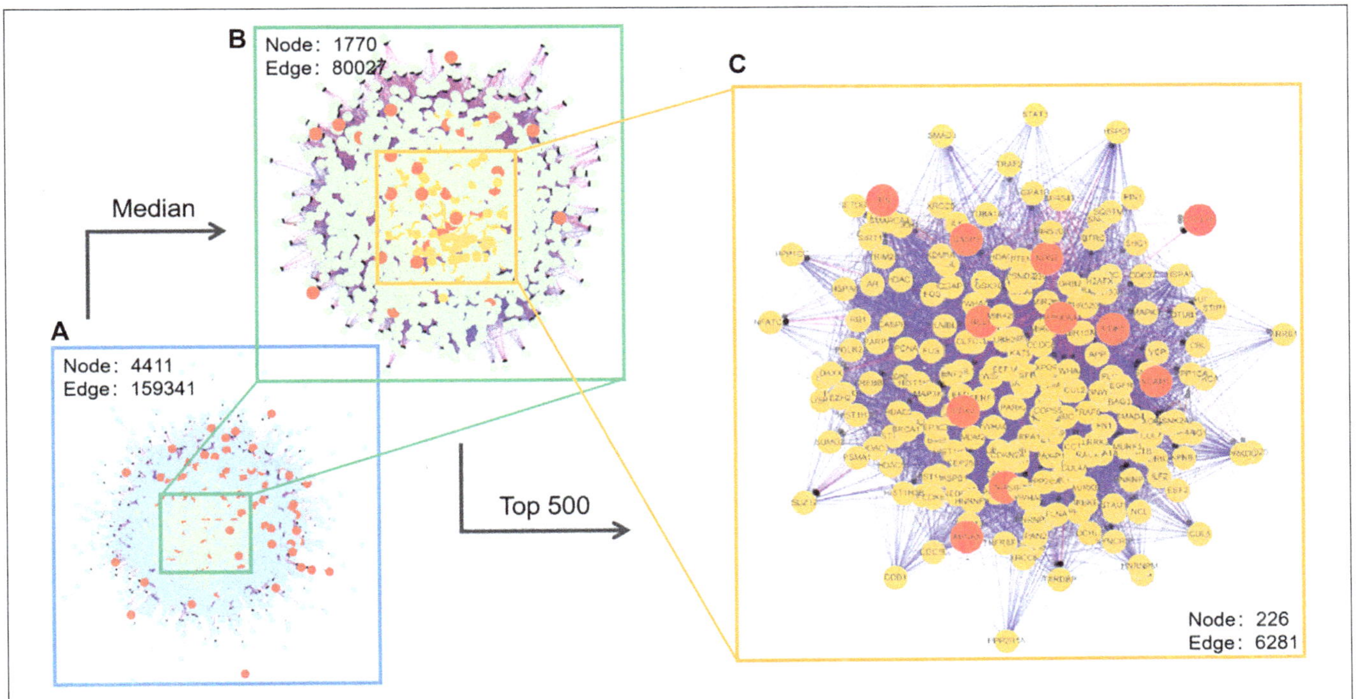

FIGURE 3 | Interaction network of Astragalus polysaccharide targets (with magnified median figure and the top 500 points).

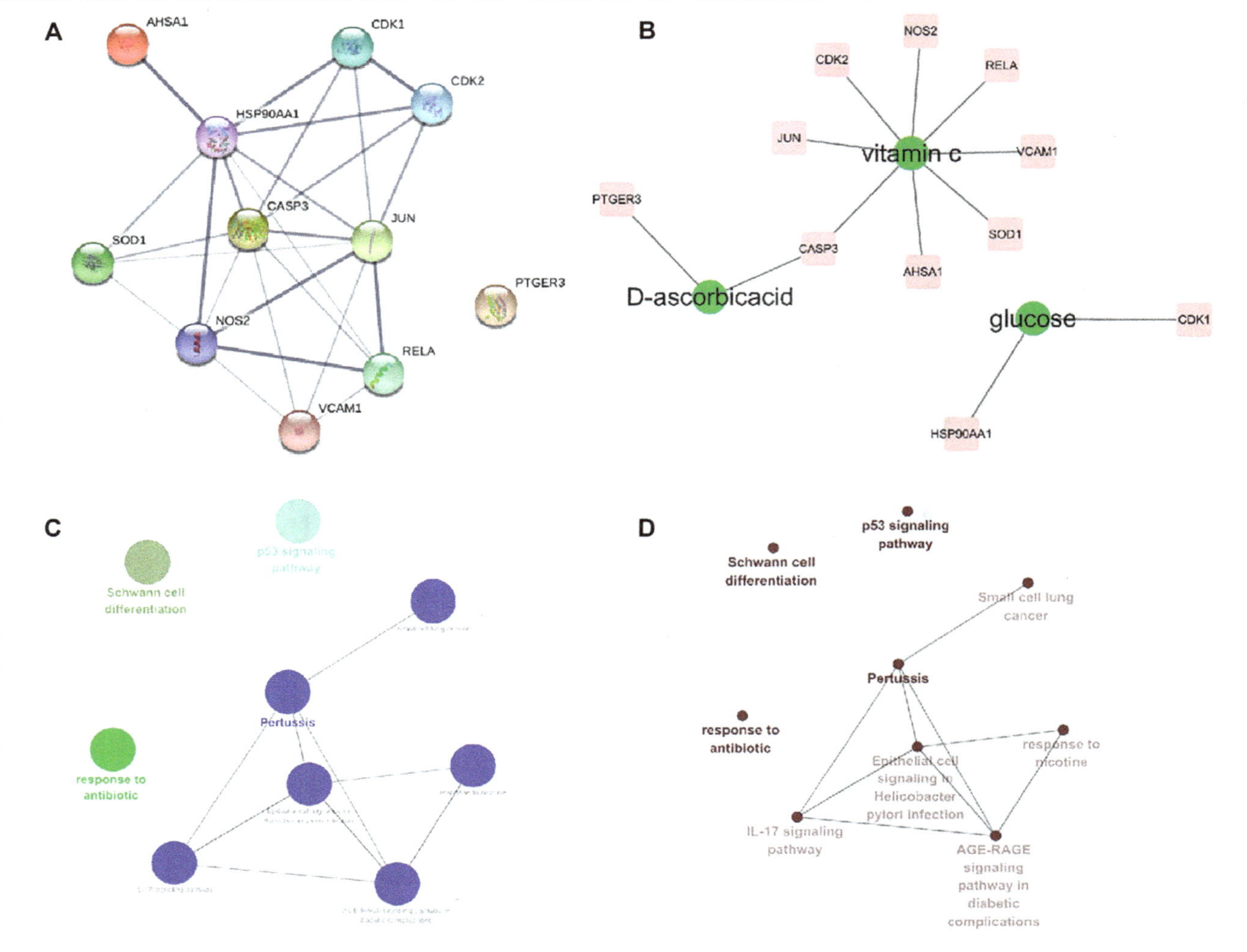

FIGURE 4 | Interaction network of core targets and pathway enrichment analysis. **(A)** Interaction network of core targets. **(B)** Core target component network **(C,D)** Core targets pathway enrichment network.

correlation with Astragalus polysaccharides in treating pulmonary fibrosis. Therefore, we regard these 11 targets as the potential core targets of Astragalus polysaccharides in treating pulmonary fibrosis.

Construction and Enrichment Analysis of Core Target Network

We have further constructed PPI network for these 11 core targets, and found that JUN, CASP3 and HSP90AA1 have higher degrees in the network, suggesting that they may play a key role in the treatment (**Figure 4A**). In addition, we also screened out three components of Astragalus polysaccharides that act on the 11 core targets (D-ascorbicacid, Vitamin C, Glucose) (**Figure 4B**). And ClueGO was used to construct pathways enrichment network for the core targets, and the pathways enrichment includes Schwann cell differentiation, p53 signaling pathway, response to antibiotic, Pertussis, Small cell lung cancer, IL-17 signaling pathway, Epithelial cell signaling in *Helicobacter pylori* infection, response to nicotine, AGE-RAGE signaling pathway in diabetic complications. Among them, four types were obtained by clustering (**Figures 4C,D**).

Molecular Docking

Up to now, only pirfenidone and Nidanib have been approved by FDA to treat pulmonary fibrosis in the world, and these two drugs have a good clinical effect on pulmonary fibrosis. According to previous reports, pirfenidone can inhibit targets such as IL6 and TNFα, and through the previous component target network construction, we found the polysaccharide component (Vitamin C) that acts on these two targets, so we follow up with the docking scores of pirfenidone with IL6 and TNFα as reference values. The results show that the affinity scores of Vitamin C, an active compound in Astragalus polysaccharides, with these two targets are similar to

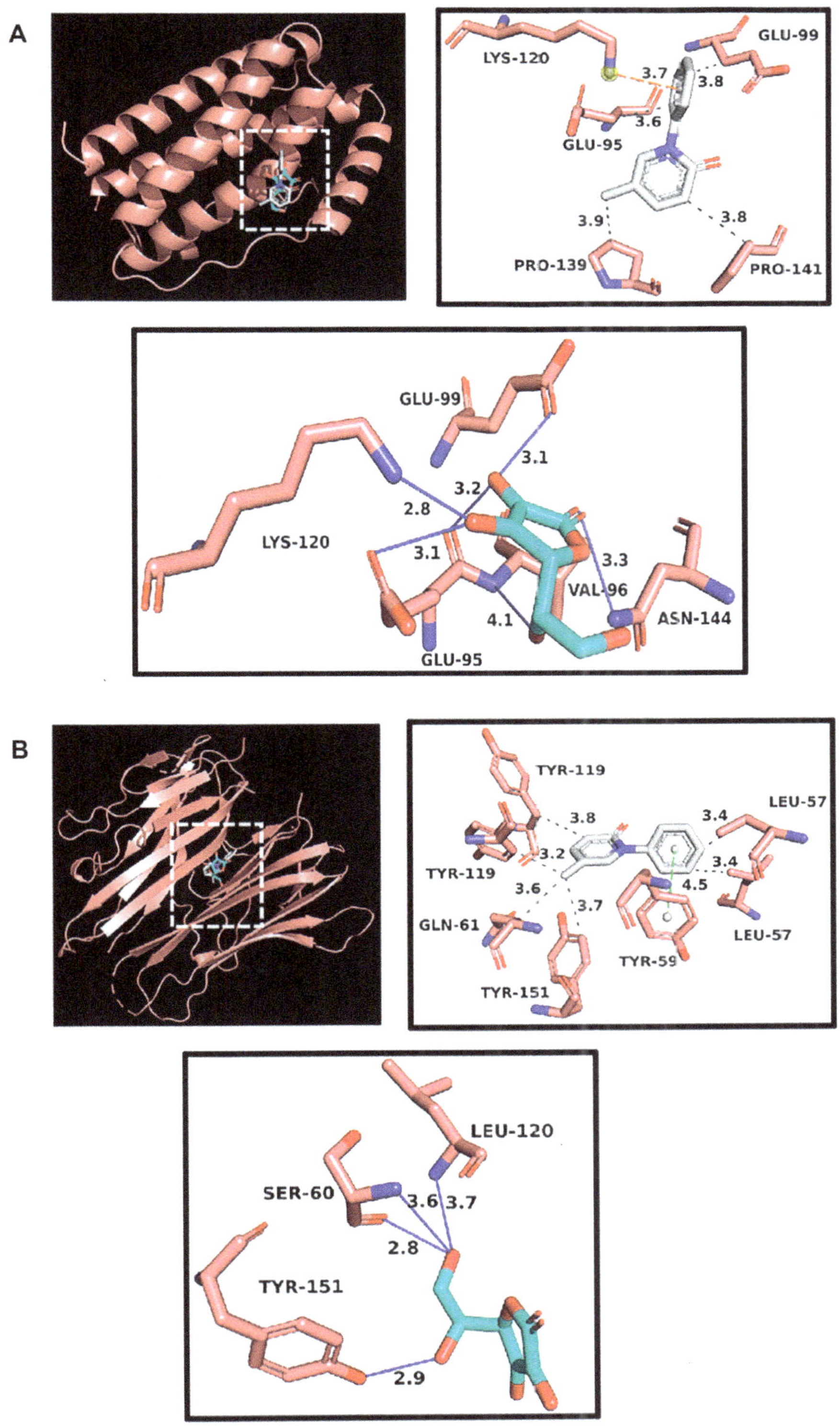

FIGURE 5 | (A) Docking display of pirfenidone and Vitamin C with IL6 respectively. Gray compound represents pirfenidone, and blue compounds represent Vitamin C. **(B)** Docking display of pirfenidone and Vitamin C with TNFα respectively. Gray compound represents pirfenidone, and blue compounds represent Vitamin C.

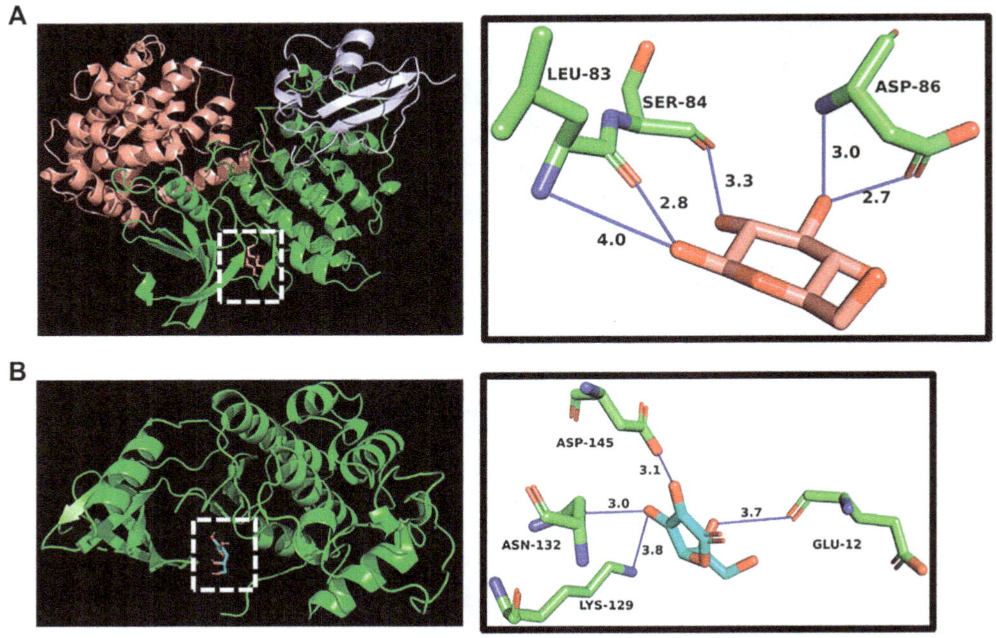

FIGURE 6 | (A) Docking display of CDK1 and glucose. **(B)** Docking display of CDK2 and Vitamin C.

those of pirfenidone, indicating that the key active substances in Astragalus polysaccharides may play an anti-pulmonary fibrosis role, and the molecular docking is shown in **Figure 5**. In addition, we have docked two core targets, CDK1 and CDK2, and docked the Glucose and Vitamin C acting on these two targets into the active pockets of small molecule inhibitors of CDK1 and CDK2, respectively. CDK1 and CDK2 belong to cyclin-dependent protein kinases, which are important factors in cell cycle regulation. It has been reported that lung fibrosis can be controlled to some extent by inhibiting CDKs. It was found that the affinity was similar to the docking scores of IL6 and TNFα, indicating that these key active components may play a key role in the treatment of pulmonary fibrosis (**Figure 6**).

DISCUSSION

For a long time, the treatment of pulmonary fibrosis has been a difficult problem in the world. Except for lung transplantation, there is still a lack of very effective treatment drugs and methods (Kistler et al., 2014). At present, the western medicines used clinically to treat pulmonary fibrosis, such as pirfenidone and Nidanib, can only slow down the decline rate of pulmonary function in patients with mild to moderate pulmonary fibrosis, but the adverse reactions are obvious and expensive. The clinical mortality rate of pulmonary fibrosis is not lower than that of tumor, and the incidence rate is increasing year by year. Due to the pandemic of COVID-19, the incidence rate will further increase (Hutchinson et al., 2015; George et al., 2020). However, there is no ideal therapeutic drug at present, and the pathogenesis is not completely clear and complicated. Therefore, it is very meaningful to find more effective therapeutic targets and drug research and development. In recent years, with the deepening of research on pulmonary fibrosis, the exploration of treating pulmonary fibrosis with traditional Chinese medicine has gradually increased, and great progress has been made in treating pulmonary fibrosis with traditional Chinese medicine, which has attracted much attention because of its multi-channels, multi-targets, few side effects and remarkable curative effect (Ji et al., 2020; Yu et al., 2020). Astragalus polysaccharide is an important active substance in Astragalus membranaceus. Studies have shown that Astragalus polysaccharide has anti-fibrosis pharmacological activities (Li et al., 2011). However, the components of Astragalus polysaccharides are complex, and at present, there is a lack of research on the mechanism of Astragalus polysaccharides against pulmonary fibrosis, and the mechanism of Astragalus polysaccharides against pulmonary fibrosis is still unclear. In this study, the core pharmacodynamic substances and targets were preliminarily determined by network pharmacology, and the core targets were enriched by GO and KEGG pathways. Finally, the molecular docking study of these core active components and core targets was carried out by AutoDock Vina to verify the analysis results of network pharmacology. Ten kinds of active ingredients in Astragalus polysaccharides were screened out, among which Ascorbicacid, Glucose and D-Ascorbicacid are the core targets in the network, suggesting that these active ingredients play an important role in the treatment of pulmonary fibrosis by Astragalus polysaccharides. By analyzing the target interaction network VCAM1,RELA,CDK2,JUN,CDK1,HSP90AA1,NOS2,

SOD1,CASP3,AHSA1, PTGER3 are at the core of the network, which can be regarded as the key targets of Astragalus polysaccharides in treating pulmonary fibrosis.

Marcia Rodrigues et al.' s research shows that Asorbicacid can treat pulmonary fibrosis caused by paraquat poisoning, and the results of animal experiments show that Asorbic acid mainly treats pulmonary fibrosis by reducing the number of macrophages, neutrophils and lymphocytes in fibrotic mice, reducing the levels of IL-6, TGF-β and IL-17 and increasing the activity of antioxidant enzymes in lung homogenate (Rodrigues da Silva et al., 2018). It was suggested that glucose metabolism may be beneficial to prevent myofibroblast differentiation in idiopathic pulmonary fibrosis (Azuelos, 2020). VCAM1 is upregulated in idiopathic pulmonary fibrosis, which can induce TGF-β1, and its main mechanism is to inhibit the proliferation of fibroblasts by reducing G2/M and S phases of cell cycle (Agassandian et al., 2015). Previous studies have shown that the phosphorylation of RELA on Ser536 will affect hepatic myofibroblasts. For pulmonary fibrosis, current studies have shown that the phosphorylation of RELA on Ser536 may be the core regulator of pulmonary fibroblasts (Moles et al., 2013). JNK is a member of mitogen-related protein kinase family. Studies have shown that JNK plays an important role in pulmonary fibrosis, in which JNK1 promotes collagen deposition and leads to further development of pulmonary fibrosis (Alcorn et al., 2009).

Through GO enrichment analysis of the key targets of effective components of Astragalus membranaceus, it is confirmed that Astragalus membranaceus has certain influence on many biological processes, such as response to hypoxia, aging, positive regulation of cell division, response to antibiotic, inflammatory response, negative regulation of apoptotic process, etc. Pathways related to pulmonary fibrosis in KEGG pathway mainly include Pathways in cancer, Malaria, TNF signaling pathway, Non-alcoholic fatty liver disease (NAFLD), Rheumatoid arthritis, NF- kappa B signaling pathway, Pertussis, Tuberculosis, Herpes simplex infection, Hepatitis B, Small cell lung cancer etc.

The results of molecular docking show that the binding properties of the main active components of Astragalus polysaccharides to the key targets selected from the research results are similar to those of the control drug pirfenidone, which indicates that the key active components of Astragalus polysaccharides can stably bind to receptors and play an anti-pulmonary fibrosis role. The molecular docking prediction results provide further evidence for the active components of Astragalus polysaccharide to act on specific targets to treat pulmonary fibrosis.

In this study, a "compound-target" network was established by the method of network pharmacology, and the relationship between pulmonary fibrosis, active components of Astragalus polysaccharides and their targets was studied as a whole. The key compounds and core targets of Astragalus polysaccharides for treating lung cancer and their action pathways were screened, and the multi-component, multi-target and multi-pathway action mechanism of anti-lung cancer was preliminarily discussed, which provided important theoretical clues and basis for further in-depth study on the medicinal material basis and action mechanism of Astragalus polysaccharides for treating pulmonary fibrosis. In this paper, the mechanism of action of Astragalus polysaccharide is discussed based on its chemical components and targets, but it cannot fully reflect the influence of metabolites of Astragalus polysaccharide on the mechanism of action. Therefore, the results of this study still have some limitations, and it is necessary to further verify the results of pharmacological prediction analysis based on network.

AUTHOR CONTRIBUTIONS

PB contributed to conception and design of the study. WZ organized the database. ST wrote the first draft of the manuscript. All authors contributed to manuscript revision, read, and approved the submitted version.

REFERENCES

Agassandian, M., Tedrow, J. R., Sembrat, J., Kass, D. J., Zhang, Y., Goncharova, E. A., et al. (2015). VCAM-1 Is a TGF-B1 Inducible Gene Upregulated in Idiopathic Pulmonary Fibrosis. *Cell Signal* 27 (12), 2467–2473. doi:10.1016/j.cellsig.2015.09.003

Alcorn, J. F., van der Velden, J., Brown, A. L., McElhinney, B., Irvin, C. G., and Janssen-Heininger, Y. M. (2009). c-Jun N-Terminal Kinase 1 Is Required for the Development of Pulmonary Fibrosis. *Am. J. Respir. Cel Mol Biol* 40 (4), 422–432. doi:10.1165/rcmb.2008-0174OC

Azuelos, I. (2020). Glucose Metabolism in Idiopathic Pulmonary Fibrosis. London: University College London. Thesis.

Block, K. I., and Mead, M. N. (2003). Immune System Effects of Echinacea, Ginseng, and astragalus: a Review. *Integr. Cancer Ther.* 2 (3), 247–267. doi:10.1177/1534735403256419

Datta, A., Scotton, C. J., and Chambers, R. C. (2011). Novel Therapeutic Approaches for Pulmonary Fibrosis. *Br. J. Pharmacol.* 163 (1), 141–172. doi:10.1111/j.1476-5381.2011.01247.x

Di Cesare Mannelli, L., Pacini, A., Micheli, L., Femia, A. P., Maresca, M., Zanardelli, M., et al (2017). Astragali Radix: Could it Be an Adjuvant for Oxaliplatin-Induced Neuropathy? *Sci. Rep.* 7, 42021–42113. doi:10.1038/srep42021

George, P. M., Wells, A. U., and Jenkins, R. G. (2020). Pulmonary Fibrosis and COVID-19: the Potential Role for Antifibrotic Therapy. *Lancet Respir. Med.* 8 (8), 807–815. doi:10.1016/S2213-2600(20)30225-3

Huang, da. W., Sherman, B. T., and Lempicki, R. A. (2009). Systematic and Integrative Analysis of Large Gene Lists Using DAVID Bioinformatics Resources. *Nat. Protoc.* 4 (1), 44–57. doi:10.1038/nprot.2008.211

Hutchinson, J., Fogarty, A., Hubbard, R., and McKeever, T. (2015). Global Incidence and Mortality of Idiopathic Pulmonary Fibrosis: a Systematic Review. *Eur. Respir. J.* 46 (3), 795–806. doi:10.1183/09031936.00185114

Ji, K., Ma, J., Wang, L., Li, N., Dong, S., Shi, L., et al. (2020). Efficacy and Safety of Traditional Chinese Medicine in Idiopathic Pulmonary Fibrosis: a Meta-Analysis. *Evidence-Based Complement. Altern. Med.* 2020, 1752387. doi:10.1155/2020/1752387

King, T. E., Jr, Bradford, W. Z., Castro-Bernardini, S., Fagan, E. A., Glaspole, I., Glassberg, M. K., et al. (2014). A Phase 3 Trial of Pirfenidone in Patients with

Idiopathic Pulmonary Fibrosis. *N. Engl. J. Med.* 370 (22), 2083–2092. doi:10.1056/NEJMoa1402582

King, T. E., Jr, Pardo, A., and Selman, M. (2011). Idiopathic Pulmonary Fibrosis. *Lancet* 378 (9807), 1949–1961. doi:10.1016/S0140-6736(11)60052-4

Kistler, K. D., Nalysnyk, L., Rotella, P., and Esser, D. (2014). Lung Transplantation in Idiopathic Pulmonary Fibrosis: a Systematic Review of the Literature. *BMC Pulm. Med.* 14, 139–212. doi:10.1186/1471-2466-14-139

Lederer, D. J., and Martinez, F. J. (2018). Idiopathic Pulmonary Fibrosis. *N. Engl. J. Med.* 378 (19), 1811–1823. doi:10.1056/nejmra1705751

Li, J., Li, j. Y., Chen, J. J., and Lu, L. C. (2011). Effects of Astragalus Polysaccharides on Level of Cytokines and Pathological Structure of Lung Tissue in Rat Model of Pulmoanry Fibrosis. *Lishizhen Med. Materia Med. Res.* 22 (7), 1684–1685. doi:10.1016/j.carbpol.2020.116740

Li, Q., Cheng, T., Wang, Y., and Bryant, S. H. (2010). PubChem as a Public Resource for Drug Discovery. *Drug Discov. Today* 15 (23-24), 1052–1057. doi:10.1016/j.drudis.2010.10.003

Lopes, C. T., Franz, M., Kazi, F., Donaldson, S. L., Morris, Q., and Bader, G. D. (2010). Cytoscape Web: an Interactive Web-Based Network Browser. *Bioinformatics* 26 (18), 2347–2348. doi:10.1093/bioinformatics/btq430

Ma, L., Wang, R., and Miao, M. (2020). Medication Rule of Chinese Materia Medica in Treatment of Pulmonary Fibrosis Based on Data Mining [Chinese]. *Chin. Traditional Herbal Drugs* 51, 1406–1411. doi:10.7501/j.issn.0253-2670.2020.06.005

Moles, A., Sanchez, A. M., Banks, P. S., Murphy, L. B., Luli, S., Borthwick, L., et al. (2013). Inhibition of RelA-Ser536 Phosphorylation by a Competing Peptide Reduces Mouse Liver Fibrosis without Blocking the Innate Immune Response. *Hepatology* 57 (2), 817–828. doi:10.1002/hep.26068

Mora, A. L., Rojas, M., Pardo, A., and Selman, M. (2017). Emerging Therapies for Idiopathic Pulmonary Fibrosis, a Progressive Age-Related Disease. *Nat. Rev. Drug Discov.* 16 (11), 755–772. doi:10.1038/nrd.2017.170

Morris, G. M., and Lim-Wilby, M. (2008). Molecular Docking, in Molecular Modeling of Proteins. *Methods Mol. Biol.*, 443 365–382. doi:10.1007/978-1-59745-177-2_19

Raghu, G., Collard, H. R., Egan, J. J., Martinez, F. J., Behr, J., Brown, K. K., et al. (2011). An Official ATS/ERS/JRS/ALAT Statement: Idiopathic Pulmonary Fibrosis: Evidence-Based Guidelines for Diagnosis and Management. *Am. J. Respir. Crit. Care Med.* 183 (6), 788–824. doi:10.1164/rccm.2009-040GL

Renzoni, E., Srihari, V., and Sestini, P. (2014). Pathogenesis of Idiopathic Pulmonary Fibrosis: Review of Recent Findings. *F1000prime Rep.* 6, 69. doi:10.12703/P6-69

Richeldi, L., du Bois, R. M., Raghu, G., Azuma, A., Brown, K. K., Costabel, U., et al. (2014). Efficacy and Safety of Nintedanib in Idiopathic Pulmonary Fibrosis. *N. Engl. J. Med.* 370 (22), 2071–2082. doi:10.1056/NEJMoa1402584

Rodrigues da Silva, M., Schapochnik, A., Peres Leal, M., Esteves, J., Bichels Hebeda, C., Sandri, S., et al. (2018). Beneficial Effects of Ascorbic Acid to Treat Lung Fibrosis Induced by Paraquat. *PLoS One* 13, e0205535. doi:10.1371/journal.pone.0205535

Ru, J., Li, P., Wang, J., Zhou, W., Li, B., Huang, C., et al. (2014). TCMSP: a Database of Systems Pharmacology for Drug Discovery from Herbal Medicines. *J. Cheminform* 6 (1), 13–16. doi:10.1186/1758-2946-6-13

Safran, M., Solomon, I., Shmueli, O., Lapidot, M., Shen-Orr, S., Adato, A., et al. (2002). GeneCards 2002: towards a Complete, Object-Oriented, Human Gene Compendium. *Bioinformatics* 18 (11), 1542–1543. doi:10.1093/bioinformatics/18.11.1542

Shahrajabian, M., Sun, W., and Cheng, Q. (2019). *A Review of astragalus Species as Foodstuffs, Dietary Supplements, a Traditional Chinese Medicine and a Part of Modern Pharmaceutical Science. Appl. Ecol. Environ. Res.* 17, 13371–13382.doi:10.15666/aeer/1706_1337113382

Shahzad, M., Shabbir, A., Wojcikowski, K., Wohlmuth, H., and Gobe, G. C. (2016). The Antioxidant Effects of Radix Astragali (Astragalus Membranaceus and Related Species) in Protecting Tissues from Injury and Disease. *Curr. Drug Targets* 17 (12), 1331–1340. doi:10.2174/1389450116666150907104742

Trott, O., and Olson, A. J. (2010). AutoDock Vina: Improving the Speed and Accuracy of Docking with a New Scoring Function, Efficient Optimization, and Multithreading. *J. Comput. Chem.* 31 (2), 455–461. doi:10.1002/jcc.21334

Vancheri, C., and du Bois, R. M. (2013). A Progression-free End-point for Idiopathic Pulmonary Fibrosis Trials: Lessons from Cancer. *Eur. Respir. J.* 41 (2), 262–269. doi:10.1183/09031936.00115112

Wang, J., Jia, J., Song, L., Gong, X., Xu, J., Yang, M., et al. (2019). *Extraction, Structure, and Pharmacological Activities of Astragalus Polysaccharides. Appl. Sci.* 9 (1), 122. doi:10.3390/app9010122

Wuyts, W. A., Wijsenbeek, M., Bondue, B., Bouros, D., Bresser, P., Robalo Cordeiro, C., et al. (2020). Idiopathic Pulmonary Fibrosis: Best Practice in Monitoring and Managing a Relentless Fibrotic Disease. *Respiration* 99 (1), 73–82. doi:10.1159/000504763

Yu, X. Q., Yang, S. G., Xie, Y., and Li, J. S. (2020). Traditional Chinese Medicine in the Treatment of Idiopathic Pulmonary Fibrosis Based on Syndrome Differentiation: Study Protocol of an Exploratory Trial. *J. Integr. Med.* 18 (2), 163–168. doi:10.1016/j.joim.2019.12.005

Zaman, T., and Lee, J. S. (2018). Risk Factors for the Development of Idiopathic Pulmonary Fibrosis: a Review. *Curr. Pulmonol Rep.* 7 (4), 118–125. doi:10.1007/s13665-018-0210-7

Zhang, R., Zhu, X., Bai, H., and Ning, K. (2019). Network Pharmacology Databases for Traditional Chinese Medicine: Review and Assessment. *Front. Pharmacol.* 10, 123. doi:10.3389/fphar.2019.00123

Zhao, G. Z., Guo, Y. H., Li, B., Hu, J., Chen, T. F., Di, H. R., et al. (2017). Research Progress of Traditional Chinese Medicine in Prevention and Treatment of Sepsis. *Zhongguo Zhong Yao Za Zhi* 42 (8), 1423–1429. doi:10.19540/j.cnki.cjcmm.2017.0038

Zheng, Y., Ren, W., Zhang, L., Zhang, Y., Liu, D., and Liu, Y. (2020). A Review of the Pharmacological Action of Astragalus Polysaccharide. *Front. Pharmacol.* 11, 349. doi:10.3389/fphar.2020.00349

Zhou, R., Chen, H., Chen, J., Chen, X., Wen, Y., and Xu, L. (2018). Extract from Astragalus Membranaceus Inhibit Breast Cancer Cells Proliferation via PI3K/AKT/mTOR Signaling Pathway. *BMC Complement. Altern. Med.* 18 (1), 83–88. doi:10.1186/s12906-018-2148-2

Zhou, Y., Tong, X., Ren, S., Wang, X., Chen, J., Mu, Y., et al. (2016). Synergistic Anti-liver Fibrosis Actions of Total astragalus Saponins and Glycyrrhizic Acid via TGF-β1/Smads Signaling Pathway Modulation. *J. Ethnopharmacol* 190, 83–90. doi:10.1016/j.jep.2016.06.011

Zoete, V., Daina, A., Bovigny, C., and Michielin, O. (2016). SwissSimilarity: a Web Tool for Low to Ultra High Throughput Ligand-Based Virtual Screening. *ACS Publications* 56, 1399–1404. doi:10.1021/acs.jcim.6b00174

4

Targeting Oxidative Stress as a Therapeutic Approach for Idiopathic Pulmonary Fibrosis

Cristina Estornut[1], Javier Milara[1,2,3†]*, María Amparo Bayarri[1], Nada Belhadj[1] and Julio Cortijo[1,2,3,4†]*

[1]Department of Pharmacology, Faculty of Medicine, University of Valencia, Valencia, Spain, [2]Pharmacy Unit, University General Hospital Consortium, Valencia, Spain, [3]CIBERES, Health Institute Carlos III, Valencia, Spain, [4]Research and Teaching Unit, University General Hospital Consortium, Valencia, Spain

***Correspondence:**
Cristina Estornut
cristina.estna@gmail.com
Javier Milara
xmilara@hotmail.com

†These authors share senior authorship

Idiopathic pulmonary fibrosis (IPF) is a chronic interstitial lung disease characterized by an abnormal reepithelialisation, an excessive tissue remodelling and a progressive fibrosis within the alveolar wall that are not due to infection or cancer. Oxidative stress has been proposed as a key molecular process in pulmonary fibrosis development and different components of the redox system are altered in the cellular actors participating in lung fibrosis. To this respect, several activators of the antioxidant machinery and inhibitors of the oxidant species and pathways have been assayed in preclinical *in vitro* and *in vivo* models and in different clinical trials. This review discusses the role of oxidative stress in the development and progression of IPF and its underlying mechanisms as well as the evidence of oxidative stress in human IPF. Finally, we analyze the mechanism of action, the efficacy and the current status of different drugs developed to inhibit the oxidative stress as anti-fibrotic therapy in IPF.

Keywords: IPF—idiopathic pulmonary fibrosis, fibrosis, oxidative stress, ROS—reactive oxygen species, antioxidant therapy

INTRODUCTION

Idiopathic Pulmonary Fibrosis

Among all the idiopathic interstitial pneumonias, the most common form is idiopathic pulmonary fibrosis (IPF), whose incidence is estimated to be ranged between 2.8 and 9.3 per 100,000 people per year in North America and Europe (Barratt et al., 2018). IPF occurs primarily in older adults, mainly in men; it is characterised by chronic and progressive fibrosis related to a decrease in pulmonary function, progressive respiratory distress, and a remarkable poor prognosis. It is generally nonresponsive to traditional therapies such as anti-inflammatory and immunomodulatory treatment (Richeldi et al., 1941; Day, 2008; Barratt et al., 2018; Lederer and Martinez, 2018).

As the disease progresses, some pathological changes appear, including fibrotic lesions and accumulation of fibroblast in focal zones called "fibroblast foci," which causes the characteristic "honeycomb" appearance. The etiologic stimulus that initiates the disease and the underlying mechanism of pulmonary fibrosis are still unknown or poorly understood. Current studies suggest that fibrosis may result from the presence of continuous stimuli (both endogenous and exogenous) or injury followed by an aberrant wound healing process and a dysregulated repair/remodelling of the lung (Kinnula et al., 2005; Kliment and Oury, 2010).

Lung fibrosis is associated with accumulation of fibroblasts, myofibroblast activation or differentiation, alveolar reepithelization, extracellular matrix (ECM) dysregulation, oxidative stress, and inflammation (Phan, 2002; Manni and Oury, 2014). Thus, fibrosis development is mediated by interactions between various cell types such as fibroblasts; myofibroblasts; epithelial cells, especially type I and II alveolar epithelial cells (AECs); mesothelial and mesenchymal cells, as well as immune system cells. Although most studies have focused on the fibrotic process and the proliferation of fibroblast and myofibroblast, several studies suggest that increased oxidative stress may play a major role in the development and progression of IPF (Bocchino et al., 2010; Liguori et al., 2018; Cameli et al., 2020).

This review addresses the importance of the balance of oxidants/antioxidants in the pathogenesis of pulmonary fibrosis as well as the evidence of oxidative stress in human IPF with emphasis on the pharmacological approach targeting oxidative stress.

Oxidative Stress in Idiopathic Pulmonary Fibrosis

Oxidative stress arises as a result of an imbalance between reactive oxygen species (ROS) and reactive nitrogen species (RNS) production and antioxidant defence that leads to cellular dysfunction and tissue damage (Hosseinzadeh et al., 2018b). ROS are highly reactive oxygen metabolites; some examples are superoxide anion ($O_2^{\bullet-}$), hydroxyl radical ($HO^{\bullet}$), and hydrogen peroxide (H_2O_2). RNS are molecules derived from the reaction between nitric oxide (NO) and O_2 and derivates, one example is peroxynitrite. RNS can generate oxidative stress but also the named nitrosative stress (Thomas et al., 2008; Otoupalova et al., 2020). Lungs, due to their anatomy, location, and function, are particularly susceptible to oxidative stress (Crapo, 2003; Kinnula et al., 2005; Hosseinzadeh et al., 2018b).

Exogenous oxidizing agents such as cigarette smoke, toxins, hyperoxia, asbestos fibres, drugs and radiation also induce the production of ROS/RNS. Exogenous or endogenous generated ROS/RNS may directly damage the alveolar epithelium, favouring fibrotic interstitial lung responses (Kinnula et al., 2005). In addition to directly damaging the lung epithelium, ROS/RNS may also favour the development of pulmonary fibrosis by altering the expression of mediators implicated in the pathogenesis of IPF, such as the pro-fibrotic growth factor, transforming growth factor β (TGF-β). This growth factor is known to be modulated by ROS, indeed, experimental studies have evidenced that ROS can increase the secretion of TGF-β from epithelial cells and directly activate it (Barcellos-Hoff and Dix, 1996; Bellocq et al., 1999; Pociask et al., 2004). In turn, TGF-β stimulates the proliferation of fibroblasts and its differentiation into myofibroblasts (Thannickal et al., 2003). Oxidants may also alter the nature of surrounding ECM (Larios et al., 2001). Both ROS and RNS play an important role in the regulation of ECM, degradation and turnover (Fu et al., 2003; Nelson and Melendez, 2004). In lungs, alveolar inflammatory cells including lymphocytes, macrophages and neutrophils also produce ROS/RNS. In IPF patients, in addition to these inflammatory cells, fibroblasts and myofibroblast produce high levels of ROS/RNS in response to cytokines and growth factors and are involved in the underlying mechanism of fibrosis development **Table 1** (Bergeron et al., 2003; Waghray et al., 2005).

The main producers of ROS/RNS include nicotinamide adenine dinucleotide phosphate oxidases (NADPH oxidases, NOXs), myeloperoxidase (MPO), xanthine oxidase, nitric oxide synthase (NOS), and the mitochondrial electron transport chain (Kinnula et al., 2005; Hosseinzadeh et al., 2018b). From the family members of the NOX, the isoforms Nox1, Nox2 and Nox4 have been found to be implicated in the pathogenesis of pulmonary fibrosis but not Nox3 (Masamune et al., 2008; Griffith et al., 2009; Amara et al., 2010). Nox4 is ubiquitously expressed in various cell types of lung tissues including macrophages and structural cells such as smooth muscle cells, endothelial cells, mesenchymal cells, and epithelial cells (Lee et al., 2010a; Harijith et al., 2017). In IPF patients, Nox4 is strongly expressed in fibroblast foci and increases the expression of α-smooth muscle actin (α-SMA), fibronectin and procollagen, which are the most characteristic profibrotic molecules (Griffith et al., 2009; Hecker et al., 2009; Amara et al., 2010). Furthermore, Nox4 plays a critical role in myofibroblast tissue repair functions and fibrogenesis (Hecker et al., 2009). It is well known that TGF-β induces Nox4-dependent ROS production, which, in turn, promotes fibroblast migration (Amara et al., 2010) and this ROS production is also involved in the acquisition of pro-fibrotic myofibroblast phenotypes, including differentiation, contraction, apoptotic resistance, and ECM deposition (Hecker et al., 2009; Cameli et al., 2020). Nox4 expression is also increased in IPF senescent fibroblasts/myofibroblasts (Jarman et al., 2014) and ROS generated by Nox4 promotes senescence and the apoptosis-resistant phenotype (Hecker et al., 2014). Hyperplastic type II AECs from IPF patients' lungs highly express this NOX isoform (Amara et al., 2010) and Nox4-dependent ROS generation induces epithelial-to-mesenchymal transition (EMT) in alveolar epithelial cells (Hecker et al., 2009; Cameli et al., 2020). Other studies demonstrate that Nox4 is implicated in the profibrotic polarization of macrophages and the genetic removal of Nox4 in macrophages reduces ECM deposition protecting from induced pulmonary fibrosis (He et al., 2019). In addition, Nox4, along with Nox1, Nox2, is also expressed in vascular smooth muscle cells (VSMCs) (Huetsch et al., 2019). A study has reported that Nox4 is highly expressed in thickened pulmonary arteries in IPF patients (Pache et al., 2011). It has been proved that VSMCs are activated by TGF-β1 to induce Nox4, leading to increased VSMCs proliferation (Sturrock et al., 2006). Nox4 expression may be altered in VSMCs and is likely to mediate vascular remodelling that may generate pulmonary hypertension in lungs from IPF patients (Kato and Hecker, 2020). Vascular endothelial cells also express Nox4 (Bernard et al., 2014), ROS generated by Nox4 is implicated in the regulation of endothelial cell motility and angiogenesis. Furthermore, Nox4 expression is higher at sites of

TABLE 1 | Summary of the molecules of the redox system and the implicated process in the IPF participating cells.

Cell	Redox system molecule	Implicated process	Reference
(myo)fibroblasts	NOX4	↑αSMA ↑fibronectin ↑procollagen ↑migration ↑profibrotic phenotype ↑senescence ↓apoptosis	Hecker et al. (2009); Griffith et al. (2009); Amara et al. (2010); Hecker et al. (2014); Jarman et al. (2014); Cameli et al. (2020)
	iNOS (NO)	↑TGFβ ↑collagen ↑HSP47 ↑ECM-degrading enzymes	Zeidler et al. (2004); Hsu et al. (2007); Kliment and Oury. (2010)
	mtROS	↑profibrotic genes	Jain et al. (2013)
	Nrf2	↓fibrotic progression	Artaud-Macari et al. (2013)
Epithelial cells	NOX4	↑EMT	Hecker et al. (2009); Cameli et al. (2020)
	mtROS	↑senescence ↑apoptosis	Yoon et al. (2005); Panduri et al. (2009); Taslidere et al. (2014); Rangarajan et al. (2017)
	H_2O_2	Mimics TGFβ	Rhyu et al. (2005)
	Catalase	↓H_2O_2 ↓fibroblast activation	Waghray et al. (2005)
	SOD	↓ECM oxidative degradation	Petersen et al. (2004)
Inflammatory cells	NOX2 and NOX4	↑ECM deposition	He et al. (2019)
VSMCs	NOX4	↑proliferation ↑remodelling	Sturrock et al. (2006); Kato and Hecker. (2020)
Endothelial cells	NOX 2 and NOX4	↑angiogenesis	Teng et al. (2012); Jarman et al. (2014)

αSMA, α-smooth muscle actin; ECM, extracellular matrix; EMT, epithelial-to-mesenchimal transition; HSP47, heat-shock protein 47; iNOS, inducible NOS; mtROS, mitochondrial ROS; NO, nitric oxide: NOS, nitric oxide synthase; NOX, NADPH, oxidases; Nrf2, nuclear factor erythroid 2-related factor 2; SOD, superoxide dismutase; TGFβ, transforming growth factor β.

angiogenesis within fibrotic regions and adjacent to fibrotic foci (Jarman et al., 2014).

Whereas Nox4 is mainly expressed in fibroblasts and epithelial cells, Nox2, is primarily expressed by neutrophils and macrophages and, to a lesser extent, in structural cells (mesenchymal cells, smooth muscle cells, endothelial cells, and airway epithelial cells) (Harijith et al., 2017). In IPF patients, neutrophils show an increased expression of Nox2 subunits (Kato and Hecker, 2020) and genetic removal of some of these subunits partially protects from the development of fibrosis in lung fibrosis mice models (Manoury et al., 2005; Kato and Hecker, 2020). Nox2-mediated ROS in vascular endothelial cells is implicated in autophagy induction, which contributes to impaired angiogenesis (Teng et al., 2012).

In lungs, NOS is the major enzyme producer of NO. The NOS family includes three isoforms: endothelial (eNOS), neuronal (nNOS) and inducible (iNOS) (Ricciardolo et al., 2004). RNS are mostly generated by iNOS, which is expressed by a huge variety of cells from the respiratory system. In normal conditions, NO has biological roles such as the relaxation of smooth muscle cells in pulmonary and cardiovascular system, however high levels of $NO^\bullet$ and NO-derived species may interact with different molecules and modify their function (Ricciardolo et al., 2006). In IPF, the high levels of iNOS expression and nitrotyrosine production in fibroblasts, as well as epithelial cells and macrophages, leads to unusual nitrosative stress. This nitrostive stress modifies different proteins in the lungs facilitating fibrogenesis and progression of the disease (Saleh et al., 1997).

Different studies have demonstrated that NO signal pathway may enhance TGF-β expression in lung fibroblasts and increase the expression of collagen type I and heat-shock protein (HSP) 47 (Hsu et al., 2007; Kliment and Oury, 2010). Further studies have demonstrated NO also seems to promote the expression of ECM-degrading enzymes in fibroblasts (Zeidler et al., 2004; Kliment and Oury, 2010). Additionally, endothelial cells may be involved in lung fibrosis through the production of the free radical NO (Michiels, 2003).

As we have mentioned, mitochondria is a major source of ROS production due to the uncoupling of the electron transport chain (Osborn-Heaford et al., 2012) and this production increases with senescence and ageing (Lee et al., 2002; Kurundkar and Thannickal, 2016). ROS generated by mitochondria are released into the cytosol and have been proved to be crucial in mediating pulmonary fibrosis (Cheresh et al., 2013). The pro-fibrotic factor, TGF-β1, enhances mitochondrial ROS, which have been proven to induce the expression of pro-fibrotic genes during myofibroblast differentiation. Pulmonary fibroblasts from IPF patients show a higher generation of mitochondrial ROS and inhibition of the generation of mitochondrial ROS decreases pro-fibrotic gene expression (Jain et al., 2013). Mitochondrial ROS generation is also increased in bleomycin-induced pulmonary fibrosis (Kim et al., 2016). Additionally, the epithelial cell damage occurring in IPF is linked with increased mitochondrial ROS (Kuwano et al., 2003). In turn, TGF-β1 induces mitochondrial ROS generation through mitochondrial complex IV inhibition in lung epithelial cells (Yoon et al., 2005). Furthermore, upregulation of mitochondrial ROS by TGF-β1 induce senescence in lung epithelial cells (Yoon et al., 2005; Taslidere et al., 2014). It has been suggested that mitochondrial impairment represents a key process for epithelial cell apoptosis in lung fibrosis (Panduri et al., 2009; Rangarajan et al., 2017).

The lung counteracts the damage induced by ROS with a wide variety of antioxidant defences. This endogenous antioxidant system includes small-molecular-weight antioxidants [vitamin E, melatonin, glutathione (GSH), uric acid, etc], classic antioxidant enzymes [superoxide dismutases (SODs), catalase, and glutathione peroxidase (GPx)], other antioxidant enzymes [peroxiredoxins (PRXs), thioredoxins (TRXs)], phase II detoxifying enzymes [glutathione-S-transferase (GST) isozymes, NADP(H), quinone oxidoreductase (NQO1), etc], stress-response proteins [heme oxygenase (HO)-1, ferritin, etc.], mucins (MUC), and metal binding proteins (lactoferrin, transferrin, metallothionein, etc) (Walters et al., 2008). The nuclear factor erythroid 2-related factor 2 (Nrf2) induces the expression of most of the antioxidant and detoxifying enzymes, which makes this factor essential for activating the antioxidant defence system. Under normal conditions, Nrf2 is sequestered in the cytoplasm by binding to Kelch like-ECH-associated protein 1 (KEAP1). In response to stress signals, Nrf2 is released from KEAP1 and translocated into the nucleus, where induces the expression of hundreds of antioxidant genes. Additionally, Nrf2 regulates the expression of genes involved in inflammatory and fibrotic responses (Hybertson et al., 2011). Fibroblasts and myofibroblasts from IPF patients express lower levels of Nrf2 when compared to controls fibroblasts. Activators of Nrf2 inhibit TGF-β1-induced pro-fibrotic effects in IPF fibroblasts and attenuate pulmonary fibrosis in animal models (Artaud-Macari et al., 2013).

In lungs, these antioxidant enzymes are expressed by the bronchial and alveolar epithelial cells and macrophages (Kinnula et al., 2005) and different studies suggest that overexpression of some of these antioxidant enzymes may protect against pulmonary fibrosis (Kang et al., 2003; Gao et al., 2008).

AECs in the lungs produce catalase, which exerts its activity via reducing H_2O_2 and, therefore, inhibits H_2O_2-mediated fibroblast activation in IPF lungs (Waghray et al., 2005). As well as epithelial cells, inflammatory cells also express the antioxidant enzyme catalase. It has been reported that intratracheal administration of catalase in asbestos-treated mice prevents the development of pulmonary fibrosis by inhibiting the generation of H_2O_2 in inflammatory cells (Murthy et al., 2009).

All three isoforms of superoxide dismutase, including extracellular-SOD (EC-SOD), are highly expressed in the lungs. In addition, they play a critical role in induced pulmonary fibrosis models by preventing oxidative stress (Bowler et al., 2002; Rabbani et al., 2005). It has been evidenced that EC-SOD exerts anti-fibrotic effects in lungs through prevention of oxidative degradation of ECM, avoiding the destructive effects of ECM degradation products on pulmonary epithelial and mesenchymal cells (Petersen et al., 2004).

Reduced GSH, a low-molecular weight antioxidant, is synthesized by bronchial epithelial cells and alveolar macrophages. Different studies supported that TGF-β1 suppresses gene expression of glutamate cysteine ligases (GCL), an enzyme implicated in the biosynthesis of GSH, in alveolar epithelial cells (Arsalane et al., 1997; Jardine et al., 2002). Overexpression of the active form of TGF-β1 in mice induces lung fibrosis, and it is associated with downregulation of GCL gene expression, decreased GSH levels in BALF, and increased oxidative stress (Liu et al., 2012).

Evidence of Oxidative Stress Biomarkers in IPF Patients

Given the accepted role of oxidative stress in IPF, it is essential to investigate the presence of oxidative stress biomarkers. These biomarkers could provide clues about the disease progression and prognosis as well as be useful in the clinical assessment of the patients. It was in 1987 when the presence of oxidative stress biomarkers was first described (Cantin et al., 1987) in IPF patients. Since then, several researchers have investigated oxidative stress indicators in this pathology, as is resumed in **Table 2**.

GSH is one of the antioxidant small molecule par excellence and one of the most measured biomarkers. Levels of this antioxidant molecule and its oxidized form, GSSG, have been measured as indicators of oxidative stress in multiple diseases. Regarding IPF, most of the studies reported lower levels of total GHS (reduced (GSH) + oxidized (GSSG), tGSH) and reduced GSH in IPF patients than in controls (Cantin et al., 1989; Borok et al., 1991; Meyer et al., 1994; Rahman et al., 1999; Beeh et al., 2002; Muramatsu et al., 2016; Veith et al., 2017), just two studies found no differences in GSH or tGSH between IPF patients and controls (Meyer et al., 1994; Markart et al., 2009). GSSG levels are found to be similar between IPF patients and controls (Rahman et al., 1999; Veith et al., 2017) or higher in IPF (Markart et al., 2009; Muramatsu et al., 2016). Ratios between the different forms of GSH have also been measured and are shown in **Table 2**. Most of the studies found no correlation between GSH forms and lung function. However, Beeh et al. (2002) found an inverse relationship between GSH sputum levels and disease severity and a positive correlation between GSH and vital capacity (VC %), Muramatsu et al. (2016) also found an inverse correlation between the change in GSSG and the change in forced vital capacity (FVC).

Another marker for oxidative stress is lipid peroxidation, usually determined through levels of thiobarbituric acid reactive substances (TBARS), and among all the lipid oxidation products the most studied is the malondialdehyde (MDA). These biomarkers were found to be higher in IPF patients when compared to healthy controls (Jack et al., 1996; Rahman et al., 1999). Jack et al. (1996) also found a significant negative correlation between the changes in lipid peroxidation and the changes in VC (%). Isoprostanes are free radical–catalyzed prostaglandin isomers whose generation reflects lipid peroxidation *in vivo* and, thus, are biomarkers of oxidative stress (Lawson et al., 1999). Concentrations of isoprostanes, especially 8-isoprostane, have been found to be higher in IPF patients compared to controls (Psathakis et al., 2006; Jackson et al., 2010; Chow et al., 2012; Malli et al., 2013; Shimizu et al., 2014). In addition, carbonyl proteins serve as markers of oxidized proteins and concentrations have been found to be higher in IPF patients than in healthy in controls (Lenz et al., 1996; Lenz et al., 2004; Rottoli et al., 2005; Bargagli et al., 2007).

TABLE 2 | Summary of the oxidative stress biomarkers analysed in different biological specimens of IPF patients.

Specimen	Comparison (n)	Biomarker	Lung function/severity disease correlation	Reference
ELF	IPF (15) vs. Ctrl (19)	↓tGSH ↔GSH/GSH + GSSG	No correlation	Cantin et al. (1989)
ELF	IPF (10) vs. Ctrl (19)	↓tGSH ↓GSH	N/A	Borok et al. (1991)
ELF BALF	IPF (17) vs. Ctrl (14)	↓tGSH ↔tGSH	No correlation	Meyer et al. (1994)
BALF	IPF (12) vs. Ctrl (31)	↓GSH ↔GSSG ↓GSH/GSSG	N/A	Rahman et al. (1999)
Sputum Plasma	IPF (16) vs. Ctrl (15)	↓tGSH	↑disease severity ↓VC	Beeh et al. (2002)
BALF	IPF (16) vs. Ctrl (20)	↔GSH ↑GSSG	No correlation	Markart et al. (2009)
Blood	IPF (22) vs. Ctrl (29)	↓tGSH ↓tGSH/GSSG ↑GSSG	No correlation ↓FVC	Muramatsu et al. (2016)
Blood	IPF (11) vs. Ctrl (9)	↓GSH ↔GSSG	N/A	Veith et al. (2017)
Serum	IPF (37) vs. Ctrl (6)	↑lipid peroxidation ↑TBARS	↑disease severity ↓VC No correlation	Jack et al. (1996)
Plasma BALF	IPF (12) vs. Ctrl (31)	↑MDA ↓TEAC	N/A	Rahman et al. (1999)
BALF	IPF non-smokers (14) vs Ctrl non-smokers (9)	↑Carbonyl proteins	N/A	Lenz et al. (1996)
BALF	IPF (9) vs. Ctrl (5)	↑Carbonyl proteins	N/A	Lenz et al. (2004)
BALF	IPF (13) vs. Ctrl (5)	↑Carbonyl proteins	N/A	Rottoli et al. (2005)
BALF	IPF (15) vs. Ctrl (8)	↑Carbonyl proteins	N/A	Bargagli et al. (2007)
EBC	IPF (16) vs. Ctrl (15)	↑8-isoprostane ↑H_2O_2	No correlation ↓DLCO	Psathakis et al. (2006)
Plasma and urine	IPF (29) vs. Ctrl (6)	↑Pl-isoprostanes ↔Ur- H_2O_2	N/A	Jackson et al. (2010)
	IPF at rest (29) vs. IPF after physical exercise	↔Pl-isoprostanes ↓Pl-TAC ↑Ur-isoprostanes ↔Ur- H_2O_2		
EBC	IPF (20) vs. Ctrl (20)	↑8-isoprostane ↔ NOx ↔ H_2O_2 ↑3-NT	No correlation ↓FVE1, ↓FVC, ↓VC, ↓TLC	Chow et al. (2012)
Serum and BALF	IPF (16) vs. Ctrl (17)	↑8-isoprostane	N/A	Malli et al. (2013)
EBC	IPF (6) vs. Ctrl (6)	↑8-isoPGF2α	N/A	Shimizu et al. (2014)
Plasma	IPF (21) vs. Ctrl (12)	↑hydroperoxides	↑dyspnea severity ↓ FVC ↓DLCO	Daniil et al. (2006)
Serum	IPF (43) vs. Ctrl (30)	↑hydroperoxides	↓FVC ↓DLCO ↑acute exacerbation	Matsuzawa et al. (2015)
BALF	IPF (16) vs. Ctrl (20)	↑uric acid ↑ascorbic acid ↑vitamin A ↑vitamin E	N/A	Markart et al. (2009)
Blood	IPF (11) vs. Ctrl (9)	↓uric acid (not sig) ↓ascorbic acid (not sig) ↓TEAC	N/A	Veith et al. (2017)
Lung tissue	IPF (10) vs. Ctrl (5)	↔ECSOD	N/A	Kinnula et al., 2006
	IPF fibrotic areas vs IPF normal areas	↓ECSOD		
Lung tissue	IPF (10) vs. Ctrl (310)	↔PrxII	N/A	Vuorinen et al. (2008)
Lung tissue	IPF (7) vs. Ctrl (7)	↔NRF2 ↑SRX1	N/A	Mazur et al. (2010)
	IPF hyperplastic epithelium vs IPF normal epithelium	↑NRF2 ↑KEAP1		

3-NT, 3-nitrotyrosine; BALF, bronchoalveolar lavage fluid; Ctrl, control; DLCO, diffusing capacity of the lungs for carbon monoxide; EBC, expired breath condensate; ECSOD, Extracellular Superoxide Dismutase; ELF, epithelial lining fluid; FEV, forced expiratory volume; FVC, forced vital capacity; GSH, glutathione; GSSG, oxidized glutathione; IPF, idiopathic pulmonary fibrosis; KEAP1, Kelch like-ECH-associated protein 1; MDA, malondialdehyde; N/A, not available; not sig, not significative; NOx, NADPH, oxidases; NRF2, nuclear factor erythroid 2-related factor 2; Pl, plasma; PrxII, peroxiredoxin II; SRX1, sulfiredoxin-1; TAC, total antioxidant capacity; TBARS, thiobarbituric acid reactive substances; TEAC, trolox equivalent antioxidant capacity; tGSH, total glutathione; Ur, urine.

Some studies have also measured the levels of H_2O_2 and in some cases, concentrations of this marker are higher in IPF patients, and a negative correlation between H_2O_2 and diffusing capacity of the lungs for carbon monoxide (DLCO) was observed (Psathakis et al., 2006). Other studies, on the other hand, reported no differences between groups (Jackson et al., 2010; Chow et al., 2012).

Hydroperoxide measurements, though are less common, are also used as oxidative stress biomarkers. Concentrations of these biomarkers are significantly higher in IPF patients than in controls. It has also been found a significant positive correlation between concentrations of hydroperoxides and severity of dyspnea or acute exacerbation and a negative correlation between the concentrations of hydroperoxides, FVC, and DLCO (Daniil et al., 2006; Matsuzawa et al., 2015).

Small-molecular-weight antioxidant molecules play a significant role in lung antioxidant defences. These small molecules include GSH, as we have mentioned above, but also other molecules such as vitamins and acid uric, which are also used as oxidative stress biomarkers. A study performed by Markart et al. (2009) reported significantly higher levels of uric acid, ascorbic acid (vitamin C), retinol (vitamin A), and tocopherol (vitamin E) in IPF patients when compared to healthy controls. However, a more recent study has reported that concentrations of uric acid and vitamin C were slightly, but not significantly, lower in IPF patients than in controls (Veith et al., 2017).

The antioxidant capacity can be also measured as an oxidative stress biomarker and, in some studies, it has been found to be significantly lower in IPF patients (Rahman et al., 1999; Jackson et al., 2010; Veith et al., 2017). Another molecule useful in oxidative stress measurements is 3-nitrotyrosine (3-NT) and it has been found to be higher in IPF patients compared to controls. Additionally, it is reported that there is an inverse correlation between 3-NT concentrations and forced expiratory volume (FEV1) (%), FVC (%), VC (%), and total lung capacity (TLC, %) (Chow et al., 2012).

When the biological specimen used is lung tissue, the studied oxidative stress biomarker is usually the expression of proteins or transcription factors implicated in different antioxidant pathways, such as the antioxidant enzyme SOD or the transcription factor Nrf2. ECSOD expression was found to be significantly lower in fibrotic areas when compared to non-fibrotic areas (Kinnula et al., 2006). Furthermore, regarding the antioxidant enzyme peroxiredoxin (PRX) II, it was found that there was no major Prx II oxidation in IPF lungs compared with the normal lung (Vuorinen et al., 2008). On the other hand, Mazur et al. (2010) analysed the Nrf2 –sulfiredoxin-1 (SRX1) pathway. The authors found non-specific cell variability in the expression of the Nrf2 pathway in healthy and fibrotic lungs. By contrast, the expression of SRX1 was increased in IPF compared to controls. Furthermore, the morphometric evaluation revealed that Nrf2 and KEAP1 were significantly increased in the hyperplastic alveolar epithelium compared to the normal alveolar epithelium (Mazur et al., 2010).

A huge number of oxidative stress biomarkers have been described in patients with IPF. Here we have just highlighted the most commonly analysed. The evaluation of these biomarkers could help in the clinical assessment of patients with IPF.

ANTIOXIDANT THERAPY IN IDIOPATHIC PULMONARY FIBROSIS

Considering oxidative stress plays a central role in the development and progression of IPF, antioxidant therapies have been proposed for many years. There are a few publications that review the use of antioxidant molecules or NOX inhibitors, naturals and synthetics, as potential therapeutics for lung fibrosis (Kinnula et al., 2005; Day, 2008; Kato and Hecker, 2020; Wang et al., 2021). In this review, we have selected the most advanced studies that include *in vitro, in vivo* and human evidence that could be translated into future treatments of IPF Summarized in **Table 3**.

NOX Inhibitors

Diphenyleneiodonium

Diphenyleneiodonium (DPI) is a potent inhibitor of NOX, which specifically and irreversibly binds to flavin, the membranous component of the NOX. It is the most commonly used and well-studied Nox inhibitor; however, its irreversible binding, lack of specific, poor solubility and toxicity *in vivo* do not make it the suitable candidate for a therapeutic option (O'Donnell et al., 1993; Kato and Hecker, 2020) (**Figure 1**).

Even so, DPI has been reported to inhibit collagen type I deposition and proliferation of pulmonary cells after stimulation with IPF sera (Fois et al., 2018). Another study has demonstrated that DPI decreases MPO activity, iNOS expression, intracellular ROS levels, the number of inflammatory cells, and cytokines TNF-α and IL-6 in lipopolysaccharide (LPS)-induced acute lung injury rats (Kim et al., 2019).

VAS2870

Vas2870 was first described as a Nox2 inhibitor but later was described as a pan-NADPH oxidase inhibitor, with no selectivity for any NOX isoform (Wingler et al., 2012). It has been used in different cell models, but it has shown off-target effects due to its unspecific redox mode of action (Kato and Hecker, 2020). However, VAS2870 has been proved to reduce ROS generation restore epithelium barrier integrity and preserve cell viability in LPS-induced injury in alveolar epithelial cells (Li et al., 2020). It has also been reported to protect human pulmonary microvascular endothelial cells against LPS-induced inflammation through inhibiting the generation of ROS (Li et al., 2020); to inhibit phenotypic changes in fibrotic cells, including α-SMA and vimentin expression (Choi et al., 2016); and to suppress growth factor-mediated ROS liberation and migration in VSMC (ten Freyhaus et al., 2006) (**Figure 1**).

GKT137831 and GKT136901

GKT137831 and GKT136901 were developed by Genkyotex (Geneva, Switzerland) through a high-throughput screening approach to discover small-molecule inhibitors targeting NOX enzymes (Laleu et al., 2010). Both small molecules are Nox4/

TABLE 3 | Summary of potential therapeutic antioxidants for IPF reviewed in this study.

Drug	Class	Mechanism of action	Clinical trial identifier NCT	Reference
DPI	NOX inhibitor	Pan-NOXs inhibitor		O'Donnell et al. (1993); Kato and Hecker. (2020)
Vas2870	NOX inhibitor	Pan-NOXs inhibitor		Kato and Hecker, (2020)
GKT137831	NOX inhibitor	NOX4/NOX1 dual inhibitor	NCT03865927	Gaggini et al. (2011)
GKT136901	NOX inhibitor	NOX4/NOX1 dual inhibitors		Gaggini et al. (2011)
Apocynin	NOX inhibitor	NOX2 inhibitor ROS scavenger		Heumüller et al. (2008); Augsburger et al. (2019)
Metformin	NOX inhibitor Anti-diabetic	NOX4 inhibitor		Sato et al. (2016); Rangarajan et al. (2018)
NAC	Antioxidant enhancer	ROS scavenger GSH precursor ---| NFkB ↑ Nrf2	NCT00639496 NCT00650091 UMIN000015508 NCT02707640 NCT04300920 NCT03720483	Watchorn et al. (1998); Parmentier et al. (1999); Cuzzocrea et al. (2001); Sugiura et al. (2009); Ji et al. (2010)
Quercetin	Antioxidant enhancer Senolytic	ROS scavenger ↑ Nrf2	NCT02874989	Tanigawa et al. (2007); Veith et al. (2017); Cazzola et al. (2018); Sellarés and Rojas. (2019)
Salvianolic acid B	Antioxidant enhancer	ROS scavenger ↑ Nrf2 ---| NOX2,4	NCT03274544	Xiao et al. (2020)
EGCG	Antioxidant enhancer	ROS scavenger ↑ Nrf2 ↓Inflammatory mediators ↓Lipid peroxidation	NCT03928847	Salah et al. (1995); Nanjo et al. (1999); Nagai et al. (2002a); Negishi et al. (2004); Zhang et al. (2007a); Sriram et al. (2009a)
Tanshinone IIA and Sodium tanshinone IIA sulfonate	Antioxidant enhancer	ROS scavenger ↑ Nrf2 ↑GSH ---| NOX4		Zhang and Wang. (2007); An et al. (2019)
Resveratrol	Antioxidant enhancer	ROS scavenger ↑ Nrf2		Zhu et al. (2017)
Sulforaphane	Antioxidant enhancer	↑ Nrf2		Elbarbry and Elrody. (2011) Kim and Park. (2016)
Melatonin	Antioxidant enhancer	ROS scavenger ↑ Nrf2 ↓Inflammatory mediators		Swiderska-Kolacz et al. (2006); Reiter et al. (2007); Santofimia-Castaño et al. (2015); Goc et al. (2017)
Curcumin	Antioxidant enhancer	ROS scavenger ↑ Nrf2 ↑ Antioxidant molecules		Lee et al. (2010b); Zhou et al. (2011); Lelli et al. (2017)
Pirfenidone	Antifibrotic Antioxidant enhancer	ROS scavenger ↑ Nrf2 ↑ Antioxidant molecules ↓ Lipid peroxidation ↓Inflammatory mediators	NCT00287716 NCT00287729 NCT01366209	Giri et al. (1999); Misra and Rabideau. (2000); Nakazato et al. (2002); Oku et al. (2008); Ma et al. (2021)
Thalidomide	Antiemetic Antioxidant enhancer	↑ Antioxidant molecules	NCT00162760 NCT00600028	Amirshahrokh. (2013); Dong et al. (2017)
Crocin	Antioxidant enhancer	↑ Nrf2 ↑ Antioxidant molecules		Zaghloul et al. (2019); Mehrabani et al. (2020)
Isorhamnetin	Antioxidant enhancer	ROS scavenger ↑ Nrf2		Chi et al. (2016); Zheng et al. (2019); Luo et al. (2019); Ren et al. (2021)
Echinochrome A	Antioxidant enhancer	↑ Antioxidant molecules ↓Inflammatory mediators		Lebed'ko et al. (2015)

(Continued on following page)

TABLE 3 | (*Continued*) Summary of potential therapeutic antioxidants for IPF reviewed in this study.

Drug	Class	Mechanism of action	Clinical trial identifier NCT	Reference
AEOL 10150	Catalytic antioxidant mimetics	Mimics SOD Mimics CAT		Rabbani et al. (2007); Garofalo et al. (2014); MacVittie et al. (2017); Zhang et al. (2018b)
AEOL 10113	Catalytic antioxidant mimetics	Mimics SOD		Vujaskovic et al. (2002)
MnTBAP	Catalytic antioxidant mimetics	Mimics SOD		Oury et al. (2001); Venkatadri et al. (2017)

CAT, catalase; DPI, Diphenyleneiodonium; EGCG, Epigallocatechin gallate; NAC, n-acetyl cysteine; NFκβ, nuclear factor kappa beta; NOX, NADPH, oxidase; NRF2, nuclear factor erythroid 2-related factor 2; ROS, reactive oxygen species; SOD, superoxide dismutase.

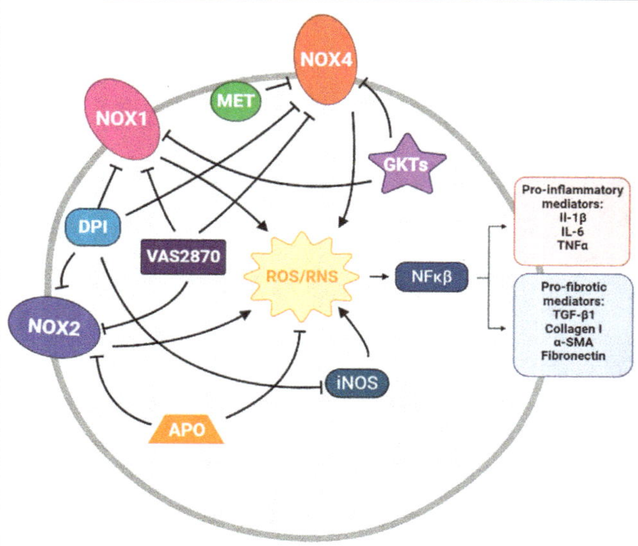

FIGURE 1 | Simplified diagram of the principal molecular mechanisms of the NOX inhibitors Diphenyleneiodonium (DPI), VAS2870, GKT137831 and GKT136901 (GKTs), Apocynin (APO) and Metformin (MET). αSMA: alpha smooth muscle actin; IL-1β: interleuquina 1beta; IL-6: interleuquina 6; iNOS: inducible nitrogen oxide synthase; NFκβ: nuclear factor kappa beta; NOX1,2,4: NADPH oxidases; ROS/RNS: reactive oxygen species/reactive nitrogen species; TGF-β1: transforming growth factor beta 1; TNFα: tumoral necrosis factor alpha Created with Biorender.com.

Nox1 dual inhibitors. GKT137831 has been demonstrated to have strong antifibrotic activity at a low dose with much better efficacy than pirfenidone in curative model of bleomycin-induced pulmonary fibrosis in mice, as it is reported by the company (Gaggini et al., 2011). These Genkyotex compounds have also been reported to have protective effects in different pre-clinical *in vitro* and *in vivo* studies (Carnesecchi et al., 2011; Green et al., 2012; Jiang et al., 2012; Wan et al., 2016; Tanaka et al., 2017; Cui et al., 2018) (**Figure 1**).

In 2010, GKT137831 was granted orphan drug status for the treatment of IPF by the European Commission and is currently in clinical trials for IPF. A phase 2 clinical trial of GKT137831 [GKT137831 in IPF Patients With Idiopathic Pulmonary Fibrosis (GKT137831)] has recently started and it is a placebo-controlled, multicentre, randomized trial to test GKT137831 in ambulatory patients with IPF. The primary outcome is the reduction of the circulating concentrations of o,o'-dityrosine, an oxidative stress biomarker. Changes in concentrations of the collagen degradation and FVC are some of the secondary outcomes (ClinicalTrials.gov Identifier: NCT03865927).

Other NOX Inhibitors

Some other molecules are also claimed to be NOX inhibitors. It is the case of apocynin, a natural organic compound obtained from plants, that was found to have therapeutic effects in animal models of various diseases (Virdis et al., 2016). In particular, it shows a protective and therapeutic effect on bleomycin-induced lung fibrosis in rats (Kilic et al., 2015). However, although this compound is usually defined as a Nox2 inhibitor, several studies have reported that apocynin would have intrinsic antioxidant properties rather than be a Nox inhibitor (Heumüller et al., 2008; Augsburger et al., 2019). On the other hand, we have metformin, an anti-diabetic drug not known primarily for its antioxidant potential, but a recent study has demonstrated that treatment with metformin inhibits TGF-β1–induced Nox4 expression, ROS generation and myofibroblast differentiation in lung fibroblasts *in vitro* and also attenuates bleomycin-induced lung fibrosis (Sato et al., 2016; Rangarajan et al., 2018). Despite the lack of clinical trials regarding the efficacy of metformin in the treatment of IPF, there is a retrospective study in humans treated with pirfenidone along with metformin; however, its results are not particularly promising (Spagnolo et al., 2018). Only future trials could provide more clues about this (**Figure 1**).

On the other hand, numerous groups are currently working on the finding or development of new NOX inhibitors that may become a therapeutic option in treating IPF.

Antioxidant Enhancers and Reactive Oxygen Species Scavenger

N-Acetyl Cysteine

N-acetyl cysteine (NAC) is an L-cysteine derived aminoacid with powerful reductive capacity. This aminothiol is not only a GSH

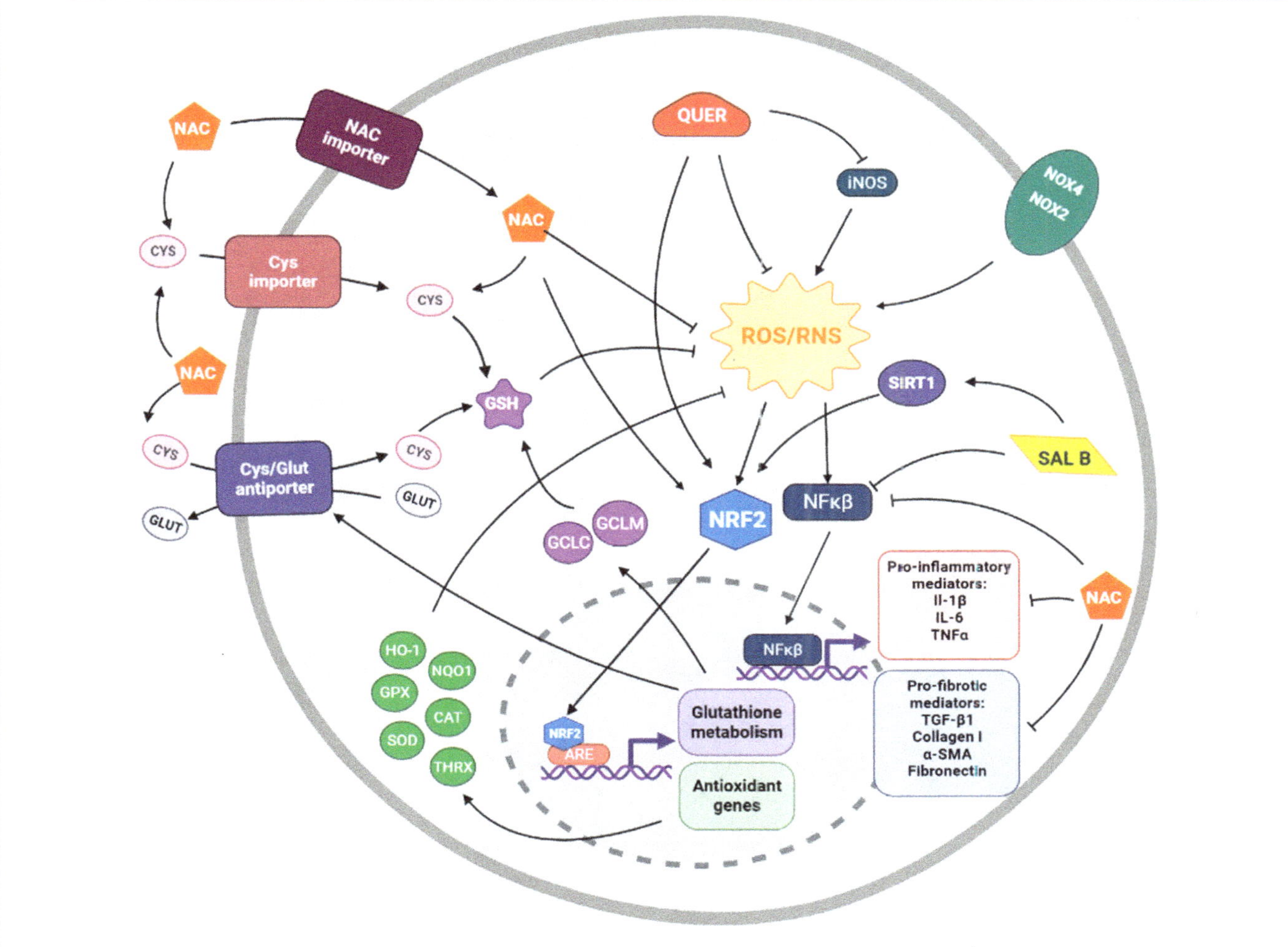

FIGURE 2 | Simplified diagram of the principal molecular mechanisms of the antioxidant enhancers n-acetyl cysteine (NAC), Quercetin (QUER) and Salvianolic acid B (SAL B). αSMA: alpha smooth muscle actin; ARE: antioxidant responsive element; CAT: catalase; CYS: cysteine; GCLC: glutamate cysteine ligase catalytic subunit; GCLM: glutamate cysteine ligase modifier subunit; GLUT: glutamate; GPX: glutathione peroxidase; GSH: glutathione; HO-1: heme oxygenase 1; IL-1β: interleuquina 1beta; IL-6: interleuquina 6; iNOS: inducible nitrogen oxide synthase; NFκβ: nuclear factor kappa beta; NOX1,2,4: NADPH oxidases; NQO1: NAD(P)H:quinone oxidoreductase 1; NRF2: nuclear factor erythroid 2-related factor 2; ROS/RNS: reactive oxygen species/reactive nitrogen species; TGF-β1: transforming growth factor beta 1; TNFα: tumoral necrosis factor alpha; SIRT: sirtuine 1; SOD: supeoxide dismutase Created with Biorender.com.

precursor but also presents a direct ROS-scavenging capacity and may induce Nrf2 expression (Cuzzocrea et al., 2001; Sugiura et al., 2009; Ji et al., 2010). These properties have made NAC a broadly used potent antioxidant (**Figure 2**).

In vitro *Cellular Studies*

Several *in vitro* assays have demonstrated that NAC prevents GSH depletion in various cell types such as macrophages, epithelial cells, and fibroblasts (Watchorn et al., 1998; Parmentier et al., 1999; Liu et al., 2004; Felton et al., 2009). NAC has also been reported to inhibit collagen production and EMT in TGF-β1-stimulated murine embryo fibroblasts and rat alveolar epithelial cells, respectively (Liu et al., 2004; Felton et al., 2009). A further study found that NAC significantly diminishes TGF-β1-induced fibronectin and VEGF production as well as α-SMA expression in human lung fibroblasts (Sugiura et al., 2009). These studies implied that NAC may affect the TGF-β1-induced tissue remodelling or fibrotic process *in vitro*.

Numerous studies have demonstrated that NAC inhibits the production of different inflammatory mediators such as tumour necrosis factor alpha (TFNα), interleukin-8 (IL-8) and matrix metalloproteinase-9 (MMP-9) in epithelial cells, macrophages, and lymphocytes from patients with IPF (Watchorn et al., 1998; Parmentier et al., 1999; Cu et al., 2009; Radomska-Leśniewska et al., 2010).

In vivo *Animal Studies*

The first study that demonstrated the antifibrotic effect of NAC was performed by Shahzeidi et al. (1991). They showed that NAC inhibits collagen accumulation in lungs from rats with bleomycin-induced lung fibrosis (Shahzeidi et al., 1991). Since then, several studies have reported that NAC inhibits several

TABLE 4 | Summary of clinical trials of antioxidant therapies of IPF.

Drugs	Identifier (acronym)	Study desing, sample size	Primary endpoint	Secondary endpoints	Outcome	Observations
GKT137831 (400 mg b.i.d) Vs.Placebo	NCT03865927	Phase 2 Randomized Double-Blind Parallel Assignment Placebo-Controlled n = 60	Changes in concentrations of circulating o,o'-dityrosine at 24 weeks	Changes in concentrations of the collagen degradation product FVC, 6MWD at 24 weeks	Recruiting	
NAC (oral 600 mg t.i.d) + prednisone + azathioprine Vs. Placebo + prednisone + azathioprine	NCT00639496 (IFIGENIA)	Phase 3 Randomized Double-Blind Parallel Assignment Placebo-Controlled n = 184	Changes in VC and DLCO at 6 and 12 months	CRP-score at 6 and 12 months	Completed. Three-drug therapy preserved VC and DLCO	
NAC (oral 600 mg t.i.d) + prednisolone + azathioprine Vs. NAC (oral 600 mg t.i.d) + placebo Vs. placebo	NCT00650091 (PANTHER)	Phase 3 Randomized Double-Blind Parallel Assignment Placebo-Controlled n = 264	Changes in FVC at 60 weeks	The time-to-death or a 10% decline in FVC, acute exacerbations, respiratory infections at 60 weeks	Completed. NAC offered no significant benefit	Three-drug regimen was stopped due to safety concerns
NAC (inhaled 352.4 mg b.i.d) + pirfenidone Vs. placebo + pirfenidone	UMIN000015508	Phase 3 Randomized Open-label Parallel Assignment Placebo-Controlled n = 150	Changes in FVC at 48 weeks	Changes in 6MWD, VC, TLC, DLCO at 48 weeks	Completed. Combination therapy did not bring any clinical benefit	
NAC (oral 600 mg t.i.d) + pirfenidone Vs. Placebo + pirfenidone	NCT02707640 (PANORAMA)	Phase 2 Randomized Double-Blind Parallel Assignment Placebo-Controlled n = 123	Assessment of adverse events at 24 weeks	Changes in FVC, DLCO, 6MWD at 24 weeks	Completed. NAC does not alter tolerability profile of pirfenidone and is unlikely to be beneficial	
NAC (oral 600 mg t.i.d) Vs. Placebo	NCT04300920 (PRECISIONS)	Phase 3 Randomized Double-Blind Parallel Assignment Placebo-Controlled n = 200	10% relative decline FVC, first respiratory hospitalization, lung transplant or death from any cause at 24 months	Time to first all-cause hospitalization, annualized rate of respiratory hospitalizations, changes in DLCO at 24 months	Recruiting	
NAC (inhaled) Vs. placebo	NCT03720483	Phase 1/2 Randomized Open-label Crossover Assignment, n = 0	Changes in FVC at week 10 and 18	Changes in DLCO at week 10 and 18	Withdrawn	The study encountered challenges during startup due to the COVID-19 epidemic and was withdrawn
Dasatinib (100 mg/d) + Quercetin (1250 mg/d) Vs. Placebo	NCT02874989	Phase 1 Randomized Open-label Parallel Assignment, Placebo-Controlled n = 26	Retention rates and completion rates for planned clinical assessments (e.g., percentage of pro-inflammatory expressing cells, blood pressure, weight, heart rate) at 4 weeks	Safety and change in functional and reported health measures	Completed. Senolytics improved 6MWD	
PROLUNG (contains Salvianolic acid B)	NCT03720483	Open-label Single Group Assignment n = 6	Change in FVC at 6 months	Changes in SGRQ score, SF-36 score, WHOQOL-BREF score and in adverse events over 6 months	Terminated	Difficulty in recruiting eligible patients

(Continued on following page)

TABLE 4 | (*Continued*) Summary of clinical trials of antioxidant therapies of IPF.

Drugs	Identifier (acronym)	Study desing, sample size	Primary endpoint	Secondary endpoints	Outcome	Observations
EGCG (600 mg daily)	NCT03928847	Early Phase I Open-label Single Group Assignment $n = 35$	LOXL2 activity and TGFbeta1 signaling biomarkers such as Snail1 and pSmad3 at 2 weeks	Maximum plasma concentration of EGCG 0, 2, 4, 12 h post dose and adverse events at 2 weeks	Recruiting	
Pirfenidone (1197 or 2403 mg in divided doses t.i.d) Vs. placebo	NCT00287716 (CAPACITY: study 004	Phase 3 Randomized Double-Blind Parallel Assignment Placebo-Controlled $n = 435$	Changes in FVC at 72 weeks	PFS, changes in 6MWD, SpO2, DLCO, dyspnea score and worsening of IPF at 72 weeks	Completed. Improvement in lung function, in PFS, and in the associated death	
Pirfenidone (2403 mg in divided doses t.i.d) Vs. placebo	NCT00287729 (CAPACITY: study 006)	Phase 3 Randomized Double-Blind Parallel Assignment Placebo-Controlled $n = 344$	Changes in FVC at 72 weeks	PFS, changes in 6MWD, SpO2, DLCO, dyspnea score and worsening of IPF at 72 weeks	Completed. Improvement in lung function, in PFS, and in the associated death	
Thalidomide (400 mg daily)	NCT00162760	Phase 2 Non-Randomized Open-label Single Group Assignment $n = 19$	Safety, feasibility and efficacy of thalidomide administered daily for 1 year	changes in pulmonary function tests, radiographs, dyspnea scales and quality of life measures	Completed. No results available	
Thalidomide (50–100 mg daily) Vs. Placebo	NCT00600028	Phase 3 Randomized Double-Blind Crossover Assignment Placebo-Controlled $n = 344$	Suppression of cough measured by the CQLQ at 6 months	Suppression of cough measured by the VAS at 6 months	Completed. Thalidomide improved cough and respiratory quality of life	

6MWD, 6-min walk distance; b.i.d, bis in die, twice a day; CQLQ, Cough Quality of Life Questionnaire; CRP -score, clinical, radiologic and physiologic score; DLCO, diffusion capacity for CO; EGCG, Epigallocatechin-3-gallate; FVC, forced vital capacity; NAC, N-acetylcysteine; PFS, progression-free survival; SF-36, 36-Item Short Form Survey; SGRQ, St. George's Respiratory Questionnaire; SpO2, oxygen saturation by pulse oximetry; t.i.d, ter in die, three times a day; TLC, total lung capacity; VAS, visual analog scale of cough; VC, vital capacity; WHOQOL-BREF, world Health Organization Quality of Life abbreviated version.

profibrotic mechanisms in bleomycin-induced fibrosis murine models (Myllärniemi and Kaarteenaho, 2015). For instance, aerosolized administration of NAC attenuated bleomycin-induced lung fibrosis in mice *via* the decrease of the amounts of hydroxyproline, fibrosis and several cytokines' levels (Hagiwara et al., 2000). Further studies performed by our group showed that treatment with NAC, in bleomycin-exposed rats, decreased the augmented collagen deposition and the inflammatory cells numbers. It also increased GSH levels and decreased MUC5a expression, fibrotic areas, TNF-α levels and MPO activity (Cortijo et al., 2001; Mata et al., 2003; Serrano-Mollar et al., 2003).

More recent animal studies on NAC using lung fibrosis murine models have been performed. In 2012, a study revealed that NAC treatment reversed lysyl oxidase activity to normal levels and increased GSH levels in the lung of bleomycin-induced rats, inhibiting TGF-β1 and α-SMA expression, thus attenuating pulmonary fibrosis (Li et al., 2012). A posterior study demonstrated that administration of NAC-pre-treated human mesenchymal stem cells to nude mice with bleomycin-induced lung injury decreased the pathological grade of lung inflammation and fibrosis, hydroxyproline content and numbers of neutrophils and inflammatory cytokines in BALF and apoptotic cells (Wang et al., 2013). The therapeutic potential of NAC in pulmonary fibrosis was also studied in rats exposed to silica particles. It was demonstrated that NAC treated silica-exposed rats showed significantly lower fibrosis scores, as well as lower levels of hydroxyproline amounts and MDA. NAC also attenuated silica-induced increments in TNF-α, IL-8, high-sensitivity C-reactive protein and ROS content (Zhang et al., 2013; Zhang et al., 2014a).

Human Clinical Trials

In contrast to most cases of drug development, animal and human trials with NAC were conducted even earlier than *in vitro* ones. *In vitro* assays have shown, indeed, that NAC reduces fibrotic and remodelling processes in fibrosis models. Nevertheless, previously, *in vivo* animal trials had already suggested that NAC could be a good candidate for clinical trials. All clinical trials regarding NAC are summarized in **Table 4**.

In the 1990s, several open-label studies were conducted to analyse the efficacy of the short-term treatment of NAC in patients with various types of pulmonary fibrosis. These studies reported that total GSH levels increased and pulmonary function tests significantly improved after therapy with NAC (Meyer et al., 1994; Meyer et al., 1995; Behr et al., 1997).

The first clinical trial that assesses the effectiveness of NAC in IPF therapy was the IFIGENIA, which purpose was to determine whether NAC added to prednisone and azathioprine was more effective than the standard therapy with prednisone plus azathioprine. This study showed the three-drug therapy preserved VC and DLCO in IPF patients better than standard therapy (Demedts et al., 2005) (ClinicalTrials.gov Identifier: NCT00639496).

In the IFIGENIA trial, all patients received the combination of the three drugs but none, NAC alone. Thus, in order to study the effectiveness of NAC monotherapy for the treatment of IPF, it was conducted the PANTHER trial. Initially, subjects who have IPF were randomly assigned to receive: 1) three-drug regimen (NAC, prednisolone, and azathioprine), 2) NAC and placebo, or 3) placebo. After performing a midpoint analysis of the study, the three-drug regimen was stopped due to safety concerns. For this reason, the entire study was interrupted for 3 months but later continued. The primary outcome was the change in FVC over 60 weeks. Results showed that acetylcysteine offered no significant benefit concerning the preservation of FVC in patients with IPF when compared with placebo (Izumi et al., 2012; Martinez et al., 2014) (ClinicalTrials.gov number, NCT00650091).

Following this line, a phase III clinical trial evaluating the efficacy and safety of combined therapy with pirfenidone and inhaled NAC for IPF was conducted in Japan. The primary outcome was a change in FVC. Data showed there was no difference between the two groups in the change in FVC. Therefore, combination therapy did not bring any clinical benefit (Sakamoto et al., 2021) (University Hospital Medical Information Network registration number UMIN000015508). In addition to this study, a similar phase II trial was conducted, the PANORAMA study. The aim was to assess the safety and tolerability of NAC in IPF patients receiving background pirfenidone therapy. Again, findings suggested that the addition of NAC to pirfenidone does not substantially alter the tolerability profile of pirfenidone and is unlikely to be beneficial in IPF (Behr et al., 2016) (ClinicalTrials.gov Identifier: NCT02707640).

In 2015, a post hoc exploratory analysis of subjects enrolled in the PANTHER-IPF clinical trial was conducted to determine whether specific polymorphisms in toll-interacting protein (*TOLLIP*) and *MUC5B* genes modified the efficacy of NAC. These genes have been associated with IPF susceptibility and survival. TOLLIP encodes toll-interacting protein (TOLLIP), which is inhibitory of toll-like receptors, which are, in turn, responsible for the activation of inflammatory, oxidative and immune response pathways. This post hoc study showed that NAC might improve prognosis in genetically predisposed individuals, specifically, those carrying an rs3750920 (TOLLIP) TT genotype (Oldham et al., 2015). In order to assess this hypothesis, it has been proposed a genotype-stratified clinical trial: the PRECISIONS trial. The purpose of this study is to compare the effect of NAC plus standard care in patients diagnosed with IPF who have the TOLLIP rs3750920 TT genotype and it will compare the time to a composite endpoint of relative decline in lung function. Recruitment is ongoing and the study is estimated to finish in 2025. Thus, no results are published yet (ClinicalTrials.gov Identifier: NCT04300920).

Furthermore, a further phase I/II open label pilot study has been recently proposed to investigate the safety and tolerability of inhaled NAC in patients with IPF. It is titled "Pilot Study to Evaluate Inhaled N-Acetylcysteine in Pulmonary Fibrosis." The primary outcomes are changes in pulmonary function: FVC and DLCO. This study faced different challenges during enrolment due to the COVID-19 epidemic and it is withdrawn at this moment. It is estimated to start at the beginning of 2022 and finish at the end of 2023 (ClinicalTrials.gov Identifier: NCT03720483).

Quercetin

The antioxidant quercetin (3,3′,4′,5,7-pentahydroxyflavone) is a polyphenolic plant flavonoid ubiquitously present in vegetables and fruit as well as tea and red wine (Formica and Regelson, 1995; D'Andrea, 2015). It is a potent direct ROS scavenger but, also, indirectly, exerts its antioxidant function *via* activating the Nrf2 pathway and inducing Nrf2-regulated genes, such as NQO1, HO-1, GPX1, etc. (Tanigawa et al., 2007; Veith et al., 2017). However, quercetin has not only strong antioxidant but also anti-inflammatory capacities (Boots et al., 2008; Impellizzeri et al., 2015) (**Figure 2**).

Quercetin is also known as a senolytic drug, which induces selective elimination of senescent cells. It is usually used in combination with dasatinib, a tyrosine kinase inhibitor used in the treatment of some cancers (Cazzola et al., 2018; Sellarés and Rojas, 2019).

In vitro *Cellular Studies*

Different studies have reported that quercetin induces expression of HO-1 in macrophages, preventing H_2O_2-induced apoptosis (Chow et al., 2005) and in mouse fibroblasts and normal human lung fibroblasts suppressing TGF-β-induced collagen production (Nakamura et al., 2011). Quercetin was also reported to inhibit the liberation of inflammatory cytokines such as TNF-α, IL8 and IL6 in macrophages (Manjeet and Ghosh, 1999) and alveolar epithelial cells (Geraets et al., 2007; Gauliard et al., 2008).

Furthermore, several investigations have demonstrated that quercetin has antifibrotic properties and inhibit skin, liver, or kidney fibrosis (Lee et al., 2003; Phan et al., 2003; Ren et al., 2016). In lung cells, quercetin has been reported to inhibit proliferation and expression of TBFβ1 in human embryonic lung fibroblasts activated by silicotic alveolar macrophages (Peng et al., 2013). Quercetin also suppresses bleomycin-induced EMT and intracellular level of ROS in alveolar type II-like cells (Takano et al., 2020). It has also been that this flavonoid ameliorates pulmonary fibrosis in TGF-β-treated human embryonic lung fibroblast (Zhang et al., 2018c).

Finally, quercetin along with dasatinib have been proved to be a powerful senolytic cocktail. Studies *in vitro* and *ex vivo* using primary fibrotic mouse alveolar epithelial type II and primary human fibroblasts demonstrated that treatment with this senolytic combination attenuates fibrotic mediator expression, such as senescence-associated secretory phenotype factor and extracellular matrix markers (Lehmann et al., 2017; Schafer et al., 2017).

In vivo *Animal Studies*

Several studies have highlighted the protective effect of quercetin in various pulmonary fibrosis models, exercising anti-inflammatory and antifibrotic effects. In 2008, a study demonstrated that quercetin, although not influencing collagen deposition, attenuates the pulmonary oxidative stress and inflammatory in bleomycin-induced lung fibrosis hamster model (Martinez et al., 2008). Liposomal quercetin was demonstrated to attenuate bleomycin-induced pulmonary fibrosis *in vivo* by the suppression of inflammatory cytokines (TNF-α, IL-1β, and IL-6) and the diminish of total cells and macrophage counts in BALF. Moreover, treatment with liposomal quercetin produced a significant reduction of hydroxyproline content and apparently lessened areas of lung fibrosis and collagen deposition (Baowen et al., 2010). Furthermore, quercetin treatment was shown to reduce the expression of collagen, fibronectin, and MMP-7, decrease the level of inflammatory cytokines such as TNF-α and enhance Nrf2-induced pulmonary antioxidant defences (Verma et al., 2013; Boots et al., 2020). Thus, this demonstrates quercetin exerts anti-fibrogenic and anti-inflammatory effects, possibly *via* modulation of the redox balance by inducing Nrf2.

The effect of quercetin was also studied on pulmonary fibrosis induced by silica particles in rat models. Quercetin was demonstrated to reduce hydroxyproline content, and increase catalase and GPx activity (Liu et al., 2014a). Quercetin and dihydroquercetin also showed a protective effect against inflammatory processes associated with pulmonary fibrosis in bleomycin mice models. It was reported inhibition of oedema formation and body weight loss, as well as amelioration of polymorphonuclear infiltration into the lung tissue and reduction of the number of inflammatory cells in BALF. Moreover, these polyphenols suppressed iNOS, preventing oxidative and nitrosative lung injury (Impellizzeri et al., 2015). Moreover, these polyphenols suppressed iNOS, preventing oxidative and nitrosative lung injury (Impellizzeri et al., 2015).

The effects of quercetin have also been studied in combination with other compounds. Schafer et al. (2017) demonstrated that the combination of quercetin with dasatinib, the senolytic cocktail, attenuates bleomycin-mediated lung injury in mice. Quercetin has also been combined with gallic acid, another potent natural antioxidant, to investigate their protective effect against bleomycin-induced pulmonary fibrosis in rats. The combination treatment demonstrated a remarkable decrease in lung hydroxyproline and TNF-α level and an increase in catalase activity. The combination treatment also significantly enhanced lung SOD activity and GSH level and decreased NO and IL-6 levels (Mehrzadi et al., 2020).

Human Clinical Trials

As mentioned in the previous paragraphs, quercetin is able to reduce oxidative stress and fibrotic processes such as EMT in different IPF effector cells. In addition, several *in vivo* studies have reported that quercetin has antifibrotic and anti-inflammatory effects through modulation of the redox balance probably by activation of Nrf2, among others. However, there are no human clinical trials testing quercetin treatment in IPF patients. On the other hand, the beneficial effect of quercetin supplementation on markers of oxidative stress and inflammation in other interstitial lung diseases, such as sarcoidosis, has been studied in different clinical trials (Boots et al., 2009; Boots et al., 2011) (ClinicalTrials.gov Identifier: NCT00402623 and NCT00512967).

Nevertheless, since *in vitro* and *in vivo* studies have demonstrated that the senolytic cocktail of quercetin and dasitinib is effective in IPF models, between 2016 and 2018, it was performed the first-in-human, small scale, pilot clinical trial to assess the feasibility, acceptability, best methods, and measurement characteristics of potential study outcomes for the senolytic drug combination dasatinib and quercetin in stable IPF patients. It was titled "Targeting Pro-Inflammatory Cells in Idiopathic Pulmonary Fibrosis: a Human Trial (IPF)" The primary endpoints were retention rates and completion rates for planned clinical assessments. Secondary endpoints were safety and change in functional and reported health measures. This first-in-humans open-label pilot study provided initial evidence that senolytics may improve the 6-min walk distance in IPF (Justice et al., 2019) (ClinicalTrials.gov identifier: NCT02874989) Summarized in **Table 4**.

Salvianolic Acid B

Salvianolic acid B (Sal B) is one most active phenolic acids extracted from *Salvia miltiorrhiza*, Danshen. It shows strong antioxidant, anti-inflammatory, antifibrotic, and anti-apoptotic capacities (Cao et al., 2012). It can exert its antioxidant effects by directly scavenging ROS or by increasing the expression of different antioxidant enzymes such as SOD, GPx, and HO-1 or inhibiting the expression of Nox2 and Nox4; being the regulation of the Nrf2 pathway the core target of these antioxidant mechanisms (Xiao et al., 2020) (**Figure 2**).

In vitro *Cellular Studies*

Sal B was found to inhibit TGF-β1-induced cell proliferation, differentiation, expression collagen type I, endogenous TGF-β1 production, and α-SMA expression in lung fibroblasts (Jiang et al., 2009; Zhang et al., 2011; Zhang et al., 2014b; Liu et al., 2016c), as well as EMT of alveolar epithelial cells (Liu et al., 2016c). A recent study has demonstrated that Sal B exerts an anti-inflammatory role by protecting endothelial cells from oxidative stress injury (Liu et al., 2018b). A further study has also demonstrated that Sal B inhibits LPS-induced inflammation *in vitro*, by down-regulating the protein expression of pro-inflammatory cytokine such as IL-1β and TNF- α (Jiang et al., 2020). Sal B treatment was also reported to reduce ROS production and inhibit myofibroblast transdifferentiation *via* the up-regulation of the Nrf2 pathway in human lung fibroblasts (Liu et al., 2018a).

In vivo *Animal Studies*

Results from various bleomycin-induced pulmonary fibrosis *in vivo* studies showed that Sal B treatment ameliorates lung fibrosis, inhibits inflammatory cell infiltration and diminishes inflammatory cytokine production. It also reduces collagen accumulation and α-SMA expression, increases the expression of Nrf2 and protects endothelial cells against oxidative stress injury and inhibits endothelial cell apoptosis (Liu et al., 2015; Liu et al., 2016c; Liu et al., 2018b; Zhang et al., 2021). Sal B was also reported to protect against paraquat-induced pulmonary fibrosis by mediating Nrf2/Nox4 redox balance, as increased Nrf2 expression and reduced Nox4 one, and TGF-β1/Smad3 signalling (Liu et al., 2016a).

Human Clinical Trials

As we have reviewed above, Sal B has been reported to reduce different fibrotic processes such as proliferation, TGF-β1 expression, EMT or myofibroblast transdifferentiation in *in vitro* models of fibrosis. *In vivo* studies have also demonstrated that Sal B protects from fibrosis and inflammation in bleomycin and paraquat models probably by upregulating Nrf2. As it is usual in this kind of compound, there is no clinical trial testing the effects of Sal B on its own.

Nevertheless, in 2017 it was started an open label clinical trial of Chinese herbal medicine for IPF ("The Effectiveness of an Empirical Chinese Medicine Formulation for Idiopathic Pulmonary Fibrosis: an Open Label Clinical Trial"), whose aim was to determine whether treatment with the herbal formula PROLUNG could improve IPF symptoms, respiratory function and the quality of life compared with pretreatment baseline. The primary outcome was the annual rate of change in FVC. The PROLUNG formula contained, among others, Radix *Salviae Miltiorrhizae,* the main bioactive compound of which is Sal B. Unfortunately, the trial was terminated in 2021 due to difficulties recruiting eligible patients (ClinicalTrials.gov Identifier: NCT03274544) Summarized in **Table 4**.

Epigallocatechin Gallate

Epigallocatechin gallate (EGCG) is a polyphenol, the ester from epigallocatechin and gallic acid, and the major biological component of green tea, even though it can be also found in some other vegetables such as onions, hazelnuts and plums (Tsai et al., 2019). EGCG has a potent radical scavenging activity towards both superoxide and hydroxyl radicals, as well as, peroxyl radicals, nitric oxide, carbon-centered ROS and lipid oxidation products (Salah et al., 1995; Nanjo et al., 1999; Zhang et al., 2007a). Several studies have shown that EGCG acts not only as an antioxidant but also as an antiapoptotic, anti-inflammatory and antifibrotic agent (Nagai et al., 2002a; Sriram et al., 2009b; Oz, 2017; Minnelli et al., 2018). Another study suggests that EGCG can act as an antioxidant directly but also indirectly by increasing the activity of other antioxidants or enzymes (Negishi et al., 2004; Zhang et al., 2007a). This catechin may also participate in the regulation of mitochondrial metabolism (Shi et al., 2018b) (**Figure 3**).

In vitro *Cellular Studies*

The protective role of EGCG was investigated *in vitro* inducing fibroblast cell lines with TGF-β1. Simultaneous treatment with EGCG inhibited the increased fibroblast proliferation, reduced hydroxyproline levels and decreased expression of MMP-2 and -9, *p*-Smad, α-SMA and type I collagen. Thus, EGCG inhibited fibroblast activation and collagen accumulation by inhibiting TGF-β1 signalling (Sriram et al., 2015). Another experimental study explored the effect of EGCG on gene expression in pulmonary fibroblasts from IPF patients. The gene expression changes observed were mainly involved in the biosynthesis and metabolism of cholesterol, suggesting that EGCG may exercise its effects through regulation of the cholesterol-associated genes (Tsai et al., 2019).

Despite there are not many *in vitro* studies that explore the therapeutic potential of EGCG in pulmonary fibrosis, there are several that investigate its effects in inflammatory processes. For instance, EGCG is shown to inhibit neutrophil elastase and elastase-mediated activation of MMP-9 (Sartor et al., 2002). Another *in vitro* study has also revealed that EGCG suppresses ROS activity and inhibits apoptosis and chemokine-induced chemotaxis in activated neutrophils (Donà et al., 2003). In addition, EGCG is demonstrated to reduce neutrophil transmigration through monolayers of endothelial cells (Hofbauer et al., 1999).

In vivo *Animal Studies*

In 2003, Donà et al. (2003) demonstrated that both oral EGCG and green tea extract block neutrophil recruitment and neutrophil-mediated angiogenesis *in vivo* in an inflammatory angiogenesis mouse model induced by macrophage inflammatory protein-2 and LPS. They also showed that oral administration of green tea extract reduced inflammatory cell infiltration and the patchy fibrosis in pulmonary fibrosis and inflammation mouse model induced by intratracheal instillation of fluorescein isothiocyanate (FITC) (Donà et al., 2003).

Further studies demonstrated that EGCG administration alleviates the oxidative stress generated during bleomycin-induced pulmonary fibrosis in rat models. Furthermore, administration of this compound improved body weight and enzymic and non-enzymic antioxidants. It also decreased levels of ROS, lipid peroxidation, hydroxyproline, and the activity of myeloperoxidase. On the other hand, it increased cell counts. EGCG treatment also decreased the increased expression of nuclear factor-kB, TNF-α, IL-1b, MMP-2, and 9, TGF-β1, Smads, and α-SMA; restored the activities of antioxidant enzymes such as GST and NQO1; and induced Nrf2 (Sriram et al., 2008; Sriram et al., 2009a; Sriram et al., 2015).

A study from 2014 showed that EGCG treatment provides antioxidant, anti-inflammatory, and anti-proliferative effects that protect against irradiation-induced pulmonary fibrosis in rats. Treatment with EGCG reduced mortality rates and lung index scores; improved histological changes in the lung; reduced collagen depositions and MDA content; enhanced SOD

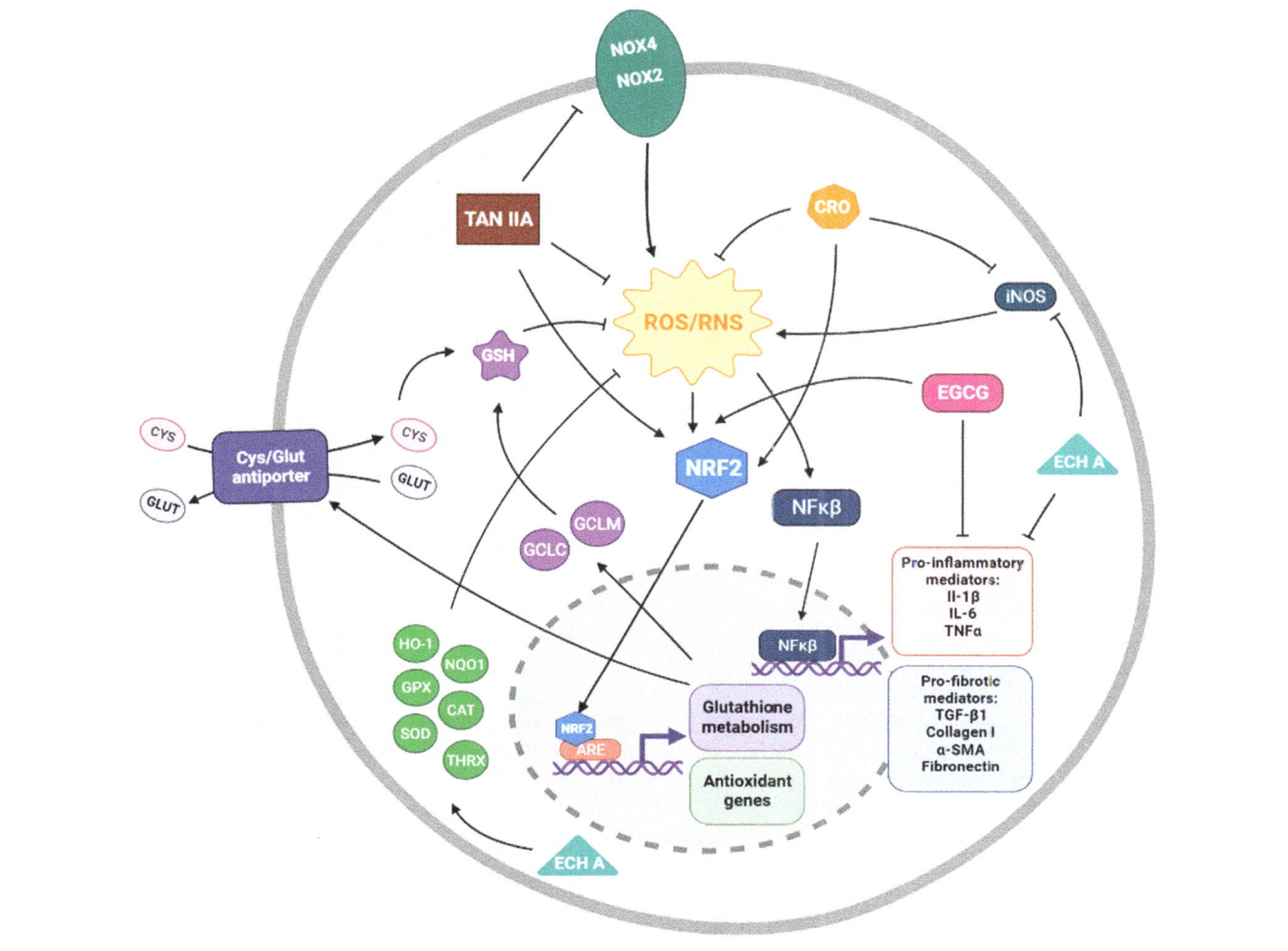

FIGURE 3 | Simplified diagram of the principal molecular mechanisms of the antioxidant enhancers Epigallocatechin (EGCG), Tanshinone IIA (TAN IIA), Crocin (CRO) and Echinochrome A (ECH A). αSMA: alpha smooth muscle actin; ARE: antioxidant responsive element; CAT: catalase; CYS: cysteine; GCLC: glutamate cysteine ligase catalytic subunit; GCLM: glutamate cysteine ligase modifier subunit; GLUT: glutamate; GPX: glutathione peroxidase; GSH: glutathione; HO-1: heme oxygenase 1; IL-1β: interleuquina 1beta; IL-6: interleuquina 6; iNOS: inducible nitrogen oxide synthase; NFκβ: nuclear factor kappa beta; NOX1,2,4: NADPH oxidases; NQO1: NAD(P)H:quinone oxidoreductase 1; NRF2: nuclear factor erythroid 2-related factor 2; ROS/RNS: reactive oxygen species/reactive nitrogen species; TGF-β1: transforming growth factor beta 1; TNFα: tumoral necrosis factor alpha; SIRT: sirtuine 1; SOD: supeoxide dismutase Created with Biorender.com.

activity; inhibited (myo) fibroblast proliferation; protected alveolar epithelial type II (AE2) cells; and regulated serum levels of TGF-β1, IL-6, IL-10, and TNF-α. Treatment with EGCG also activated Nrf2 and its downstream antioxidant enzymes HO-1 and NQO-1 (You et al., 2014).

Human Clinical Trials

It has been demonstrated, as we have reviewed above, in *in vitro* studies that treatment with EGCG inhibits fibroblast proliferation, among others fibrotic processes, and, mainly, inflammatory processes. In several *in vivo* assays, it has been reported that EGCG provides antioxidant, anti-inflammatory and antifibrotic protection in different IPF models mainly via activation of the Nrf2 pathway.

Based on of these preclinical studies, in 2018, started an open label trial to test the effects of oral EGCG treatment on lung tissues and serum samples obtained from 20 patients with IPF and it is titled "Fibroblast Specific Inhibition of LOXL2 and TGFbeta1 Signaling in Patients With Pulmonary Fibrosis." Half of the patients were given orally EGCG before they underwent biopsy, and the other half did not receive the treatment. EGCG treatment reversed profibrotic biomarkers in their diagnostic biopsies: type I collagen, snail family transcriptional repressor and phosphorylated SMAD3 levels were significantly lower in treated patients. This study is in an early phase; therefore, future results are expected in coming years (Chapman et al., 2020) (ClinicalTrials.gov Identifier: NCT03928847) Summarized in **Table 4**.

The same authors that conducted the open label study extended these findings to advanced pulmonary fibrosis using cultured precision-cut lung slices from explants of IPF patients undergoing transplantation. They discovered EGCG attenuate

TGF-β1 signalling and new collagen accumulation and activated MMP-dependent collagen I turnover (Wei et al., 2021).

Tanshinone IIA and Sodium Tanshinone IIA Sulfonate

Tanshinone IIA (TanIIA) is an active compound in *Salvia miltiorrhizae* Bunge, also known as Danshen, with numerous pharmacological activities, including antioxidant, anti-inflammatory, anticancer, and cardio-cerebrovascular protection activities (Cai et al., 2016). Due to the strong liposubility of TIIA, some researchers use its water-soluble derivative form, Sodium tanshinone IIA sulfonate (STS), which is reported to have superior bio-availability and similar pharmacological activity to TanIIA (Chen et al., 2016; Chen et al., 2017). It has also been reported that TanIIa exerts its cytoprotective effect through inhibition of ROS via activation of the Nrf2 pathway (Zhang and Wang, 2007) (**Figure 3**).

In vitro *Cellular Studies*

TanIIA was reported to suppress TGF-β1-induced EMT and collagen I production in lung alveolar epithelial cells (Tang et al., 2015). Another study demonstrated in mouse embryonic fibroblasts that TanIIA inhibits myofibroblast activation through restoring redox homeostasis by activating Nrf2 and suppressing Nox4. Additionally, it was demonstrated TanIIA may activate Nrf2/GSH signalling to restrain myofibroblast proliferation by limiting glutamate availability to support cell growth (An et al., 2019). A more recent study has demonstrated that TanIIA inhibits silica-induced EMT and reduces oxidative stress *via* activation of the Nrf2 pathway in human alveolar epithelial cells and human bronchial epithelial cells (Feng et al., 2020b).

Similarly, STS was reported to ameliorate silica-induced cell proliferation and oxidative stress *via* activation of the Nrf2 and thioredoxin system in a coculture model of macrophages and pulmonary fibroblasts (Zhu et al., 2016). More recently, *in vitro* studies with pulmonary fibroblasts have reported that STS inhibits inflammation *via* downregulation of IL-1β and TNF-α. Additionally, STS was reported to inhibit TGF-β1-induced proliferation and α-SMA and collagen I overexpression in pulmonary fibroblasts (Jiang et al., 2020).

In vivo *Animal Studies*

Wu et al. (2014) showed that TanIIA treatment attenuates bleomycin-induced pulmonary fibrosis and inflammation and decreases expression of TGF-β1 *via* modulating angiotensin-converting enzyme 2/angiotensin-(1–7) axis in rats. Later, other studies demonstrated that TanIIA mitigates bleomycin-induced pulmonary fibrosis, myofibroblast activation, collagen deposition, inflammatory cell infiltration and pro-inflammatory cytokine release in murine models (He et al., 2015; Tang et al., 2015; An et al., 2019). Additionally, it was also reported that TanIIA treatment reduces oxidative stress biomarker MDA levels and inhibits COX-2-associated oxidative reaction and iNOS-derived NO production (He et al., 2015). Furthermore, several studies have demonstrated that TanIIA attenuates silica-induced pulmonary fibrosis in rats via TGF-β1/Smad signalling suppression, Nox4 inhibition and Nrf2/ARE signalling activation. They also reported an Nrf2-mediated inhibition of EMT and a decrease in oxidative stress biomarkers (Feng et al., 2019; Feng et al., 2020a; Feng et al., 2020b).

In 1994, Wang, He and Zhang studied the effects of STS treatment against bleomycin-induced pulmonary fibrosis in rats. They revealed STS decreases levels of lipid peroxides and hydroxyproline, ameliorating fibrosis (Wang et al., 1994). More recent studies have demonstrated that STS reduces ROS and MDA production and collagen deposition, thereby attenuating silica-induced pulmonary fibrosis in rats, *via* activation of the Nrf2 and thioredoxin system (Zhu et al., 2016; Zhu et al., 2020).

Human Clinical Trials

Despite the promising preclinical results that have demonstrated TanIIA activates the Nrf2 pathway and ameliorates different fibrotic processes in IPF models, there are no clinical trials on TanIIA. On the other hand, there are some clinical trials on STS regarding various diseases but none regarding pulmonary fibrosis.

Resveratrol

Resveratrol (3,5,4-trihydroxystilbene) is a nonflavonoid polyphenolic compound found in multiple plant species, including grapes and peanuts. Resveratrol has been reported to exert a vast number of health benefits, such as antioxidant, anti-inflammatory, antifibrotic, antiviral, and anticancer activities, through many different mechanisms of action (Tomé-Carneiro et al., 2013; Ma and Li, 2020). Several studies have highlighted the therapeutic effects of resveratrol against lung diseases mainly by decreasing oxidant stress and inhibiting inflammatory responses (Conte et al., 2015; Ma and Li, 2020). One of the protective mechanisms of resveratrol par excellence is the activation of the Nrf2 pathway and, therefore, the induction of the expression of several antioxidants enzymes and the regulation of GSH homeostasis (Zhu et al., 2017) (**Figure 4**).

In vitro *Cellular Studies*

Resveratrol was demonstrated to inhibit both fibroblast proliferation and differentiation into myofibroblast. In addition, different results demonstrated that resveratrol represses TGF-β1-induced collagen production, lung fibroblast proliferation (both normal and IPF lung fibroblasts) and attenuates α-SMA expression (Fagone et al., 2011). He et al. (2012) demonstrated that resveratrol suppresses oxidative stress and fibrogenic responses induced by paraquat (a fibrosis inducer herbicide) through activation of the Nrf2 pathway and, thus, inducing cytoprotective genes, such as HO-1 and NQO1. A posterior study showed resveratrol was able to repress and reverse myofibroblasts TGF-β- and/or CXCL12-mediated transformation (Mehrzadi et al., 2020). Resveratrol was also reported to inhibit the liberation of inflammatory cytokines such as IL-8 and IL-6 in lung epithelial cells (Gauliard et al., 2008).

In vivo *Animal Studies*

Resveratrol has been shown to produce antifibrotic effects in murine models of various diseases such as renal, cardiac, and

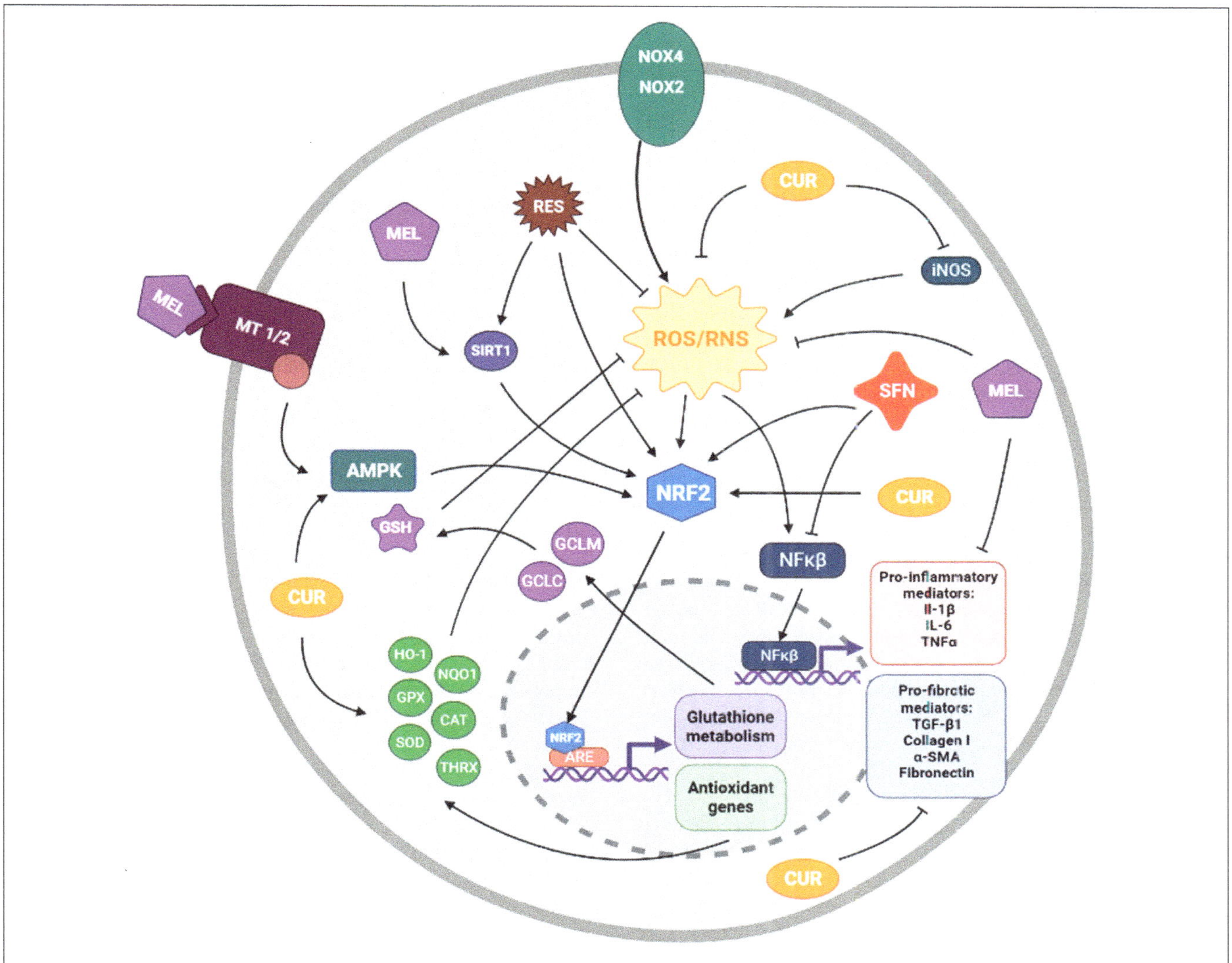

FIGURE 4 | Simplified diagram of the principal molecular mechanisms of the antioxidant enhancers Resveratrol (RES), Sulforaphane (SFN), Melatonin (MEL) and Curcumin (CUR). αSMA: alpha smooth muscle actin; AMPK: AMP-activated protein kinase; ARE: antioxidant responsive element CAT: catalase; CYS: cysteine; GCLC: glutamate cysteine ligase catalytic subunit; GCLM: glutamate cysteine ligase modifier subunit; GLUT: glutamate; GPX: glutathione peroxidase; GSH: glutathione; HO-1: heme oxygenase 1; IL-1β: interleuquina 1beta; IL-6: interleuquina 6; iNOS: inducible nitrogen oxide synthase; NFκβ: nuclear factor kappa beta; NOX1,2,4: NADPH oxidases; NQO1: NAD(P)H:quinone oxidoreductase 1; NRF2: nuclear factor erythroid 2-related factor 2; ROS/RNS: reactive oxygen species/reactive nitrogen species; TGF-β1: transforming growth factor beta 1; TNFα: tumoral necrosis factor alpha; SIRT: sirtuine 1 SOD: supeoxide dismutase Created with Biorender.com.

hepatic fibrosis (Conte et al., 2015). In the context of pulmonary fibrosis, resveratrol was demonstrated to ameliorate oxidative injury and fibrosis induced by bleomycin due to its antioxidant properties (Sener et al., 2007). Similarly, posteriors studies confirmed the promising potential of resveratrol on the treatment of fibrosis in the same bleomycin-induced pulmonary fibrosis rat model (Akgedik et al., 2012; Wang et al., 2018). Further studies demonstrated that treatment with resveratrol ameliorates LPS-induced EMT and pulmonary fibrosis through suppression of oxidative stress and TGF-β1/Smad signalling pathway (Zhang et al., 2015). Additionally, resveratrol has been reported to abolish bleomycin- and particulate matter-induced lung inflammation and fibrosis (Impellizzeri et al., 2015; Ding et al., 2019).

Human Clinical Trials

It has been demonstrated resveratrol is able to inhibit several fibrotic processes through suppression of oxidative stress in *in vitro* and *in vivo* assays, as we have explained above. Nevertheless, it seems the obtained results have not provided sufficient preclinical evidence to consider resveratrol a good candidate for human trials. Indeed, none of the clinical trials on resveratrol registered in https://clinicaltrials.gov regards lung diseases.

Sulforaphane

Sulforaphane (SFN) is an organosulfur compound, mainly found in cruciferous vegetables, with indirect antioxidant activity *via* the Nrf2-mediated induction of phase II detoxifying enzymes (Elbarbry and Elrody, 2011; Kim and Park, 2016) (**Figure 4**).

In vitro *Cellular Studies*

SFN treatment was reported to decrease oxidants and to induce Nrf2 expression, antioxidants, and myofibroblast dedifferentiation in normal and IPF fibroblasts (Artaud-Macari et al., 2013). Various studies in human and rat alveolar epithelial cells have also demonstrated that activation of the Nrf2 antioxidant pathway by SFN protects against ROS production and TGF-β1-induced EMT (Zhou et al., 2016; Zhang et al., 2018d; Qu et al., 2019). SFN has also been proved to attenuate TGF-β1-induced expression of fibrosis-related proteins, such as fibronectin, collagen I, collagen IV, and α-SMA in human alveolar epithelial cells and human fibroblasts (Kyung et al., 2018; Liu et al., 2021).

In vivo *Animal Studies*

Several studies have reported that SFN has antifibrotic and antioxidant activity in various animal models (Elbarbry and Elrody, 2011). SFN treatment of bleomycin-induced pulmonary fibrosis attenuates fibrosis, apoptosis and lung oxidative stress by increasing the expression of antioxidant enzymes, NQO1, HO-1, SOD and catalase, *via* upregulation of Nrf2 gene expression (Yan et al., 2017). Another study reported that SFN decreases bleomycin-induced fibronectin expression, TGF-β1 expression, and the levels of collagen I in bleomycin-induced pulmonary fibrosis mouse model (Kyung et al., 2018).

Human Clinical Trials

As we have mentioned above, several *in vitro* and *in vivo* studies using SFN have reported promising results in pulmonary fibrosis models *via* the activation of Nrf2, which is its main target. Nevertheless, there are no clinical trials on IPF. On the other hand, SFN has been used in several clinical trials to treat a wide variety of diseases such as cancer, neurological disorders, asthma, allergies and Chronic Obstructive Pulmonary Disease (COPD).

Melatonin

Melatonin (N-acetyl-5-methoxytryptamine) is the main secretory product of the pineal gland and, along with its metabolites, is a potent antioxidant with lipophilic and hydrophilic characteristics (Reiter et al., 2016; Hosseinzadeh et al., 2018b). Melatonin can exert its antioxidant effects by either directly scavenging ROS and RNS or by indirectly up-regulating the expression and activities of endogenous antioxidants (Reiter et al., 2016). The antioxidant actions of melatonin are both receptor-dependent and independent (Reiter et al., 2007). In addition to regulating oxidative stress, melatonin modulates a variety of molecular pathways such as circadian biology, inflammation, proliferation, apoptosis and cellular injury (Wang, 2009; Jin et al., 2014; Vriend and Reiter, 2015; Hosseinzadeh et al., 2018a). Several studies have revealed that melatonin is able to induce the expression of GSH and various antioxidant enzymes such as catalase, SOD, and GPx, as well as to activate the Nrf2 signalling pathway (Swiderska-Kołacz et al., 2006; Santofimia-Castaño et al., 2015; Goc et al., 2017) (**Figure 4**).

In vitro *Cellular Studies*

Various studies have reported that melatonin treatment upregulates Nrf2 expression, reduces ROS production and MDA levels, and prevents LPS- or TGF-β1-induced EMT in alveolar epithelial cells (Yu et al., 2016; Ding et al., 2020). Melatonin has also been reported to inhibit the expression of TGF-β1, collagen I and SMAD3 phosphorylation in pulmonary cells exposed to cigarette smoke and LPS (Shin et al., 2017). Different studies have also demonstrated that melatonin suppresses acrolein-induced IL-8 production in human pulmonary fibroblasts (Kim et al., 2012) and inhibits TGF-β1-induced fibrogenesis in mouse lung fibroblasts (Zhao et al., 2018). It also attenuates chromium-induced lung injury by reducing the production of oxidative stress and inflammatory mediators and by inhibiting cell apoptosis *via* activation of the Nrf2 signalling pathway in mouse lung epithelial cells (Han et al., 2019). Additionally, it has been reported that lipid-core nanocapsules of melatonin reduced oxidative DNA damage detected in alveolar epithelial cells treated with paraquat (Charão et al., 2015).

In vivo *Animal Studies*

Several studies have investigated the effects of melatonin on bleomycin-induced pulmonary fibrosis in murine models and have found that melatonin prevents lung fibrosis development by suppressing oxidative stress and protein and lipid peroxidation (Arslan et al., 2002; Genovese et al., 2005; Yildirim et al., 2006; Karimfar et al., 2015; Zhao et al., 2018). Melatonin has also been reported to inhibit endoplasmic reticulum stress and EMT in bleomycin-induced pulmonary fibrosis in mice (Zhao et al., 2014). Furthermore, treatment with melatonin has been shown to attenuate chromium-induced lung injury *via* activating the Nrf2 pathway in rats (Han et al., 2019) and also to reduce leukocyte and macrophage inflammation and fibrosis in carbon tetrachloride-induced oxidative lung damage in rats (Taslidere et al., 2014).

Human Clinical Trials

Despite the several *in vitro* and *in vivo* assays demonstrating that melatonin reduces different processes involved in fibrosis, such as apoptosis or fibrogenesis, there are no clinical trials regarding pulmonary fibrosis.

Curcumin

Curcumin (diferuloylmethane) is a polyphenol compound, contained in the spice turmeric and isolated from the rhizome of the plant Curcuma longa. Curcumin has been found to have a multitude of pharmacological properties such as anticancer, antiviral, antiarthritic, anti-amyloid, antioxidant, and anti-inflammatory properties. The underlying mechanisms of these effects appear to involve the regulation of various molecular targets, including transcription factors, growth factors, inflammatory cytokines, protein kinases and other enzymes. Curcumin exerts its antioxidant activities directly, by scavenging superoxide anion and hydroxyl radicals, and indirectly by, among others, activating the Nrf2 pathway and inducing the expression of different antioxidant enzymes such as

HO-1 (Lee et al., 2010b; Zhou et al., 2011; Lelli et al., 2017) (**Figure 4**).

In vitro *Cellular Studies*

Several studies demonstrated that curcumin inhibits collagen I deposition, expression of α-SMA and vimentin, as well as proliferation and differentiation in TGF-β-induced human and mouse lung fibroblasts or IPF fibroblasts (Smith et al., 2010; Liu et al., 2016b; Chen et al., 2019; Saidi et al., 2019; Chun-Bin et al., 2020). Curcumin has also been reported to protect lung mesenchymal stem cells from H_2O_2 and to block the radiation-induced generation of ROS by upregulating the expression of Nrf2 and HO-1 (Lee et al., 2010b; Ke et al., 2020).

In vivo *Animal Studies*

Numerous *in vivo* experiments have demonstrated the antifibrotic potential of curcumin. Treatment with curcumin has been reported to inhibit the release of inflammatory cytokines, the expression of fibronectin, vimentin and TGF-β1, the hydroxyproline content, the ECM accumulation, the collagen I and IV deposition, the production of TNF-α, superoxide, NO and MDA as well as to raise the expression of SOD and GPX in bleomycin-induced pulmonary fibrosis murine models (Punithavathi et al., 2000; Zhou et al., 2006a; Zhou et al., 2006b; Zhang et al., 2007b; Xu et al., 2007; Chen et al., 2008; Zhao et al., 2008; Smith et al., 2010; Durairaj et al., 2020).

Other pulmonary fibrosis models such as paraquat-, silica particles-, radiation-, aspiration material- and amiodarone-induced models have revealed that curcumin is able to reduce the levels of TGF-β1, TNF-α, IL-6 and collagen type I, and to decrease the generation of ROS, hydroxyproline content, MDA and MPO and iNOS activity, to increase the activity of SOD, GPx and HO-1 (Thresiamma et al., 1998; Punithavathi et al., 2003; Xu et al., 2007; Guzel et al., 2009; Jiang et al., 2009; Lee et al., 2010b; Cho et al., 2013; Li et al., 2015; Barsan et al., 2021).

Human Clinical Trials

Curcumin has been reported to have antioxidant and antifibrotic potentials both *in vitro* and in different animal models, as we have seen before. Furthermore, it has been tested in various clinical trials for the treatment of different lung diseases, especially COPD, but none of the clinical trials regards pulmonary fibrosis.

Pirfenidone

Pirfenidone (PFD, 5-methyl-1-phenyl-2-[1H]-pyridone) is an oral broad-spectrum drug and is one of the two pharmacological treatments recommended for the treatment of IPF. Although no specific mode of action has been identified, PFD possesses antifibrotic, anti-inflammatory, and antioxidant properties (Poletti et al., 2014; Ruwanpura et al., 2020) (**Figure 5**).

In vitro *Cellular Studies*

Regarding its antifibrotic potential, cell culture experiments on human lung fibroblasts and alveolar epithelial cells have revealed that PFD is able to inhibit fibroblast proliferation, myofibroblast differentiation, collagen synthesis, fibronectin production, deposition of ECM components, and α-SMA and HSP47 expression (Nakayama et al., 2008; Conte et al., 2014; Ma et al., 2018; Molina-Molina et al., 2018). Various studies have reported that PFD may inhibit the release of proinflammatory cytokines such as IL-6, IL-8, IL-1β and TNF-α and enhance the release of the anti-inflammatory cytokine IL-10, thereby exerting its anti-inflammatory effect (Nakazato et al., 2002; Oku et al., 2002; Spond et al., 2003; Liu et al., 2017a; Ruwanpura et al., 2020).

Regarding its antioxidant properties, PFD has been reported to reduce ROS production, as it is a scavenger of hydroxyl and superoxide anion free radicals (Giri et al., 1999). It has also been reported to inhibit NADPH-dependent lipid peroxidation in sheep liver microsomes (Misra and Rabideau, 2000). A more recent study has reported that PFD improves Nrf2, HO-1 and GPX1 expression and reduces collagen I and Il-6 levels in TGF-β1-induced mouse lung fibroblasts (Liu et al., 2017b). A further study has revealed that, contrary to sera from IPF naive patients, sera from PFD treated IPF patients failed to significantly induce both ROS generation and collagen synthesis in primary human pulmonary artery smooth muscle cells, demonstrating the antioxidant properties of PFD (Fois et al., 2018). PFD has also been reported to increase the expression of SOD1, catalase and Nrf2, as well as reduce the increased level of ROS in alveolar epithelial cells exposed to cigarette smoke extract (Ma et al., 2021).

In vivo *Animal Studies*

Several studies have demonstrated the antifibrotic and anti-inflammatory effects of PFD in experimental animal models, especially in bleomycin-induced pulmonary fibrosis models. These studies revealed that PFD prevents the accumulation of hydroxyproline, collagen I and III, inflammatory cells and TGF-β1 in BALF, and/or lung tissue (Iyer et al., 1995; Iyer et al., 2000; Tian et al., 2006; Oku et al., 2008; Myllärniemi and Kaarteenaho, 2015).

In the 1990s, studies in hamster models of fibrosis indicated that PFD ameliorates bleomycin-induced lung fibrosis by suppressing oxidative stress mediators, such as MDA and MPO, and enhancing SOD activity (Iyer et al., 1995; Iyer et al., 1999). PFD has also been reported to attenuate bleomycin-induced pulmonary fibrosis in mice by improving the expression of Nrf2, HO-1 and GPx1 and reducing levels of ROS and MDA in serum, BALF and lung tissues (Liu et al., 2017b). In 2018, a study investigated the effect of PFD in paraquat-induced lung injury and fibrosis in mice and demonstrated that PFD ameliorates lung injury and fibrosis through inhibition of inflammation and oxidative stress, downregulation of profibrotic cytokines and enzymes for ROS production such as Nox1, Nox4, iNOS and through up-regulation of antioxidant enzymes such as SOD, catalase and GPx1 (Pourgholamhossein et al., 2018).

Human Clinical Trials

The antioxidant and antifibrotic potential of PFD has been extensively demonstrated both *in vitro* and *in vivo* models of IPF, even though we have only highlighted the results regarding its antioxidant potential. The significant number of evidence made PFD a perfect candidate for human clinical trials.

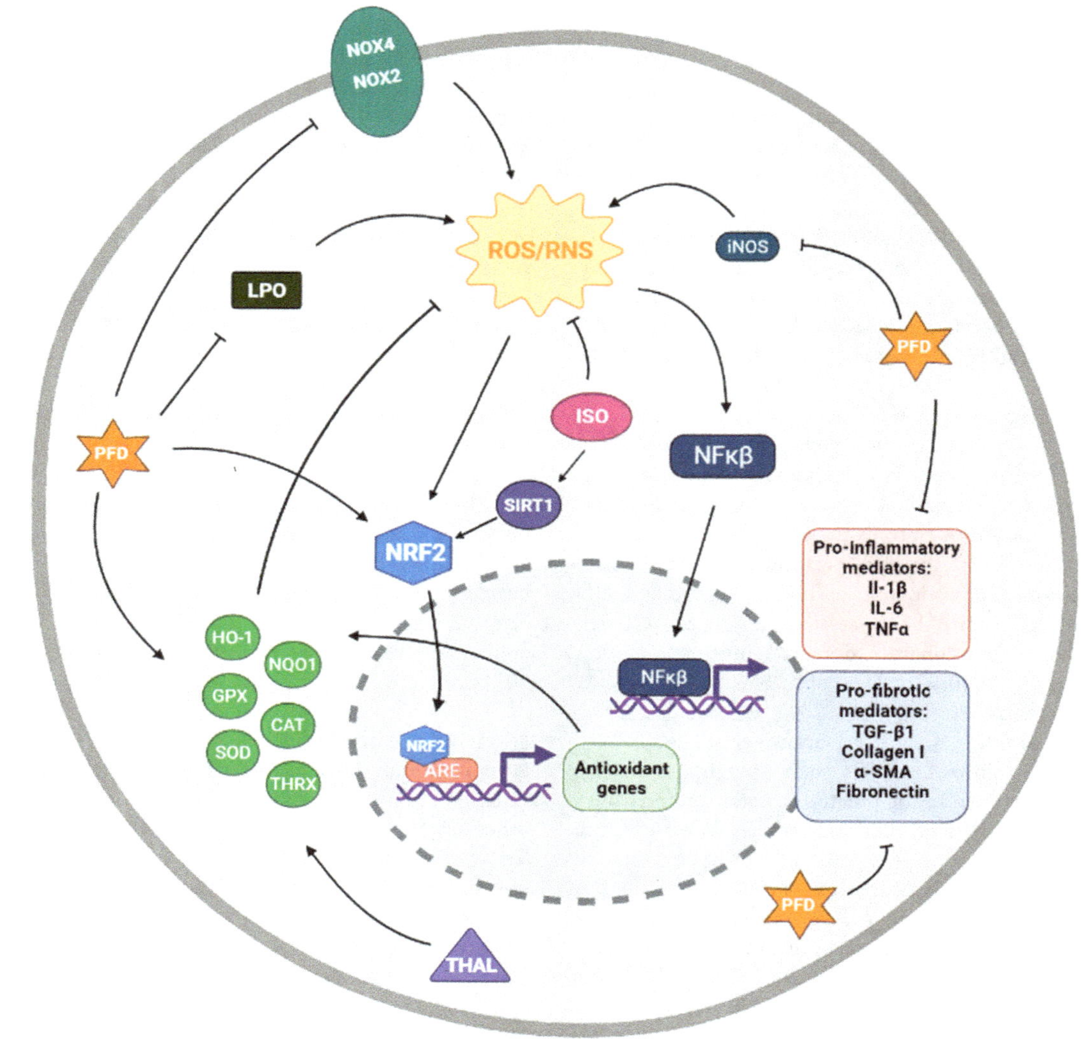

FIGURE 5 | Simplified diagram of the principal molecular mechanisms of the antioxidant enhancers Pirfenidone (PFD), Thalidomide (THAL) and Isorhamnetin (ISO). αSMA: alpha smooth muscle actin; ARE: antioxidant responsive element; CAT: catalase; CYS: cysteine; GLUT: glutamate; GPX: glutathione peroxidase; HO-1: heme oxygenase 1; IL-1β: interleuquina 1beta; IL-6: interleuquina 6; iNOS: inducible nitrogen oxide synthase; LPO: lipoperoxidation; NFκβ: nuclear factor kappa beta; NOX1,2,4: NADPH oxidases; NQO1: NAD(P)H:quinone oxidoreductase 1; NRF2: nuclear factor erythroid 2-related factor 2; ROS/RNS: reactive oxygen species/ reactive nitrogen species; TGF-β1: transforming growth factor beta 1; THRX: thioredoxin; TNFα: tumoral necrosis factor alpha; SIRT: sirtuine 1; SOD: supeoxide dismutase Created with Biorender.com.

Although there are multiple trials to test the efficacy of PFD in humans for IPF treatment, only four phase III clinical studies of PFD in IPF have been completed and reported (Liu et al., 2017a). Two open-label studies described for the first time the promising results of PFD for the treatment of IPF (Raghu et al., 1999; Nagai et al., 2002b). Later, a phase III trial was conducted in Japan and demonstrated that PFD preserves VC, the primary outcome, and improves progression-free survival time, the second outcome in mild IPF patients (Taniguchi et al., 2010).

Between 2006 and 2011 the CAPACITY (Clinical Studies Assessing Pirfenidone in idiopathic pulmonary fibrosis: Research of Efficacy and Safety Outcomes) phase III trial was conducted. This programme included two similar multinational trials (studies 004 and 006). The results of the two integrated trials showed a significant improvement in the lung function, the primary outcome, but also in progression-free survival time, in the change in FVC and in the associated death (Noble et al., 2011) (ClinicalTrials.gov Identifier: NCT00287716 and NCT00287729). Another phase III trial, ASCEND (Assessment of Pirfenidone to Confirm Efficacy and Safety in Idiopathic Pulmonary Fibrosis) study was conducted between 2011 and 2014. This trial confirmed that PFD reduces disease progression, as improved lung function, exercise tolerance, and progression-free survival (King et al., 2014) (ClinicalTrials.gov Identifier: NCT01366209) Summarized in **Table 4**.

Thalidomide

Thalidomide (Thal, α-N-phthalimido glutarimide) is a glutamic acid derivative that was initially prescribed as a sedative and antiemetic drug but it was removed from the market for its teratogenic effects (Franks et al., 2004; Sharma et al., 2007). Thal possesses various pharmacological properties, including anti-inflammatory, antifibrotic and anti-angiogenic (Chong et al., 2006; Mondello et al., 2009; Zhang et al., 2018a). Although the mechanism of action that underlies these properties is still unclear, Thal may exert its biological activities by modulating inflammatory cytokines, growth factors and nitric oxide (Sampaio et al., 1991; Franks et al., 2004; Amirshahrokhi, 2013) (**Figure 5**).

In vitro *Cellular Studies*

Thal was reported to reduce IL-18, IL-8 and TNF-α release from LPS-induced alveolar macrophages (Tavares et al., 1997; Ye et al., 2006). Additionally, several studies have demonstrated that Thal reduces the production of IL-6, TGF-β1, collagen type I and IV, α-SMA, vimentin, MMP-2 and -9, fibronectin and CTGF as well as to inhibit transdifferentiation, EMT and oxidative stress in TGF-β1-induced human and mouse lung fibroblasts (Tabata et al., 2007; Choe et al., 2010; Amirshahrokhi, 2013; Dong et al., 2017; Wu et al., 2020).

In vivo *Animal Studies*

Various investigations have revealed that Thal prevents bleomycin- or paraquat-induced pulmonary fibrosis in murine models by downregulating the expression of IL-6, IL-8, IL-1β, TNF- α, TGF-β, collagen, hydroxyproline, VEGF, *p*-JNK and α-SMA (Tabata et al., 2007; Choe et al., 2010; Amirshahrokhi, 2013; Liu et al., 2014b; Dong et al., 2017). In addition, Thal has been reported to reduce MPO, NO, MDA and ROS and to enhance the activity of SOD and thioredoxin reductase in bleomycin- or paraquat-induced pulmonary fibrosis murine models (Amirshahrokhi, 2013; Dong et al., 2017).

Human Clinical Trials

Thal is currently used in the treatment of multiple myeloma, but its use in other diseases is restricted due to its teratogenic effects (Cavallo et al., 2007). Nevertheless, since various preclinical studies demonstrated IPF is able to reduce different fibrotic processes, in 2005 it was started an open label phase II trial. This clinical trial aimed to determine whether Thal can stop the progression of fibrosis in IPF patients ("Treatment of Idiopathic Pulmonary Fibrosis With Thalidomide"). It was conducted between 2005 and 2010 and the primary outcome was to determine the safety, feasibility and efficacy of Thal. However, there are no results available about this study, probably because these are not promising results (ClinicalTrials.gov Identifier: NCT00162760).

On the other hand, there is a phase III trial testing the efficacy of Thal in suppressing the chronic cough of IPF ("Treatment of Chronic Cough in Idiopathic Pulmonary Fibrosis With Thalidomide"). The primary endpoint was the cough-specific quality of life measured by the Cough Quality of Life Questionnaire (CQLQ) and results showed that Thal improved cough and respiratory quality of life in IPF patients (Horton et al., 2012) (ClinicalTrials.gov Identifier: NCT00600028) Summarized in **Table 4**.

Other Antioxidant Molecules

The antioxidant compounds reviewed above are the most studies ones of a large list of molecules able to enhance the antioxidant defence system against the fibrotic process. However, some antioxidant compounds have promising therapeutic results.

For instance, crocin, a natural antioxidant molecule, remarkably decreases TNF-α, MDA, TGF-β1 and NO levels, up-regulates Nrf2 and HO-1 and attenuates fibrosis in the lungs of bleomycin-exposed rats (Zaghloul et al., 2019; Mehrabani et al., 2020) (**Figure 3**). Another recently studied antioxidant is isorhamnetin, a flavonol aglycone isolated from the traditional Chinese medicine *Hippophae rhamnoides L.* (Shi et al., 2018a). Isorhamnetin has been demonstrated to inhibit bleomycin-induced collagen deposition, reduce type I collagen and α-SMA expression, and alleviate EMT and endoplasmic reticulum stress *in vivo* and *in vitro* (Zheng et al., 2019; Luo et al., 2019), as well as to decrease the expression of inflammatory cytokines (Ren et al., 2021; Chi et al., 2016) (**Figure 5**). Apart from these, another antioxidant molecule is echinochrome A, a quinoid pigment of marine invertebrates that exhibits potent antioxidant properties (Lebedev et al., 2005). It has been reported to have a direct cytoprotective effect under conditions of oxidative stress in pulmonary fibroblasts (Sazonova et al., 2020) and to reduce the severity of bleomycin-induced oxidative stress in the lungs of murine models (Lebed'ko et al., 2015) (**Figure 3**).

These are just a few examples of the studied antioxidant compounds but, indeed, the number of antioxidant components able to decrease fibrotic process through suppression of oxidative stress is countless and growing.

Superoxide Dismutase Mimetics

As we have mentioned above, SOD enzymes play a critical role in the antioxidant defence of the respiratory system. Thus, several of studies have investigated whether SOD enzymes administration can protect against oxidative stress and ameliorate some lung diseases. Treatment with SODs, encapsulated SODs, liposomal SOD preparations, and recombinant manganese superoxide dismutase, MnSOD, resulted to offer antioxidant protection in fibrosis models; however, these compounds developed some immunogenic complications (Kinnula and Crapo, 2003). Thereby, further studies have opted for synthetic small-molecular-weight SOD mimetics. These molecules include salen compounds, macrocyclics and metalloporphyrins and have been found to have antioxidant and anti-inflammatory properties (Salvemini et al., 2002).

AEOL 10150 is a broad-spectrum metalloporphyrin SOD mimic and several studies have shown that this agent protects lung tissues from radiation-induced injury in murine and primate models. It also reduces macrophages accumulation, oxidative stress, and collagen deposition (Rabbani et al., 2007; Garofalo et al., 2014; MacVittie et al., 2017; Zhang et al., 2018b). The metalloporphyrin AEOL 10113 has also been reported to reduce

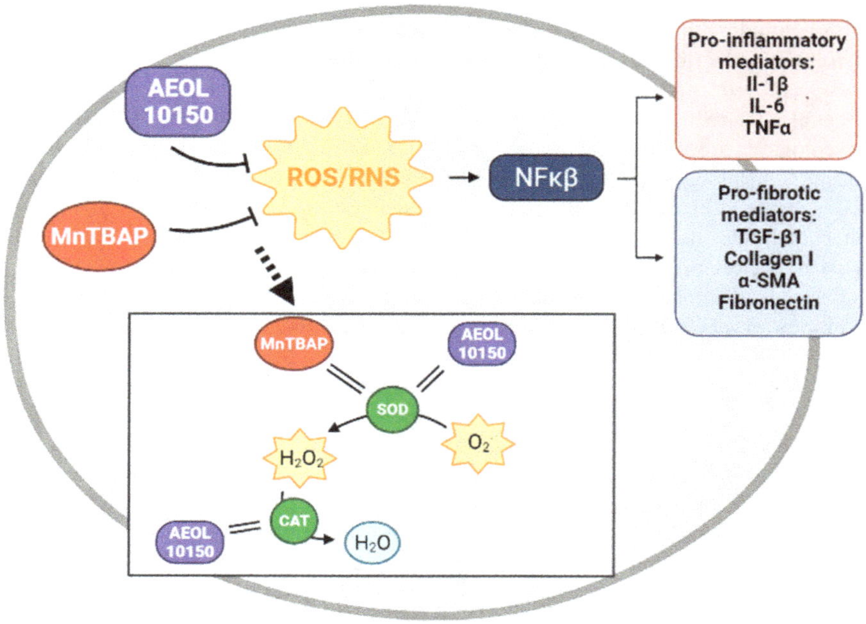

FIGURE 6 | Simplified diagram of the principal molecular mechanisms of the SOD mimetics AEL10150 and MnTBAP. αSMA: alpha smooth muscle actin; CAT: catalase; IL-1β: interleuquina 1beta; IL-6: interleuquina 6; NFκβ: nuclear factor kappa beta; ROS/RNS: reactive oxygen species/reactive nitrogen species; TGF-β1: transforming growth factor beta 1; TNFα: tumoral necrosis factor alpha; SOD: supeoxide dismutase Created with Biorender.com.

TGF-β levels and collagen deposition and to have a protective effect from radiation-induced lung injury (Vujaskovic et al., 2002). MnTBAP is another metalloporphyrin SOD mimic that has been demonstrated to attenuate bleomycin-induced pulmonary fibrosis in *in vitro* and *in vivo* models (Oury et al., 2001; Venkatadri et al., 2017). These compounds have; however, not yet been tested in human lung fibrosis (**Figure 6**).

PITFALLS OF ANTIOXIDANT THERAPIES IN IDIOPATHIC PULMONARY FIBROSIS

In this review, we have classified the antioxidant drugs into three classes: NOX inhibitors, antioxidants enhancers and ROS scavengers, and SOD mimetics. We have described the *in vitro* and *in vivo* results obtained with each drug in the treatment of pulmonary fibrosis. As well as a description of existing clinical trials, if any.

Although all these compounds may seem promising drugs for the treatment of fibrosis, most of them have critical drawbacks, as we will describe below.

Regarding the NOX inhibitors molecules, the classical molecules DPI and Vas2870 have been proven to be useful drugs in preclinical assays to elucidate the role of oxidative stress, specifically NOx molecules, in the development and progression of pulmonary fibrosis and could be helpful in the development of new drugs. However, both compounds have resulted not been suitable options for the treatment of IPF due to their lack of specificity, toxicity, and off-target effects, as they may have unpredictable effects in humans.

In contrast to DPI and Vas2870, the GKTs designed inhibitors are specific for Nox4/Nox1. As we have mentioned, the isoforms Nox1 and Nox4 are implicated in the pathogenesis of IPF. Nox4, in particular, is overexpressed in most of the cells implicated in the pathophysiology of IPF, such as (myo)fibroblasts and epithelial cells, and it contributes to the alteration of different processes such as migration, senescence, differentiation and EMT among others. It is, therefore, logical to think that Nox4 and Nox1 are promising drug targets for IPF. The specificity of these small molecules helps in avoiding off-target effects and in the determination of the effective dose, which is usually lower than in the case of broad-spectrum drugs. Preclinical assays both *in vitro* and *in vivo* have provided excellent results, or so the company has reported. Indeed, the GKT37831 compound has completed a phase I clinical trial with enough good results and a phase II clinical trial is ongoing. Thus, this small molecule is probably the most promising option for the treatment of IPF.

Apocynin had been considered as a NOX inhibitor for a long time; however, it has been recently demonstrated that it is a ROS scavenger. Therefore, like many other natural ROS scavengers, such as flavonoids, it has demonstrated beneficial effects in *in vitro* and *in vivo* models, but there is a lack of evidence for its efficacy in humans. The last NOX inhibitor mentioned in this review is metformin. In this case, *in vitro* and *in vivo* assays have shown that metformin is able to attenuate or reverse lung fibrosis processes; however, retrospective human clinical studies have reported that metformin is ineffective for the treatment of pulmonary fibrosis in diabetics patients with IPF.

Antioxidant enhancers and ROS scavengers are usually more tolerated than NOX inhibitors, but, on the other hand, their efficacy is also lower.

Among all the antioxidant enhancers, NAC is probably one of the most studied for the treatment of pulmonary fibrosis. Its promising results both *in vitro* and *in vivo* suggested that it could be an appropriate option for treating the oxidative stress occurring in IPF. Indeed, it has been reported to be effective in the treatment of other diseases such as Chronic Obstructive Pulmonary Disease (COPD) or bronchitis. However, the successive clinical trials have not reported successful results. On the other hand, the PRECISIONS trial has opened the door to a much more personalised therapy, based on the genetic characteristics of each patient and, probably, it is the key for the treatment of such diseases as IPF, which is characterised by the existence of several phenotypes. Additionally, another recently proposed study aims to test the effectiveness of NAC administered by inhalation. The change in the administration could improve its effectiveness as the drug would act directly in the lungs, where the damage is occurring. However, given all the results, treatment with NAC alone would be very unlikely to be effective in curbing fibrosis.

Many of the antioxidant compounds studied in this review are natural flavonoid or polyphenols compounds such as Quercetin, Sal B, EGCG, TanIIA and STS, resveratrol and curcumin. These compounds have shown a strong antioxidant and, in many cases, anti-inflammatory power in *in vitro* and *in vivo* preclinical fibrotic models however their clinical utility as antifibrotic agents is more than questionable. Natural compounds like these are usually very well tolerated with no toxic effects, but, on the other hand, they are less effective than other chemical derived drugs. Furthermore, they have no specific mode of action: they can have a multitude of targets or be ROS scavengers by themselves. The lower efficacy together with the lack of specificity makes it difficult to establish an effective dose to reach an acceptable clinical efficacy. Therefore, these drugs are more indicated for prevention than for treatment of diseases such as IPF and they could be useful in combination with other antifibrotic drugs.

Despite de several *in vitro* and *in vivo* assays demonstrating the benefit of using these kinds of antioxidants to treat diseases such as IPF, the reality is that the use of antioxidants in clinical trials has shown to be predominately ineffective (Steinhubl, 2008). The lack of benefit in clinical trials could have different explanations. The easiest explanation is that the chosen compound is not adequate for the disease. Another potential explanation may be that although the compound is adequate, it is tested at inappropriate doses or for inadequate durations (Steinhubl, 2008; M Davies and G Holt, 2018). In most cases, antioxidant compounds need unrealistic doses to have a physiological effect, indeed, it has been reported that they would be present at greater than 10^{13} molecules per cell (M Davies and G Holt, 2018). This could be not only because their efficacy is often lower than other drugs, but also because their consumption by ROS is more rapid. Furthermore, it seems illogical to use antioxidant therapies over just a few years to reverse the results of several decades of oxidative stress.

In this review, we also mentioned other three natural compounds, crocin, isorhamnetin and echinocrome A. These three compounds have shown a high antioxidant potential and, since they are natural, are unlikely to generate toxic effects. However, *in vitro* and *in vivo* assays with these compounds are scarce, thus, further evidence of their efficacy in fibrotic processes would be needed before they could be considered for clinical trials.

We consider that some of the antioxidants reviewed here deserve special mention, as is the case of SFN. This compound is a natural derivative, but unlike other drugs of this type, has more specific molecular targets. This is an advantage in establishing a dose that achieves sufficient efficacy in humans. One of its most important targets is Nrf2, a key factor in antioxidant defences and highly implicated in diseases related to oxidative stress, for instance, its expression is decreased in some IPF effector cells. Therefore, SFN, since it activates Nrf2, would be a possible candidate for human clinical trials regarding IPF, although more preclinical *in vitro* and *in vivo* trials may be needed beforehand.

Another drug that we would like to discuss separately is melatonin, as its origin is different from the rest. Melatonin is a hormone that has been shown to have strong antifibrotic effects due to its antioxidant and anti-inflammatory potential. As it is a hormone produced by the body itself, its use as a drug must be well controlled. Thus, concentration and dose (single or chronic) may be carefully studied. Chronic treatment with melatonin may have the opposite of the desired effects, so it may not be a good option for the treatment of fibrosis, since is a chronic disease. Furthermore, melatonin is heavily involved in circadian rhythms and altering its levels in the body can have detrimental effects. On the other hand, its use could be useful at specific times during the treatment of fibrosis.

In this review, we have also mentioned the PFD, one of the antifibrotic drugs par excellence and one of the two currently approved drugs for the treatment of IPF. As we have reviewed here, several *in vitro* and *in vivo* studies have shown that PFD has potent antioxidant effects. However, probably, a large part of these effects is due to its main antifibrotic effect. PFD has several mechanisms of action, many of which are still unknown. Due to the difficulty in determining its specific mechanisms of action, it cannot be said PFD to be a pure antioxidant drug or to have a main antioxidant power.

Another of the drugs already used in clinical practice that we have discussed in this review is Thal. In this case, Thal, in addition to its teratogenicity, which severely limits its use, has been reported ineffective in treating IPF in humans in different clinical trials. Although preclinical studies may suggest that it has anti-fibrotic effects, the reality is that the use of thalidomide for the treatment of IPF is out of the question. Thal is being tested to treat the chronic cough associated with IPF, however, four clinical studies are currently underway investigating P2X3-receptor antagonists as potential antitussives, the results are promising and they are safer than Thal (Dicpinigaitis et al., 2020). Therefore, it would also make no sense to use Thal to treat chronic cough when these antagonists are safer and more effective.

Finally, we have discussed some recently designed SOD mimetics, such as AEOL10150, AEOL 10113 and MnTBAP. These compounds, in contrast to most of the seen above, have a more specific mechanism of action, making it easier to determine the most effective concentration. Furthermore, the use of designed compounds that mimic a biological molecule avoid the complications arising from the use of the biological molecule itself, that, in this case, would be, primarily, the SOD molecule. These compounds, together with the synthetic NOX-inhibitors GKTs, are possibly the ones with the most promising future. However, more research is needed on these compounds before they can be considered suitable for clinical trials.

CONCLUDING REMARKS

Idiopathic pulmonary fibrosis is the major idiopathic interstitial pneumonia with no cause identified and it is characterized by cellular proliferation, interstitial inflammation, and a chronic and progressive fibrosis. It usually does not respond to traditional therapies such as anti-inflammatory and immunomodulatory treatments. Several studies have suggested that increased oxidative stress may play a central role in the development and progression of IPF; indeed, cellular participants in lung fibrosis show, in most cases, an imbalance between oxidants and antioxidants. In addition, the massive number of oxidative stress biomarkers described in patients with IPF have evidenced the involvement of ROS in the pathogenesis of the disease. Regarding this, several ROS scavengers and modulators of the antioxidant machinery have been tested as potential therapeutics for lung fibrosis in preclinical *in vitro* and *in vivo* models and in different clinical trials. In this review, we have highlighted the role of oxidative stress in the pathology of lung fibrosis and its underlying mechanisms. However, the principal aim of this review is to analyze the mechanism of action, the efficacy, and the current status of different drugs able to protect against oxidative stress and act as antifibrotic therapy in IPF. Several more antioxidant molecules can be considered as potential therapeutics for lung diseases but have not been included in this review due to the lack of enough experimental evidence in lung fibrosis; however, they can be consulted in different reviews (Kinnula et al., 2005; Day, 2008; Kato and Hecker, 2020; Wang et al., 2021).

Despite the evidence of the significance of oxidative stress in the progression and development of IPF, as well as the anti-fibrotic effect that many antioxidants have been reported to have, it is unlikely that antioxidant monotherapy will be able to reverse or halt IPF progression, as its efficacy is partial. However, the use of antioxidant drugs may serve to improve some aspects of the disease and may be useful in combination with anti-fibrotic drugs. This situation is not unique to IPF but also occurs with other complex diseases such as cancer (Hayes et al., 2020), where antioxidant drug treatments have been used also mainly for prevention or supplementation (Ozben, 2015; Athreya and Xavier, 2017).

Therefore, antioxidant therapies in IPF should probably be focused on complementing other more efficient antifibrotic therapies.

AUTHOR CONTRIBUTIONS

Conceived and designed revision: CE, JM, MAB, and JC; Analyzed the data: CE, JM, MAB, and JC; Contributed to the writing of the manuscript: CE, JM, MAB, and JC. Revision and final approval of the manuscript: CE, JM, MAB, and JC.

REFERENCES

Akgedik, R., Akgedik, S., Karamanlı, H., Uysal, S., Bozkurt, B., Ozol, D., et al. (2012). Effect of Resveratrol on Treatment of Bleomycin-Induced Pulmonary Fibrosis in Rats. *Inflammation* 35, 1732–1741. doi:10.1007/s10753-012-9491-0

Amara, N., Goven, D., Prost, F., Muloway, R., Crestani, B., and Boczkowski, J. (2010). NOX4/NADPH Oxidase Expression Is Increased in Pulmonary Fibroblasts from Patients with Idiopathic Pulmonary Fibrosis and Mediates TGFbeta1-Induced Fibroblast Differentiation into Myofibroblasts. *Thorax* 65, 733–738. doi:10.1136/thx.2009.113456

Amirshahrokhi, K. (2013). Anti-inflammatory Effect of Thalidomide in Paraquat-Induced Pulmonary Injury in Mice. *Int. Immunopharmacol* 17, 210–215. doi:10.1016/j.intimp.2013.06.005

An, L., Peng, L. Y., Sun, N. Y., Yang, Y. L., Zhang, X. W., Li, B., et al. (2019). Tanshinone IIA Activates Nuclear Factor-Erythroid 2-Related Factor 2 to Restrain Pulmonary Fibrosis via Regulation of Redox Homeostasis and Glutaminolysis. *Antioxid. Redox Signal.* 30, 1831–1848. doi:10.1089/ars.2018.7569

Arsalane, K., Dubois, C. M., Muanza, T., Bégin, R., Boudreau, F., Asselin, C., et al. (1997). Transforming Growth Factor-Beta1 Is a Potent Inhibitor of Glutathione Synthesis in the Lung Epithelial Cell Line A549: Transcriptional Effect on the GSH Rate-Limiting Enzyme Gamma-Glutamylcysteine Synthetase. *Am. J. Respir. Cel Mol Biol* 17, 599–607. doi:10.1165/ajrcmb.17.5.2833

Arslan, S. O., Zerin, M., Vural, H., and Coskun, A. (2002). The Effect of Melatonin on Bleomycin-Induced Pulmonary Fibrosis in Rats. *J. Pineal Res.* 32, 21–25. doi:10.1034/j.1600-079x.2002.10796.x

Artaud-Macari, E., Goven, D., Brayer, S., Hamimi, A., Besnard, V., Marchal-Somme, J., et al. (2013). Nuclear Factor Erythroid 2-related Factor 2 Nuclear Translocation Induces Myofibroblastic Dedifferentiation in Idiopathic Pulmonary Fibrosis. *Antioxid. Redox Signal.* 18, 66–79. doi:10.1089/ars.2011.4240

Athreya, K., and Xavier, M. F. (2017). Antioxidants in the Treatment of Cancer. *Nutr. Cancer* 69, 1099–1104. doi:10.1080/01635581.2017.1362445

Augsburger, F., Filippova, A., Rasti, D., Seredenina, T., Lam, M., Maghzal, G., et al. (2019). Pharmacological Characterization of the Seven Human NOX Isoforms and Their Inhibitors. *Redox Biol.* 26, 101272. doi:10.1016/j.redox.2019.101272

Baowen, Q., Yulin, Z., Xin, W., Wenjing, X., Hao, Z., Zhizhi, C., et al. (2010). A Further Investigation Concerning Correlation between Anti-fibrotic Effect of

Liposomal Quercetin and Inflammatory Cytokines in Pulmonary Fibrosis. *Eur. J. Pharmacol.* 642, 134–139. doi:10.1016/j.ejphar.2010.05.019

Barcellos-Hoff, M. H., and Dix, T. A. (1996). Redox-mediated Activation of Latent Transforming Growth Factor-Beta 1. *Mol. Endocrinol.* 10, 1077–1083. doi:10.1210/mend.10.9.8885242

Bargagli, E., Penza, F., Vagaggini, C., Magi, B., Perari, M. G., and Rottoli, P. (2007). Analysis of Carbonylated Proteins in Bronchoalveolar Lavage of Patients with Diffuse Lung Diseases. *Lung* 185, 139–144. doi:10.1007/s00408-007-9001-6

Barratt, S. L., Creamer, A., Hayton, C., and Chaudhuri, N. (2018). Idiopathic Pulmonary Fibrosis (IPF): An Overview. *J. Clin. Med.* 7, 201. doi:10.3390/jcm7080201

Barsan, M., Rajnoveanu, A. G., Cocarla, A., Bolfa, P., Login, C. C., Socaciu, A. I., et al. (2021). A Study of Oxidative Stress and Pulmonary Damage after Silica Instillation in Rats and the Effect of Curcumin Administration. *Med. Pr* 72, 239–247. doi:10.13075/mp.5893.01050

Beeh, K. M., Beier, J., Haas, I. C., Kornmann, O., Micke, P., and Buhl, R. (2002). Glutathione Deficiency of the Lower Respiratory Tract in Patients with Idiopathic Pulmonary Fibrosis. *Eur. Respir. J.* 19, 1119–1123. doi:10.1183/09031936.02.00262402

Behr, J., Bendstrup, E., Crestani, B., Günther, A., Olschewski, H., Sköld, C. M., et al. (2016). Safety and Tolerability of Acetylcysteine and Pirfenidone Combination Therapy in Idiopathic Pulmonary Fibrosis: a Randomised, Double-Blind, Placebo-Controlled, Phase 2 Trial. *Lancet Respir. Med.* 4, 445–453. doi:10.1016/S2213-2600(16)30044-3

Behr, J., Maier, K., Degenkolb, B., Krombach, F., and Vogelmeier, C. (1997). Antioxidative and Clinical Effects of High-Dose N-Acetylcysteine in Fibrosing Alveolitis. Adjunctive Therapy to Maintenance Immunosuppression. *Am. J. Respir. Crit. Care Med.* 156, 1897–1901. doi:10.1164/ajrccm.156.6.9706065

Bellocq, A., Azoulay, E., Marullo, S., Flahault, A., Fouqueray, B., Philippe, C., et al. (1999). Reactive Oxygen and Nitrogen Intermediates Increase Transforming Growth Factor-Beta1 Release from Human Epithelial Alveolar Cells through Two Different Mechanisms. *Am. J. Respir. Cel Mol Biol* 21, 128–136. doi:10.1165/ajrcmb.21.1.3379

Bergeron, A., Soler, P., Kambouchner, M., Loiseau, P., Milleron, B., Valeyre, D., et al. (2003). Cytokine Profiles in Idiopathic Pulmonary Fibrosis Suggest an Important Role for TGF-Beta and IL-10. *Eur. Respir. J.* 22, 69–76. doi:10.1183/09031936.03.00014703

Bernard, K., Hecker, L., Luckhardt, T. R., Cheng, G., and Thannickal, V. J. (2014). NADPH Oxidases in Lung Health and Disease. *Antioxid. Redox Signal.* 20, 2838–2853. doi:10.1089/ars.2013.5608

Bocchino, M., Agnese, S., Fagone, E., Svegliati, S., Grieco, D., Vancheri, C., et al. (2010). Reactive Oxygen Species Are Required for Maintenance and Differentiation of Primary Lung Fibroblasts in Idiopathic Pulmonary Fibrosis. *PLoS One* 5, e14003. doi:10.1371/journal.pone.0014003

Boots, A. W., Drent, M., de Boer, V. C., Bast, A., Haenen, G. R., and Haenen, Guido. R. M. M. (2011). Quercetin Reduces Markers of Oxidative Stress and Inflammation in Sarcoidosis. *Clin. Nutr.* 30, 506–512. doi:10.1016/j.clnu.2011.01.010

Boots, A. W., Drent, M., Swennen, E. L., Moonen, H. J., Bast, A., and Haenen, G. R. (2009). Antioxidant Status Associated with Inflammation in Sarcoidosis: a Potential Role for Antioxidants. *Respir. Med.* 103, 364–372. doi:10.1016/j.rmed.2008.10.007

Boots, A. W., Veith, C., Albrecht, C., Bartholome, R., Drittij, M. J., Claessen, S. M. H., et al. (2020). The Dietary Antioxidant Quercetin Reduces Hallmarks of Bleomycin-Induced Lung Fibrogenesis in Mice. *BMC Pulm. Med.* 20, 112. doi:10.1186/s12890-020-1142-x

Boots, A. W., Wilms, L. C., Swennen, E. L., Kleinjans, J. C., Bast, A., and Haenen, G. R. (2008). *In Vitro* and *Ex Vivo* Anti-inflammatory Activity of Quercetin in Healthy Volunteers. *Nutrition* 24, 703–710. doi:10.1016/j.nut.2008.03.023

Borok, Z., Buhl, R., Grimes, G. J., Bokser, A. D., Hubbard, R. C., Holroyd, K. J., et al. (1991). Effect of Glutathione Aerosol on Oxidant-Antioxidant Imbalance in Idiopathic Pulmonary Fibrosis. *Lancet* 338, 215–216. doi:10.1016/0140-6736(91)90350-x

Bowler, R. P., Nicks, M., Warnick, K., and Crapo, J. D. (2002). Role of Extracellular Superoxide Dismutase in Bleomycin-Induced Pulmonary Fibrosis. *Am. J. Physiol. Lung Cel Mol Physiol* 282, L719–L726. doi:10.1152/ajplung.00058.2001

Cai, Y., Zhang, W., Chen, Z., Shi, Z., He, C., and Chen, M. (2016). Recent Insights into the Biological Activities and Drug Delivery Systems of Tanshinones. *Int. J. Nanomedicine* 11, 121–130. doi:10.2147/IJN.S84035

Cameli, P., Carleo, A., Bergantini, L., Landi, C., Prasse, A., and Bargagli, E. (2020). Oxidant/Antioxidant Disequilibrium in Idiopathic Pulmonary Fibrosis Pathogenesis. *Inflammation* 43, 1–7. doi 10.1007/s10753-019-01059-1

Cantin, A. M., North, S. L., Fells, G. A., Hubbard, R. C., and Crystal, R. G. (1987). Oxidant-Mediated Epithelial Cell Injury in Idiopathic Pulmonary Fibrosis. *J Clin Invest* 79, 1665–1673. doi:10.1172/JCI113005

Cantin, A. M., Hubbard, R. C., and Crystal, R. G. (1989). Glutathione Deficiency in the Epithelial Lining Fluid of the Lower Respiratory Tract in Idiopathic Pulmonary Fibrosis. *Am. Rev. Respir. Dis.* 139, 370–372. doi:10.1164/ajrccm/139.2.370

Cao, W., Guo, X. W., Zheng, H. Z., Li, D. P., Jia, G. B., and Wang, J. (2012). Current Progress of Research on Pharmacologic Actions of Salvianolic Acid B. *Chin. J. Integr. Med.* 18, 316–320. doi:10.1007/s11655-012-1052-8

Carnesecchi, S., Deffert, C., Donati, Y., Basset, O., Hinz, B., Preynat-Seauve, O., et al. (2011). A Key Role for NOX4 in Epithelial Cell Death during Development of Lung Fibrosis. *Antioxid. Redox Signal.* 15, 607–619. doi:10.1089/ars.2010.3829

Cavallo, F., Boccadoro, M., and Palumbo, A. (2007). Review of Thalidomide in the Treatment of Newly Diagnosed Multiple Myeloma. *Ther. Clin. Risk Manag.* 3, 543–552.

Cazzola, M., Matera, M. G., Rogliani, P., and Calzetta, L. (2018). Senolytic Drugs in Respiratory Medicine: Is it an Appropriate Therapeutic Approach? *Expert Opin. Investig. Drugs* 27, 573–581. doi:10.1080/13543784.2018.1492548

Chapman, H. A., Wei, Y., Montas, G., Leong, D., Golden, J. A., Trinh, B. N., et al. (2020). Reversal of TGFβ1-Driven Profibrotic State in Patients with Pulmonary Fibrosis. *N. Engl. J. Med.* 382, 1068–1070. doi:10.1056/NEJMc1915189

Charão, M. F., Baierle, M., Gauer, B., Goethel, G., Fracasso, R., Paese, K., et al. (2015). Protective Effects of Melatonin-Loaded Lipid-Core Nanocapsules on Paraquat-Induced Cytotoxicity and Genotoxicity in a Pulmonary Cell Line. *Mutat. Res. Genet. Toxicol. Environ. Mutagen* 784-785, 1–9. doi:10.1016/j.mrgentox.2015.04.006

Chen, B., Zhang, D. P., and Gao, W. (2008). Effect of Curcumin on the Expression of Collagen Type I Protein and Transforming Growth Factor-Beta1 mRNA in Pulmonary Fibrosis Rats. *Zhonghua Lao Dong Wei Sheng Zhi Ye Bing Za Zhi* 26, 257–261. doi:10.17179/excli2016-485

Chen, D., Lin, X. X., Huang, W. H., Zhang, W., Tan, Z. R., Peng, J. B., et al. (2016). Sodium Tanshinone IIA Sulfonate and its Interactions with Human CYP450s. *Xenobiotica* 46, 1085–1092. doi:10.3109/00498254.2016.1152417

Chen, P. X., Zhang, Y. L., Xu, J. W., Yu, M. H., Huang, J. H., Zhao, L., et al. (2017). Sodium Tanshinone IIA Sulfonate Stimulated Cl- Secretion in Mouse Trachea. *PLoS One* 12, e0178226. doi:10.1371/journal.pone.0178226

Chen, Y. C., Chen, B. C., Huang, H. M., Lin, S. H., and Lin, C. H. (2019). Activation of PERK in ET-1- and Thrombin-induced Pulmonary Fibroblast Differentiation: Inhibitory Effects of Curcumin. *J. Cel Physiol* 234, 15977–15988. doi:10.1002/jcp.28256

Cheresh, P., Kim, S.-J., Tulasiram, S., and Kamp, D. W. (2013). Oxidative Stress and Pulmonary Fibrosis. *Biochim. Biophys. Acta (Bba) - Mol. Basis Dis.* 1832, 1028–1040. doi:10.1016/j.bbadis.2012.11.021

Chi, G., Zhong, W., Liu, Y., Lu, G., Lü, H., Wang, D., et al. (2016). Isorhamnetin Protects Mice from Lipopolysaccharide-Induced Acute Lung Injury via the Inhibition of Inflammatory Responses. *Inflamm. Res.* 65, 33–41. doi:10.1007/s00011-015-0887-9

Cho, Y. J., Yi, C. O., Jeon, B. T., Jeong, Y. Y, Kang, G. M., Lee, J. E., et al. (2013). Curcumin Attenuates Radiation-Induced Inflammation and Fibrosis in Rat Lungs. *Korean J. Physiol. Pharmacol.* 17, 267–274. doi:10.4196/kjpp.2013.17.4.267

Choe, J. Y., Jung, H. J., Park, K. Y., Kum, Y. S., Song, G. G., Hyun, D. S., et al. (2010). Anti-fibrotic Effect of Thalidomide through Inhibiting TGF-Beta-Induced ERK1/2 Pathways in Bleomycin-Induced Lung Fibrosis in Mice. *Inflamm. Res.* 59, 177–188. doi:10.1007/s00011-009-0084-9

Choi, S. H., Kim, M., Lee, H. J. Kim, E. H., Kim, C. H., and Lee, Y. J. (2016). Effects of NOX1 on Fibroblastic Changes of Endothelial Cells in Radiation-induced P-ulmonary F-ibrosis. *Mol. Med. Rep.* 13, 4135–4142. doi:10.3892/mmr.2016.5090

Chong, L. W., Hsu, Y. C., Chiu, Y. T., Yang, K. C., and Huang, Y. T. (2006). Anti-fibrotic Effects of Thalidomide on Hepatic Stellate Cells and Dimethylnitrosamine-Intoxicated Rats. *J. Biomed. Sci.* 13, 403–418. doi:10.1007/s11373-006-9079-5

Chow, J. M., Shen, S. C., Huan, S. K., Lin, H. Y., and Chen, Y. C. (2005). Quercetin, but Not Rutin and Quercitrin, Prevention of H2O2-Induced Apoptosis via Anti-oxidant Activity and Heme Oxygenase 1 Gene Expression in Macrophages. *Biochem. Pharmacol.* 69, 1839–1851. doi:10.1016/j.bcp.2005.03.017

Chow, S., Thomas, P. S., Malouf, M., and Yates, D. H. (2012). Exhaled Breath Condensate (EBC) Biomarkers in Pulmonary Fibrosis. *J. Breath Res.* 6, 016004. doi:10.1088/1752-7155/6/1/016004

Chun-Bin, S., Yi, Y., Qin-Yi, W., Yang, L., Jing-Ze, Y., Hai-Jing, X., et al. (2020). The Main Active Components of Curcuma Zedoaria Reduces Collagen Deposition in Human Lung Fibroblast via Autophagy. *Mol. Immunol.* 124, 109–116. doi:10.1016/j.molimm.2020.05.017

Conte, E., Fagone, E., Fruciano, M., Gili, E., Iemmolo, M., and Vancheri, C. (2015). Anti-inflammatory and Antifibrotic Effects of Resveratrol in the Lung. *Histol. Histopathol* 30, 523–529. doi:10.14670/HH-30.523

Conte, E., Gili, E., Fagone, E., Fruciano, M., Iemmolo, M., and Vancheri, C. (2014). Effect of Pirfenidone on Proliferation, TGF-β-Induced Myofibroblast Differentiation and Fibrogenic Activity of Primary Human Lung Fibroblasts. *Eur. J. Pharm. Sci.* 58, 13–19. doi:10.1016/j.ejps.2014.02.014

Cortijo, J., Cerdá-Nicolás, M., Serrano, A., Bioque, G., Estrela, J. M., Santangelo, F., et al. (2001). Attenuation by Oral N-Acetylcysteine of Bleomycin-Induced Lung Injury in Rats. *Eur. Respir. J.* 17, 1228–1235. doi:10.1183/09031936.01.00049701

Crapo, J. D. (2003). Oxidative Stress as an Initiator of Cytokine Release and Cell Damage. *Eur. Respir. J. Suppl.* 44, 4s–6s. doi:10.1183/09031936.03.00000203a

Cu, A., Ye, Q., Sarria, R., Nakamura, S., Guzman, J., and Costabel, U. (2009). N-acetylcysteine Inhibits TNF-Alpha, sTNFR, and TGF-Beta1 Release by Alveolar Macrophages in Idiopathic Pulmonary Fibrosis *In Vitro*. *Sarcoidosis Vasc. Diffuse Lung Dis.* 26, 147–154.

Cui, Y., Wang, Y., Li, G., Ma, W., Zhou, X. S., Wang, J., et al. (2018). The Nox1/Nox4 Inhibitor Attenuates Acute Lung Injury Induced by Ischemia-Reperfusion in Mice. *PLoS One* 13, e0209444. doi:10.1371/journal.pone.0209444

Cuzzocrea, S., Mazzon, E., Dugo, L., Serraino, I., Ciccolo, A., Centorrino, T., et al. (2001). Protective Effects of N-Acetylcysteine on Lung Injury and Red Blood Cell Modification Induced by Carrageenan in the Rat. *FASEB J.* 15, 1187–1200. doi:10.1096/fj.00-0526hyp

D'Andrea, G. (2015). Quercetin: A Flavonol with Multifaceted Therapeutic Applications? *Fitoterapia* 106, 256–271. doi:10.1016/j.fitote.2015.09.018

Daniil, Z. D., Papageorgiou, E., Koutsokera, A., Kostikas, K., Kiropoulos, T., Papaioannou, A. I., et al. (2006). Serum Levels of Oxidative Stress as a Marker of Disease Severity in Idiopathic Pulmonary Fibrosis. *Pulm. Pharmacol. Ther.* 21, 26–31. doi:10.1016/j.pupt.2006.10.005

Day, B. J. (2008). Antioxidants as Potential Therapeutics for Lung Fibrosis. *Antioxid. Redox Signaling* 10, 355–370. doi:10.1089/ars.2007.1916

Demedts, M., Behr, J., Buhl, R., Costabel, U., Dekhuijzen, R., Jansen, H. M., et al. (2005). High-dose Acetylcysteine in Idiopathic Pulmonary Fibrosis. *N. Engl. J. Med.* 353, 2229–2242. doi:10.1056/NEJMoa042976

Dicpinigaitis, P. V., McGarvey, L. P., and Canning, B. J. (2020). P2X3-Receptor Antagonists as Potential Antitussives: Summary of Current Clinical Trials in Chronic Cough. *Lung* 198, 609–616. doi:10.1007/s00408-020-00377-8

Ding, S., Wang, H., Wang, M., Bai, L., Yu, P., and Wu, W. (2019). Resveratrol Alleviates Chronic "Real-World" Ambient Particulate Matter-Induced Lung Inflammation and Fibrosis by Inhibiting NLRP3 Inflammasome Activation in Mice. *Ecotoxicol Environ. Saf.* 182, 109425. doi:10.1016/j.ecoenv.2019.109425

Ding, Z., Wu, X., Wang, Y., Ji, S., Zhang, W., Kang, J., et al. (2020). Melatonin Prevents LPS-Induced Epithelial-Mesenchymal Transition in Human Alveolar Epithelial Cells via the GSK-3β/Nrf2 Pathway. *Biomed. Pharmacother.* 132, 110827. doi:10.1016/j.biopha.2020.110827

Donà, M., Dell'Aica, I., Calabrese, F., Benelli, R., Morini, M., Albini, A., et al. (2003). Neutrophil Restraint by green tea: Inhibition of Inflammation, Associated Angiogenesis, and Pulmonary Fibrosis. *J. Immunol.* 170, 4335–4341. doi:10.4049/jimmunol.170.8.4335

Dong, X., Li, X., Li, M., Chen, M., Fan, Q., and Wei, W. (2017). Antiinflammation and Antioxidant Effects of Thalidomide on Pulmonary Fibrosis in Mice and Human Lung Fibroblasts. *Inflammation* 40, 1836–1846. doi:10.1007/s10753-017-0625-2

Durairaj, P., Venkatesan, S., Narayanan, V., and Babu, M. (2020). Protective Effects of Curcumin on Bleomycin-Induced Changes in Lung Glycoproteins. *Mol. Cel Biochem* 469, 159–167. doi:10.1007/s11010-020-03737-3

Elbarbry, F., and Elrody, N. (2011). Potential Health Benefits of Sulforaphane: A Review of the Experimental, Clinical and Epidemiological Evidences and Underlying Mechanisms. *J. Med. Plant Res.* 5, 473.

Fagone, E., Conte, E., Gili, E., Fruciano, M., Pistorio, M. P., Lo Furno, D., et al. (2011). Resveratrol Inhibits Transforming Growth Factor-β-Induced Proliferation and Differentiation of *Ex Vivo* Human Lung Fibroblasts into Myofibroblasts through ERK/Akt Inhibition and PTEN Restoration. *Exp. Lung Res.* 37, 162–174. doi:10.3109/01902148.2010.524722

Felton, V. M., Borok, Z., and Willis, B. C. (2009). N-acetylcysteine Inhibits Alveolar Epithelial-Mesenchymal Transition. *Am. J. Physiol. Lung Cel Mol Physiol* 297, L805–L812. doi:10.1152/ajplung.00009.2009

Feng, F., Cheng, P., Xu, S., Li, N., Wang, H., Zhang, Y., et al. (2020a). Tanshinone IIA Attenuates Silica-Induced Pulmonary Fibrosis via Nrf2-Mediated Inhibition of EMT and TGF-β1/Smad Signaling. *Chem. Biol. Interact* 319, 109024. doi:10.1016/j.cbi.2020.109024

Feng, F., Cheng, P., Zhang, H., Li, N., Qi, Y., Wang, H., et al. (2019). The Protective Role of Tanshinone IIA in Silicosis Rat Model via TGF-β1/Smad Signaling Suppression, NOX4 Inhibition and Nrf2/ARE Signaling Activation. *Drug Des. Devel Ther.* 13, 4275–4290. doi:10.2147/DDDT.S230572

Feng, F., Li, N., Cheng, P., Zhang, H., Wang, H., Wang, Y., et al. (2020b). Tanshinone IIA Attenuates Silica-Induced Pulmonary Fibrosis via Inhibition of TGF-B1-Smad Signaling Pathway. *Biomed. Pharmacother.* 121, 109586. doi:10.1016/j.biopha.2019.109586

Fois, A. G., Posadino, A. M., Giordo, R., Cossu, A., Agouni, A., Rizk, N. M., et al. (2018). Antioxidant Activity Mediates Pirfenidone Antifibrotic Effects in Human Pulmonary Vascular Smooth Muscle Cells Exposed to Sera of Idiopathic Pulmonary Fibrosis Patients. *Oxid Med. Cel Longev* 2018, 2639081. doi:10.1155/2018/2639081

Formica, J. V., and Regelson, W. (1995). Review of the Biology of Quercetin and Related Bioflavonoids. *Food Chem. Toxicol.* 33, 1061–1080. doi:10.1016/0278-6915(95)00077-1

Franks, M. E., Macpherson, G. R., and Figg, W. D. (2004). Thalidomide. *The Lancet* 363, 1802–1811. doi:10.1016/S0140-6736(04)16308-3

Fu, X., Kassim, S. Y., Parks, W. C., and Heinecke, J. W. (2003). Hypochlorous Acid Generated by Myeloperoxidase Modifies Adjacent Tryptophan and glycine Residues in the Catalytic Domain of Matrix Metalloproteinase-7 (Matrilysin): an Oxidative Mechanism for Restraining Proteolytic Activity during Inflammation. *J. Biol. Chem.* 278, 28403–28409. doi:10.1074/jbc.M304739200

Gaggini, F., Laleu, B., Orchard, M., Fioraso-Cartier, L., Cagnon, L., Houngninou-Molango, S., et al. (2011). Design, Synthesis and Biological Activity of Original Pyrazolo-Pyrido-Diazepine, -pyrazine and -oxazine Dione Derivatives as Novel Dual Nox4/Nox1 Inhibitors. *Bioorg. Med. Chem.* 19, 6989–6999. doi:10.1016/j.bmc.2011.10.016

Gao, F., Kinnula, V. L., Myllärniemi, M., and Oury, T. D. (2008). Extracellular Superoxide Dismutase in Pulmonary Fibrosis. *Antioxid. Redox Signaling* 10, 343–354. doi:10.1089/ars.2007.1908

Garofalo, M. C., Ward, A. A., Farese, A. M., Bennett, A., Taylor-Howell, C., Cui, W., et al. (2014). A Pilot Study in Rhesus Macaques to Assess the Treatment Efficacy of a Small Molecular Weight Catalytic Metalloporphyrin Antioxidant (AEOL 10150) in Mitigating Radiation-Induced Lung Damage. *Health Phys.* 106, 73–83. doi:10.1097/HP.0b013e3182a4d967

Gauliard, B., Grieve, D., Wilson, R., Crozier, A., Jenkins, C., Mullen, W. D., et al. (2008). The Effects of Dietary Phenolic Compounds on Cytokine and Antioxidant Production by A549 Cells. *J. Med. Food* 11, 382–384. doi:10.1089/jmf.2007.593

Genovese, T., Di Paola, R., Mazzon, E., Muià, C., Caputi, A. P., and Cuzzocrea, S. (2005). Melatonin Limits Lung Injury in Bleomycin Treated Mice. *J. Pineal Res.* 39, 105–112. doi:10.1111/j.1600-079X.2005.00229.x

Geraets, L., Moonen, H. J., Brauers, K., Wouters, E. F., Bast, A., and Hageman, G. J. (2007). Dietary Flavones and Flavonoles Are Inhibitors of poly(ADP-Ribose)

polymerase-1 in Pulmonary Epithelial Cells. *J. Nutr.* 137, 2190–2195. doi:10.1093/jn/137.10.2190

Giri, S. N., Leonard, S., Shi, X., Margolin, S. B., and Vallyathan, V. (1999). Effects of Pirfenidone on the Generation of Reactive Oxygen Species *In Vitro. J. Environ. Pathol. Toxicol. Oncol.* 18, 169–177.

Goc, Z., Szaroma, W., Kapusta, E., and Dziubek, K. (2017). Protective Effects of Melatonin on the Activity of SOD, CAT, GSH-Px and GSH Content in Organs of Mice after Administration of SNP. *Chin. J. Physiol.* 60, 1–10. doi:10.4077/CJP.2017.BAF435

Green, D. E., Murphy, T. C., Kang, B. Y., Kleinhenz, J. M., Szyndralewiez, C., Page, P., et al. (2012). The Nox4 Inhibitor GKT137831 Attenuates Hypoxia-Induced Pulmonary Vascular Cell Proliferation. *Am. J. Respir. Cel Mol Biol* 47, 718–726. doi:10.1165/rcmb.2011-0418OC

Griffith, B., Pendyala, S., Hecker, L., Lee, P. J., Natarajan, V., and Thannickal, V. J. (2009). NOX Enzymes and Pulmonary Disease. *Antioxid. Redox Signal* 11, 2505–2516. doi:10.1089/ars.2009.2599

Guzel, A., Kanter, M., Aksu, B., Basaran, U. N., Yalçin, O., Guzel, A., et al. (2009). Preventive Effects of Curcumin on Different Aspiration Material-Induced Lung Injury in Rats. *Pediatr. Surg. Int.* 25, 83–92. doi:10.1007/s00383-008-2282-x

Hagiwara, S. I., Ishii, Y., and Kitamura, S. (2000). Aerosolized Administration of N-Acetylcysteine Attenuates Lung Fibrosis Induced by Bleomycin in Mice. *Am. J. Respir. Crit. Care Med.* 162, 225–231. doi:10.1164/ajrccm.162.1.9903129

Han, B., Li, S., Lv, Y., Yang, D., Li, J., Yang, Q., et al. (2019). Dietary Melatonin Attenuates Chromium-Induced Lung Injury via Activating the Sirt1/Pgc-1α/Nrf2 Pathway. *Food Funct.* 10, 5555–5565. doi:10.1039/c9fo01152h

Harijith, A., Natarajan, V., and Fu, P. (2017). The Role of Nicotinamide Adenine Dinucleotide Phosphate Oxidases in Lung Architecture Remodeling. *Antioxidants (Basel)* 6, 104. doi:10.3390/antiox6040104

Hayes, J. D., Dinkova-Kostova, A. T., and Tew, K. D. (2020). Oxidative Stress in Cancer. *Cancer Cell* 38, 167–197. doi:10.1016/j.ccell.2020.06.001

He, C., Larson-Casey, J. L., Davis, D., Hanumanthu, V. S., Longhini, A. L. F., Thannickal, V. J., et al. (2019). NOX4 Modulates Macrophage Phenotype and Mitochondrial Biogenesis in Asbestosis. *JCI Insight* 4, e126551. doi:10.1172/jci.insight.126551

He, H., Tang, H., Gao, L., Wu, Y., Feng, Z., Lin, H., et al. (2015). Tanshinone IIA Attenuates Bleomycin-Induced Pulmonary Fibrosis in Rats. *Mol. Med. Rep.* 11, 4190–4196. doi:10.3892/mmr.2015.3333

He, X., Wang, L., Szklarz, G., Bi, Y., and Ma, Q. (2012). Resveratrol Inhibits Paraquat-Induced Oxidative Stress and Fibrogenic Response by Activating the Nuclear Factor Erythroid 2-related Factor 2 Pathway. *J. Pharmacol. Exp. Ther.* 342, 81–90. doi:10.1124/jpet.112.194142

Hecker, L., Logsdon, N. J., Kurundkar, D., Kurundkar, A., Bernard, K., Hock, T., et al. (2014). Reversal of Persistent Fibrosis in Aging by Targeting Nox4-Nrf2 Redox Imbalance. *Sci. Transl Med.* 6, 231ra47. doi:10.1126/scitranslmed.3008182

Hecker, L., Vittal, R., Jones, T., Jagirdar, R., Luckhardt, T. R., Horowitz, J. C., et al. (2009). NADPH Oxidase-4 Mediates Myofibroblast Activation and Fibrogenic Responses to Lung Injury. *Nat. Med.* 15, 1077–1081. doi:10.1038/nm.2005

Heumüller, S., Wind, S., Barbosa-Sicard, E., Schmidt, H. H., Busse, R., Schröder, K., et al. (2008). Apocynin Is Not an Inhibitor of Vascular NADPH Oxidases but an Antioxidant. *Hypertension* 51, 211–217. doi:10.1161/HYPERTENSIONAHA.107.100214

Hofbauer, R., Frass, M., Gmeiner, B., Handler, S., Speiser, W., and Kapiotis, S. (1999). The green tea Extract Epigallocatechin Gallate Is Able to Reduce Neutrophil Transmigration through Monolayers of Endothelial Cells. *Wien Klin Wochenschr* 111, 278–282.

Horton, M. R., Santopietro, V., Mathew, L., Horton, K. M., Polito, A. J., Liu, M. C., et al. (2012). Thalidomide for the Treatment of Cough in Idiopathic Pulmonary Fibrosis: a Randomized Trial. *Ann. Intern. Med.* 157, 398–406. doi:10.7326/0003-4819-157-6-201209180-00003

Hosseinzadeh, A., Javad-Moosavi, S. A., Reiter, R. J., Hemati, K., Ghaznavi, H., and Mehrzadi, S. (2018a). Idiopathic Pulmonary Fibrosis (IPF) Signaling Pathways and Protective Roles of Melatonin. *Life Sci.* 201, 17–29. doi:10.1016/j.lfs.2018.03.032

Hosseinzadeh, A., Javad-Moosavi, S. A., Reiter, R. J., Yarahmadi, R., Ghaznavi, H., and Mehrzadi, S. (2018b). Oxidative/nitrosative Stress, Autophagy and Apoptosis as Therapeutic Targets of Melatonin in Idiopathic Pulmonary Fibrosis. *Expert Opin. Ther. Targets* 22, 1049–1061. doi:10.1080/14728222.2018.1541318

Hsu, Y. C., Wang, L. F., and Chien, Y. W. (2007). Nitric Oxide in the Pathogenesis of Diffuse Pulmonary Fibrosis. *Free Radic. Biol. Med.* 42, 599–607. doi:10.1016/j.freeradbiomed.2006.11.031

Huetsch, J. C., Suresh, K., and Shimoda, L. A. (2019). Regulation of Smooth Muscle Cell Proliferation by NADPH Oxidases in Pulmonary Hypertension. *Antioxidants (Basel)* 8, 56. doi:10.3390/antiox8030056

Hybertson, B. M., Gao, B., Bose, S. K., and McCord, J. M. (2011). Oxidative Stress in Health and Disease: the Therapeutic Potential of Nrf2 Activation. *Mol. Aspects Med.* 32, 234–246. doi:10.1016/j.mam.2011.10.006

Impellizzeri, D., Talero, E., Siracusa, R., Alcaide, A., Cordaro, M., Maria Zubelia, J., et al. (2015). Protective Effect of Polyphenols in an Inflammatory Process Associated with Experimental Pulmonary Fibrosis in Mice. *Br. J. Nutr.* 114, 853–865. doi:10.1017/S0007114515002597

Iyer, S. N., Gurujeyalakshmi, G., and Giri, S. N. (1999). Effects of Pirfenidone on Transforming Growth Factor-Beta Gene Expression at the Transcriptional Level in Bleomycin Hamster Model of Lung Fibrosis. *J. Pharmacol. Exp. Ther.* 291, 367–373.

Iyer, S. N., Hyde, D. M., and Giri, S. N. (2000). Anti-inflammatory Effect of Pirfenidone in the Bleomycin-Hamster Model of Lung Inflammation. *Inflammation* 24, 477–491. doi:10.1023/a 1007068313370

Iyer, S. N., Wild, J. S., Schiedt, M. J., Hyde, D. M., Margolin, S. B., and Giri, S. N. (1995). Dietary Intake of Pirfenidone Ameliorates Bleomycin-Induced Lung Fibrosis in Hamsters. *J. Lab Clin. Med.* 125, 779–785.

Izumi, S., Iikura, M., and Hirano, S. (2012). Prednisone, Azathioprine, and N-Acetylcysteine for Pulmonary Fibrosis. *N. Engl. J. Med.* 367, 870–871. doi:10.1056/NEJMc1207471

Jack, C. I., Jackson, M. J., Johnston, I. D., and Hind, C. R. (1996). Serum Indicators of Free Radical Activity in Idiopathic Pulmonary Fibrosis. *Am. J. Respir. Crit. Care Med.* 153, 1918–1923. doi:10.1164/ajrccm.153.6.8665056

Jackson, R., Ramos, C., Gupta, C., and Gomez-Marin, O. (2010). Exercise Decreases Plasma Antioxidant Capacity and Increases Urinary Isoprostanes of IPF Patients. *Respir. Med.* 104, 1919–1928. doi:10.1016/j.rmed.2010.07.021

Jain, M., Rivera, S., Monclus, E. A., Synenki, L., Zirk, A., Eisenbart, J., et al. (2013). Mitochondrial Reactive Oxygen Species Regulate Transforming Growth Factor-β Signaling. *J. Biol. Chem.* 288, 770–777. doi:10.1074/jbc.M112.431973

Jardine, H., MacNee, W., Donaldson, K., and Rahman, I. (2002). Molecular Mechanism of Transforming Growth Factor (TGF)-beta1-induced Glutathione Depletion in Alveolar Epithelial Cells. Involvement of AP-1/ARE and Fra-1. *J. Biol. Chem.* 277, 21158–21166. doi:10.1074/jbc.M112145200

Jarman, E. R., Khambata, V. S., Cope, C., Jones, P., Roger, J., Ye, L. Y., et al. (2014). An Inhibitor of NADPH Oxidase-4 Attenuates Established Pulmonary Fibrosis in a Rodent Disease Model. *Am. J. Respir. Cell Mol Biol* 50, 158–169. doi:10.1165/rcmb.2013-0174OC

Ji, L., Liu, R., Zhang, X. D., Chen, H. L., Bai, H., Wang, X., et al. (2010). N-acetylcysteine Attenuates Phosgene-Induced Acute Lung Injury via Up-Regulation of Nrf2 Expression. *Inhal Toxicol.* 22, 535–542. doi:10.3109/08958370903525183

Jiang, J. X., Chen, X., Serizawa, N., Szyndralewiez, C., Page, P., Schröder, K., et al. (2012). Liver Fibrosis and Hepatocyte Apoptosis Are Attenuated by GKT137831, a Novel NOX4/NOX1 Inhibitor *In Vivo. Free Radic. Biol. Med.* 53, 289–296. doi:10.1016/j.freeradbiomed.2012.05.007

Jiang, L., Wang, J., Ju, J., and Dai, J. (2020). Salvianolic Acid B and Sodium Tanshinone II A Sulfonate Prevent Pulmonary Fibrosis through Anti-inflammatory and Anti-fibrotic Process. *Eur. J. Pharmacol.* 883, 173352. doi:10.1016/j.ejphar.2020.173352

Jiang, Z. Y., Zou, L., Shi, S. S., Lu, Y. R., Dong, J., Yang, C. H., et al. (2009). Effects of Curcumin on TNF-Alpha and TGF-Beta1 in Serum and Lung Tissue of SiO2-Induced Fibrosis in Mice. *Xi Bao Yu Fen Zi Mian Yi Xue Za Zhi* 25, 399–401.

Jin, H., Wang, Y., Zhou, L., Liu, L., Zhang, P., Deng, W., et al. (2014). Melatonin Attenuates Hypoxic Pulmonary Hypertension by Inhibiting the Inflammation and the Proliferation of Pulmonary Arterial Smooth Muscle Cells. *J. Pineal Res.* 57, 442–450. doi:10.1111/jpi.12184

Justice, J. N., Nambiar, A. M., Tchkonia, T., LeBrasseur, N. K., Pascual, R., Hashmi, S. K., et al. (2019). Senolytics in Idiopathic Pulmonary Fibrosis: Results from a First-In-Human, Open-Label, Pilot Study. *EBioMedicine* 40, 554–563. doi:10.1016/j.ebiom.2018.12.052

Kang, S. K., Rabbani, Z. N., Folz, R. J., Golson, M. L., Huang, H., Yu, D., et al. (2003). Overexpression of Extracellular Superoxide Dismutase Protects Mice from Radiation-Induced Lung Injury. *Int. J. Radiat. Oncol. Biol. Phys.* 57, 1056–1066. doi:10.1016/s0360-3016(03)01369-5

Karimfar, M. H., Rostami, S., Haghani, K., Bakhtiyari, S., and Noori-Zadeh, A. (2015). Melatonin Alleviates Bleomycin-Induced Pulmonary Fibrosis in Mice. *J. Biol. Regul. Homeost Agents* 29, 327–334.

Kato, K., and Hecker, L. (2020). NADPH Oxidases: Pathophysiology and Therapeutic Potential in Age-Associated Pulmonary Fibrosis. *Redox Biol.* 33, 101541. doi:10.1016/j.redox.2020.101541

Ke, S., Zhang, Y., Lan, Z., Li, S., Zhu, W., and Liu, L. (2020). Curcumin Protects Murine Lung Mesenchymal Stem Cells from H2O2 by Modulating the Akt/Nrf2/HO-1 Pathway. *J. Int. Med. Res.* 48, 300060520910665. doi:10.1177/0300060520910665

Kilic, T., Parlakpinar, H., Taslidere, E., Yildiz, S., Polat, A., Vardi, N., et al. (2015). Protective and Therapeutic Effect of Apocynin on Bleomycin-Induced Lung Fibrosis in Rats. *Inflammation* 38, 1166–1180. doi:10.1007/s10753-014-0081-1

Kim, G. D., Lee, S. E., Kim, T. H., Jin, Y. H., Park, Y. S., and Park, C. S. (2012). Melatonin Suppresses Acrolein-Induced IL-8 Production in Human Pulmonary Fibroblasts. *J. Pineal Res.* 52, 356–364. doi:10.1111/j.1600-079X.2011.00950.x

Kim, J. K., and Park, S. U. (2016). Current Potential Health Benefits of Sulforaphane. *EXCLI J.* 15, 571–577. doi:10.17179/excli2016-485

Kim, S. J., Cheresh, P., Jablonski, R. P., Morales-Nebreda, L., Cheng, Y., Hogan, E., et al. (2016). Mitochondrial Catalase Overexpressed Transgenic Mice Are Protected against Lung Fibrosis in Part via Preventing Alveolar Epithelial Cell Mitochondrial DNA Damage. *Free Radic. Biol. Med.* 101, 482–490. doi:10.1016/j.freeradbiomed.2016.11.007

Kim, S. K., Rho, S. J., Kim, S. H., Kim, S. Y., Song, S. H., Yoo, J. Y., et al. (2019). Protective Effects of Diphenyleneiodonium, an NADPH Oxidase Inhibitor, on Lipopolysaccharide-Induced Acute Lung Injury. *Clin. Exp. Pharmacol. Physiol.* 46, 153–162. doi:10.1111/1440-1681.13050

King, T. E., Bradford, W. Z., Castro-Bernardini, S., Fagan, E. A., Glaspole, I., Glassberg, M. K., et al. (2014). A Phase 3 Trial of Pirfenidone in Patients with Idiopathic Pulmonary Fibrosis. *N. Engl. J. Med.* 370, 2083–2092. doi:10.1056/NEJMoa1402582

Kinnula, V. L., and Crapo, J. D. (2003). Superoxide Dismutases in the Lung and Human Lung Diseases. *Am. J. Respir. Crit. Care Med.* 167, 1600–1619. doi:10.1164/rccm.200212-1479SO

Kinnula, V. L., Fattman, C. L., Tan, R. J., and Oury, T. D. (2005). Oxidative Stress in Pulmonary Fibrosis: a Possible Role for Redox Modulatory Therapy. *Am. J. Respir. Crit. Care Med.* 172, 417–422. doi:10.1164/rccm.200501-017PP

Kinnula, V. L., Hodgson, U. A., Lakari, E. K., Tan, R. J., Sormunen, R. T., Soini, Y. M., et al. (2006). Extracellular Superoxide Dismutase Has a Highly Specific Localization in Idiopathic Pulmonary Fibrosis/usual Interstitial Pneumonia. *Histopathology* 49, 66–74. doi:10.1111/j.1365-2559.2006.02470.x

Kliment, C. R., and Oury, T. D. (2010). Oxidative Stress, Extracellular Matrix Targets, and Idiopathic Pulmonary Fibrosis. *Free Radic. Biol. Med.* 49, 707–717. doi:10.1016/j.freeradbiomed.2010.04.036

Kurundkar, A., and Thannickal, V. J. (2016). Redox Mechanisms in Age-Related Lung Fibrosis. *Redox Biol.* 9, 67–76. doi:10.1016/j.redox.2016.06.005

Kuwano, K., Nakashima, N., Inoshima, I., Hagimoto, N., Fujita, M., Yoshimi, M., et al. (2003). Oxidative Stress in Lung Epithelial Cells from Patients with Idiopathic Interstitial Pneumonias. *Eur. Respir. J.* 21, 232–240. doi:10.1183/09031936.03.00063203

Kyung, S. Y., Kim, D. Y., Yoon, J. Y., Son, E. S., Kim, Y. J., Park, J. W., et al. (2018). Sulforaphane Attenuates Pulmonary Fibrosis by Inhibiting the Epithelial-Mesenchymal Transition. *BMC Pharmacol. Toxicol.* 19, 13. doi:10.1186/s40360-018-0204-7

Laleu, B., Gaggini, F., Orchard, M., Fioraso-Cartier, L., Cagnon, L., Houngninou-Molango, S., et al. (2010). First in Class, Potent, and Orally Bioavailable NADPH Oxidase Isoform 4 (Nox4) Inhibitors for the Treatment of Idiopathic Pulmonary Fibrosis. *J. Med. Chem.* 53, 7715–7730. doi:10.1021/jm100773e

Larios, J. M., Budhiraja, R., Fanburg, B. L., and Thannickal, V. J. (2001). Oxidative Protein Cross-Linking Reactions Involving L-Tyrosine in Transforming Growth Factor-Beta1-Stimulated Fibroblasts. *J. Biol. Chem.* 276, 17437–17441. doi:10.1074/jbc.M100426200

Lawson, J. A., FitzGerald, G. A., and Rokach, J. (1999). Isoprostanes: Formation, Analysis and Use As Indices of Lipid Peroxidation in Vivo. *J Biol Chem.* 274, 24441–24444. doi:10.1074/jbc.274.35.24441

Lebed'ko, O. A., Ryzhavskii, B. Y., and Demidova, O. V. (2015). Effect of Antioxidant Echinochrome A on Bleomycin-Induced Pulmonary Fibrosis. *Bull Exp. Biol. Med.* 159, 351–354. doi:10.1007/s10517-015-2960-3

Lebedev, A. V., Ivanova, M. V., and Levitsky, D. O. (2005). Echinochrome, a Naturally Occurring Iron Chelator and Free Radical Scavenger in Artificial and Natural Membrane Systems. *Life Sci.* 76, 863–875. doi:10.1016/j.lfs.2004.10.007

Lederer, D. J., and Martinez, F. J. (2018). Idiopathic Pulmonary Fibrosis. *N. Engl. J. Med.* 378, 1811–1823. doi:10.1056/NEJMra1705751

Lee, C. F., Qiao, M., Schröder, K., Zhao, Q., and Asmis, R. (2010a). Nox4 Is a Novel Inducible Source of Reactive Oxygen Species in Monocytes and Macrophages and Mediates Oxidized Low Density Lipoprotein-Induced Macrophage Death. *Circ. Res.* 106, 1489–1497. doi:10.1161/CIRCRESAHA.109.215392

Lee, E. S., Lee, H. E., Shin, J. Y., Yoon, S., and Moon, J. O. (2003). The Flavonoid Quercetin Inhibits Dimethylnitrosamine-Induced Liver Damage in Rats. *J. Pharm. Pharmacol.* 55, 1169–1174. doi:10.1211/0022357021396

Lee, H. C., Yin, P. H., Chi, C. W., and Wei, Y. H. (2002). Increase in Mitochondrial Mass in Human Fibroblasts under Oxidative Stress and during Replicative Cell Senescence. *J. Biomed. Sci.* 9, 517–526. doi:10.1007/BF02254978

Lee, J. C., Kinniry, P. A., Arguiri, E., Serota, M., Kanterakis, S., Chatterjee, S., et al. (2010b). Dietary Curcumin Increases Antioxidant Defenses in Lung, Ameliorates Radiation-Induced Pulmonary Fibrosis, and Improves Survival in Mice. *Radiat. Res.* 173, 590–601. doi:10.1667/RR1522.1

Lehmann, M., Korfei, M., Mutze, K., Klee, S., Skronska-Wasek, W., Alsafadi, H. N., et al. (2017). Senolytic Drugs Target Alveolar Epithelial Cell Function and Attenuate Experimental Lung Fibrosis *Ex Vivo*. *Eur. Respir. J.* 50, 1602367. doi:10.1183/13993003.02367-2016

Lelli, D., Sahebkar, A., Johnston, T. P., and Pedone, C. (2017). Curcumin Use in Pulmonary Diseases: State of the Art and Future Perspectives. *Pharmacol. Res.* 115, 133–148. doi:10.1016/j.phrs.2016.11.017

Lenz, A. G., Costabel, U., and Maier, K. L. (1996). Oxidized BAL Fluid Proteins in Patients with Interstitial Lung Diseases. *Eur. Respir. J.* 9, 307–312. doi:10.1183/09031936.96.09020307

Lenz, A. G., Hinze-Heyn, H., Schneider, A., Behr, J., Häussinger, K., Heindi, S., et al. (2004). Influence of Inflammatory Mechanisms on the Redox Balance in Interstitial Lung Diseases. *Respir. Med.* 98, 737–745. doi:10.1016/j.rmed.2004.02.007

Li, D., Cong, Z., Yang, C., and Zhu, X. (2020). Inhibition of LPS-Induced Nox2 Activation by VAS2870 Protects Alveolar Epithelial Cells through Eliminating ROS and Restoring Tight Junctions. *Biochem. Biophys. Res. Commun.* 524, 575–581. doi:10.1016/j.bbrc.2020.01.134

Li, H., Liu, B., Li, P., Feng, L., Ma, H., Xuan, S., et al. (2015). Inhibitory Effects of Curcumin on Inflammatory Cytokines in Rats with Paraquat Poisoning. *Zhonghua Lao Dong Wei Sheng Zhi Ye Bing Za Zhi* 33, 689–692.

Li, S., Yang, X., Li, W., Li, J., Su, X., Chen, L., et al. (2012). N-acetylcysteine Downregulation of Lysyl Oxidase Activity Alleviating Bleomycin-Induced Pulmonary Fibrosis in Rats. *Respiration* 84, 509–517. doi:10.1159/000340041

Liguori, I., Russo, G., Curcio, F., Bulli, G., Aran, L., Della-Morte, D., et al. (2018). Oxidative Stress, Aging, and Diseases. *Clin. Interv. Aging* 13, 757–772. doi:10.2147/CIA.S158513

Liu, B., Cao, B., Zhang, D., Xiao, N., Chen, H., Li, G. Q., et al. (2016a). Salvianolic Acid B Protects against Paraquat-Induced Pulmonary Injury by Mediating Nrf2/Nox4 Redox Balance and TGF-β1/Smad3 Signaling. *Toxicol. Appl. Pharmacol.* 309, 111–120. doi:10.1016/j.taap.2016.08.004

Liu, D., Gong, L., Zhu, H., Pu, S., Wu, Y., Zhang, W., et al. (2016b). Curcumin Inhibits Transforming Growth Factor β Induced Differentiation of Mouse Lung Fibroblasts to Myofibroblasts. *Front Pharmacol.* 7, 419. doi:10.3389/fphar.2016.00419

Liu, M., Xu, H., Zhang, L., Zhang, C., Yang, L., Ma, E., et al. (2018a). Salvianolic Acid B Inhibits Myofibroblast Transdifferentiation in Experimental Pulmonary Fibrosis via the Up-Regulation of Nrf2. *Biochem. Biophys. Res. Commun.* 495, 325–331. doi:10.1016/j.bbrc.2017.11.014

Liu, M., Zheng, M., Xu, H., Liu, L., Li, Y., Xiao, W., et al. (2015). Anti-pulmonary Fibrotic Activity of Salvianolic Acid B Was Screened by a Novel Method Based on the Cyto-Biophysical Properties. *Biochem. Biophys. Res. Commun.* 468, 214–220. doi:10.1016/j.bbrc.2015.10.127

Liu, N., Cao, F., Li, Q., Zhang, Y., Zhang, Z., and Guan, W. (2014a). Study of Quercetin on Pulmonary Fibrosis by Silica Particles. *Wei Sheng Yan Jiu* 43, 814–818.

Liu, P., Luo, G., Dodson, M., Schmidlin, C. J., Wei, Y., Kerimoglu, B., et al. (2021). The NRF2-Loc344887 Signaling axis Suppresses Pulmonary Fibrosis. *Redox Biol.* 38, 101766. doi:10.1016/j.redox.2020.101766

Liu, Q., Chu, H., Ma, Y., Wu, T., Qian, F., Ren, X., et al. (2016c). Salvianolic Acid B Attenuates Experimental Pulmonary Fibrosis through Inhibition of the TGF-β Signaling Pathway. *Sci. Rep.* 6, 27610. doi:10.1038/srep27610

Liu, Q., Shi, X., Tang, L., Xu, W., Jiang, S., Ding, W., et al. (2018b). Salvianolic Acid B Attenuates Experimental Pulmonary Inflammation by Protecting Endothelial Cells against Oxidative Stress Injury. *Eur. J. Pharmacol.* 840, 9–19. doi:10.1016/j.ejphar.2018.09.030

Liu, R. M., Liu, Y., Forman, H. J., Olman, M., and Tarpey, M. M. (2004). Glutathione Regulates Transforming Growth Factor-Beta-Stimulated Collagen Production in Fibroblasts. *Am. J. Physiol. Lung Cell Mol Physiol* 286, L121–L128. doi:10.1152/ajplung.00231.2003

Liu, R. M., Vayalil, P. K., Ballinger, C., Dickinson, D. A., Huang, W. T., Wang, S., et al. (2012). Transforming Growth Factor β Suppresses Glutamate-Cysteine Ligase Gene Expression and Induces Oxidative Stress in a Lung Fibrosis Model. *Free Radic. Biol. Med.* 53, 554–563. doi:10.1016/j.freeradbiomed.2012.05.016

Liu, X., Qian, L., Nan, H., Cui, M., Hao, X., and Du, Y. (2014b). Function of the Transforming Growth Factor-B1/c-Jun N-Terminal Kinase Signaling Pathway in the Action of Thalidomide on a Rat Model of Pulmonary Fibrosis. *Exp. Ther. Med.* 7, 669–674. doi:10.3892/etm.2013.1457

Liu, Y., Lu, F., Kang, L., Wang, Z., and Wang, Y. (2017b). Pirfenidone Attenuates Bleomycin-Induced Pulmonary Fibrosis in Mice by Regulating Nrf2/Bach1 Equilibrium. *BMC Pulm. Med.* 17, 63. doi:10.1186/s12890-017-0405-7

Liu, Y. M., Nepali, K., and Liou, J. P. (2017a). Idiopathic Pulmonary Fibrosis: Current Status, Recent Progress, and Emerging Targets. *J. Med. Chem.* 60, 527–553. doi:10.1021/acs.jmedchem.6b00935

Luo, W., Liu, Q., Jiang, N., Li, M., and Shi, L. (2019). Isorhamnetin Inhibited Migration and Invasion via Suppression of Akt/ERK-Mediated Epithelial-To-Mesenchymal Transition (EMT) in A549 Human Non-small-cell Lung Cancer Cells. *Biosci. Rep.* 39, BSR20190159. doi:10.1042/BSR20190159

M Davies, A., and G Holt, A. (2018). Why Antioxidant Therapies Have Failed in Clinical Trials. *J. Theor. Biol.* 457, 1–5. doi:10.1016/j.jtbi.2018.08.014

Ma, B. N., and Li, X. J. (2020). Resveratrol Extracted from Chinese Herbal Medicines: A Novel Therapeutic Strategy for Lung Diseases. *Chin. Herb Med.* 12, 349–358. doi:10.1016/j.chmed.2020.07.003

Ma, Y., Luo, L., Liu, X., Li, H., Zeng, Z., He, X., et al. (2021). Pirfenidone Mediates Cigarette Smoke Extract Induced Inflammation and Oxidative Stress *In Vitro* and *In Vivo*. *Int. Immunopharmacol* 96, 107593. doi:10.1016/j.intimp.2021.107593

Ma, Z., Zhao, C., Chen, Q., Yu, C., Zhang, H., Zhang, Z., et al. (2018). Antifibrotic Effects of a Novel Pirfenidone Derivative *In Vitro* and *In Vivo*. *Pulm. Pharmacol. Ther.* 53, 100–106. doi:10.1016/j.pupt.2018.10.006

MacVittie, T. J., Gibbs, A., Farese, A. M., Barrow, K., Bennett, A., Taylor-Howell, C., et al. (2017). AEOL 10150 Mitigates Radiation-Induced Lung Injury in the Nonhuman Primate: Morbidity and Mortality Are Administration Schedule-dependent. *Radiat. Res.* 187, 298–318. doi:10.1667/RR4413.1

Malli, F., Bardaka, F., Tsilioni, I., Karetsi, E., Gourgoulianis, K. I., and Daniil, Z. (2013). 8-isoprostane Levels in Serum and Bronchoalveolar Lavage in Idiopathic Pulmonary Fibrosis and Sarcoidosis. *Food Chem. Toxicol.* 61, 160–163. doi:10.1016/j.fct.2013.05.016

Manjeet K, R., and Ghosh, B. (1999). Quercetin Inhibits LPS-Induced Nitric Oxide and Tumor Necrosis Factor-Alpha Production in Murine Macrophages. *Int. J. Immunopharmacol* 21, 435–443. doi:10.1016/s0192-0561(99)00024-7

Manni, M. L., and Oury, T. D. (2014). "Oxidative Stress and Pulmonary Fibrosis," in Systems Biology Of Free Radicals And Antioxidants*Anonymous* (Berlin, Heidelberg: Springer Berlin Heidelberg), 1611–1631. doi:10.1007/978-3-642-30018-9_122

Manoury, B., Nenan, S., Leclerc, O., Guenon, I., Boichot, E., Planquois, J. M., et al. (2005). The Absence of Reactive Oxygen Species Production Protects Mice against Bleomycin-Induced Pulmonary Fibrosis. *Respir. Res.* 6, 11. doi:10.1186/1465-9921-6-11

Markart, P., Luboeinski, T., Korfei, M., Schmidt, R., Wygrecka, M., Mahavadi, P., et al. (2009). Alveolar Oxidative Stress Is Associated with Elevated Levels of Nonenzymatic Low-Molecular-Weight Antioxidants in Patients with Different Forms of Chronic Fibrosing Interstitial Lung Diseases. *Antioxid. Redox Signal.* 11, 227–240. doi:10.1089/ars.2008.2105

Martinez, F. J., Martinez, F. J., de Andrade, J. A., Anstrom, K. J., King, T. E., and Raghu, G. (2014). Randomized Trial of Acetylcysteine in Idiopathic Pulmonary Fibrosis. *N. Engl. J. Med.* 370, 2093–2101. doi:10.1056/NEJMoa1401739

Martinez, J. A., Ramos, S. G., Meirelles, M. S., Verceze, A. V., Arantes, M. R., and Vannucchi, H. (2008). Effects of Quercetin on Bleomycin-Induced Lung Injury: a Preliminary Study. *J. Bras Pneumol* 34, 445–452. doi:10.1590/s1806-37132008000700003

Masamune, A., Watanabe, T., Kikuta, K., Satoh, K., and Shimosegawa, T. (2008). NADPH Oxidase Plays a Crucial Role in the Activation of Pancreatic Stellate Cells. *Am. J. Physiol. Gastrointest. Liver Physiol.* 294, G99–G108. doi:10.1152/ajpgi.00272.2007

Mata, M., Ruíz, A., Cerdá, M., Martinez-Losa, M., Cortijo, J., Santangelo, F., et al. (2003). Oral N-Acetylcysteine Reduces Bleomycin-Induced Lung Damage and Mucin Muc5ac Expression in Rats. *Eur. Respir. J.* 22, 900–905. doi:10.1183/09031936.03.00018003

Matsuzawa, Y., Kawashima, T., Kuwabara, R., Hayakawa, S., Irie, T., Yoshida, T., et al. (2015). Change in Serum Marker of Oxidative Stress in the Progression of Idiopathic Pulmonary Fibrosis. *Pulm. Pharmacol. Ther.* 32, 1–6. doi:10.1016/j.pupt.2015.03.005

Mazur, W., Lindholm, P., Vuorinen, K., Myllärniemi, M., Salmenkivi, K., and Kinnula, V. L. (2010). Cell-specific Elevation of NRF2 and Sulfiredoxin-1 as Markers of Oxidative Stress in the Lungs of Idiopathic Pulmonary Fibrosis and Non-specific Interstitial Pneumonia. *APMIS* 118, 703–712. doi:10.1111/j.1600-0463.2010.02646.x

Mehrabani, M., Goudarzi, M., Mehrzadi, S., Siahpoosh, A., Mohammadi, M., Khalili, H., et al. (2020). Crocin: a Protective Natural Antioxidant against Pulmonary Fibrosis Induced by Bleomycin. *Pharmacol. Rep.* 72, 992–1001. doi:10.1007/s43440-019-00023-y

Mehrzadi, S., Hosseini, P., Mehrabani, M., Siahpoosh, A., Goudarzi, M., Khalili, H., et al. (2020). Attenuation of Bleomycin-Induced Pulmonary Fibrosis in Wistar Rats by Combination Treatment of Two Natural Phenolic Compounds: Quercetin and Gallic Acid. *Nutr. Cancer* 73, 2039–2049. doi:10.1080/01635581.2020.1820053

Meyer, A., Buhl, R., Kampf, S., and Magnussen, H. (1995). Intravenous N-Acetylcysteine and Lung Glutathione of Patients with Pulmonary Fibrosis and Normals. *Am. J. Respir. Crit. Care Med.* 152, 1055–1060. doi:10.1164/ajrccm.152.3.7663783

Meyer, A., Buhl, R., and Magnussen, H. (1994). The Effect of Oral N-Acetylcysteine on Lung Glutathione Levels in Idiopathic Pulmonary Fibrosis. *Eur. Respir. J.* 7, 431–436. doi:10.1183/09031936.94.07030431

Michiels, C. (2003). Endothelial Cell Functions. *J. Cel Physiol* 196, 430–443. doi:10.1002/jcp.10333

Minnelli, C., Moretti, P., Fulgenzi, G., Mariani, P., Laudadio, E., Armeni, T., et al. (2018). A Poloxamer-407 Modified Liposome Encapsulating Epigallocatechin-3-Gallate in the Presence of Magnesium: Characterization and Protective Effect against Oxidative Damage. *Int. J. Pharm.* 552, 225–234. doi:10.1016/j.ijpharm.2018.10.004

Misra, H. P., and Rabideau, C. (2000). Pirfenidone Inhibits NADPH-dependent Microsomal Lipid Peroxidation and Scavenges Hydroxyl Radicals. *Mol. Cel Biochem* 204, 119–126. doi:10.1023/a:1007023532508

Molina-Molina, M., Machahua-Huamani, C., Vicens-Zygmunt, V., Llatjós, R., Escobar, I., Sala-Llinas, E., et al. (2018). Anti-fibrotic Effects of Pirfenidone and Rapamycin in Primary IPF Fibroblasts and Human Alveolar Epithelial Cells. *BMC Pulm. Med.* 18, 63. doi:10.1186/s12890-018-0626-4

Mondello, S., Mazzon, E., Di Paola, R., Crisafulli, C., Mondello, P., Buemi, M., et al. (2009). Thalidomide Suppresses Sclerosing Encapsulating Peritonitis in a Rat Experimental Model. *Shock* 32, 332–339. doi:10.1097/SHK.0b013e3181994974

Muramatsu, Y., Sugino, K., Ishida, F., Tatebe, J., Morita, T., and Homma, S. (2016). Effect of Inhaled N-Acetylcysteine Monotherapy on Lung Function and Redox Balance in Idiopathic Pulmonary Fibrosis. *Respir. Investig.* 54, 170–178. doi:10.1016/j.resinv.2015.11.004

Murthy, S., Adamcakova-Dodd, A., Perry, S. S., Tephly, L. A., Keller, R. M., Metwali, N., et al. (2009). Modulation of Reactive Oxygen Species by Rac1 or

Catalase Prevents Asbestos-Induced Pulmonary Fibrosis. *Am. J. Physiol. Lung Cel Mol Physiol* 297, L846–L855. doi:10.1152/ajplung.90590.2008

Myllärniemi, M., and Kaarteenaho, R. (2015). Pharmacological Treatment of Idiopathic Pulmonary Fibrosis - Preclinical and Clinical Studies of Pirfenidone, Nintedanib, and N-Acetylcysteine. *Eur. Clin. Respir. J.* 2, 26385. doi:10.3402/ecrj.v2.26385

Nagai, K., Jiang, M. H., Hada, J., Nagata, T., Yajima, Y., Yamamoto, S., et al. (2002a). Epigallocatechin Gallate Protects against NO Stress-Induced Neuronal Damage after Ischemia by Acting as an Anti-oxidant. *Brain Res.* 956, 319–322. doi:10.1016/s0006-8993(02)03564-3

Nagai, S., Hamada, K., Shigematsu, M., Taniyama, M., Yamauchi, S., and Izumi, T. (2002b). Open-label Compassionate Use One Year-Treatment with Pirfenidone to Patients with Chronic Pulmonary Fibrosis. *Intern. Med.* 41, 1118–1123. doi:10.2169/internalmedicine.41.1118

Nakamura, T., Matsushima, M., Hayashi, Y., Shibasaki, M., Imaizumi, K., Hashimoto, N., et al. (2011). Attenuation of Transforming Growth Factor-β-Stimulated Collagen Production in Fibroblasts by Quercetin-Induced Heme Oxygenase-1. *Am. J. Respir. Cel Mol Biol* 44, 614–620. doi:10.1165/rcmb.2010-0338OC

Nakayama, S., Mukae, H., Sakamoto, N., Kakugawa, T., Yoshioka, S., Soda, H., et al. (2008). Pirfenidone Inhibits the Expression of HSP47 in TGF-Beta1-Stimulated Human Lung Fibroblasts. *Life Sci.* 82, 210–217. doi:10.1016/j.lfs.2007.11.003

Nakazato, H., Oku, H., Yamane, S., Tsuruta, Y., and Suzuki, R. (2002). A Novel Anti-fibrotic Agent Pirfenidone Suppresses Tumor Necrosis Factor-Alpha at the Translational Level. *Eur. J. Pharmacol.* 446, 177–185. doi:10.1016/s0014-2999(02)01758-2

Nanjo, F., Mori, M., Goto, K., and Hara, Y. (1999). Radical Scavenging Activity of tea Catechins and Their Related Compounds. *Biosci. Biotechnol. Biochem.* 63, 1621–1623. doi:10.1271/bbb.63.1621

Negishi, H., Xu, J. W., Ikeda, K., Njelekela, M., Nara, Y., and Yamori, Y. (2004). Black and green tea Polyphenols Attenuate Blood Pressure Increases in Stroke-Prone Spontaneously Hypertensive Rats. *J. Nutr.* 134, 38–42. doi:10.1093/jn/134.1.38

Nelson, K. K., and Melendez, J. A. (2004). Mitochondrial Redox Control of Matrix Metalloproteinases. *Free Radic. Biol. Med.* 37, 768–784. doi:10.1016/j.freeradbiomed.2004.06.008

Noble, P. W., Albera, C., Bradford, W. Z., Costabel, U., Glassberg, M. K., Kardatzke, D., et al. (2011). Pirfenidone in Patients with Idiopathic Pulmonary Fibrosis (CAPACITY): Two Randomised Trials. *Lancet* 377, 1760–1769. doi:10.1016/S0140-6736(11)60405-4

O'Donnell, B. V., Tew, D. G., Jones, O. T., and England, P. J. (1993). Studies on the Inhibitory Mechanism of Iodonium Compounds with Special Reference to Neutrophil NADPH Oxidase. *Biochem. J.* 290, 41–49. doi:10.1042/bj2900041

Oku, H., Nakazato, H., Horikawa, T., Tsuruta, Y., and Suzuki, R. (2002). Pirfenidone Suppresses Tumor Necrosis Factor-Alpha, Enhances Interleukin-10 and Protects Mice from Endotoxic Shock. *Eur. J. Pharmacol.* 446, 167–176. doi:10.1016/s0014-29990201757-0

Oku, H., Shimizu, T., Kawabata, T., Nagira, M., Hikita, I., Ueyama, A., et al. (2008). Antifibrotic Action of Pirfenidone and Prednisolone: Different Effects on Pulmonary Cytokines and Growth Factors in Bleomycin-Induced Murine Pulmonary Fibrosis. *Eur. J. Pharmacol.* 590, 400–408. doi:10.1016/j.ejphar.2008.06.046

Oldham, J. M., Ma, S. F., Martinez, F. J., Anstrom, K. J., Raghu, G., Schwartz, D. A., et al. (2015). TOLLIP, MUC5B, and the Response to N-Acetylcysteine Among Individuals with Idiopathic Pulmonary Fibrosis. *Am. J. Respir. Crit. Care Med.* 192, 1475–1482. doi:10.1164/rccm.201505-1010OC

Osborn-Heaford, H. L., Ryan, A. J., Murthy, S., Racila, A.-M., He, C., Sieren, J. C., et al. (2012). Mitochondrial Rac1 GTPase Import and Electron Transfer from Cytochrome C Are Required for Pulmonary Fibrosis. *J. Biol. Chemistry* 287, 3301–3312. doi:10.1074/jbc.M111.308387

Otoupalova, E., Smith, S., Cheng, G., and Thannickal, V. J. (2020). Oxidative Stress in Pulmonary Fibrosis. *Compr. Physiol.* 10, 509–547. doi:10.1002/cphy.c190017

Oury, T. D., Thakker, K., Menache, M., Chang, L. Y., Crapo, J. D., and Day, B. J. (2001). Attenuation of Bleomycin-Induced Pulmonary Fibrosis by a Catalytic Antioxidant Metalloporphyrin. *Am. J. Respir. Cel Mol Biol* 25, 164–169. doi:10.1165/ajrcmb.25.2.4235

Oz, H. S. (2017). Chronic Inflammatory Diseases and Green Tea Polyphenols. *Nutrients* 9, 561. doi:10.3390/nu9060561

Ozben, T. (2015). Antioxidant Supplementation on Cancer Risk and during Cancer Therapy: an Update. *Curr. Top. Med. Chem.* 15, 170–178. doi:10.2174/1568026615666141209160918

Pache, J. C., Carnesecchi, S., Deffert, C., Donati, Y., Herrmann, F. R., Barazzone-Argiroffo, C., et al. (2011). NOX-4 Is Expressed in Thickened Pulmonary Arteries in Idiopathic Pulmonary Fibrosis. *Nat. Med.* 17, 31–33. doi:10.1038/nm0111-31

Panduri, V., Liu, G., Surapureddi, S., Kondapalli, J., Soberanes, S., de Souza-Pinto, N. C., et al. (2009). Role of Mitochondrial hOGG1 and Aconitase in Oxidant-Induced Lung Epithelial Cell Apoptosis. *Free Radic. Biol. Med.* 47, 750–759. doi:10.1016/j.freeradbiomed.2009.06.010

Parmentier, M., Drost, E., and Hirani, N. (1999). Thiol Antioxidantsinhibit Neutrophil Chemotaxis by Decreasing Release of IL-8 from Macrophages and Pulmonary Epithelial Cells. *Am J. Respir. Crit. Care. Med.*, 159, A286, (New York, NY: Amer Lung Assoc).

Peng, H., Liu, Y., Wang, J., Zhao, X., and Wang, X. (2013). Effect of Quercetin on the Expression of TGF-Beta1 in Human Embryonic Lung Fibroblasts Activated by the Silicotic Alveolar Macrophages. *Wei Sheng Yan Jiu* 42, 99–102.

Petersen, S. V., Oury, T. D., Ostergaard, L., Valnickova, Z., Wegrzyn, J., Thøgersen, I. B., et al. (2004). Extracellular Superoxide Dismutase (EC-SOD) Binds to Type I Collagen and Protects against Oxidative Fragmentation. *J. Biol. Chem.* 279, 13705–13710. doi:10.1074/jbc.M310217200

Phan, S. H. (2002). The Myofibroblast in Pulmonary Fibrosis. *Chest* 122, 286S–289S. doi:10.1378/chest.122.6_suppl.286s

Phan, T. T., Lim, I. J., Sun, L., Chan, S. Y., Bay, B. H., Tan, E. K., et al. (2003). Quercetin Inhibits Fibronectin Production by Keloid-Derived Fibroblasts. Implication for the Treatment of Excessive Scars. *J. Dermatol. Sci.* 33, 192–194. doi:10.1016/j.jdermsci.2003.08.008

Pociask, D. A., Sime, P. J., and Brody, A. R. (2004). Asbestos-derived Reactive Oxygen Species Activate TGF-Beta1. *Lab. Invest.* 84, 1013–1023. doi:10.1038/labinvest.3700109

Poletti, V., Ravaglia, C., and Tomassetti, S. (2014). Pirfenidone for the Treatment of Idiopathic Pulmonary Fibrosis. *Expert Rev. Respir. Med.* 8, 539–545. doi:10.1586/17476348.2014.915750

Pourgholamhossein, F., Rasooli, R., Pournamdari, M., Pourgholi, L., Samareh-Fekri, M., Ghazi-Khansari, M., et al. (2018). Pirfenidone Protects against Paraquat-Induced Lung Injury and Fibrosis in Mice by Modulation of Inflammation, Oxidative Stress, and Gene Expression. *Food Chem. Toxicol.* 112, 39–46. doi:10.1016/j.fct.2017.12.034

Psathakis, K., Mermigkis, D., Papatheodorou, G., Loukides, S., Panagou, P., Polychronopoulos, V., et al. (2006). Exhaled Markers of Oxidative Stress in Idiopathic Pulmonary Fibrosis. *Eur. J. Clin. Invest.* 36, 362–367. doi:10.1111/j.1365-2362.2006.01636.x

Punithavathi, D., Venkatesan, N., and Babu, M. (2000). Curcumin Inhibition of Bleomycin-Induced Pulmonary Fibrosis in Rats. *Br. J. Pharmacol.* 131, 169–172. doi:10.1038/sj.bjp.0703578

Punithavathi, D., Venkatesan, N., and Babu, M. (2003). Protective Effects of Curcumin against Amiodarone-Induced Pulmonary Fibrosis in Rats. *Br. J. Pharmacol.* 139, 1342–1350. doi:10.1038/sj.bjp.0705362

Qu, J., Zhang, Z., Zhang, P., Zheng, C., Zhou, W., Cui, W., et al. (2019). Downregulation of HMGB1 Is Required for the Protective Role of Nrf2 in EMT-Mediated PF. *J. Cel Physiol* 234, 8862–8872. doi:10.1002/jcp.27548

Rabbani, Z. N., Anscher, M. S., Folz, R. J., Archer, E., Huang, H., Chen, L., et al. (2005). Overexpression of Extracellular Superoxide Dismutase Reduces Acute Radiation Induced Lung Toxicity. *BMC Cancer* 5, 59. doi:10.1186/1471-2407-5-59

Rabbani, Z. N., Batinic-Haberle, I., Anscher, M. S., Huang, J., Day, B. J., Alexander, E., et al. (2007). Long-term Administration of a Small Molecular Weight Catalytic Metalloporphyrin Antioxidant, AEOL 10150, Protects Lungs from Radiation-Induced Injury. *Int. J. Radiat. Oncol. Biol. Phys.* 67, 573–580. doi:10.1016/j.ijrobp.2006.09.053

Radomska-Leśniewska, D. M., Skopińska-Różewska, E., Jankowska-Steifer, E., Sobiecka, M., Sadowska, A. M., Hevelke, A., et al. (2010). N-acetylcysteine Inhibits IL-8 and MMP-9 Release and ICAM-1 Expression by Bronchoalveolar Cells from Interstitial Lung Disease Patients. *Pharmacol. Rep.* 62, 131–138. doi:10.1016/s1734-1140(10)70250-4

Raghu, G., Johnson, W. C., Lockhart, D., and Mageto, Y. (1999). Treatment of Idiopathic Pulmonary Fibrosis with a New Antifibrotic Agent, Pirfenidone:

Results of a Prospective, Open-Label Phase II Study. *Am. J. Respir. Crit. Care Med.* 159, 1061–1069. doi:10.1164/ajrccm.159.4.9805017

Rahman, I., Skwarska, E., Henry, M., Davis, M., O'Connor, C. M., FitzGerald, M. X., et al. (1999). Systemic and Pulmonary Oxidative Stress in Idiopathic Pulmonary Fibrosis. *Free Radic. Biol. Med.* 27, 60–68. doi:10.1016/s0891-5849(99)00035-0

Rangarajan, S., Bernard, K., and Thannickal, V. J. (2017). Mitochondrial Dysfunction in Pulmonary Fibrosis. *Ann. Am. Thorac. Soc.* 14, S383–S388. doi:10.1513/AnnalsATS.201705-370AW

Rangarajan, S., Bone, N. B., Zmijewska, A. A., Jiang, S., Park, D. W., Bernard, K., et al. (2018). Metformin Reverses Established Lung Fibrosis in a Bleomycin Model. *Nat. Med.* 24, 1121–1127. doi:10.1038/s41591-018-0087-6

Reiter, R. J., Mayo, J. C., Tan, D. X., Sainz, R. M., Alatorre-Jimenez, M., and Qin, L. (2016). Melatonin as an Antioxidant: under Promises but over Delivers. *J. Pineal Res.* 61, 253–278. doi:10.1111/jpi.12360

Reiter, R. J., Tan, D. X., Manchester, L. C., Pilar Terron, M., Flores, L. J., and Koppisepi, S. (2007). Medical Implications of Melatonin: Receptor-Mediated and Receptor-independent Actions. *Adv. Med. Sci.* 52, 11–28.

Ren, J., Li, J., Liu, X., Feng, Y., Gui, Y., Yang, J., et al. (2016). Quercetin Inhibits Fibroblast Activation and Kidney Fibrosis Involving the Suppression of Mammalian Target of Rapamycin and β-catenin Signaling. *Sci. Rep.* 6, 23968. doi:10.1038/srep23968

Ren, X., Han, L., Li, Y., Zhao, H., Zhang, Z., Zhuang, Y., et al. (2021). Isorhamnetin Attenuates TNF-α-Induced Inflammation, Proliferation, and Migration in Human Bronchial Epithelial Cells via MAPK and NF-Kb Pathways. *Anat. Rec. (Hoboken)* 304, 901–913. doi:10.1002/ar.24506

Rhyu, D. Y., Yang, Y., Ha, H., Lee, G. T., Song, J. S., Uh, S. T., et al. (2005). Role of Reactive Oxygen Species in TGF-Beta1-Induced Mitogen-Activated Protein Kinase Activation and Epithelial-Mesenchymal Transition in Renal Tubular Epithelial Cells. *J. Am. Soc. Nephrol.* 16, 667–675. doi:10.1681/ASN.2004050425

Ricciardolo, F. L., Di Stefano, A., Sabatini, F., and Folkerts, G. (2006). Reactive Nitrogen Species in the Respiratory Tract. *Eur. J. Pharmacol.* 533, 240–252. doi:10.1016/j.ejphar.2005.12.057

Ricciardolo, F. L., Sterk, P. J., Gaston, B., and Folkerts, G. (2004). Nitric Oxide in Health and Disease of the Respiratory System. *Physiol. Rev.* 84, 731–765. doi:10.1152/physrev.00034.2003

Richeldi, L., Collard, H. R., and Jones, M. G. (1941). Idiopathic Pulmonary Fibrosis. *Lancet* 389, 1941–1952.

Rottoli, P., Magi, B., Cianti, R., Bargagli, E., Vagaggini, C., Nikiforakis, N., et al. (2005). Carbonylated Proteins in Bronchoalveolar Lavage of Patients with Sarcoidosis, Pulmonary Fibrosis Associated with Systemic Sclerosis and Idiopathic Pulmonary Fibrosis. *Proteomics* 5, 2612–2618. doi:10.1002/pmic.200401206

Ruwanpura, S. M., Thomas, B. J., and Bardin, P. G. (2020). Pirfenidone: Molecular Mechanisms and Potential Clinical Applications in Lung Disease. *Am. J. Respir. Cel Mol Biol* 62, 413–422. doi:10.1165/rcmb.2019-0328TR

Saidi, A., Kasabova, M., Vanderlynden, L., Wartenberg, M., Kara-Ali, G. H., Marc, D., et al. (2019). Curcumin Inhibits the TGF-β1-dependent Differentiation of Lung Fibroblasts via PPARγ-Driven Upregulation of Cathepsins B and L. *Sci. Rep.* 9, 491. doi:10.1038/s41598-018-36858-3

Sakamoto, S., Kataoka, K., Kondoh, Y., Kato, M., Okamoto, M., Mukae, H., et al. (2021). Pirfenidone Plus Inhaled N-Acetylcysteine for Idiopathic Pulmonary Fibrosis: a Randomised Trial. *Eur. Respir. J.* 57, 2000348. doi:10.1183/13993003.00348-2020

Salah, N., Miller, N. J., Paganga, G., Tijburg, L., Bolwell, G. P., and Rice-Evans, C. (1995). Polyphenolic Flavanols as Scavengers of Aqueous Phase Radicals and as Chain-Breaking Antioxidants. *Arch. Biochem. Biophys.* 322, 339–346. doi:10.1006/abbi.1995.1473

Saleh, D., Barnes, P. J., and Giaid, A. (1997). Increased Production of the Potent Oxidant Peroxynitrite in the Lungs of Patients with Idiopathic Pulmonary Fibrosis. *Am. J. Respir. Crit. Care Med.* 155, 1763–1769. doi:10.1164/ajrccm.155.5.9154889

Salvemini, D., Riley, D. P., and Cuzzocrea, S. (2002). SOD Mimetics Are Coming of Age. *Nat. Rev. Drug Discov.* 1, 367–374. doi:10.1038/nrd796

Sampaio, E. P., Sarno, E. N., Galilly, R., Cohn, Z. A., and Kaplan, G. (1991). Thalidomide Selectively Inhibits Tumor Necrosis Factor Alpha Production by Stimulated Human Monocytes. *J. Exp. Med.* 173, 699–703. doi:10.1084/jem.173.3.699

Santofimia-Castaño, P., Clea Ruy, D., Garcia-Sanchez, L., Jimenez-Blasco, D., Fernandez-Bermejo, M., Bolaños, J. P., et al. (2015). Melatonin Induces the Expression of Nrf2-Regulated Antioxidant Enzymes via PKC and Ca2+ Influx Activation in Mouse Pancreatic Acinar Cells. *Free Radic. Biol. Med.* 87, 226–236. doi:10.1016/j.freeradbiomed.2015.06.033

Sartor, L., Pezzato, E., and Garbisa, S. (2002) Epigallocatechin-3-gallate Inhibits Leukocyte Elastase: Potential of the Phyto-Factor in Hindering Inflammation, Emphysema, and Invasion. *J. Leukoc. Biol.* 71, 73–79.

Sato, N., Takasaka, N., Yoshida, M., Tsubouchi, K., Minagawa, S., Araya, J., et al. (2016). Metformin Attenuates Lung Fibrosis Development via NOX4 Suppression. *Respir. Res.* 17, 107. doi:10.1186/s12931-016-0420-x

Sazonova, E. N., Kuznetsova, M. S., Vasileva, E. A., Mishchenko, N. P., Tsimbalist, N. A., and Lebed'ko, O. A. (2020). Cytoprotective Effect of Echinochrome A in Primary Culture of Pulmonary Fibroblasts from Albino Rats under Conditions of Oxidative Stress. *Bull. Exp. Biol. Med.* 169, 582–585. doi:10.1007/s10517-020-04933-3

Schafer, M. J., White, T. A., Iijima, K., Haak, A. J., Ligresti, G., Atkinson, E. J., et al. (2017). Cellular Senescence Mediates Fibrotic Pulmonary Disease. *Nat. Commun.* 8, 14532. doi:10.1038/ncomms14532

Sellarés, J., and Rojas, M. (2019). Quercetin in Idiopathic Pulmonary Fibrosis: Another Brick in the Senolytic Wall. *Am. J. Respir. Cell Mol Biol* 60, 3–4. doi:10.1165/rcmb.2018-0267ED

Sener, G., Topaloğlu, N., Sehirli, A. O., Ercan, F., and Gedik, N. (2007). Resveratrol Alleviates Bleomycin-Induced Lung Injury in Rats. *Pulm. Pharmacol. Ther.* 20, 642–649. doi:10.1016/j.pupt.2006.07.003

Serrano-Mollar, A., Closa, D., Prats, N., Blesa, S., Martinez-Losa, M., Cortijo, J., et al. (2003). *In Vivo* antioxidant Treatment Protects against Bleomycin-Induced Lung Damage in Rats. *Br. J. Pharmacol.* 138, 1037–1048. doi:10.1038/sj.bjp.0705138

Shahzeidi, S., Sarnstrand, B., Jeffery, P. K., McAnulty, R. J., and Laurent, G. J. (1991). Oral N-Acetylcysteine Reduces Bleomycin-Induced Collagen Deposition in the Lungs of Mice. *Eur. Respir. J.* 4, 845–852.

Sharma, N. L., Sharma, V. C., Mahajan, V. K., Shanker, V., Ranjan, N., and Gupta, M. (2007). Thalidomide: an Experience in Therapeutic Outcome and Adverse Reactions. *J. Dermatolog Treat* 18, 335–340. doi:10.1080/09546630701386993

Shi, H., He, J., Li, X., Han, J., Wu, R., Wang, D., et al. (2018a). Isorhamnetin, the Active Constituent of a Chinese Herb Hippophae Rhamnoides L, Is a Potent Suppressor of Dendritic-Cell Maturation and Trafficking. *Int. Immunopharmacol* 55, 216–222. doi:10.1016/j.intimp.2017.12.014

Shi, W., Li, L., Ding, Y., Yang, K., Chen, Z., Fan, X., et al. (2018b). The Critical Role of Epigallocatechin Gallate in Regulating Mitochondrial Metabolism. *Future Med. Chem.* 10, 795–809. doi:10.4155/fmc-2017-0204

Shimizu, Y., Dobashi, K., Sano, T., and Yamada, M. (2014). ROCK Activation in Lung of Idiopathic Pulmonary Fibrosis with Oxidative Stress. *Int. J. Immunopathol Pharmacol.* 27, 37–44. doi:10.1177/039463201402700106

Shin, N. R., Park, J. W., Lee, I. C., Ko, J. W., Park, S. H., Kim, J. S., et al. (2017). Melatonin Suppresses Fibrotic Responses Induced by Cigarette Smoke via Downregulation of TGF-B1. *Oncotarget* 8, 95692–95703. doi:10.18632/oncotarget.21680

Smith, M. R., Gangireddy, S. R., Narala, V. R., Hogaboam, C. M., Standiford, T. J., Christensen, P. J., et al. (2010). Curcumin Inhibits Fibrosis-Related Effects in IPF Fibroblasts and in Mice Following Bleomycin-Induced Lung Injury. *Am. J. Physiol. Lung Cell Mol Physiol* 298, L616–L625. doi:10.1152/ajplung.00002.2009

Spagnolo, P., Kreuter, M., Maher, T. M., Wuyts, W., Bonella, F., Corte, T. J., et al. (2018). Metformin Does Not Affect Clinically Relevant Outcomes in Patients with Idiopathic Pulmonary Fibrosis. *Respiration* 96, 314–322. doi:10.1159/000489668

Spond, J., Case, N., Chapman, R. W., Crawley, Y., Egan, R. W., Fine, J., et al. (2003). Inhibition of Experimental Acute Pulmonary Inflammation by Pirfenidone. *Pulm. Pharmacol. Ther.* 16, 207–214. doi:10.1016/S1094-5539(03)00026-9

Sriram, N., Kalayarasan, S., Manikandan, R., Arumugam, M., and Sudhandiran, G. (2015). Epigallocatechin Gallate Attenuates Fibroblast Proliferation and Excessive Collagen Production by Effectively Intervening TGF-B1 Signalling. *Clin. Exp. Pharmacol. Physiol.* 42, 849–859. doi:10.1111/1440-1681.12428

Sriram, N., Kalayarasan, S., and Sudhandiran, G. (2008). Enhancement of Antioxidant Defense System by Epigallocatechin-3-Gallate during Bleomycin Induced Experimental Pulmonary Fibrosis. *Biol. Pharm. Bull* 31, 1306–1311. doi:10.1248/bpb.31.1306

Sriram, N., Kalayarasan, S., and Sudhandiran, G. (2009a). Epigallocatechin-3-gallate Augments Antioxidant Activities and Inhibits Inflammation during Bleomycin-Induced Experimental Pulmonary Fibrosis through Nrf2-Keap1 Signaling. *Pulm. Pharmacol. Ther.* 22, 221–236. doi:10.1016/j.pupt.2008.12.010

Sriram, N., Kalayarasan, S., and Sudhandiran, G. (2009b). Epigallocatechin-3-gallate Exhibits Anti-fibrotic Effect by Attenuating Bleomycin-Induced Glycoconjugates, Lysosomal Hydrolases and Ultrastructural Changes in Rat Model Pulmonary Fibrosis. *Chem. Biol. Interact* 180, 271–280. doi:10.1016/j.cbi.2009.02.017

Steinhubl, S. R. (2008). Why Have Antioxidants Failed in Clinical Trials? *Am. J. Cardiol.* 101, 14D–19D. doi:10.1016/j.amjcard.2008.02.003

Sturrock, A., Cahill, B., Norman, K., Huecksteadt, T. P., Hill, K., Sanders, K., et al. (2006). Transforming Growth Factor-Beta1 Induces Nox4 NAD(P)H Oxidase and Reactive Oxygen Species-dependent Proliferation in Human Pulmonary Artery Smooth Muscle Cells. *Am. J. Physiol. Lung Cell Mol Physiol* 290, L661–L673. doi:10.1152/ajplung.00269.2005

Sugiura, H., Ichikawa, T., Liu, X., Kobayashi, T., Wang, X. Q., Kawasaki, S., et al. (2009). N-acetyl-L-cysteine Inhibits TGF-Beta1-Induced Profibrotic Responses in Fibroblasts. *Pulm. Pharmacol. Ther.* 22, 487–491. doi:10.1016/j.pupt.2009.04.002

Swiderska-Kołacz, G., Klusek, J., and Kołataj, A. (2006). The Effect of Melatonin on Glutathione and Glutathione Transferase and Glutathione Peroxidase Activities in the Mouse Liver and Kidney *In Vivo*. *Neuro Endocrinol. Lett.* 27, 365–368.

Tabata, C., Tabata, R., Kadokawa, Y., Hisamori, S., Takahashi, M., Mishima, M., et al. (2007). Thalidomide Prevents Bleomycin-Induced Pulmonary Fibrosis in Mice. *J. Immunol.* 179, 708–714. doi:10.4049/jimmunol.179.1.708

Takano, M., Deguchi, J., Senoo, S., Izumi, M., Kawami, M., and Yumoto, R. (2020). Suppressive Effect of Quercetin against Bleomycin-Induced Epithelial-Mesenchymal Transition in Alveolar Epithelial Cells. *Drug Metab. Pharmacokinet.* 35, 522–526. doi:10.1016/j.dmpk.2020.08.001

Tanaka, T., Saito, Y., Matsuda, K., Kamio, K., Abe, S., Kubota, K., et al. (2017). Cyclic Mechanical Stretch-Induced Oxidative Stress Occurs via a NOX-dependent Mechanism in Type II Alveolar Epithelial Cells. *Respir. Physiol. Neurobiol.* 242, 108–116. doi:10.1016/j.resp.2017.04.007

Tang, H., He, H., Ji, H., Gao, L., Mao, J., Liu, J., et al. (2015). Tanshinone IIA Ameliorates Bleomycin-Induced Pulmonary Fibrosis and Inhibits Transforming Growth Factor-beta-β-dependent Epithelial to Mesenchymal Transition. *J. Surg. Res.* 197, 167–175. doi:10.1016/j.jss.2015.02.062

Tanigawa, S., Fujii, M., and Hou, D. X. (2007). Action of Nrf2 and Keap1 in ARE-Mediated NQO1 Expression by Quercetin. *Free Radic. Biol. Med.* 42, 1690–1703. doi:10.1016/j.freeradbiomed.2007.02.017

Taniguchi, H., Ebina, M., Kondoh, Y., Ogura, T., Azuma, A., Suga, M., et al. (2010). Pirfenidone in Idiopathic Pulmonary Fibrosis. *Eur. Respir. J.* 35, 821–829. doi:10.1183/09031936.00005209

Taslidere, E., Esrefoglu, M., Elbe, H., Cetin, A., and Ates, B. (2014). Protective Effects of Melatonin and Quercetin on Experimental Lung Injury Induced by Carbon Tetrachloride in Rats. *Exp. Lung Res.* 40, 59–65. doi:10.3109/01902148.2013.866181

Tavares, J. L., Wangoo, A., Dilworth, P., Marshall, B., Kotecha, S., and Shaw, R. J. (1997). Thalidomide Reduces Tumour Necrosis Factor-Alpha Production by Human Alveolar Macrophages. *Respir. Med.* 91, 31–39. doi:10.1016/s0954-6111(97)90134-7

ten Freyhaus, H., Huntgeburth, M., Wingler, K., Schnitker, J., Bäumer, A. T., Vantler, M., et al. (2006). Novel Nox Inhibitor VAS2870 Attenuates PDGF-dependent Smooth Muscle Cell Chemotaxis, but Not Proliferation. *Cardiovasc. Res.* 71, 331–341. doi:10.1016/j.cardiores.2006.01.022

Teng, R. J., Du, J., Welak, S., Guan, T., Eis, A., Shi, Y., et al. (2012). Cross Talk between NADPH Oxidase and Autophagy in Pulmonary Artery Endothelial Cells with Intrauterine Persistent Pulmonary Hypertension. *Am. J. Physiol. Lung Cell Mol Physiol* 302, L651–L663. doi:10.1152/ajplung.00177.2011

Thannickal, V. J., Lee, D. Y., White, E. S., Cui, Z., Larios, J. M., Chacon, R., et al. (2003). Myofibroblast Differentiation by Transforming Growth Factor-Beta1 Is Dependent on Cell Adhesion and Integrin Signaling via Focal Adhesion Kinase. *J. Biol. Chem.* 278, 12384–12389. doi:10.1074/jbc.M208544200

Thomas, D. D., Ridnour, L. A., Isenberg, J. S., Flores-Santana, W., Switzer, C. H., Donzelli, S., et al. (2008). The Chemical Biology of Nitric Oxide: Implications in Cellular Signaling. *Free Radic. Biol. Med.* 45, 18–31. doi:10.1016/j.freeradbiomed.2008.03.020

Thresiamma, K. C., George, J., and Kuttan, R. (1998). Protective Effect of Curcumin, Ellagic Acid and Bixin on Radiation Induced Genotoxicity. *J. Exp. Clin. Cancer Res.* 17, 431–434.

Tian, X. L., Yao, W., Guo, Z. J., Gu, L., and Zhu, Y. J. (2006). Low Dose Pirfenidone Suppresses Transforming Growth Factor Beta-1 and Tissue Inhibitor of Metalloproteinase-1, and Protects Rats from Lung Fibrosis Induced by Bleomycina. *Chin Med. Sci. J.* 21, 145–151.

Tomé-Carneiro, J., Larrosa, M., González-Sarrías, A., Tomás-Barberán, F., García-Conesa, M., and Espín, J. (2013). Resveratrol and Clinical Trials: The Crossroad from *In Vitro* Studies to Human Evidence. *Cpd* 19, 6064–6093. doi:10.2174/13816128113199990407

Tsai, M. J., Chang, W. A., Liao, S. H., Chang, K. F., Sheu, C. C., and Kuo, P. L. (2019). The Effects of Epigallocatechin Gallate (EGCG) on Pulmonary Fibroblasts of Idiopathic Pulmonary Fibrosis (IPF)-A Next-Generation Sequencing and Bioinformatic Approach. *Int. J. Mol. Sci.* 20, 1958. doi:10.3390/ijms20081958

Veith, C., Drent, M., Bast, A., van Schooten, F. J., and Boots, A. W. (2017). The Disturbed Redox-Balance in Pulmonary Fibrosis Is Modulated by the Plant Flavonoid Quercetin. *Toxicol. Appl. Pharmacol.* 336, 40–48. doi:10.1016/j.taap.2017.10.001

Venkatadri, R., Iyer, A. K., Ramesh, V., Wright, C., Castro, C. A., Yakisich, J. S., et al. (2017). MnTBAP Inhibits Bleomycin-Induced Pulmonary Fibrosis by Regulating VEGF and Wnt Signaling. *J. Cell Physiol* 232, 506–516. doi:10.1002/jcp.25608

Verma, R., Kushwah, L., Gohel, D., Patel, M., Marvania, T., and Balakrishnan, S. (2013). Evaluating the Ameliorative Potential of Quercetin against the Bleomycin-Induced Pulmonary Fibrosis in Wistar Rats. *Pulm. Med.* 2013, 921724. doi:10.1155/2013/921724

Virdis, A., Gesi, M., and Taddei, S. (2016). Impact of Apocynin on Vascular Disease in Hypertension. *Vascul Pharmacol.* 87, 1–5. doi:10.1016/j.vph.2016.08.006

Vriend, J., and Reiter, R. J. (2015). Melatonin Feedback on Clock Genes: a Theory Involving the Proteasome. *J. Pineal Res.* 58, 1–11. doi:10.1111/jpi.12189

Vujaskovic, Z., Batinic-Haberle, I., Rabbani, Z. N., Feng, Q. F., Kang, S. K., Spasojevic, I., et al. (2002). A Small Molecular Weight Catalytic Metalloporphyrin Antioxidant with Superoxide Dismutase (SOD) Mimetic Properties Protects Lungs from Radiation-Induced Injury. *Free Radic. Biol. Med.* 33, 857–863. doi:10.1016/s0891-5849(02)00980-2

Vuorinen, K., Ohlmeier, S., Leppäranta, O., Salmenkivi, K., Myllärniemi, M., and Kinnula, V. L. (2008). Peroxiredoxin II Expression and its Association with Oxidative Stress and Cell Proliferation in Human Idiopathic Pulmonary Fibrosis. *J. Histochem. Cytochem.* 56, 951–959. doi:10.1369/jhc.2008.951806

Waghray, M., Cui, Z., Horowitz, J. C., Subramanian, I. M., Martinez, F. J., Toews, G. B., et al. (2005). Hydrogen Peroxide Is a Diffusible Paracrine Signal for the Induction of Epithelial Cell Death by Activated Myofibroblasts. *FASEB j.* 19, 1–16. doi:10.1096/fj.04-2882fje

Walters, D. M., Cho, H. Y., and Kleeberger, S. R. (2008). Oxidative Stress and Antioxidants in the Pathogenesis of Pulmonary Fibrosis: a Potential Role for Nrf2. *Antioxid. Redox Signal* 10, 321–332. doi:10.1089/ars.2007.1901

Wan, W. Y., Hollins, F., Haste, L., Woodman, L., Hirst, R. A., Bolton, S., et al. (2016). NADPH Oxidase-4 Overexpression Is Associated with Epithelial Ciliary Dysfunction in Neutrophilic Asthma. *Chest* 149, 1445–1459. doi:10.1016/j.chest.2016.01.024

Wang, C. M., He, Q. Z., and Zhang, R. X. (1994). Effects of Tanshionone to Bleomycin Induced Pulmonary Fibrosis of Rats on Histological Changes and Production of Lipid Peroxides and Hydroxyproline. *Zhonghua Jie He He Hu Xi Za Zhi* 17, 308320–320.

Wang, J., He, F., Chen, L., Li, Q., Jin, S., Zheng, H., et al. (2018). Resveratrol Inhibits Pulmonary Fibrosis by Regulating miR-21 through MAPK/AP-1 Pathways. *Biomed. Pharmacother.* 105, 37–44. doi:10.1016/j.biopha.2018.05.104

Wang, L., Li, S., Yao, Y., Yin, W., and Ye, T. (2021). The Role of Natural Products in the Prevention and Treatment of Pulmonary Fibrosis: a Review. *Food Funct.* 12, 990–1007. doi:10.1039/D0FO03001E

Wang, Q., Zhu, H., Zhou, W. G., Guo, X. C., Wu, M. J., Xu, Z. Y., et al. (2013). N-acetylcysteine-pretreated Human Embryonic Mesenchymal Stem Cell

Administration Protects against Bleomycin-Induced Lung Injury. *Am. J. Med. Sci.* 346, 113–122. doi:10.1097/MAJ.0b013e318266e8d8

Wang, X. (2009). The Antiapoptotic Activity of Melatonin in Neurodegenerative Diseases. *CNS Neurosci. Ther.* 15, 345–357. doi:10.1111/j.1755-5949.2009.00105.x

Watchorn, T., Mulier, B., and MacNee, W. (1998). Does Increasingintracellular Glutathione Inhibit Cytokine-Induced Nitric Oxide Release and NF-kB Activation. *Am J Respir Crit Care Med*, 157, A889.

Wei, Y., Dong, W., Jackson, J., Ho, T. C., Le Saux, C. J., Brumwell, A., et al. (2021). Blocking LOXL2 and TGFβ1 Signalling Induces Collagen I Turnover in Precision-Cut Lung Slices Derived from Patients with Idiopathic Pulmonary Fibrosis. *Thorax* 76, 729–732. doi:10.1136/thoraxjnl-2020-215745

Wingler, K., Altenhoefer, S. A., Kleikers, P. W., Radermacher, K. A., Kleinschnitz, C., and Schmidt, H. H. (2012). VAS2870 Is a Pan-NADPH Oxidase Inhibitor. *Cell Mol Life Sci* 69, 3159–3160. doi:10.1007/s00018-012-1107-1

Wu, H., Li, Y., Wang, Y., Xu, D., Li, C., Liu, M., et al. (2014). Tanshinone IIA Attenuates Bleomycin-Induced Pulmonary Fibrosis via Modulating Angiotensin-Converting Enzyme 2/Angiotensin-(1-7) axis in Rats. *Int. J. Med. Sci.* 11, 578–586. doi:10.7150/ijms.8365

Wu, Y., Liu, L., Zhang, J., Huang, L., Huang, S., and He, J. (2020). Thalidomide Inhibits the Gene Promoter of Connective Tissue Growth Factor in Human Embryonic Lung Fibroblasts. *Ann. Palliat. Med.* 9, 2516–2523. doi:10.21037/apm-19-398

Xiao, Z., Liu, W., Mu, Y. P., Zhang, H., Wang, X. N., Zhao, C. Q., et al. (2020). Pharmacological Effects of Salvianolic Acid B against Oxidative Damage. *Front Pharmacol.* 11, 572373. doi:10.3389/fphar.2020.572373

Xu, M., Deng, B., Chow, Y. L., Zhao, Z. Z., and Hu, B. (2007). Effects of Curcumin in Treatment of Experimental Pulmonary Fibrosis: a Comparison with Hydrocortisone. *J. Ethnopharmacol* 112, 292–299. doi:10.1016/j.jep.2007.03.011

Yan, B., Ma, Z., Shi, S., Hu, Y., Ma, T., Rong, G., et al. (2017). Sulforaphane Prevents Bleomycin-induced P-ulmonary F-ibrosis in M-ice by I-nhibiting O-xidative S-tress via N-uclear F-actor E-rythroid 2-related F-actor-2 A-ctivation. *Mol. Med. Rep.* 15, 4005–4014. doi:10.3892/mmr.2017.6546

Ye, Q., Chen, B., Tong, Z., Nakamura, S., Sarria, R., Costabel, U., et al. (2006). Thalidomide Reduces IL-18, IL-8 and TNF-Alpha Release from Alveolar Macrophages in Interstitial Lung Disease. *Eur. Respir. J.* 28, 824–831. doi:10.1183/09031936.06.00131505

Yildirim, Z., Kotuk, M., Erdogan, H., Iraz, M., Yagmurca, M., Kuku, I., et al. (2006). Preventive Effect of Melatonin on Bleomycin-Induced Lung Fibrosis in Rats. *J. Pineal Res.* 40, 27–33. doi:10.1111/j.1600-079X.2005.00272.x

Yoon, Y. S., Lee, J. H., Hwang, S. C., Choi, K. S., and Yoon, G. (2005). TGF Beta1 Induces Prolonged Mitochondrial ROS Generation through Decreased Complex IV Activity with Senescent Arrest in Mv1Lu Cells. *Oncogene* 24, 1895–1903. doi:10.1038/sj.onc.1208262

You, H., Wei, L., Sun, W. L., Wang, L., Yang, Z. L., Liu, Y., et al. (2014). The green tea Extract Epigallocatechin-3-Gallate Inhibits Irradiation-Induced Pulmonary Fibrosis in Adult Rats. *Int. J. Mol. Med.* 34, 92–102. doi:10.3892/ijmm.2014.1745

Yu, N., Sun, Y. T., Su, X. M., He, M., Dai, B., and Kang, J. (2016). Melatonin Attenuates TGFβ1-Induced Epithelial-Mesenchymal Transition in Lung Alveolar Epithelial Cells. *Mol. Med. Rep.* 14, 5567–5572. doi:10.3892/mmr.2016.5950

Zaghloul, M. S., Said, E., Suddek, G. M., and Salem, H. A. (2019). Crocin Attenuates Lung Inflammation and Pulmonary Vascular Dysfunction in a Rat Model of Bleomycin-Induced Pulmonary Fibrosis. *Life Sci.* 235, 116794. doi:10.1016/j.lfs.2019.116794

Zeidler, P., Hubbs, A., Battelli, L., and Castranova, V. (2004). Role of Inducible Nitric Oxide Synthase-Derived Nitric Oxide in Silica-Induced Pulmonary Inflammation and Fibrosis. *J. Toxicol. Environ. Health A.* 67, 1001–1026. doi:10.1080/15287390490447296

Zhang, B., Safa, R., Rusciano, D., and Osborne, N. N. (2007a). Epigallocatechin Gallate, an Active Ingredient from green tea, Attenuates Damaging Influences to the Retina Caused by Ischemia/reperfusion. *Brain Res.* 1159, 40–53. doi:10.1016/j.brainres.2007.05.029

Zhang, D. P., Qiu, H., Zhuang, Y., and Meng, F. Q. (2007b). The Effect of Curcumin on Bleomycin-Induced Pulmonary Fibrosis in Rats. *Zhonghua Jie He He Hu Xi Za Zhi* 30, 197–201.

Zhang, H., Yang, Y., Wang, Y., Wang, B., and Li, R. (2018a). Renal-protective Effect of Thalidomide in Streptozotocin-Induced Diabetic Rats through Anti-inflammatory Pathway. *Drug Des. Devel Ther.* 12, 89–98. doi:10.2147/DDDT.S149298

Zhang, H., Yin, G., Jiang, H., and Zhang, C. (2013). High-dose N-Acetylcysteine Decreases Silica-Induced Lung Fibrosis in the Rat. *J. Int. Med. Res.* 41, 1179–1186. doi:10.1177/0300060513488503

Zhang, H. S., and Wang, S. Q. (2007). Nrf2 Is Involved in the Effect of Tanshinone IIA on Intracellular Redox Status in Human Aortic Smooth Muscle Cells. *Biochem. Pharmacol.* 73, 1358–1366. doi:10.1016/j.bcp.2007.01.004

Zhang, L., He, Y. L., Li, Q. Z., Hao, X. H., Zhang, Z. F., Yuan, J. X., et al. (2014a). N-acetylcysteine Alleviated Silica-Induced Lung Fibrosis in Rats by Down-Regulation of ROS and Mitochondrial Apoptosis Signaling. *Toxicol. Mech. Methods* 24, 212–219. doi:10.3109/15376516.2013.879974

Zhang, M., Cao, S. R., Zhang, R., Jin, J. L., and Zhu, Y. F. (2014b). The Inhibitory Effect of Salvianolic Acid B on TGF-B1-Induced Proliferation and Differentiation in Lung Fibroblasts. *Exp. Lung Res.* 40, 172–185. doi:10.3109/01902148.2014.895070

Zhang, M., Feng, Z. S., and Deng, Z. T. (2011). Effect of Salvianolic Acid B on TGF-Beta1-Induced Human Embryonic Lung Fibroblast's Biological Behavior. *Zhongguo Zhong Xi Yi Jie He Za Zhi* 31, 1401–1404.

Zhang, T., Liu, M., Gao, Y., Li, H., Song, L., Hou, H., et al. (2021). Salvianolic Acid B Inhalation Solution Enhances Antifibrotic and Anticoagulant Effects in a Rat Model of Pulmonary Fibrosis. *Biomed. Pharmacother.* 138, 111475. doi:10.1016/j.biopha.2021.111475

Zhang, X., Cai, Y., Zhang, W., and Chen, X. (2018c). Quercetin Ameliorates Pulmonary Fibrosis by Inhibiting SphK1/S1P Signaling. *Biochem. Cell Biol* 96, 742–751. doi:10.1139/bcb-2017-0302

Zhang, X. R., Zhou, W. X., and Zhang, Y. X. (2018b). Improvements in SOD Mimic AEOL-10150, a Potent Broad-Spectrum Antioxidant. *Mil. Med. Res.* 5, 30. doi:10.1186/s40779-018-0176-3

Zhang, Y. Q., Liu, Y. J., Mao, Y. F., Dong, W W., Zhu, X. Y., and Jiang, L. (2015). Resveratrol Ameliorates Lipopolysaccharide-Induced Epithelial Mesenchymal Transition and Pulmonary Fibrosis through Suppression of Oxidative Stress and Transforming Growth Factor-B1 Signaling. *Clin. Nutr.* 34, 752–760. doi:10.1016/j.clnu.2014.08.014

Zhang, Z., Qu, J., Zheng, C., Zhang, P., Zhou, W., Cui, W., et al. (2018d). Nrf2 Antioxidant Pathway Suppresses Numb-Mediated Epithelial-Mesenchymal Transition during Pulmonary Fibrosis. *Cell Death Dis* 9, 83. doi:10.1038/s41419-017-0198-x

Zhao, C. J., Niu, J. Z., Wang, J. F., Zhou, G., and Tang, B. H. (2008). Effects of Curcumin on Bleomycin-Induced Damages in Pulmonary Functions in Rats. *Zhongguo Zhong Yao Za Zhi* 33, 1434–1438.

Zhao, H., Wu, Q. Q., Cao, L. F, Qing, H. Y., Zhang, C., Chen, Y. H., et al. (2014). Melatonin Inhibits Endoplasmic Reticulum Stress and Epithelial-Mesenchymal Transition during Bleomycin-Induced Pulmonary Fibrosis in Mice. *PLoS One* 9, e97266. doi:10.1371/journal.pone.0097266

Zhao, X., Sun, J., Su, W., Shan, H., Zhang, B., Wang, Y., et al. (2018). Melatonin Protects against Lung Fibrosis by Regulating the Hippo/YAP Pathway. *Int. J. Mol. Sci.* 19, 1118. doi:10.3390/ijms19041118

Zheng, Q., Tong, M., Ou, B., Liu, C., Hu, C, and Yang, Y. (2019). Isorhamnetin Protects against Bleomycin-Induced Pulmonary Fibrosis by Inhibiting Endoplasmic Reticulum Stress and Epithelial-Mesenchymal Transition. *Int. J. Mol. Med.* 43, 117–126. doi:10.3892/ijmm.2018.3965

Zhou, G., Niu, J. Z., Wang, J. F., Chen, W. T., Liu, T. X., Li, Y. S., et al. (2006a). Experimental Study on Effect of Curcumin on Inhibiting Injury of Free Radical in Pulmonary Fibrosis Rats. *Zhongguo Zhong Yao Za Zhi* 31, 669–672.

Zhou, G., Wang, J. F., Niu, J. Z., Lu, Y. S., Chen, W. T., Li, Z. H., et al. (2006b). Experimental Study on Protective Effects of Curcumin on Exaggerated Extracellular Matrix Accumulation of Pulmonary Fibrosis Rats. *Zhongguo Zhong Yao Za Zhi* 31, 570–573.

Zhou, H., Beevers, C. S., and Huang, S. (2011). The Targets of Curcumin. *Curr. Drug Targets* 12, 332–347. doi:10.2174/138945011794815356

Zhou, W., Mo, X., Cui, W., Zhang, Z., Li, D., Li, L., et al. (2016). Nrf2 Inhibits Epithelial-Mesenchymal Transition by Suppressing Snail Expression during Pulmonary Fibrosis. *Sci. Rep.* 6, 38646. doi:10.1038/srep38646

Zhu, X.-d., Lei, X.-p., and Dong, W.-b. (2017). Resveratrol as a Potential Therapeutic Drug for Respiratory System Diseases. *Dddt* 11, 3591–3598. doi:10.2147/DDDT.S148868

Zhu, Z., Li, Q., Xu, C., Zhao, J., Li, S., Wang, Y., et al. (2020). Sodium Tanshinone IIA Sulfonate Attenuates Silica-Induced Pulmonary Fibrosis in Rats via Activation of the Nrf2 and Thioredoxin System. *Environ. Toxicol. Pharmacol.* 80, 103461. doi:10.1016/j.etap.2020.103461

Zhu, Z., Wang, Y., Liang, D., Yang, G., Chen, L., Niu, P., et al. (2016). Sodium Tanshinone IIA Sulfonate Suppresses Pulmonary Fibroblast Proliferation and Activation Induced by Silica: Role of the Nrf2/Trx Pathway. *Toxicol. Res. (Camb)* 5, 116–125. doi:10.1039/c5tx00291e

5

The Interaction between Pulmonary Fibrosis and COVID-19 and the Application of Related Anti-Fibrotic Drugs

Hao Shen[1,2†], Nu Zhang[3†], Yuqing Liu[4], Xuerong Yang[1,2], Yuanyuan He[1,2], Qi Li[1,2], Xiaoyan Shen[1,2], Yulian Zhu[5] and Yong Yang[1,2]**

[1]Department of Pharmacy, Sichuan Academy of Medical Sciences and Sichuan Provincial People's Hospital, School of Medicine, University of Electronic Science and Technology of China, Chengdu, China, [2]Personalized Drug Therapy Key Laboratory of Sichuan Province, School of Medicine, University of Electronic Science and Technology of China, Chengdu, China, [3]Department of Pharmacy, People's Hospital of Fushun County, Fushun, China, [4]School of Basic Medicine and Clinical Pharmacy, China Pharmaceutical University, Nanjing, China, [5]Department of Pharmacy, Ziyang People's Hospital, Ziyang, China

***Correspondence:**
Yulian Zhu
1054507078@qq.com
Yong Yang
yyxpower@163.com

†These authors have contributed equally to this work

COVID-19 is a highly contagious respiratory disease, which mainly affects the lungs. Critically ill patients are easily complicated by cytokine storms, acute respiratory distress syndrome (ARDS), and respiratory failure, which seriously threaten their lives. Pulmonary fibrosis (PF) is a common interstitial lung disease, and its pathogenesis may involve the participation of a variety of immune cells and inflammatory factors. Current studies have shown that patients with COVID-19 may be complicated by pulmonary fibrosis, and patients with pulmonary fibrosis may also be at higher risk of contracting COVID-19 than healthy people. Pulmonary fibrosis is an important risk factor leading to the aggravation of COVID-19 disease. COVID-19 complicated by cytokine storm and ARDS mechanism pathways are similar to the pathogenesis of pulmonary fibrosis. The potential interaction between pulmonary fibrosis and COVID-19 can cause acute exacerbation of the patient's condition, but the potential mechanism between the two has not been fully elucidated. Most of the drug treatment programs for COVID-19-related pulmonary fibrosis are currently formulated about the relevant guidelines for idiopathic pulmonary fibrosis (IPF), and there is no clear drug treatment program recommendation. This article aims to summarize the relevant mechanism pathways of COVID-19 and pulmonary fibrosis, explore the interrelationships and possible mechanisms, and discuss the value and risks of existing and potential COVID-19-related pulmonary fibrosis treatment drugs, to provide reference for anti-fibrosis treatment for patients.

Keywords: pulmonary fibrosis, COVID-19, mechanism, interaction, drug, treatment

INTRODUCTION

Severe Acute Respiratory Syndrome Coronavirus type 2 (SARS-COV-2) belongs to the coronavirus subfamily, named coronavirus disease 2019 by the World Health Organization. It is more infectious than Severe Acute respiratory syndrome (SARS) and Middle East Respiratory Syndrome (MERS). Unfortunately, it first broke out in Wuhan, China, in December 2019. Patients infected with SARS-COV-2 may be asymptomatic or present with severe symptoms such as acute respiratory distress syndrome (ARDS) and pulmonary fibrosis. Pulmonary fibrosis (PF) is a common interstitial lung disease, and its pathogenesis may involve the joint participation of various immune cells and inflammatory factors. It is characterized by excessive deposition of extracellular matrix (ECM) in the lung interstitium, which destroys typical parenchymal structure and leads to progressive loss of lung function. Of these, idiopathic pulmonary fibrosis (IPF) is the most common the most severe form, with a median survival of only 2–3 years for untreated patients (Sharif, 2017). The risk factors of idiopathic pulmonary fibrosis and COVID-19 have a lot in common, such as age, sex, smoking history, hypertension, diabetes, obesity, and so on (Li HH. et al., 2021). Both diseases start from lung injury. COVID-19 can lead to more severe ARDS, while IPF usually progresses slowly, and the incidence is hidden.

According to an international multicenter study, the survival rate of hospitalized patients for COVID-19 complicated with idiopathic pulmonary fibrosis or non-idiopathic pulmonary fibrosis was significantly lower than that of patients without pulmonary fibrosis, that is, patients with Interstitial lung diseases (ILD), especially those with fibrotic ILD, faced a higher risk of death after infection with COVID-19 (Drake et al., 2020). A cohort study, which brought into 8,256,161 COVID-19 patients with respiratory diseases, proposed that compared with patients without respiratory diseases, patients with respiratory diseases had a higher risk of hospitalization due to new corona pneumonia (Aveyard et al., 2021). And COVID-19 and IPF have similar risk factors (George et al., 2020). It means that pulmonary fibrosis may be associated with the occurrence of severe COVID-19. COVID-19 Patients with idiopathic pulmonary fibrosis may have a poor prognosis and high mortality.

All ILD, especially IPF, is characterized by acute exacerbation. The pathobiology of acute exacerbation of IPF may be related to inherent defects, an internal acceleration of potential fibrotic conditions, or a response to hidden external events leading to acute lung injury (ALI) and histopathological diffuse alveolar injury (DAD), which make the lungs of IPF patients more vulnerable to external injury than non-IPF. And respiratory failure caused by an acute exacerbation of IPF is related to higher hospital mortality, more than 50% in most cases (Collard et al., 2016). A comparative study in Shanghai (Weng et al., 2019) found that inflammatory cytokines (IL-6, IFN-γ, MIG, IL-17, and IL-9), which play a crucial role in anti-infective responses, were significantly higher in acute exacerbation of IPF than in stable IPF and control groups. And the experimental data showed that the ratio of serum LGM and neutrophils in patients with acute exacerbation of IPF were significantly higher than those with stable IPF. It means that the acute phase of IPF can be triggered by viral infections and greatly enhanced anti-infective immune responses. The COVID-19 Pneumonia and PF are serious diseases characterized by lung injury and repair (Jenkins, 2020). Infection, which is one of the critical causes of ALI, can also cause acute exacerbation of IPF (Weng et al., 2019). Therefore, COVID-19 infection may lead to ALI, accelerate the occurrence of PF, and acute exacerbation of IPF, which may eventually lead to respiratory failure and death. A pre-discharge study of patients with COVID-19 infection suggested that hospitalized COVID-19 patients with basic pulmonary fibrosis diseases may increase their tolerance to low oxygen saturation of the blood (SpO_2) compared with those without basic pulmonary fibrosis diseases in the absence of subjective dyspnea (Fuglebjerg et al., 2020). It may lead to more unobvious clinical symptoms in COVID-19 patients with PF than those without, and miss the best time to rescue. In general, COVID-19 infection may aggravate PF and increase the risk of death in patients with that.

Therefore, according to various clinical studies, patients with IPF are at high risk of dying from COVID-19, which may lead to the development of pulmonary fibrosis through either virus-induced ALI or cytokine-mediated alveolar damage (Jenkins, 2020). The purpose of this paper is to summarize relevant studies in the existing literature and provide a treatment basis for patients with comorbidity of COVID-19 and IPF.

The Interaction Mechanism Between COVID-19 and Pulmonary Fibrosis

The Route of Infection of SARS-COV-2

Angiotensin converting enzyme 2 (ACE2) is a zinc metalloproteinase, belonging to type I transmembrane protein, whose N-terminal domain-containing carboxypeptidase catalytic site is extracellular and C-terminal tail is intracellular (Donoghue et al., 2000). Spike "S" protein is an exogenous protein expressed in novel Coronavirus and is the key site of virus infection (Huang et al., 2020). When SARS-CoV-2 infects the host cell, its spike "S" protein completes the adsorption process by binding to ACE2 on the host cell, and another cytokine serine protease TMPRSS2 is used to initiate spike "S" protein, both of which eventually lead to the virus invading the target cell (Hoffmann et al., 2020). After entering the cell, the virus unshells, biosynthesizes, assembles, and releases in the cell, eventually causing the host cell to rupture and die. ACE2 gene was widely expressed, including alveolar, trachea, and bronchial epithelial cells, with the highest expression in nasal luminal epithelial cells and decreased expression throughout the lower respiratory tract. Interestingly, this decline parallels a significant decrease in the gradient of SARS-COV-2 infection from upper to lower respiratory tract epithelial cells (Hoffmann et al., 2020; Hou et al., 2020). This creates favorable conditions for the adsorption and invasion of SARS-CoV-2. One of the physiological functions of ACE2 is to convert angiotensin II (Ang II) into angiotensin 1–7 (Ang 1-7), which plays an essential role in controlling cardiovascular and blood pressure (Donoghue et al., 2000). Importantly, Ang II has a fibrotic effect by upregulating the level of pro-fibrosis cytokine transforming growth factor-β1 (TGF-β1), which is involved in transforming fibroblasts into myofibroblasts and extensive collagen deposition (Haulica et al., 2004). However, Ang 1-7 exerts vasodilation, reduces cytokine secretion, inflammation, cardiopulmonary protection, and anti-fibrosis by binding to Mas receptors (Shenoy et al., 2010; He and Garmire, 2020; Sanchis-Gomar et al., 2020). In general, the high affinity of the spike "S" protein on the SARS-CoV-2 envelope to the ACE2 receptor can down-regulate the level of ACE2, increase the level of Ang II and decrease the level of Ang1-7, thus promoting inflammation and pulmonary fibrosis.

Given the difficulty in controlling the high infectivity of SARS-COV-2, we have to suspect that other pathways may infect SARS-COV-2 *in vitro* besides ACE2. CD147, a type II transmembrane protein, is associated with SARS-COV-2 infection (Aguiar et al., 2020; Wang et al., 2020). Wang et al. (2020) showed an interaction between CD147 and the spike "S" protein of SARS-COV-2. They blocked CD147 by CD147 antibody, and the results showed that the amplification of SARS-COV-2 could be inhibited. Thus, they revealed a new viral entry pathway, the CD147-spike protein pathway. Studies have confirmed that, in addition to ACE2 and CD147, SARS-CoV-2 can enter host cells by binding to some other receptors. Recent research hotspots include Cathepsin L1 (Aguiar et al., 2020), integrins αvβ3 and αvβ6 (Calver et al., 2021), and even low-density lipoprotein receptor class A domain containing 3 (LDLRAD3) and C-type lectin domain family 4 member G (CLEC4G) (Zhu et al., 2021). The pathologic consequences of SARS-COV-2 binding to these receptors are uncertain. Still, the effects may greatly contribute to the progression of viral infection and disease, making treatment more difficult.

The Status Quo of IPF

A survey covering 22 studies in 12 countries estimated the incidence and prevalence of IPF at 0.09–1.30 and 0.33–4.51 per population, respectively (Maher et al., 2021). The occurrence and development of IPF are closely related to aging, genetic background (premature shortening of leukocyte telomere), and epigenetic modification (Fraga et al., 2005; Yang et al., 2019; Duckworth et al., 2021). It is highly correlated with a variety of external factors, including smoking, air pollution, microaspiration, and viral infection, which can lead to repeated damage and repair of alveolar cells (Baccarelli et al., 2009; Launay et al., 2009; Wootton et al., 2011) In the susceptibility stage of pulmonary fibrosis, gene mutations or mutations, epithelial cell replacement lead to telomere shortening, and environmental factors eventually lead to epithelial cell dysfunction (Nunes, 2003). In the initiation stage, molecular mediators of epithelial cell dysfunction such as ER stress; excessive transforming growth factor-β (TGF-β) activation; and growth factor, chemokine, or Wnt secretion lead to EMT, fibrocyte recruitment, and fibroblast differentiation (Nunes, 2003). These molecular mediators will lead to progressive stages in which pathological mesenchymal cells release abnormal types and amounts of stromal proteins that reshape the lung and form scar lung (Nunes, 2003).

COVID-19 Secondary Pulmonary Fibrosis

Multiple Shreds of Evidences of Pulmonary Fibrosis Secondary to COVID-19

A number of studies have directly or indirectly proved that patients infected with SARS-CoV-2 would develop pulmonary fibrosis. CT scans of patients infected with COVID-19 show ground glass shadows that are prone to progression to patchy fibrosis (Ojha et al., 2020). Fibrotic changes in the lungs were found in the autopsy of patients who died of COVID-19 (Liu et al., 2020; Yao et al., 2020). In addition, the factors involved in pulmonary fibrosis such as TGF-β, interleukin-6 (IL-6), and tumor necrosis factor-α (TNF-α) were increased in patients infected with COVID-19. In addition, a meta-analysis of more than 50,000 hospitalized COVID-19 patients showed that the incidence of ARDS was 14.8% (Sun et al., 2020). And more importantly, ARDS patients were very prone to pulmonary fibrosis. Mechanical ventilation, an essential treatment during ARDS, promotes direct penetration of high concentrations of SARS-COV-2 into the lower respiratory tract, potentially causing acute lung injury. Perhaps the underlying mechanisms are epithelial-to-mesenchymal transformation (EMT), changes in cell morphology, and the release of pro-fibrotic mediators such as TGF-β(Gaikwad et al., 2020).

Mechanisms of Pulmonary Fibrosis in COVID-19

The abnormal immune system can lead to cytokine storm, resulting in increase plasma concentrations of interleukin 1β, 2, 7, and 10, monocyte chemotactic protein 1, granulocyte-colony stimulating factor, macrophage inflammatory protein 1α, interferon -γ -inducible protein 10 (IP-10), and TNF-α(Hui and Zumla, 2019; Huang et al., 2020; Li et al., 2020). It has been identified that galectin-3 (Gal3) expressed by macrophages, epithelial and alveolar cells in the lung plays a key role in the pro-inflammatory response of microglia (Reyfman et al., 2019). Gal3 binds to and activates TREM2 and TLR4 (Burguillos et al., 2015; Boza-Serrano et al., 2019), both of which have been associated with pulmonary disease, including fibrosis.

Cytokine storm is considered an important factor in accelerating disease progression, leading to severe illness and death. It is one of the main causes of ARDS and multiple organ failure (Chousterman et al., 2017). Due to the abnormal release of matrix metalloproteinases during ARDS, not only the epithelium and endothelium are severely damaged, but also the ECM cross-linking is enhanced, resulting in the change of the structure and composition of interstitial ECM in pulmonary fibrosis (Zemans et al., 2009; Nkyimbeng et al., 2013; Craig et al., 2015; Philp et al., 2018). When alveolar epithelial cells are injured, type II alveolar epithelial cells (ATII cells) proliferate and differentiate into I alveolar cells (ATI cells) to repair the damaged alveoli (Aspal and Zemans, 2020). The evidence supports that the aging and loss of ATII cells are involved in the pathogenesis of IPF(Sisson et al., 2010; Yao et al., 2021). Then, there is reason, to suspect that ATII is also highly associated with fibrosis in virus-infected patients. In addition, alveolar epithelial cells can secrete a series of inflammatory factors, soluble mediators, and remodeling factors, which are closely related to the process of IPF. For example, TGF-β, a factor that stimulates the formation of pulmonary fibrosis, can be activated by the cell membrane integrin of epithelial cells (Jenkins et al., 2006; Tatler and Jenkins, 2012). TGF-β acts on the mesenchymal cells, leading to proliferation and differentiation of fibroblasts into contractile myofibroblasts, and thus causing abnormal production and deposition of extracellular matrix proteins in fibroblasts (Xu et al., 2003; Tatler et al., 2016; Sibinska et al., 2017).

Unfortunately, there is new evidence that SARS-COV-2 can bind to cell surface integrins αvβ3 and αvβ6, facilitating their internalization into lung epithelial cells, which in turn accelerates the activity of TGF-β(Calver et al., 2021). This troublesome activation mechanism seems to make the disease harder to control. Except for TGF-β, platelet-derived growth factor (PDGF), connective tissue growth factor (CTGF), interleukin-6 (IL-6), and other cytokines expression increase, also play a certain role in the fibrosis process (Antoniades et al., 1990; Crestani et al., 1994; Pan et al., 2001). Endothelial cells, when injured, transform to a mesenchymal state (EndMT), with an increase in abnormal types and amounts of mesenchymal protein secretion, and at the same time, matrix metalloproteinases degrade the basement membrane collagen that lies beneath the endothelial cells (Gaikwad et al., 2020). These physiological reactions will eventually lead to abnormal accumulation of fibroblasts and myofibroblasts, excessive deposition of matrix proteins in the interstitium of the lung. Then the structure and composition of lung interstitium were changed. Finally, lung tissue sclerosis leads to impaired physiological function and presents a series of clinical symptoms.

Risk Factors

When infected with the COVID-19, people may show different symptoms, ranging from asymptomatic to mild such as fever, cough, muscle soreness, or fatigue, and some may become severe like ARDS. Respectively, the proportion of severe and critical cases is as high as 14 and 5% (Wu and McGoogan, 2020). So it is very important to effectively identify the risk factors that promote the development of the disease. Studies have shown that age is an important factor in developing diseases and even death (Zhou et al., 2020; Zhang JJ. et al., 2021). In addition, some studies have shown that male and other chronic diseases, including hypertension, diabetes, obesity, cardiovascular and respiratory diseases, can be positive in the disease leading to exacerbation and death (Zhang J. et al., 2020; Ebinger et al., 2020; Sun et al., 2020). It's worth noting that pulmonary fibrosis plays an important role in the infection of COVID-19.

Predictive Factors of Pulmonary Fibrosis Secondary to COVID-19

There have been many clinical studies on predictors of pulmonary fibrosis secondary to COVID-19. The focus of the study is mainly in two aspects: on the one hand, the level of cytokines including Krebs von den Lungen-6(KL-6), and on the other hand, the CT imaging features.

A growing number of studies support a significant correlation between elevated KL-6 levels and the development of pulmonary fibrosis (Crisan-Dabija et al., 2021; Peng et al., 2021; Xue et al., 2021). For example, a clinical study involving 289 COVID-19 patients finds that KL-6, which is rising earlier than the fibrotic-like change of CT imaging in the lungs, could predict not only the onset of pulmonary fibrosis, but also whether it was reversible (Xue et al., 2021). This is good for both clinicians and COVID-19 patients. However, not all COVID-19 patients have been found a significant association between KL-6 and pulmonary fibrosis. Early in the disease, when extensive lung injury occurs, repair mechanisms of pulmonary epithelial cell is synchronously activated which causing the elevated level of KL-6 (Major et al., 2020). Some studies find that KL-6 were not significantly elevated in some COVID-19 patients with secondary pulmonary fibrosis, possibly because the time when found the occurance of pulmonary fibrosis is later than the time when repair mechanisms was activated and KL-6 was released in large quantities (Xue et al., 2021). In addition, studies have shown that c-reactive protein (CRP), interleukin-6(IL-6), D-dimer and hepatic cytokines (HGF) and C-X-C motif chemokine 13 (CXCL13) are associated with the occurrence of pulmonary fibrosis in patients with COVID-19 (Francone et al., 2020; Yu et al., 2020; Perreau et al., 2021). A study identified two new specific monocyte subsets in patients with severe disease COVID-19:Mono 0 and Mono 5, showing pro-fibrotic and pro-inflammatory characteristics (Zhang Y. et al., 2021). Unfortunately, these studies are all implement in single-center with small sample. Follow-up evaluation of COVID-19 patients from multiple centers is needed to support this conclusion.

Due to inadequate predictive performance of cytokines, radiological assessment may be a method to assess the extent of lung damage caused by COVID-19 and predict the occurrence of pulmonary fibrosis. The features of CT imagine such as interstitial thickening, irregular interfacial, coarse reticular pattern and parenchymal band may be predictive factors of pulmonary fibrosis, and irregular interfacial and parenchymal band can predict the early formation of pulmonary fibrosis (Yu et al., 2020). Multivariable analysis identified age of greater than 50 years, heart rate greater than 100 beats per minute at admission, duration of hospital stay greater than or equal to 17 days, acute respiratory distress syndrome, noninvasive mechanical ventilation, and baseline lung severity score as independent predictors for fibrotic-like changes in the lung at 6 months (Caruso et al., 2021; Han et al., 2021). Similarly, these studies lack rigorous and high-quality evidence. So we can't make specific recommendations. But based on the above evidence, for patients with advanced age, severe illness, long hospitalization and high CT scores, we should strengthen follow-up after discharge, pay attention to the changes of lung function and carry out health education for them. In the future, more high-quality multi-center large sample data are needed to prove the reliability of these conclusions.

Whether IPF Patients Are More Susceptible to COVID-19

In recent years, great progress has been made in understanding the pathogenesis of pulmonary fibrosis. Factors like genetics, environmental and aging are involved in the initiation of the fibrosis process. Genome-wide studies have identified many genes associated with the development of IPF, including MUC5B, TERT, FAM13A, DSP, and AKAP13 (John et al., 2021).

Endothelial dysfunction is joint in the IPF, and in patients with pulmonary fibrosis, the level of vascular endothelial growth factor (VEGF) in bronchoalveolar lavage fluid (BALF) is reduced (Koyama et al., 2002). Evidence suggests that the patients with IPF may exhibit susceptibility to SARS-COV-2 due to immune-induced microvascular injury and endothelial cell necrosis (Magro et al., 2006).

Early studies have found that ACE2 is a protective protein that has a positive effect on physiological functions. The regulatory feedback axis composed of ACE2, its product Ang 1-7, and Ang 1-7 receptor plays an important role in pulmonary fibrosis (Li HH. et al., 2021).

Another study (Crisan-Dabija et al., 2020) showed a significant genetic association between IPF patients and elevated expression of AKAP13. This Rho guanine nucleotide exchange factor that regulates the activation of RhoA, which is a molecule that plays an important role in pro-fibrotic signaling pathways. The activation of RhoA drives the fibrotic phenotype, then promotes pulmonary fibrosis. In animal models (pulmonary artery endothelial cells) (Monaghan-Benson et al., 2018), activation of the RhoA/ROCK down-regulates the expression of ACE2, resulting in an imbalance of the renin-angiotensin system (RAS). SARS-COV-2 is known to bind and inhibit ACE2 protein through the affinity and efficiency of its S-spike protein. Given this, IPF patients may be at higher risk.

Studies on pulmonary fibrosis tissue from patients with IPF have shown an increased expression of ACE2 in fibroblasts (Aloufi et al., 2021; Li HH. et al., 2021), and fibroblasts have been identified to carry viral particles of SARS-COV-2 in COVID-19 patients. An *in vitro* study (Li HH. et al., 2021) found that ACE2 and TMPRSS2 were significantly upregulated in the fibroblasts of the IPF and co-expressed in fibroblast-specific protein 1(FSP-1)+ lung fibroblasts. The increased expression of ACE2 in fibroblasts may be related to the feedback regulation of cells. Still, its failure to play a protective role may be related to the activity of receptors, so more studies are needed to explore its specific regulatory mechanism. ACE2, as a protective factor, is widely believed to regulate cell inflammation and apoptosis. The strong affinity between SARS-COV-2 and ACE2 will lead to a decrease in ACE2, while the reduced lung function of IPF patients may increase the possibility of disease aggravation after infection. As for whether the patients with IPF are more sensitive to SARS-COV-2, further clinical studies are needed to find its possible mechanism.

POTENTIAL AGENTS FOR PULMONARY FIBROSIS ASSOCIATED WITH SARS-COV-2 INFECTION

Antiviral Agents

Coronavirus infection could directly promote pulmonary fibrosis. The nucleocapsid protein of Severe Acute Respiratory Syndrome Coronavirus type 1 (SARS-CoV-1) is reported to directly enhance TGF-β signaling, which could strongly promote fibrosis (Zhao et al., 2008). And the nucleocapsid protein of SARS-CoV-2 is over 90% similar to that of SARS-CoV-1 (Tilocca et al., 2020). Therefore, it is critical to reduce the viral load and thus the duration of viral pneumonia in order to prevent fibrosis. Remdesivir is a nucleotide analogue that could selectively block RNA polymerase, thus preventing viral replication. *In vitro* and animal models, remdesivir was found to be effective against SARS-CoV-1 and Middle East respiratory syndrome coronavirus (MERS-CoV). Due to its potential efficacy, the Food and Drug Administration (FDA) has granted remdesivir emergency use authorization for the treatment of COVID-19 (Singh et al., 2020). However, many clinical trials are still underway and its safety must be verified. In addition, the guanine nucleoside analogue ribavirin and the viral assembly inhibitor lopinavir/ritonavir are recommended by *The COVID-19 Diagnostic and Treatment Protocol (Trial Version 8)*, issued by the National Health Commission of the People's Republic of China. It is reported that lopinavir/ritonavir in combination with interferon-1β or ribavirin might be effective against coronaviruses (Arabi et al., 2020; Dhama et al., 2020). And the recommendation for ribavirin and lopinavir/ritonavir is mainly based on the experience in the treatment of SARS (Chu et al., 2004). The study by Yuan et al. also confirmed that virus-targeted antiviral drugs remdesivir, lopinavir and interferon antiviral drugs IFN-β, especially IFN-β 1b and IFN-β 1a, have strong inhibition effect on viral replication of SARS-COV-2 and significantly reduced viral load. EC50 of remdecivir, lopinavir, IFN-β 1b and IFN-β 1a were 1.04μM, 11.6μM, 31.2 IU/ml and 70.8 IU/ml, respectively (Yuan et al., 2020). Among 4000 COVID-19 patients in the Solidarity trial published by WHO, mortality ratios were 1.16 (95% CI, 0.96–1.39) in the IFN-β 1a plus ritonavir group and 1.12 (95% CI, 0.83–1.51) in the IFN-β 1a alone group (Consortium, 2021). The results showed no effect on mortality reduction of IFN-β 1a. A number of clinical studies have shown that the IFN-β 1b combination has potential value in clinical improvement time, nucleic acid negative conversion time and mortality of COVID-19 patients compared to the control group (using antiviral treatment regimen excluding IFN-β), and no serious adverse reactions have been observed (Hung et al., 2020). However, due to the small sample size, open label randomized controlled trial design and other reasons, it has not yet been able to fully confirm its efficacy and safety, and more high-quality RCT experiments are still needed to evaluate its benefits.

Although SARS-CoV-2 has many similarities with SARS-CoV, the current clinical experience in the treatment of COVID-19 is limited. In addition, the RNA viruses mutate rapidly. The use of antiviral drugs in the early stage of diseases with rapid viral replication is more important than in the middle and late stages with higher levels of inflammatory factors. With the aggravation of the disease, COVID-19 patients are prone to liver and kidney function damage to varying degrees. Currently recommended antiviral drugs also have potential harm to liver and kidney function, which should be paid attention to in clinical use (Wu J. et al., 2020; Pei et al., 2020). Therefore, the use of antiviral drugs has limitations.

Anti-Fibrosis Drugs

Multiple studies (Noble et al., 2011; Richeldi et al., 2011; Richeldi et al., 2014; Myllarniemi and Kaarteenaho, 2015; Margaritopoulos et al., 2016) have shown that currently available anti-fibrosis drugs nintedanib and pirfenidone can significantly reduce the decline rate of pulmonary function and forced vital capacity (FVC), mitigate the trend of acute exacerbation of fibrosis, and reduced the death rate through inhibiting the production of collagen in activated fibroblasts.

Nintedanib and pirfenidone may alleviate pulmonary fibrosis caused by COVID-19 infection through multiple mechanisms (Umemura et al., 2021). Chronic lung injury caused by overactivity of epidermal growth factor receptor (EGFR) mediated related pathways is one of the main causes of COVID-19 induced fibrosis (Venkataraman and Frieman, 2017). Nintedanib is an EGFR inhibitor that helps prevent excessive fibrotic responses in SARS and COVID-19 (Quartuccio et al., 2020). In addition, studies have found that proteins inhibited by nintedanib are causally related to increased ACE2 expression (Rao et al., 2020). Nintedanib may reduce the expression of ACE2 by inhibiting the expression of related proteins and reducing the body's response to SARS-CoV-2. Susceptibility. Pirfenidone may inhibit lung damage caused by cytokine storms after SARS-COV-2 infection by significantly reducing serum and lung IL-6 levels (Liu et al., 2017; Zhang C. et al., 2020).

There are still little data on the safety and effectiveness of nintedanib, and pirfenidone in COVID-19 patients with PF, and most clinical trials have yet to be completed. A clinical study designed to observe the efficacy and safety of nintedanib in patients with ARDS induced by COVID found that the application of nintedanib to mechanically ventilated patients with severe new coronary pneumonia can obtain a higher P/F value (according to PaO_2/FiO_2 evaluates the severity of the disease) and shorter mechanical ventilation time. In addition, CT volume measurements showed that the percentage of high-density areas in the nintedanib group was significantly lower than that in the control group when patients were not treated with mechanical ventilation. This study suggests that using nintedanib may provide potential benefits for reducing lung injury caused by COVID-19 (Umemura et al., 2021). No clinical data are available on pirfenidone for the treatment of PF in patients with SARS-COV-2 infection.

In addition, as of October 2021, pirfenidone and nintedanib are only marketed in oral form and cannot be used in intubated and mechanically ventilated patients, apparently limiting their use in ICU (George et al., 2020). Moreover, for most patients in the National Health System (NHS), nintedanib or pirfenidone is more expensive to treat. The average adjusted annual costs for patients receiving pirfenidone and nintedanib are 40,000 and 29,000 dollars (Corral et al., 2020).

At present, several clinical trials of pirfenidone inhalation in the treatment of pulmonary fibrosis have been reported. Several studies have shown that pirfenidone has a higher safety as an inhaled delivery agent for the treatment of pulmonary fibrosis. First, inhaled pirfenidone may eliminate the gastrointestinal adverse effects that often occur when administered orally. Second, inhaled powder preparations of pirfenidone have higher photostability and lower risk of phototoxicity compared to oral preparations (Onoue et al., 2013). Third, lower systemic exposure *via* inhaled administration may reduce the risk of hepatic dysfunction due to pirfenidone. A clinical trial evaluating the pharmacokinetics and safety of inhaled pirfenidone solution showed that aerosol pirfenidone was well tolerated in normal volunteers, smokers, and patients with IPF, and no clinically relevant adverse effects related to respiratory rate, spirometry, or oxygenation were observed (Khoo et al., 2020). The main drug-related adverse effect was mild and intermittent cough in a small number of subjects. Furthermore, this study found that systemic pirfenidone exposure at the 100 mg nebulized dose was on average 15 times lower than that reported for the oral licensed dose. And the Capacity 004 phase 3 study of oral pirfenidone demonstrated that adverse events were dose related, not idiosyncratic (Noble et al., 2011).

In addition,a dose/response was demonstrated for the decrease of FVC % predicted and progression-free survival in the CAPACITY 004 trial. And the epithelial lining fluid (ELF) Cmax was reported to be on average 35-fold higher for the 100 mg pirfenidone inhalation dose than the approved oral dose (Khoo et al., 2020). Moreover, a mouse IPF model using bleomycin showed that the efficacy of inhaled pirfenidone was related to peak ELF concentrations rather than AUC(Surber et al., 2014). A recent study using a rat model of paraquat-induced pulmonary fibrosis also showed that the efficacy of inhaled pirfenidone and oral administration was similar, but the inhaled dose was significantly lower than the oral dose (Rasooli et al., 2018). Therefore, the higher local concentration provided by aerosol administration may also lead to the improvement of efficacy. In addition, inhaled pirfenidone offers a new option for patients who are not covenient for oral administration, including patients who are intubated and mechanically ventilated. In summary, further studies of inhaled pirfenidone are necessary to test its long-term safety and efficacy.

At present, there is no clinical trial of inhaled pirfenidone in COVID-19 patients. Although it is mentioned in the literature (George et al., 2020) that "An inhaled formulation of pirfenidone is under evaluation in patients with COVID-19 (NCT04282902)", in fact, pirfenidone is administered orally in this clinical trial (NCT04282902).

On March 24, 2020, Unco Arendy Therapeutics announced that it is studying OATD-01, a CHIT1 inhibitor, to help treat pulmonary fibrosis in COVID-19 patients. It may have anti-inflammatory activity and may delay the development of pulmonary fibrosis. Studies are currently underway to determine whether patients who have died from COVID-19 have increased CHIT1 expression in their lung tissues, which may lead to a positive effect of OATD-01 on the pulmonary fibrotic development of the disease (Dymek et al., 2018).

Corticosteroids

Corticosteroids are not recommended for routine use of IPF in several guidelines. Still, systemic Corticosteroids can be used for short-term use in acute exacerbations of IPF to exert anti-inflammatory and immunosuppressive effects of the lung, which can inhibit inflammatory cell infiltration and fibroblast proliferation, reduce alveolar inflammation, and delay the progression of pulmonary fibrosis (Raghu et al., 2015; Homma et al., 2018). As important pathogenesis of acute exacerbation of pulmonary fibrosis, viral infection can easily cause acute lung injury in patients. In addition, patients with the pre-existing progressive pulmonary interstitial disease will have a diffuse pulmonary alveolar injury in severe cases, which is clinically manifested as dyspnea (Collard et al., 2016). This is similar to the lung characteristics seen in critical type COVID-19 patients. Therefore, Corticosteroids can be used to prevent the acute progression of pulmonary fibrosis in PF patients who are prone to severe and critical type COVID-19. The World Health Organization guidelines do not recommend stopping the original systemic Corticosteroids therapy for non-severe COVID-19 patients who have received systemic Corticosteroids therapy. If non-severe COVID-19 patients have clinical symptoms such as increased respiratory rate, respiratory distress, or hypoxemia (similar to symptoms of acute exacerbation of pulmonary fibrosis), systemic corticosteroid therapy is recommended. Systemic Corticosteroids are recommended to treat of severe and critically type COVID-19 patients (Lamontagne et al., 2021).

However, the impact of Corticosteroids on the prognosis of other viral pneumonia still needs clinical attention (Stockman et al., 2006; Arabi et al., 2018). Corticosteroids can delay the clearance of blood and respiratory viruses in SARS/MERS patients (Stockman et al., 2006; Arabi et al., 2018). Corticosteroids do not affect on improving survival, and are accompanied by steroid-related adverse events such as femoral head necrosis, hyperglycemia, and psychosis (Stockman et al., 2006; Arabi et al., 2018). A meta-analysis involving influenza pneumonia patients reported that Corticosteroid use was associated with an increased risk of mortality and secondary infection (Ni et al., 2019). However, Wu et al. said that treatment with methylprednisolone was associated with a reduced risk of death in COVID-19 patients who developed ARDS (Wu C. et al., 2020). Long-term use of low-dose corticosteroids can prevent lung remodeling in ARDS survivors (Gentile et al., 2020). Still, the risk-benefit ratio should be evaluated before use, especially in patients with diabetes, hypertension, and chronic heart failure (Villar et al., 2020). Corticosteroids may delay the clearance of viral RNA and lead to an increased risk of secondary infection (Lee et al., 2004; Arabi et al., 2018), which plays a critical role in the development of fibrosis. Therefore, the use of Corticosteroids should be more cautious. Long-term effects should be emphasized as well as therapeutic products.

Spironolactone

Spironolactone is an antihypertensive and antiandrogen drug, and it has been reported that it may have important significance in the prevention of pulmonary fibrosis (Zannad et al., 2000; Barut et al., 2016; Yavas et al., 2019). The mechanisms that may have potential benefits for COVID-19 are: 1) increase the circulating level of ACE2 and prevent SARS-COV-2 from entering cells; 2) Block the mineralocorticoid receptors; 3) Down-regulation of TMPRSS2; 4) Anti-inflammatory, antioxidant, anti-fibrosis, and antiviral properties (Cadegiani et al., 2020; Kotfis et al., 2021). ACE2 and TMPRSS2 are key regulators of SARS-COV-2 cell entry. It has been reported that the elevation of the physiological corticosteroid receptor activator aldosterone is associated with fibrosis and a high inflammatory response (Stone et al., 2020; Salama et al., 2021). Therefore, spironolactone has potential value in preventing or reducing pulmonary fibrosis after COVID-19. In addition, Atalay et al. confirmed the effectiveness of spironolactone in treating ALI in rats (Atalay et al., 2010). And Lieber et al. found that spironolactone can reduce acute pneumonia caused by bleomycin or lipopolysaccharide (Lieber et al., 2013). Still, related experiments were performed on animal models such as rats or other rodents, and its conclusions have apparent limitations. In addition, there is currently a lack of direct clinical research results showing that mineralocorticoid receptor antagonists are beneficial for pulmonary fibrosis after viral infection. In the future, further trials are needed to evaluate the potential benefits of spironolactone to COVID-19 and to clarify its mechanism further.

Cytokine Inhibitors

Tocilizumab

Tocilizumab is a humanized monoclonal antibody against IL-6, which can bind to the soluble IL-6 receptor on the cell membrane and inhibit the function of IL-6 (Gautret et al., 2020). IL-6 is not only the main therapeutic target for the treatment of COVID-19 complicated by cytokine storm syndrome (Wan et al., 2020), it is also a pro-fibrotic factor produced in the Th2-type immune response. Studies have observed that fibroblasts induce fibroblasts to transform into myofibroblasts by secreting IL-6, which promotes the occurrence and development of pulmonary fibrosis (Kobayashi et al., 2015). At present, whether tocilizumab can be used in the treatment of new crowns is still controversial. The multicenter trial results showed that tocilizumab reduced the risk of COVID-19 hospitalized patients progressing to mechanical ventilation or death on the 28th day (Salama et al., 2021). A randomized trial in Brazil stopped early due to a significant increase in deaths within 15 days in the tocilizumab treatment group compared with the placebo group (Veiga et al., 2021). Another North American study showed that tocilizumab did not prevent intubation or death of early COVID-19 hospitalized patients. However, there is currently a lack of clinical studies evaluating the long-term prognostic effect of tocilizumab in avoiding or reducing COVID-19-related pulmonary fibrosis.

TGF-β1 Inhibitors

Histone Deacetylase Inhibitors

HDAC inhibitors have been reported to show good anti-fibrotic effects mainly through suppressing TGF-β1 signaling (Atalay et al., 2010). Fibroblasts to myofibroblasts differentiation generally mediated by TGF-β1 require HDAC4 (Glenisson et al., 2007). Several studies (Glenisson et al., 2007; Barter et al., 2010; Korfei et al., 2015) have shown that HDAC could epigenetically regulate TGF-β-mediated gene expression, which leads to pulmonary fibrosis. Therefore, it is possible to treat pulmonary fibrosis with HDAC inhibitors. HDAC inhibitor tubastatin successfully ameliorated pulmonary fibrosis in murine bleomycin-induced pulmonary fibrosis model, particularly triggered by TGF-β(Saito et al., 2017). In addition, a study has demonstrated that panobinostat is superior to pirfenidone against IPF-derived fibroblasts (Korfei et al., 2018).

Murthy et al.(Murthy et al., 2021) said that COVID-19 recovered patients who show unresolved patchy areas of opacification, interstitial thickening and early signs of fibrosis during the follow-up chest CT after discharge should be considered for HDAC inhibitors treatment to reduce the possibility of the development of pulmonary fibrosis. Early treatment with HDAC inhibitors for the secondary/late consequences of SARS-CoV-2 infection will help reduce complications/mortality and improve the quality of life of patients for COVID-19 recovered patients.

CD147 Inhibitors

SARS-CoV-2 invades host cells through the CD147 receptor, which is present in multiple cell types of the lung and is highly expressed in type II alveolar cells and macrophages at the edge of the fibrotic zone. A phase 2 clinical trial to prevent COVID-19 by blocking CD147 is underway in China (Ulrich and Pillat, 2020), which is testing a humanized form of the CD147-specific antibody meplazumab. Furthermore, transient transfection of normal human lung fibroblasts to overexpress CD147 could significantly increase TGF-β1-induced cell proliferation and the expression of α-smooth muscle actin, a marker of myofibroblasts (Guillot et al., 2006), thus anti-CD147 antibodies could inhibit TGF-β1-induced proliferation and differentiation of fibroblasts into myofibroblasts that are induced by TGF-β1. Therefore, blocking CD147 is potentially valuable for the prevention of the pulmonary fibrosis due to COVID-19.

Poly-(ADP-Ribose) Polymerase Inhibitor

SARS-CoV-2 infection can induce PARP activation in lung tissue of asthmatic patients; different preclinical animal models (Ghonim et al., 2015a; Carlile et al., 2016) showed that PARPI attenuated pulmonary fibrosis caused by SARS-CoV-2 pulmonary inflammation. Its possible mechanism of improving COVID-19 pulmonary fibrosis is to protect cells from death by preventing cytokine storms (excessive activation of macrophages) (Curtin et al., 2020). Several animal model studies (Ghonim et al., 2015b) (Sethi et al., 2019; Sahu et al., 2020) have shown that PARPI, including Olaparib, can reduce the expression of IL-6 and IL-1β in many organs like the lung. Therefore, PARPI can be applied as a potential treatment for pulmonary fibrosis caused by SARS-CoV-2 infection.

Propolis

SARS-CoV-2 invasion to host cells can be prevented or reduced by Propolis extract and its components reducing TMPRSS2 expression and ACE2 anchoring (Kaur et al., 2020). Furthermore, propolis block kinase PAK-1, which increases during lung inflammation and fibrosis (Berretta et al., 2020), and PAK1 inhibitors were reported to rescue the immune system and help resist virus infection (Maruta and He, 2020). Propolis, comprising its components, can help prevent immunosuppression in the early stage of the disease and reduce the host's excessive inflammatory response by blocking excessive IL-6, IL-2, and JAK signals in the later stage (Nile et al., 2020).

Galectin-3 Inhibitor

One of the main stages of COVID-19 is the excessive inflammation stage, during which immune cells release Gal3 (Boza-Serrano et al., 2019). And it has been reported that the level of Gal3 in proliferative T cells of COVID-19 patients is elevated (Liao et al., 2020). Gal3 is a carbohydrate-binding protein expressed by macrophages, epithelial cells, and alveolar cells in the lung (Reyfman et al., 2019). Gal3 binds and activates TLR4 and TREM2, a process associated with lung diseases and pulmonary fibrosis (Boza-Serrano et al., 2019). TREM2 is expressed by macrophages and is associated with fibrosis (Liao et al., 2020). TLR, which is essential for the antiviral response, can lead to solid inflammation associated with the expression of interferon-related genes, interleukins, chemokines, and Gal3 (Guo et al., 2020). The Gal3 inhibitor TD139 provided by Galecto Biotech has proven safe and effective for patients with IPF (NCT03832946). The clinical trials using TD139 for the treatment of COVID-19 patients are still under study (NCT04473053).

Chinese Medicine Treatment Strategy for Pulmonary Fibrosis in Convalescent Sequelae of COVID-19

Current studies have proved that traditional Chinese medicine prescription is effective in the treatment of pulmonary fibrosis, and the combination of Chinese and Western medicine is obviously superior to western medicine alone therapy in delaying the decline of pulmonary function and improving the quality of life (Gan et al., 2020). In the theory of traditional Chinese medicine, COVID-19 is caused by damp toxin and epidemic gas, and the disease location is mainly in the lung as well as the spleen and stomach. Active intervention of traditional Chinese medicine in the early stage of recovery can promote the absorption of pulmonary lesions and improve pulmonary function.

Based on the studies on traditional Chinese medicine treatment of IPF and SARS-associated pulmonary fibrosis, there are many traditional Chinese medicine prescriptions that can significantly relieve the symptoms of pulmonary fibrosis and improve lung function. Huaxian Decoction is a classic prescription for the treatment of pulmonary fibrosis, which is anti-inflammatory effect may be mediated by inhibition of inflammatory factor TNF-α、TGF-β, and inhibit NF-κB activation of inflammatory signaling pathways, thus effectively alleviate inflammatory reaction, reduce clinical symptoms, improve lung function, and reduce the levels of serum laminin, hyaluronic acid and other pulmonary fibrosis indicators (Chen et al., 2016; Gan et al., 2020). Yiqi Huoxue Guben decoction can delay the decline of lung function, improve respiratory symptoms, improve activity endurance and improve the quality of life (Gan et al., 2020). Huqihuoxue Decoction can inhibit the expression of TGF-β and its protein, reduce the lung collagen deposition in patients with idiopathic pulmonary fibrosis, thus relieve the symptoms of patients. Peiyuan Quyu decoction can improve the clinical symptoms and lung function index of phlegm-stasis IPF, alleviate the progression of acute exacerbation of the disease, and significantly improve exercise endurance (Changhui, 2019). Qingjin Yifei decoction can reduce the expression of VEGF mRNA and PDGF, thereby reducing capillary permeability, dilating pulmonary artery veins, and improving vascular remodeling.

After the treatment of COVID-19 in the acute stage, the clinical outcomes of TCM dialectics mainly divided into three categories: For those with residual pathogens accompanied by qi and Yin deficiency syndrome, should be treated to nourish qi and Yin, and supplemented with the prescription of invigorating qi and promoting blood circulation, which is suitable for shengmai Decoction, Shashen Maimendong Decoction and Wuye Lugen Decoction; For those with deficiency of lung and spleen, the method is to replenish qi and strengthen the spleen, aromatize and remove dampness, and add or subtract Liujunzi Decoction; For those with qi deficiency, blood stasis and obstruction of lung collaterals, supplementing qi, activating blood circulation and collaterals are the main treatment methods, which can be combined with Buyang Huanwu Decoction and Xuanpu Hua Decoction (Gan et al., 2020).

ADJUSTMENT OF THE DRUG TREATMENT REGIMEN FOR PF PATIENTS INFECTED WITH COVID-19

The current drug treatment methods for PF, especially IPF, mainly include anti-fibrosis therapy, antacid therapy (proton pump inhibitors, H_2 receptor antagonists), hormone therapy, immunomodulatory therapy. When patients with pulmonary fibrosis are infected with SARS-COV-2, the original anti-fibrosis treatment plan should be adjusted according to the antiviral treatment plan and pathophysiological state of the patient. The suggestions and precautions of drug adjustment for anti-fibrosis therapy, anti-acid therapy, and immunomodulatory therapy are discussed.

Anti-Fibrosis Therapy

National Institute for Health and Clinical Excellence (NICE) and British Thoracic Society (BTS) guidelines recommend that patients receiving anti-fibrosis therapy should not stop using pirfenidone and nintedanib. There is currently no evidence that the use of pirfenidone and nintedanib increases the risk of SARS-CoV-2 infection or COVID-19 aggravation.

The following points should be noted in the application of nintedanib and pirfenidone. The two drugs often have gastrointestinal side effects that are similar to the symptoms of COVID-19 (diarrhea, fatigue, loss of appetite) and should be carefully differentiated in clinical use. Secondly, these two drugs have certain hepatotoxicity. COVID-19 patients, especially in severe cases, often report liver damage (George et al., 2020). The liver function of COVID-19 should be closely monitored during use, and anti-fibrosis drugs should be stopped in time if patients develop acute liver function damage. Thirdly, studies have shown that patients with COVID-19 have an increased risk of venous vascular embolism, especially pulmonary embolism. At the same time, viral infection leads to the acute progression of original pulmonary fibrosis. Meanwhile, viral infection leads to the sharp progression of pulmonary fibrosis, and the body is prone to hypercoagulability due to an imbalance between coagulation and fibrinolysis (Abou-Ismail et al., 2021). At this time, if the anticoagulant warfarin is used, attention should be paid to discontinue the use of nintedanib for anti-fibrosis therapy. It is a vascular endothelial growth factor receptor (VEGFR) inhibitor. The simultaneous use of anticoagulants will increase the risk of bleeding in patients. Finally, pirfenidone is strictly prohibited for patients with severely impaired renal function. If the patient's glomerular filtration rate (eGFR) is less than 30 ml/min/1.73 m^2, pirfenidone should be discontinued (George et al., 2020).

Antacid Therapy

Gastroesophageal reflux is a risk factor of pulmonary inflammation caused by aspiration or slight aspiration of acidic or non-acidic reflux substances into the lungs, and it is also an important mechanism of pulmonary fibrosis caused or aggravated by sustained lung injury (Trachalaki et al., 2021). Gastroesophageal reflux can be observed in 90% of patients with idiopathic fibrosis, regardless of the presence of gastrointestinal symptoms (Tobin et al., 1998). The ATS/ERS/JRS/ALAT clinical practice guidelines are weak recommendations for the use of conventional antacid therapy (PPI or H_2 receptor antagonists) in patients with pulmonary fibrosis, suggesting that conventional antacid therapy may improve pulmonary function and survival in patients with pulmonary fibrosis, and may reduce the cost of treatment for the progression of pulmonary fibrosis (Raghu et al., 2015). A clinical study analyzed the impact of throat reflux disease (a subtype of gastroesophageal reflux disease) on COVID-19 hospitalized patients. Among the 95 hospitalized patients, 37 patients had throat reflux disease (reflux symptom index, RSI >13). The median RSI score of severe and critical COVID-19 patients was significantly higher than that of ordinary patients, which suggesting that throat reflux disease may be a risk factor for severe or critical COVID-19 patients (Jiang et al., 2020). Anti-acid therapy is indeed indicated for COVID-19 patients. However, the results of a meta-analysis showed that conventional PPI treatment of COVID-19 is related to the prolonged hospital stay of patients, and it is more likely to lead to severe consequences such as admission to the intensive care unit, mechanical ventilation, acute respiratory distress syndrome or death (Li GF. et al., 2021). Recent studies have shown that famotidine can improve the clinical symptoms of non-hospitalized COVID-19 patients (Janowitz et al., 2020), and is associated with lower mortality and lower risk of death from endotracheal intubation in hospitalized patients (Mather et al., 2020). Its mechanism may be related to H_2 receptor-mediated immunomodulatory effect on mast cell histamine-cytokine crosstalk (Mather et al., 2020). Therefore, FOR COVID-19 patients, especially those in critical condition, PPI should be used cautiously, and famotidine can be considered the first choice.

Immunomodulatory Therapy

Convalescent plasma, COVID-19 human immunoglobulin, and tocilizumab are recommended for COVID-19 immunotherapy acc according to the Chinese Diagnosis and Treatment Protocol for Novel Coronavirus Pneumonia (Trial Edition 8). Tocilizumab can treat patients with extensive bilateral lung disease or severe patients with elevated IL-6 levels. However, the guidelines issued by the National Institutes of Health (NIH) indicate that there is insufficient research evidence for IL-6 inhibitors for the treatment of COVID-19. One study suggested that the TGF-β pathway in the pathogenesis of IPF could be mediated by IL-6 (Epstein Shochet et al., 2020). Tocilizumab does suggest that it can be used in patients with pulmonary fibrosis complicated with COVID-19, which has potential value in inhibiting the progression of pulmonary fibrosis and preventing cytokine storms arising from immune imbalance through immunomodulatory effects. Milo Gatti et al. conducted a pharmacovigilance evaluation on tocilizumab. The results of the study found that it easily leads to liver damage in patients. In severe cases, acute liver failure, fulminant hepatitis, and liver necrosis can occur. Severe and critically COVID-19 patients have varying degrees of liver and kidney damage. The benefit to risk ratio should be fully considered, and the continued use of tocilizumab should be carefully considered. Mild patients can continue to use it while monitoring liver function (Gatti et al., 2021).

DISCUSSION

At present, with the COVID-19 outbreak in full swing, the number of infected people is growing and challenging to control. Any progress in scientific research requires the accumulation of time. Even though scientific researchers around the world are dedicated to studying the novel coronavirus infection, the progress and outcome of COVID-19, and related treatment drugs, less than 2 years after the outbreak, there are still many research gaps and many mechanisms. The problem is difficult to explain clearly. Most importantly, drugs for the treatment of COVID-19 are still being explored and discussed, and we have not found the specific drugs we hoped. At present, the treatment of COVID-19 associated pulmonary fibrosis can only be based on the existing IPF treatment regimen. The study by Umemura et al. evaluated the efficacy and safety of nintedanib for pulmonary fibrosis induced by COVID-19 in ICU patients with severe COVID-19. The results showed that nintedanib combined with favipiravir can significantly reduce the mechanical ventilation time of ICU patients with COVID-19, the percentages of high-attenuation areas at liberation from mechanical ventilation. There was no statistically significant difference in 28 days mortality from the control group (Umemura et al., 2021). In terms of safety, there were no statistically significant differences in severe, moderate and mild liver failure and gastrointestinal reactions in nintedanib combined with favipiravir compared with favipiravir alone, but the incidence of mild and moderate acute liver failure was slightly higher. Although statistical tests showed no statistical difference between the two groups, the sample size of the experiment was small ($n = 60$), which might lead to sampling error. Meanwhile, the subjects in this study were only ICU patients, and the benefits and risks of nintedanib in patients with mild disease cannot be evaluated for the time being. In addition to the clinical study mentioned above, few clinical trials of drug therapy for COVID-19-related pulmonary fibrosis have published its results (Kotfis et al., 2021). Therefore, it is currently impossible to accurately evaluate the efficacy and safety of anti-fibrosis drugs in the treatment of COVID-19-related pulmonary fibrosis. In the process of clinical treatment, medical staff should be more cautious, strictly control the indications for drug use, carefully select the anti-fibrosis drug treatment plan, and give priority to the safety of patients after drug use. Based on the existing clinical evidence, it is more recommended to choose the first-line anti-fibrosis drugs pirfenidone and nintedanib, which are recommended by authoritative guidelines and have sufficient evidence in medicine. Currently, there is no clear interaction between the COVID-19 antiviral drugs recommended by the mainstream internationally and nintedanib and pirfenidone. In addition, nintedanib and pirfenidone are not immunosuppressive agents themselves, and there is currently no evidence that they will prolong the clearance time of SARS-CoV-2 *in vivo* (George et al., 2020).

There are various limitations of existing drugs in clinical practice, which should be paid attention to in the process of clinical use. First of all, there is an overlap between the adverse reactions of anti-fibrosis drugs and those related to COVID-19 treatment, and the incidence of adverse reactions in patients is easy to increase when combined. For example, although nintedanib and pirfenidone are both authoritative drugs recommended to treat idiopathic pulmonary fibrosis, there is currently a lack of clinical studies on their treatment of SARS-CoV-2 infected pulmonary fibrosis. Here we emphasize the safety of the drug. The adverse reactions of nintedanib and pirfenidone (including gastrointestinal reactions and liver toxicity, etc.) coincide with the clinical symptoms of COVID-19. In addition, remdesivir, lopinavir, ritonavir, and other clinically recommended antiviral drugs are also prone to gastrointestinal reactions and liver function damage in patients (Cao et al., 2020; Spinner et al., 2020; Mahajan et al., 2021). This seems to be very detrimental to the patient. Secondly, there are contradictions between anti-fibrosis drugs and new coronary treatment-related treatments. For example, nintedanib, as a VEGFR inhibitor, is likely to increase the risk of bleeding, which seems to contradict with the increased risk of pulmonary embolism in patients with COVID-19. Therefore, in the clinical use of nintedanib and anticoagulants, the patient's condition should be thoroughly evaluated. The pros and cons should be weighed to avoid the occurrence of acute disease progression and serious adverse events. Finally, there are some similarities between the anti-fibrosis treatment plan and the COVID-19 treatment plan. Patients with COVID-19 associated pulmonary fibrosis seem to have more pointers to use drugs recommended for both diseases (such as glucocorticoids, acid-suppressing drugs). Still, the potential risks of drugs should also be paid attention. For example, current clinical evidence favors glucocorticoids to control the acute progression and prevent severe and critical illness. A meta-analysis that included patients with influenza pneumonia reported that glucocorticoid use was associated with an increased risk of mortality and secondary infection (Ni et al., 2019). Severe and critically ill COVID-19 patients are more likely to be mechanically ventilated and prone to ventilator-associated pneumonia. Glucocorticoids should be used under close observation in such patients. At the same time, glucocorticoids can delay the clearance of SARS/MERS patients from blood and respiratory viruses due to immunosuppressive effects (Stockman et al., 2006; Arabi et al., 2018). Therefore, it should be noted that larger doses of glucocorticoids may delay the clearance of SARS-CoV-2 and prolong the course of patients.

We look forward to better clinical trials of targeted drugs targeting fibrosis pathways. We look forward to researchers around the world developing new drugs with both effectiveness and safety in response to the continuing outbreak of COVID-19.

AUTHOR CONTRIBUTIONS

HS, NZ, YL, XY, YH, QL, and XS jointly reviewed the literature and wrote the manuscript. YZ and YY guided the research and revised the manuscript. All authors reviewed and approved the manuscript.

ACKNOWLEDGMENTS

We acknowledge the support from Sichuan Academy of Medical Sciences and Sichuan Provincial People's Hospital, University of Electronic Science and Technology of China, Ziyang People's Hospital, People's Hospital of Fushun County, and thank YY for his contribution to the Institute.

REFERENCES

Abou-Ismail, M. Y., Diamond, A., Kapoor, S., Arafah, Y., and Nayak, L. (2021). Corrigendum to "The Hypercoagulable State in COVID-19: Incidence, Pathophysiology, and Management" [Thromb. Res., 194, October 2020, Pages 101-115]. *Thromb. Res.* 204, 146. doi:10.1016/j.thromres.2020.11.012

Aguiar, J. A., Tremblay, B. J., Mansfield, M. J., Woody, O., Lobb, B., Banerjee, A., et al. (2020). Gene Expression and *In Situ* Protein Profiling of Candidate SARS-CoV-2 Receptors in Human Airway Epithelial Cells and Lung Tissue. *Eur. Respir. J.* 56 (3). doi:10.1183/13993003.01123-2020

Aloufi, N., Traboulsi, H., Ding, J., Fonseca, G. J., Nair, P., Huang, S. K., et al. (2021). Angiotensin-converting Enzyme 2 Expression in COPD and IPF Fibroblasts: the Forgotten Cell in COVID-19. *Am. J. Physiol. Lung Cel Mol Physiol* 320 (1), L152–L157. doi:10.1152/ajplung.00455.2020

Antoniades, H. N., Bravo, M. A., Avila, R. E., Galanopoulos, T., Neville-Golden, J., Maxwell, M., et al. (1990). Platelet-derived Growth Factor in Idiopathic Pulmonary Fibrosis. *J. Clin. Invest.* 86 (4), 1055–1064. doi:10.1172/jci114808

Arabi, Y. M., Asiri, A. Y., Assiri, A. M., Aziz Jokhdar, H. A., Alothman, A., Balkhy, H. H., et al. (2020). Treatment of Middle East Respiratory Syndrome with a Combination of Lopinavir/ritonavir and Interferon-B1b (MIRACLE Trial): Statistical Analysis Plan for a Recursive Two-Stage Group Sequential Randomized Controlled Trial. *Trials* 21 (1), 8. doi:10.1186/s13063-019-3846-x

Arabi, Y. M., Mandourah, Y., Al-Hameed, F., Sindi, A. A., Almekhlafi, G. A., Hussein, M. A., et al. (2018). Corticosteroid Therapy for Critically Ill Patients with Middle East Respiratory Syndrome. *Am. J. Respir. Crit. Care Med.* 197 (6), 757–767. doi:10.1164/rccm.201706-1172OC

Aspal, M., and Zemans, R. L. (2020). Mechanisms of ATII-To-ATI Cell Differentiation during Lung Regeneration. *Int. J. Mol. Sci.* 21 (9). doi:10.3390/ijms21093188

Atalay, C., Dogan, N., Aykan, S., Gundogdu, C., and Keles, M. S. (2010). The Efficacy of Spironolactone in the Treatment of Acute Respiratory Distress Syndrome-Induced Rats. *Singapore Med. J.* 51 (6), 501–505.

Aveyard, P., Gao, M., Lindson, N., Hartmann-Boyce, J., Watkinson, P., Young, D., et al. (2021). Association between Pre-existing Respiratory Disease and its Treatment, and Severe COVID-19: a Population Cohort Study. *Lancet Respir. Med.* 9 (8), 909–923. doi:10.1016/s2213-2600(21)00095-3

Baccarelli, A., Wright, R. O., Bollati, V., Tarantini, L., Litonjua, A. A., Suh, H. H., et al. (2009). Rapid DNA Methylation Changes after Exposure to Traffic Particles. *Am. J. Respir. Crit. Care Med.* 179 (7), 572–578. doi:10.1164/rccm.200807-1097OC

Barter, M. J., Pybus, L., Litherland, G. J., Rowan, A. D., Clark, I. M., Edwards, D. R., et al. (2010). HDAC-mediated Control of ERK- and PI3K-dependent TGF-β-Induced Extracellular Matrix-Regulating Genes. *Matrix Biol.* 29 (7), 602–612. doi:10.1016/j.matbio.2010.05.002

Barut, F., Ozacmak, V. H., Turan, I., Sayan-Ozacmak, H., and Aktunc, E. (2016). Reduction of Acute Lung Injury by Administration of Spironolactone after Intestinal Ischemia and Reperfusion in Rats. *Clin. Invest. Med.* 39 (1), E15–E24. doi:10.25011/cim.v39i1.26326

Berretta, A. A., Silveira, M. A. D., Cóndor Capcha, J. M., and De Jong, D. (2020). Propolis and its Potential against SARS-CoV-2 Infection Mechanisms and COVID-19 Disease: Running Title: Propolis against SARS-CoV-2 Infection and COVID-19. *Biomed. Pharmacother.* 131, 110622. doi:10.1016/j.biopha.2020.110622

Boza-Serrano, A., Ruiz, R., Sanchez-Varo, R., García-Revilla, J., Yang, Y., Jimenez-Ferrer, I., et al. (2019). Galectin-3, a Novel Endogenous TREM2 Ligand, Detrimentally Regulates Inflammatory Response in Alzheimer's Disease. *Acta Neuropathol.* 138 (2), 251–273. doi:10.1007/s00401-019-02013-z

Burguillos, M. A., Svensson, M., Schulte, T., Boza-Serrano, A., Garcia-Quintanilla, A., Kavanagh, E., et al. (2015). Microglia-Secreted Galectin-3 Acts as a Toll-like Receptor 4 Ligand and Contributes to Microglial Activation. *Cell Rep* 10 (9), 1626–1638. doi:10.1016/j.celrep.2015.02.012

Cadegiani, F. A., Wambier, C. G., and Goren, A. (2020). Spironolactone: An Anti-androgenic and Anti-hypertensive Drug that May Provide Protection against the Novel Coronavirus (SARS-CoV-2) Induced Acute Respiratory Distress Syndrome (ARDS) in COVID-19. *Front. Med. (Lausanne)* 7, 453. doi:10.3389/fmed.2020.00453

Calver, J., Joseph, C., John, A., Organ, L., Fainberg, H., Porte, J., et al. (2021). S31Thenovel Coronavirus SARS -CoV-2binds RGD Integrins and Upregulates Avb3 Integrins in Covid -19infected Lungs. *Thorax* 76 (Suppl. 1), A22–A23. doi:10.1136/thorax-2020-BTSabstracts.37

Cao, B., Wang, Y., Wen, D., Liu, W., Wang, J., Fan, G., et al. (2020). A Trial of Lopinavir-Ritonavir in Adults Hospitalized with Severe Covid-19. *N. Engl. J. Med.* 382 (19), 1787–1799. doi:10.1056/NEJMoa2001282

Carlile, G. W., Robert, R., Matthes, E., Yang, Q., Solari, R., Hatley, R., et al. (2016). Latonduine Analogs Restore F508del-Cystic Fibrosis Transmembrane Conductance Regulator Trafficking through the Modulation of Poly-ADP Ribose Polymerase 3 and Poly-ADP Ribose Polymerase 16 Activity. *Mol. Pharmacol.* 90 (2), 65–79. doi:10.1124/mol.115.102418

Caruso, D., Guido, G., Zerunian, M., Polidori, T., Lucertini, E., Pucciarelli, F., et al. (2021). Post-acute Sequelae of COVID-19 Pneumonia: Six-Month Chest CT Follow-Up. *RADIOLOGY* 301 (2), E396–E405. doi:10.1148/radiol.2021210834

Changhui, D. C. D. Y. Z. Q. W. C. L. (2019). Clinical Effect of Peiyuan Quyu Decoction on Treating Idiopathic Pulmonary Fibrosis with Phlegm and Stasis Blocking Collaterals. *China Med. herald* 16, 124–127+139.

Chen, F., Wang, P. L., Fan, X. S., Yu, J. H., Zhu, Y., and Zhu, Z. H. (2016). Effect of Renshen Pingfei Decoction, a Traditional Chinese Prescription, on IPF Induced by Bleomycin in Rats and Regulation of TGF-β1/Smad3. *J. Ethnopharmacol* 186, 289–297. doi:10.1016/j.jep.2016.03.051

Chousterman, B. G., Swirski, F. K., and Weber, G. F. (2017). Cytokine Storm and Sepsis Disease Pathogenesis. *Semin. Immunopathol* 39 (5), 517–528. doi:10.1007/s00281-017-0639-8

Chu, C. M., Cheng, V. C., Hung, I. F., Wong, M. M., Chan, K. H., Chan, K. S., et al. (2004). Role of Lopinavir/ritonavir in the Treatment of SARS: Initial Virological and Clinical Findings. *Thorax* 59 (3), 252–256. doi:10.1136/thorax.2003.012658

Collard, H. R., Ryerson, C. J., Corte, T. J., Jenkins, G., Kondoh, Y., Lederer, D. J., et al. (2016). Acute Exacerbation of Idiopathic Pulmonary Fibrosis. An International Working Group Report. *Am. J. Respir. Crit. Care Med.* 194 (3), 265–275. doi:10.1164/rccm.201604-0801CI

Consortium, W. H. O. S. T. (2021). Repurposed Antiviral Drugs for Covid-19 - Interim WHO Solidarity Trial Results. *N. Engl. J. Med.* 384 (6), 497–511. doi:10.1056/NEJMoa2023184

Corral, M., DeYoung, K., and Kong, A. M. (2020). Treatment Patterns, Healthcare Resource Utilization, and Costs Among Patients with Idiopathic Pulmonary Fibrosis Treated with Antifibrotic Medications in US-Based Commercial and Medicare Supplemental Claims Databases: a Retrospective Cohort Study. *BMC Pulm. Med.* 20 (1), 188. doi:10.1186/s12890-020-01224-5

Craig, V. J., Zhang, L., Hagood, J. S., and Owen, C. A. (2015). Matrix Metalloproteinases as Therapeutic Targets for Idiopathic Pulmonary Fibrosis. *Am. J. Respir. Cel Mol Biol* 53 (5), 585–600. doi:10.1165/rcmb.2015-0020TR

Crestani, B., Cornillet, P., Dehoux, M., Rolland, C., Guenounou, M., and Aubier, M. (1994). Alveolar Type II Epithelial Cells Produce Interleukin-6 *In Vitro* and *In Vivo*. Regulation by Alveolar Macrophage Secretory Products. *J. Clin. Invest.* 94 (2), 731–740. doi:10.1172/jci117392

Crisan-Dabija, R., Pavel, C. A., Popa, I. V., Tarus, A., and Burlacu, A. (2020). "A Chain Only as Strong as its Weakest Link": An Up-To-Date Literature Review on the Bidirectional Interaction of Pulmonary Fibrosis and COVID-19. *J. Proteome Res.* 19 (11), 4327–4338. doi:10.1021/acs.jproteome.0c00387

Crisan-Dabija, R., Covic, A., Brinza, C., Popa, I. V., and Burlacu, A. (2021). Involvement of KL-6 Biomarker in Interstitial Lung Disease Induced by SARS-CoV-2 Infection: A Systematic Review. *Appl. Sci.* 11 (8), 3482. doi:10.3390/app11083482

Curtin, N., Bányai, K., Thaventhiran, J., Le Quesne, J., Helyes, Z., and Bai, P. (2020). Repositioning PARP Inhibitors for SARS-CoV-2 infection(COVID-19); a New Multi-Pronged Therapy for Acute Respiratory Distress Syndrome? *Br. J. Pharmacol.* 177 (16), 3635–3645. doi:10.1111/bph.15137

Dhama, K., Sharun, K., Tiwari, R., Dadar, M., Malik, Y. S., Singh, K. P., et al. (2020). COVID-19, an Emerging Coronavirus Infection: Advances and Prospects in Designing and Developing Vaccines, Immunotherapeutics, and Therapeutics. *Hum. Vaccin. Immunother.* 16 (6), 1232–1238. doi:10.1080/21645515.2020.1735227

Donoghue, M., Hsieh, F., Baronas, E., Godbout, K., Gosselin, M., Stagliano, N., et al. (2000). A Novel Angiotensin-Converting Enzyme-Related Carboxypeptidase (ACE2) Converts Angiotensin I to Angiotensin 1-9. *Circ. Res.* 87 (5), E1–E9. doi:10.1161/01.res.87.5.e1

Drake, T. M., Docherty, A. B., Harrison, E. M., Quint, J. K., Adamali, H., Agnew, S., et al. (2020). Outcome of Hospitalization for COVID-19 in Patients with Interstitial Lung Disease: An International Multicenter Study. *Am. J. Respir. Crit. Care Med.* 202 (12), 1656–1665. doi:10.1164/rccm.202007-2794OC

Duckworth, A., Gibbons, M. A., Allen, R. J., Almond, H., Beaumont, R. N., Wood, A. R., et al. (2021). Telomere Length and Risk of Idiopathic Pulmonary Fibrosis and Chronic Obstructive Pulmonary Disease: a Mendelian Randomisation Study. *Lancet Respir. Med.* 9 (3), 285–294. doi:10.1016/s2213-2600(20)30364-7

Dymek, B., Sklepkiewicz, P., Mlacki, M., Zagozdzon, A., Koralewski, R., Mazur, M., et al. (2018). CHIT1 Is a Novel Therapeutic Target in Idiopathic Pulmonary Fibrosis (IPF): Anti-fibrotic Efficacy of OATD-01, a Potent and Selective Chitinase Inhibitor in the Mouse Model of Pulmonary Fibrosis. *Eur. Respir. J.* 52. doi:10.1183/13993003.congress-2018.OA5361

Ebinger, J. E., Achamallah, N., Ji, H., Claggett, B. L., Sun, N., Botting, P., et al. (2020). Pre-existing Traits Associated with Covid-19 Illness Severity. *Plos One* 15 (7), e0236240. doi:10.1371/journal.pone.0236240

Epstein Shochet, G., Brook, E., Bardenstein-Wald, B., and Shitrit, D. (2020). TGF-β Pathway Activation by Idiopathic Pulmonary Fibrosis (IPF) Fibroblast Derived Soluble Factors Is Mediated by IL-6 Trans-signaling. *Respir. Res.* 21 (1), 56. doi:10.1186/s12931-020-1319-0

Fraga, M. F., Ballestar, E., Paz, M. F., Ropero, S., Setien, F., Ballestar, M. L., et al. (2005). Epigenetic Differences Arise during the Lifetime of Monozygotic Twins. *Proc. Natl. Acad. Sci. U S A.* 102 (30), 10604–10609. doi:10.1073/pnas.0500398102

Francone, M., Iafrate, F., Masci, G. M., Coco, S., Cilia, F., Manganaro, L., et al. (2020). Chest CT Score in COVID-19 Patients: Correlation with Disease Severity and Short-Term Prognosis. *Eur. Radiol.* 30 (12), 6808–6817. doi:10.1007/s00330-020-07033-y

Fuglebjerg, N. J. U., Jensen, T. O., Hoyer, N., Ryrsø, C. K., Lindegaard, B., and Harboe, Z. B. (2020). Silent Hypoxia in Patients with SARS CoV-2 Infection before Hospital Discharge. *Int. J. Infect. Dis.* 99, 100–101. doi:10.1016/j.ijid.2020.07.014

Gaikwad, A. V., Eapen, M. S., McAlinden, K. D., Chia, C., Larby, J., Myers, S., et al. (2020). Endothelial to Mesenchymal Transition (EndMT) and Vascular Remodeling in Pulmonary Hypertension and Idiopathic Pulmonary Fibrosis. *Expert Rev. Respir. Med.* 14 (10), 1027–1043. doi:10.1080/17476348.2020.1795832

Gan, W., Huang, Q., Xiao, G., Luo, Y., Wang, J., Zhang, C., et al. (2020). Modified Maimendong Decoction in the Treatment of Patients with Idiopathic Pulmonary Fibrosis: Study Protocol for a Randomized Contrôlled Trial. *Medicine (Baltimore)* 99 (49), e23460. doi:10.1097/md.0000000000023460

Gatti, M., Fusaroli, M., Caraceni, P., Poluzzi, E., De Ponti, F., and Raschi, E. (2021). Serious Adverse Events with Tocilizumab: Pharmacovigilance as an Aid to Prioritize Monitoring in COVID-19. *Br. J. Clin. Pharmacol.* 87 (3), 1533–1540. doi:10.1111/bcp.14459

Gautret, P., Million, M., Jarrot, P. A., Camoin-Jau, L., Colson, P., Fenollar, F., et al. (2020). Natural History of COVID-19 and Therapeutic Options. *Expert Rev. Clin. Immunol.* 16 (12), 1159–1184. doi:10.1080/1744666x.2021.1847640

Gentile, F., Aimo, A., Forfori, F., Catapano, G., Clemente, A., Cademartiri, F., et al. (2020). COVID-19 and Risk of Pulmonary Fibrosis: the Importance of Planning Ahead. *Eur. J. Prev. Cardiol.* 27 (13), 1442–1446. doi:10.1177/2047487320932695

George, P. M., Wells, A. U., and Jenkins, R. G. (2020). Pulmonary Fibrosis and COVID-19: the Potential Role for Antifibrotic Therapy. *Lancet Respir. Med.* 8 (8), 807–815. doi:10.1016/s2213-2600(20)30225-3

Ghonim, M. A., Pyakurel, K., Ibba, S. V., Al-Khami, A. A., Wang, J., Rodriguez, P., et al. (2015a). PARP Inhibition by Olaparib or Gene Knockout Blocks Asthma-like Manifestation in Mice by Modulating CD4(+) T Cell Function. *J. Transl Med.* 13, 225. doi:10.1186/s12967-015-0583-0

Ghonim, M. A., Pyakurel, K., Ibba, S. V., Wang, J., Rodriguez, P., Al-Khami, A. A., et al. (2015b). PARP Is Activated in Human Asthma and its Inhibition by Olaparib Blocks House Dust Mite-Induced Disease in Mice. *Clin. Sci. (Lond)* 129 (11), 951–962. doi:10.1042/cs20150122

Glenisson, W., Castronovo, V., and Waltregny, D. (2007). Histone Deacetylase 4 Is Required for TGFbeta1-Induced Myofibroblastic Differentiation. *Biochim. Biophys. Acta* 1773 (10), 1572–1582. doi:10.1016/j.bbamcr.2007.05.016

Guillot, S., Delaval, P., Brinchault, G., Caulet-Maugendre, S., Depince, A., Lena, H., et al. (2006). Increased Extracellular Matrix Metalloproteinase Inducer (EMMPRIN) Expression in Pulmonary Fibrosis. *Exp. Lung Res.* 32 (3-4), 81–97. doi:10.1080/01902140600710512

Guo, Y. R., Cao, Q. D., Hong, Z. S., Tan, Y. Y., Chen, S. D., Jin, H. J., et al. (2020). The Origin, Transmission and Clinical Therapies on Coronavirus Disease 2019 (COVID-19) Outbreak - an Update on the Status. *Mil. Med. Res.* 7 (1), 11. doi:10.1186/s40779-020-00240-0

Han, X., Fan, Y., Alwalid, O., Li, N., Jia, X., Yuan, M., et al. (2021). Six-month Follow-Up Chest CT Findings after Severe COVID-19 Pneumonia. *RADIOLOGY* 299 (1), E177–E186. doi:10.1148/radiol.2021203153

Haulica, I., Bild, W., Mihaila, C., Serban, D. N., Serban, L., Boisteanu, D., et al. (2004). Comparative Study of the Inhibitory Effects of Adrenomedullin on Angiotensin II Contraction in Rat Conductance and Resistance Arteries. *J. Renin Angiotensin Aldosterone Syst.* 5 (2), 79–83. doi:10.3317/jraas.2004.014

He, B., and Garmire, L. (2020). Prediction of Repurposed Drugs for Treating Lung Injury in COVID-19. *ArXiv* 9, 609. doi:10.12688/f1000research.23996.2

Hoffmann, M., Kleine-Weber, H., Schroeder, S., Krüger, N., Herrler, T., Erichsen, S., et al. (2020). SARS-CoV-2 Cell Entry Depends on ACE2 and TMPRSS2 and Is Blocked by a Clinically Proven Protease Inhibitor. *Cell* 181 (2), 271–e8. doi:10.1016/j.cell.2020.02.052

Homma, S., Bando, M., Azuma, A., Sakamoto, S., Sugino, K., Ishii, Y., et al. (2018). Japanese Guideline for the Treatment of Idiopathic Pulmonary Fibrosis. *Respir. Investig.* 56 (4), 268–291. doi:10.1016/j.resinv.2018.03.003

Hou, Y. J., Okuda, K., Edwards, C. E., Martinez, D. R., Asakura, T., Dinnon, K. H., III, et al. (2020). SARS-CoV-2 Reverse Genetics Reveals a Variable Infection Gradient in the Respiratory Tract. *Cell* 182 (2), 429–e14. doi:10.1016/j.cell.2020.05.042

Huang, C., Wang, Y., Li, X., Ren, L., Zhao, J., Hu, Y., et al. (2020). Clinical Features of Patients Infected with 2019 Novel Coronavirus in Wuhan, China. *Lancet* 395 (10223), 497–506. doi:10.1016/s0140-6736(20)30183-5

Hui, D. S. C., and Zumla, A. (2019). Severe Acute Respiratory Syndrome: Historical, Epidemiologic, and Clinical Features. *Infect. Dis. Clin. North. Am.* 33 (4), 869–889. doi:10.1016/j.idc.2019.07.001

Hung, I. F., Lung, K. C., Tso, E. Y., Liu, R., Chung, T. W., Chu, M. Y., et al. (2020). Triple Combination of Interferon Beta-1b, Lopinavir-Ritonavir, and Ribavirin in the Treatment of Patients Admitted to Hospital with COVID-19: an Open-Label, Randomised, Phase 2 Trial. *LANCET* 395 (10238), 1695–1704. doi:10.1016/S0140-6736(20)31042-4

Janowitz, T., Gablenz, E., Pattinson, D., Wang, T. C., Conigliaro, J., Tracey, K., et al. (2020). Famotidine Use and Quantitative Symptom Tracking for COVID-19 in Non-hospitalised Patients: a Case Series. *Gut* 69 (9), 1592–1597. doi:10.1136/gutjnl-2020-321852

Jenkins, G. (2020). Demystifying Pulmonary Fibrosis. *Am. J. Physiol. Lung Cel Mol Physiol* 319 (3), L554–L559. doi:10.1152/ajplung.00365.2020

Jenkins, R. G., Su, X., Su, G., Scotton, C. J., Camerer, E., Laurent, G. J., et al. (2006). Ligation of Protease-Activated Receptor 1 Enhances Alpha(v) beta6 Integrin-dependent TGF-Beta Activation and Promotes Acute Lung Injury. *J. Clin. Invest.* 116 (6), 1606–1614. doi:10.1172/jci27183

Jiang, G., Cai, Y., Yi, X., Li, Y., Lin, Y., Li, Q., et al. (2020). The Impact of Laryngopharyngeal Reflux Disease on 95 Hospitalized Patients with COVID-19 in Wuhan, China: A Retrospective Study. *J. Med. Virol.* 92 (10), 2124–2129. doi:10.1002/jmv.25998

John, A. E., Joseph, C., Jenkins, G., and Tatler, A. L. (2021). COVID-19 and Pulmonary Fibrosis: A Potential Role for Lung Epithelial Cells and Fibroblasts. *Immunol. Rev.* 302 (1), 228–240. doi:10.1111/imr.12977

Kaur, U., Acharya, K., Mondal, R., Singh, A., Saso, L., Chakrabarti, S., et al. (2020). Should ACE2 Be Given a Chance in COVID-19 Therapeutics: A Semi-systematic Review of Strategies Enhancing ACE2. *Eur. J. Pharmacol.* 887, 173545. doi:10.1016/j.ejphar.2020.173545

Khoo, J. K., Montgomery, A. B., Otto, K. L., Surber, M., Faggian, J., Lickliter, J. D., et al. (2020). A Randomized, Double-Blinded, Placebo-Controlled, Dose-Escalation Phase 1 Study of Aerosolized Pirfenidone Delivered via the PARI Investigational eFlow Nebulizer in Volunteers and Patients with Idiopathic Pulmonary Fibrosis. *J. Aerosol Med. Pulm. Drug Deliv.* 33 (1), 15–20. doi:10.1089/jamp.2018.1507

Kobayashi, T., Tanaka, K., Fujita, T., Umezawa, H., Amano, H., Yoshioka, K., et al. (2015). Bidirectional Role of IL-6 Signal in Pathogenesis of Lung Fibrosis. *Respir. Res.* 16, 99. doi:10.1186/s12931-015-0261-z

Korfei, M., Skwarna, S., Henneke, I., MacKenzie, B., Klymenko, O., Saito, S., et al. (2015). Aberrant Expression and Activity of Histone Deacetylases in Sporadic Idiopathic Pulmonary Fibrosis. *Thorax* 70 (11), 1022–1032. doi:10.1136/thoraxjnl-2014-206411

Korfei, M., Stelmaszek, D., MacKenzie, B., Skwarna, S., Chillappagari, S., Bach, A. C., et al. (2018). Comparison of the Antifibrotic Effects of the Pan-Histone Deacetylase-Inhibitor Panobinostat versus the IPF-Drug Pirfenidone in Fibroblasts from Patients with Idiopathic Pulmonary Fibrosis. *Plos One* 13 (11), e0207915. doi:10.1371/journal.pone.0207915

Kotfis, K., Lechowicz, K., Drożdżal, S., Niedźwiedzka-Rystwej, P., Wojdacz, T. K., Grywalska, E., et al. (2021). COVID-19-The Potential Beneficial Therapeutic Effects of Spironolactone during SARS-CoV-2 Infection. *Pharmaceuticals (Basel)* 14 (1). doi:10.3390/ph14010071

Koyama, S., Sato, E., Haniuda, M., Numanami, H., Nagai, S., and Izumi, T. (2002). Decreased Level of Vascular Endothelial Growth Factor in Bronchoalveolar Lavage Fluid of normal Smokers and Patients with Pulmonary Fibrosis. *Am. J. Respir. Crit. Care Med.* 166 (3), 382–385. doi:10.1164/rccm.2103112

Lamontagne, F., Agoritsas, T., Siemieniuk, R., Rochwerg, B., Bartoszko, J., Askie, L., et al. (2021). A Living WHO Guideline on Drugs to Prevent Covid-19. *Bmj* 372, n526. doi:10.1136/bmj.n526

Launay, J. M., Del Pino, M., Chironi, G., Callebert, J., Peoc'h, K., Mégnien, J. L., et al. (2009). Smoking Induces Long-Lasting Effects through a Monoamine-Oxidase Epigenetic Regulation. *Plos One* 4 (11), e7959. doi:10.1371/journal.pone.0007959

Lee, N., Allen Chan, K. C., Hui, D. S., Ng, E. K., Wu, A., Chiu, R. W., et al. (2004). Effects of Early Corticosteroid Treatment on Plasma SARS-Associated Coronavirus RNA Concentrations in Adult Patients. *J. Clin. Virol.* 31 (4), 304–309. doi:10.1016/j.jcv.2004.07.006

Li, G., Fan, Y., Lai, Y., Han, T., Li, Z., Zhou, P., et al. (2020). Coronavirus Infections and Immune Responses. *J. Med. Virol.* 92 (4), 424–432. doi:10.1002/jmv.25685

Li, G. F., An, X. X., Yu, Y., Jiao, L. R., Canarutto, D., Yu, G., et al. (2021a). Do proton Pump Inhibitors Influence SARS-CoV-2 Related Outcomes? A Meta-Analysis. *Gut* 70 (9), 1806–1808. doi:10.1136/gutjnl-2020-323366

Li, H. H., Liu, C. C., Hsu, T. W., Lin, J. H., Hsu, J. W., Li, A. F., et al. (2021b). Upregulation of ACE2 and TMPRSS2 by Particulate Matter and Idiopathic Pulmonary Fibrosis: a Potential Role in Severe COVID-19. *Part. Fibre Toxicol.* 18 (1), 11. doi:10.1186/s12989-021-00404-3

Liao, M., Liu, Y., Yuan, J., Wen, Y., Xu, G., Zhao, J., et al. (2020). Single-cell Landscape of Bronchoalveolar Immune Cells in Patients with COVID-19. *Nat. Med.* 26(6), 842, 844-+. doi: doi:10.1038/s41591-020-0901-9

Lieber, G. B., Fernandez, X., Mingo, G. G., Jia, Y., Caniga, M., Gil, M. A., et al. (2013). Mineralocorticoid Receptor Antagonists Attenuate Pulmonary Inflammation and Bleomycin-Evoked Fibrosis in Rodent Models. *Eur. J. Pharmacol.* 718 (1-3), 290–298. doi:10.1016/j.ejphar.2013.08.019

Liu, Q., Wang, R. S., Qu, G. Q., Wang, Y. Y., Liu, P., Zhu, Y. Z., et al. (2020). Gross Examination Report of a COVID-19 Death Autopsy. *Fa yi xue za zhi* 36 (1), 21–23. doi:10.12116/j.issn.1004-5619.2020.01.005

Liu, Y., Lu, F., Kang, L., Wang, Z., and Wang, Y. (2017). Pirfenidone Attenuates Bleomycin-Induced Pulmonary Fibrosis in Mice by Regulating Nrf2/Bach1 Equilibrium. *BMC Pulm. Med.* 17, 63. doi:10.1186/s12890-017-0405-7

Magro, C. M., Waldman, W. J., Knight, D. A., Allen, J. N., Nadasdy, T., Frambach, G. E., et al. (2006). Idiopathic Pulmonary Fibrosis Related to Endothelial Injury and Antiendothelial Cell Antibodies. *Hum. Immunol.* 67 (4-5), 284–297. doi:10.1016/j.humimm.2006.02.026

Mahajan, L., Singh, A. P., and Gifty (2021). Clinical Outcomes of Using Remdesivir in Patients with Moderate to Severe COVID-19: A Prospective Randomised Study. *Indian J. Anaesth.* 65 (Suppl. 1), S41–S46. doi:10.4103/ija.IJA_149_21

Maher, T. M., Bendstrup, E., Dron, L., Langley, J., Smith, G., Khalid, J. M., et al. (2021). Global Incidence and Prevalence of Idiopathic Pulmonary Fibrosis. *Respir. Res.* 22 (1), 197. doi:10.1186/s12931-021-01791-z

Major, J., Crotta, S., Llorian, M., McCabe, T. M., Gad, H. H., Priestnall, S. L., et al. (2020). Type I and III Interferons Disrupt Lung Epithelial Repair during Recovery from Viral Infection. *SCIENCE* 369(6504), 712, 717-+. doi: doi:10.1126/science.abc2061

Margaritopoulos, G. A., Vasarmidi, E., and Antoniou, K. M. (2016). Pirfenidone in the Treatment of Idiopathic Pulmonary Fibrosis: an Evidence-Based Review of its Place in Therapy. *Core Evid.* 11, 11–22. doi:10.2147/ce.S76549

Maruta, H., and He, H. (2020). PAK1-blockers: Potential Therapeutics against COVID-19. *Med. Drug Discov.* 6, 100039. doi:10.1016/j.medidd.2020.100039

Mather, J. F., Seip, R. L., and McKay, R. G. (2020). Impact of Famotidine Use on Clinical Outcomes of Hospitalized Patients with COVID-19. *Am. J. Gastroenterol.* 115 (10), 1517–1623. doi:10.14309/ajg.0000000000000832

Monaghan-Benson, E., Wittchen, E. S., Doerschuk, C. M., and Burridge, K. (2018). A Rnd3/p190RhoGAP Pathway Regulates RhoA Activity in Idiopathic Pulmonary Fibrosis Fibroblasts. *Mol. Biol. Cel* 29 (18), 2165–2175. doi:10.1091/mbc.E17-11-0642

Myllärniemi, M., and Kaarteenaho, R. (2015). Pharmacological Treatment of Idiopathic Pulmonary Fibrosis - Preclinical and Clinical Studies of Pirfenidone, Nintedanib, and N-Acetylcysteine. *Eur. Clin. Respir. J.* 2. doi:10.3402/ecrj.v2.26385

Ni, Y. N., Chen, G., Sun, J., Liang, B. M., and Liang, Z. A. (2019). The Effect of Corticosteroids on Mortality of Patients with Influenza Pneumonia: a Systematic Review and Meta-Analysis. *Crit. Care* 23, 99. doi:10.1186/s13054-019-2395-8

Nile, S. H., Nile, A., Qiu, J., Li, L., Jia, X., and Kai, G. (2020). COVID-19: Pathogenesis, Cytokine Storm and Therapeutic Potential of Interferons. *Cytokine Growth Factor. Rev.* 53, 66–70. doi:10.1016/j.cytogfr.2020.05.002

Nkyimbeng, T., Ruppert, C., Shiomi, T., Dahal, B., Lang, G., Seeger, W., et al. (2013). Pivotal Role of Matrix Metalloproteinase 13 in Extracellular Matrix Turnover in Idiopathic Pulmonary Fibrosis. *Plos One* 8 (9), e73279. doi:10.1371/journal.pone.0073279

Noble, P. W., Albera, C., Bradford, W. Z., Costabel, U., Glassberg, M. K., Kardatzke, D., et al. (2011). Pirfenidone in Patients with Idiopathic Pulmonary Fibrosis (CAPACITY): Two Randomised Trials. *LANCET* 377 (9779), 1760–1769. doi:10.1016/S0140-6736(11)60405-4

Nunes, H. (2003). Pathogenesis of Idiopathic Pulmonary Fibrosis. *Revue Des Maladies Respiratoires* 20 (5), S100–S102.

Ojha, V., Mani, A., Pandey, N. N., Sharma, S., and Kumar, S. (2020). CT in Coronavirus Disease 2019 (COVID-19): a Systematic Review of Chest CT Findings in 4410 Adult Patients. *Eur. Radiol.* 30 (11), 6129–6138. doi:10.1007/s00330-020-06975-7

Onoue, S., Seto, Y., Kato, M., Aoki, Y., Kojo, Y., and Yamada, S. (2013). Inhalable Powder Formulation of Pirfenidone with Reduced Phototoxic Risk for Treatment of Pulmonary Fibrosis. *Pharm. Res.* 30 (6), 1586–1596. doi:10.1007/s11095-013-0997-4

P, K. M., Sivashanmugam, K., Kandasamy, M., Subbiah, R., and Ravikumar, V. (2021). Repurposing of Histone Deacetylase Inhibitors: A Promising Strategy to Combat Pulmonary Fibrosis Promoted by TGF-β Signalling in COVID-19 Survivors. *Life Sci.* 266, 118883. doi:10.1016/j.lfs.2020.118883

Pan, L. H., Yamauchi, K., Uzuki, M., Nakanishi, T., Takigawa, M., Inoue, H., et al. (2001). Type II Alveolar Epithelial Cells and Interstitial Fibroblasts Express Connective Tissue Growth Factor in IPF. *Eur. Respir. J.* 17 (6), 1220–1227. doi:10.1183/09031936.01.00074101

Pei, G., Zhang, Z., Peng, J., Liu, L., Zhang, C., Yu, C., et al. (2020). Renal Involvement and Early Prognosis in Patients with COVID-19 Pneumonia. *J. Am. Soc. Nephrol.* 31 (6), 1157–1165. doi:10.1681/ASN.2020030276

Peng, D.-H., Luo, Y., Huang, L.-J., Liao, F.-L., Liu, Y.-Y., Tang, P., et al. (2021). Correlation of Krebs von den Lungen-6 and fibronectin with pulmonary fibrosis in coronavirus disease 2019. *CLINICA CHIMICA ACTA* 517, 48–53. doi:10.1016/j.cca.2021.02.012

Perreau, M., Suffiotti, M., Marques-Vidal, P., Wiedemann, A., Levy, Y., Laouénan, C., et al. (2021). The Cytokines HGF and CXCL13 Predict the Severity and the Mortality in COVID-19 Patients. *Nat. Commun.* 12 (1), 4888. doi:10.1038/s41467-021-25191-5

Philp, C. J., Siebeke, I., Clements, D., Miller, S., Habgood, A., John, A. E., et al. (2018). Extracellular Matrix Cross-Linking Enhances Fibroblast Growth and Protects against Matrix Proteolysis in Lung Fibrosis. *Am. J. Respir. Cel Mol Biol* 58 (5), 594–603. doi:10.1165/rcmb.2016-0379OC

Quartuccio, L., Semerano, L., Benucci, M., Boissier, M. C., and De Vita, S. (2020). Urgent Avenues in the Treatment of COVID-19: Targeting Downstream Inflammation to Prevent Catastrophic Syndrome. *Jt. Bone Spine* 87 (3), 191–193. doi:10.1016/j.jbspin.2020.03.011

Raghu, G., Rochwerg, B., Zhang, Y., Garcia, C. A., Azuma, A., Behr, J., et al. (2015). An Official ATS/ERS/JRS/ALAT Clinical Practice Guideline: Treatment of Idiopathic Pulmonary Fibrosis. An Update of the 2011 Clinical Practice Guideline. *Am. J. Respir. Crit. Care Med.* 192 (5), e3–19. doi:10.1164/rccm.201506-1063ST

Rao, S., Lau, A., and So, H. C. (2020). Exploring Diseases/Traits and Blood Proteins Causally Related to Expression of ACE2, the Putative Receptor of SARS-CoV-2: A Mendelian Randomization Analysis Highlights Tentative Relevance of Diabetes-Related Traits. *Diabetes Care* 43 (7), 1416–1426. doi:10.2337/dc20-0643

Rasooli, R., Rajaian, H., Pardakhty, A., and Mandegary, A. (2018). Preference of Aerosolized Pirfenidone to Oral Intake: An Experimental Model of Pulmonary Fibrosis by Paraquat. *J. Aerosol Med. Pulm. Drug Deliv.* 31 (1), 25–32. doi:10.1089/jamp.2016.1342

Reyfman, P. A., Walter, J. M., Joshi, N., Anekalla, K. R., McQuattie-Pimentel, A. C., Chiu, S., et al. (2019). Single-Cell Transcriptomic Analysis of Human Lung Provides Insights into the Pathobiology of Pulmonary Fibrosis. *Am. J. Respir. Crit. Care Med.* 199 (12), 1517–1536. doi:10.1164/rccm.201712-2410OC

Richeldi, L., Costabel, U., Selman, M., Kim, D. S., Hansell, D. M., Nicholson, A. G., et al. (2011). Efficacy of a Tyrosine Kinase Inhibitor in Idiopathic Pulmonary Fibrosis. *N. Engl. J. Med.* 365 (12), 1079–1087. doi:10.1056/NEJMoa1103690

Richeldi, L., du Bois, R. M., Raghu, G., Azuma, A., Brown, K. K., Costabel, U., et al. (2014). Efficacy and Safety of Nintedanib in Idiopathic Pulmonary Fibrosis. *N. Engl. J. Med.* 370 (22), 2071–2082. doi:10.1056/NEJMoa1402584

Sahu, B., Narota, A., and Naura, A. S. (2020). Pharmacological Inhibition of Poly (ADP-Ribose) Polymerase by Olaparib, Prevents Acute Lung Injury Associated Cognitive Deficits Potentially through Suppression of Inflammatory Response. *Eur. J. Pharmacol.* 877, 173091. doi:10.1016/j.ejphar.2020.173091

Saito, S., Zhuang, Y., Shan, B., Danchuk, S., Luo, F., Korfei, M., et al. (2017). Tubastatin Ameliorates Pulmonary Fibrosis by Targeting the TGFβ-Pi3k-Akt Pathway. *Plos One* 12 (10), e0186615. doi:10.1371/journal.pone.0186615

Salama, C., Han, J., Yau, L., Reiss, W. G., Kramer, B., Neidhart, J. D., et al. (2021). Tocilizumab in Patients Hospitalized with Covid-19 Pneumonia. *N. Engl. J. Med.* 384 (1), 20–30. doi:10.1056/NEJMoa2030340

Sanchis-Gomar, F., Lavie, C. J., Perez-Quilis, C., Henry, B. M., and Lippi, G. (2020). Angiotensin-Converting Enzyme 2 and Antihypertensives (Angiotensin Receptor Blockers and Angiotensin-Converting Enzyme Inhibitors) in Coronavirus Disease 2019. *Mayo Clin. Proc.* 95 (6), 1222–1230. doi:10.1016/j.mayocp.2020.03.026

Sethi, G. S., Sharma, S., and Naura, A. S. (2019). PARP Inhibition by Olaparib Alleviates Chronic Asthma-Associated Remodeling Features via Modulating Inflammasome Signaling in Mice. *Iubmb Life* 71 (7), 1003–1013. doi:10.1002/iub.2048

Sharif, R. (2017). Overview of Idiopathic Pulmonary Fibrosis (IPF) and Evidence-Based Guidelines. *Am. J. Manag. Care* 23 (11 Suppl. l), S176–S182.

Shenoy, V., Ferreira, A. J., Qi, Y., Fraga-Silva, R. A., Díez-Freire, C., Dooies, A., et al. (2010). The Angiotensin-Converting Enzyme 2/Angiogenesis-(1-7)/Mas Axis Confers Cardiopulmonary Protection against Lung Fibrosis and Pulmonary Hypertension. *Am. J. Respir. Crit. Care Med.* 182 (8), 1065–1072. doi:10.1164/rccm.200912-1840OC

Sibinska, Z., Tian, X., Korfei, M., Kojonazarov, B., Kolb, J. S., Klepetko, W., et al. (2017). Amplified Canonical Transforming Growth Factor-β Signalling via Heat Shock Protein 90 in Pulmonary Fibrosis. *Eur. Respir. J.* 49 (2). doi:10.1183/13993003.01941-2015

Singh, A. K., Singh, A., Singh, R., and Misra, A. (2020). Remdesivir in COVID-19: A Critical Review of Pharmacology, Pre-clinical and Clinical Studies. *Diabetes Metab. Syndr.* 14 (4), 641–648. doi:10.1016/j.dsx.2020.05.018

Sisson, T. H., Mendez, M., Choi, K., Subbotina, N., Courey, A., Cunningham, A., et al. (2010). Targeted Injury of Type II Alveolar Epithelial Cells Induces Pulmonary Fibrosis. *Am. J. Respir. Crit. Care Med.* 181 (3), 254–263. doi:10.1164/rccm.200810-1615OC

Spinner, C. D., Gottlieb, R. L., Criner, G. J., Arribas López, J. R., Cattelan, A. M., Soriano Viladomiu, A., et al. (2020). Effect of Remdesivir vs Standard Care on Clinical Status at 11 Days in Patients with Moderate COVID-19: A Randomized Clinical Trial. *JAMA* 324 (11), 1048–1057. doi:10.1001/jama.2020.16349

Stockman, L. J., Bellamy, R., and Garner, P. (2006). SARS: Systematic Review of Treatment Effects. *Plos Med.* 3 (9), e343–1531. doi:10.1371/journal.pmed.0030343

Stone, J. H., Frigault, M. J., Serling-Boyd, N. J., Fernandes, A. D., Harvey, L., Foulkes, A. S., et al. (2020). Efficacy of Tocilizumab in Patients Hospitalized with Covid-19. *N. Engl. J. Med.* 383 (24), 2333–2344. doi:10.1056/NEJMoa2028836

Sun, P., Ren, J., Li, K., Qie, S., Liu, Z., and Xi, J. (2020). Response to: Sore Throat in COVID-19: Comment on "Clinical Characteristics of Hospitalized Patients with SARS-CoV-2 Infection: A Single Arm Meta-Analysis". *J. Med. Virol.* 92 (6), 716–718. doi:10.1002/jmv.25818

Surber, M. W., Poulin, D., McInally, K., Chapdelaine, J., Gendron, D., Tat, V., et al. (2014). Inhaled Pirfenidone Improves Animal Efficacy through Superior Pulmonary and Vascular Pharmacokinetics. *AMERICAN JOURNAL RESPIRATORY CRITICAL CARE MEDICINE* 189.

Tatler, A. L., and Jenkins, G. (2012). TGF-β Activation and Lung Fibrosis. *Proc. Am. Thorac. Soc.* 9 (3), 130–136. doi:10.1513/pats.201201-003AW

Tatler, A. L., Barnes, J., Habgood, A., Goodwin, A., McAnulty, R. J., and Jenkins, G. (2016). Caffeine Inhibits TGFβ Activation in Epithelial Cells, Interrupts Fibroblast Responses to TGFβ, and Reduces Established Fibrosis Inex Vivoprecision-Cut Lung Slices. *Thorax* 71 (6), 565–567. doi:10.1136/thoraxjnl-2015-208215

Tilocca, B., Soggiu, A., Sanguinetti, M., Musella, V., Britti, D., Bonizzi, L., et al. (2020). Comparative Computational Analysis of SARS-CoV-2 Nucleocapsid Protein Epitopes in Taxonomically Related Coronaviruses. *Microbes Infect.* 22 (4-5), 188–194. doi:10.1016/j.micinf.2020.04.002

Tobin, R. W., Pope, C. E., Pellegrini, C. A., Emond, M. J., Sillery, J., and Raghu, G. (1998). Increased Prevalence of Gastroesophageal Reflux in Patients with Idiopathic Pulmonary Fibrosis. *Am. J. Respir. Crit. Care Med.* 158 (6), 1804–1808. doi:10.1164/ajrccm.158.6.9804105

Trachalaki, A., Irfan, M., and Wells, A. U. (2021). Pharmacological Management of Idiopathic Pulmonary Fibrosis: Current and Emerging Options. *Expert Opin. Pharmacother.* 22 (2), 191–204. doi:10.1080/14656566.2020.1822326

Ulrich, H., and Pillat, M. M. (2020). CD147 as a Target for COVID-19 Treatment: Suggested Effects of Azithromycin and Stem Cell Engagement. *Stem Cel Rev Rep* 16 (3), 434–440. doi:10.1007/s12015-020-09976-7

Umemura, Y., Mitsuyama, Y., Minami, K., Nishida, T., Watanabe, A., Okada, N., et al. (2021). Efficacy and Safety of Nintedanib for Pulmonary Fibrosis in Severe

Pneumonia Induced by COVID-19: An Interventional Study. *Int. J. Infect. Dis.* 108, 454–460. doi:10.1016/j.ijid.2021.05.055

Veiga, V. C., Prats, J. A. G. G., Farias, D. L. C., Rosa, R. G., Dourado, L. K., Zampieri, F. G., et al. (2021). Effect of Tocilizumab on Clinical Outcomes at 15 Days in Patients with Severe or Critical Coronavirus Disease 2019: Randomised Controlled Trial. *Bmj* 372, n84. doi:10.1136/bmj.n84

Venkataraman, T., and Frieman, M. B. (2017). The Role of Epidermal Growth Factor Receptor (EGFR) Signaling in SARS Coronavirus-Induced Pulmonary Fibrosis. *Antivir. Res* 143, 142–150. doi:10.1016/j.antiviral.2017.03.022

Villar, J., Confalonieri, M., Pastores, S. M., and Meduri, G. U. (2020). Rationale for Prolonged Corticosteroid Treatment in the Acute Respiratory Distress Syndrome Caused by Coronavirus Disease 2019. *Crit. Care Explor* 2 (4), e0111. doi:10.1097/cce.0000000000000111

Wan, S., Yi, Q., Fan, S., Lv, J., Zhang, X., Guo, L., et al. (2020). Relationships Among Lymphocyte Subsets, Cytokines, and the Pulmonary Inflammation index in Coronavirus (COVID-19) Infected Patients. *Br. J. Haematol.* 189 (3), 428–437. doi:10.1111/bjh.16659

Wang, K., Chen, W., Zhang, Z., Deng, Y., Lian, J. Q., Du, P., et al. (2020). CD147-spike Protein Is a Novel Route for SARS-CoV-2 Infection to Host Cells. *Signal. Transduct Target. Ther.* 5 (1), 283. doi:10.1038/s41392-020-00426-x

Weng, D., Chen, X. Q., Qiu, H., Zhang, Y., Li, Q. H., Zhao, M. M., et al. (2019). The Role of Infection in Acute Exacerbation of Idiopathic Pulmonary Fibrosis. *Mediators Inflamm.* 2019, 5160694. doi:10.1155/2019/5160694

Wootton, S. C., Kim, D. S., Kondoh, Y., Chen, E., Lee, J. S., Song, J. W., et al. (2011). Viral Infection in Acute Exacerbation of Idiopathic Pulmonary Fibrosis. *Am. J. Respir. Crit. Care Med.* 183 (12), 1698–1702. doi:10.1164/rccm.201010-1752OC

Wu, C., Chen, X., Cai, Y., Xia, J., Zhou, X., Xu, S., et al. (2020a). Risk Factors Associated with Acute Respiratory Distress Syndrome and Death in Patients with Coronavirus Disease 2019 Pneumonia in Wuhan, China. *JAMA Intern. Med.* 180 (7), 934–943. doi:10.1001/jamainternmed.2020.142910.1001/jamainternmed.2020.0994

Wu, J., Song, S., Cao, H. C., and Li, L. J. (2020b). Liver Diseases in COVID-19: Etiology, Treatment and Prognosis. *World J. Gastroenterol.* 26 (19), 2286–2293. doi:10.3748/wjg.v26.i19.2286

Wu, Z., and McGoogan, J. M. (2020). Characteristics of and Important Lessons from the Coronavirus Disease 2019 (COVID-19) Outbreak in China: Summary of a Report of 72 314 Cases from the Chinese Center for Disease Control and Prevention. *JAMA* 323 (13), 1239–1242. doi:10.1001/jama.2020.2648

Xu, Y. D., Hua, J., Mui, A., O'Connor, R., Grotendorst, G., and Khalil, N. (2003). Release of Biologically Active TGF-Beta1 by Alveolar Epithelial Cells Results in Pulmonary Fibrosis. *Am. J. Physiol. Lung Cel Mol Physiol* 285 (3), L527–L539. doi:10.1152/ajplung.00298.2002

Xue, M., Zhang, T., Chen, H., Zeng, Y., Lin, R., Zhen, Y., et al. (2021). Krebs Von Den Lungen-6 as a Predictive Indicator for the Risk of Secondary Pulmonary Fibrosis and its Reversibility in COVID-19 Patients. *Int. J. Biol. Sci.* 17 (6), 1565–1573. doi:10.7150/ijbs.58825

Yang, I. V., Konigsberg, I., MacPhail, K., Li, L., Davidson, E. J., Mroz, P. M., et al. (2019). DNA Methylation Changes in Lung Immune Cells Are Associated with Granulomatous Lung Disease. *Am. J. Respir. Cel Mol Biol* 60 (1), 96–105. doi:10.1165/rcmb.2018-0177OC

Yao, C., Guan, X., Carraro, G., Parimon, T., Liu, X., Huang, G., et al. (2021). Senescence of Alveolar Type 2 Cells Drives Progressive Pulmonary Fibrosis. *Am. J. Respir. Crit. Care Med.* 203 (6), 707–717. doi:10.1164/rccm.202004-1274OC

Yao, X. H., Li, T. Y., He, Z. C., Ping, Y. F., Liu, H. W., Yu, S. C., et al. (2020). A Pathological Report of Three COVID-19 Cases by Minimal Invasive Autopsies. *Zhonghua Bing Li Xue Za Zhi* 49 (5), 411–417. doi:10.3760/cma.j.cn112151-20200312-00193

Yavas, G., Yavas, C., Celik, E., Sen, E., Ata, O., and Afsar, R. E. (2019). The Impact of Spironolactone on the Lung Injury Induced by Concomitant Trastuzumab and Thoracic Radiotherapy. *Int. J. Radiat. Res.* 17 (1), 87–95. doi:10.18869/acadpub.ijrr.17.1.87

Yu, M., Liu, Y., Xu, D., Zhang, R., Lan, L., and Xu, H. (2020). Prediction of the Development of Pulmonary Fibrosis Using Serial Thin-Section CT and Clinical Features in Patients Discharged after Treatment for COVID-19 Pneumonia. *Korean J. Radiol.* 21 (6), 746–755. doi:10.3348/kjr.2020.0215

Yuan, S., Chan, C. C., Chik, K. K., Tsang, J. O., Liang, R., Cao, J., et al. (2020). Broad-Spectrum Host-Based Antivirals Targeting the Interferon and Lipogenesis Pathways as Potential Treatment Options for the Pandemic Coronavirus Disease 2019 (COVID-19). *Viruses* 12 (6). doi:10.3390/v12060628

Zannad, F., Alla, F., Dousset, B., Perez, A., Pitt, B., and Investigators, R. (2000). Limitation of Excessive Extracellular Matrix Turnover May Contribute to Survival Benefit of Spironolactone Therapy in Patients with Congestive Heart Failure: Insights from the Randomized Aldactone Evaluation Study (RALES). Rales Investigators. *Circulation* 102 (22), 2700–2706. doi:10.1161/01.Cir.102.22.2700

Zemans, R. L., Colgan, S. P., and Downey, G. P. (2009). Transepithelial Migration of Neutrophils: Mechanisms and Implications for Acute Lung Injury. *Am. J. Respir. Cel Mol Biol* 40 (5), 519–535. doi:10.1165/rcmb.2008-0348TR

Zhang, C., Wu, Z., Li, J. W., Zhao, H., and Wang, G. Q. (2020a). Cytokine Release Syndrome in Severe COVID-19: Interleukin-6 Receptor Antagonist Tocilizumab May Be the Key to Reduce Mortality. *Int. J. Antimicrob. Agents* 55 (5), 105954. doi:10.1016/j.ijantimicag.2020.105954

Zhang, J., Wang, X., Jia, X., Li, J., Hu, K., Chen, G., et al. (2020b). Risk Factors for Disease Severity, Unimprovement, and Mortality in COVID-19 Patients in Wuhan, China. *Clin. Microbiol. Infect.* 26 (6), 767–772. doi 10.1016/j.cmi.2020.04.012

Zhang, J. J., Cao, Y. Y., Tan, G., Dong, X., Wang, B. C., Lin, J., et al. (2021a). Clinical, Radiological, and Laboratory Characteristics and Risk Factors for Severity and Mortality of 289 Hospitalized COVID-19 Patients. *Allergy* 76 (2), 533–550. doi:10.1111/all.14496

Zhang, Y., Wang, S., Xia, H., Guo, J., He, K., Huang, C., et al. (2021b). Identification of Monocytes Associated with Severe COVID-19 in the PBMCs of Severely Infected Patients through Single-Cell Transcriptome Sequencing. *Engineering.* doi:10.1016/j.eng.2021.05.009

Zhao, X., Nicholls, J. M., and Chen, Y. G. (2008). Severe Acute Respiratory Syndrome-Associated Coronavirus Nucleocapsid Protein Interacts with Smad3 and Modulates Transforming Growth Factor-Beta Signaling. *J. Biol. Chem.* 283 (6), 3272–3280. doi:10.1074/jbc.M708033200

Zhou, F., Yu, T., Du, R., Fan, G., Liu, Y., Liu, Z., et al. (2020). Clinical Course and Risk Factors for Mortality of Adult Inpatients with COVID-19 in Wuhan, China: a Retrospective Cohort Study. *Lancet* 395 (10229), 1054–1062. doi:10.1016/s0140-6736(20)30566-3

Zhu, S., Liu, Y., Zhou, Z., Zhang, Z., Xiao, X., Liu, Z., et al. (2021). Genome-wide CRISPR Activation Screen Identifies Candidate Receptors for SARS-CoV-2 Entry. *Sci. China Life Sci.* doi:10.1007/s11427-021-1990-5

6

The Effect of Cardiovascular Medications on Disease-Related Outcomes in Idiopathic Pulmonary Fibrosis

Wan-Tong Zhang[1†], Xu-Jie Wang[1†], Chun-Miao Xue[2†], Xin-Yu Ji[3], Lin Pan[2], Wei-Liang Weng[1,4], Qiu-Yan Li[1,4], Guo-Dong Hua[2*] and Bao-Chen Zhu[2*]*

[1]Xiyuan Hospital, China Academy of Chinese Medical Sciences, Beijing, China, [2]Dongzhimen Hospital, Beijing University of Chinese Medicine, Beijing, China, [3]Institute of Basic Research in Clinical Medicine, China Academy of Chinese Medical Sciences, Beijing, China, [4]National Clinical Research Center for Chinese Medicine Cardiology, Beijing, China

***Correspondence:**
Qiu-Yan Li
liqiuyan1968@sohu.com
Guo-Dong Hua
zhaojhuagd@126.com
Bao-Chen Zhu
zbcbock123@sina.com

[†]These authors have contributed equally to this work

Background: Multiple studies have revealed that idiopathic pulmonary fibrosis (IPF) patients are more at risk for cardiovascular diseases and that many IPF patients receive cardiovascular medications like statins, angiotensin-converting enzyme inhibitor (ACEI), angiotensin receptor blocker (ARB), and anticoagulants. Existing studies have reported divergent findings on the link between cardiovascular medications and fibrotic disease processes. The aim of this study is to synthesize the evidence on the efficacy of cardiovascular medications in IPF.

Methods: We searched studies reporting the effect of cardiovascular medications on IPF in the PubMed, Embase, Web of Science, Cochrane Library, and two Chinese databases (China National Knowledge Infrastructure database and China Wanfang database). We calculated survival data, forced vital capacity (FVC) decline, and IPF-related mortality to assess the efficacy of cardiovascular medications in IPF. We also estimated statistical heterogeneity by using I^2 and Cochran Q tests, and publication bias was evaluated by risk of bias tools ROBINS-I.

Results: A total of 12 studies were included in the analysis. The included studies had moderate-to-serious risk of bias. Statin use was associated with a reduction in mortality (hazard ratio (HR), 0.89; 95% CI 0.83–0.97). Meta-analysis did not demonstrate any significant relationship between statin use and the FVC decline (HR, 0.86; 95% CI 0.73–1.02), ACEI/ARB use, and survival data (HR, 0.92; 95% CI 0.73–1.15) as well as anticoagulant use and survival data (HR, 1.16; 95% CI 0.62–2.19).

Conclusion: Our study suggested that there is a consistent relationship between statin therapy and survival data in IPF population. However, there is currently insufficient evidence to conclude the effect of ACEI, ARB, and anticoagulant therapy on IPF population especially to the disease-related outcomes in IPF.

Keywords: idiopathic pulmonary fibrosis, ACEI/ARB, statin, anticoagulants, meta-analysis

INTRODUCTION

Idiopathic pulmonary fibrosis (IPF) is a specific form of interstitial lung disease (ILD) (Raghu et al., 2011), characterized by progressive decline in lung function, worsening dyspnea, and impaired health-related quality of life. It generally progresses relentlessly and carries the poorest prognosis of the chronic idiopathic interstitial pneumonias, with a median survival of 3–5 years (Bjoraker et al., 1998). The pathogenesis of IPF is poorly understood. It is hypothesized that alveolar epithelial cell injury triggers release of cytokines such as transforming growth factor beta 1 (TGF-β1), platelet-derived growth factor (PDGF), and tumor necrosis factor (TNF) α. Cardiovascular diseases (Hyldgaard et al., 2014) are common comorbidities in patients with IPF, and many patients with IPF are receiving medications to reduce cardiovascular risk such as statins, anti-hypotentive agents, and anticoagulants. Statins are well known for its lipid-lowering properties through inhibition of 3-hydroxy-3-methylglutaryl coenzyme-A (HMG-CoA) reductase (LaRosa et al., 1999). *In vitro* study on lung fibroblasts showed that simvastatin can inhibit the induction of collagen production by TGF-β (Oka et al., 2013). *In vivo* study showed that simvastatin treatment severely reduced fibrosis, bronchiole adventitial collagen, and bronchiole epithelium (Kruzliak et al., 2015). Angiotensin-converting enzyme inhibitors (ACEIs) and angiotensin receptor blockers (ARBs) are widely used in the management of cardiovascular diseases and systemic hypertension (Chobanian et al., 2003). ACEI inhibits angiotensin I from converting to angiotensin II by inhibiting the activity of angiotensin converting enzyme, thus promoting vasodilation through the kallikrein–kinin system (KKS) to achieve the purpose of lowering blood pressure (Turner and Kodali, 2020). ARB directly inhibits the binding of angiotensin II type 1 receptor (AT1) with angiotensin II receptor (Piepho, 2000). In an *in vitro* study, ACEI has potential anti-pulmonary fibrosis effect by inhibiting apoptosis of human lung epithelial cells (Uhal et al., 1998). An *in vivo* study has proven that ACEI can alleviate focal alveolar lesions, alleviate lung inflammation and pulmonary fibrosis, and improve the survival rate of pulmonary fibrosis rats (Gao et al., 2013; Molteni et al., 2007). Anticoagulants are commonly used to combat thrombotic disorders such as atrial fibrillation and strokes. Recent studies have shown a systemic prothrombotic state in people with IPF (Navaratnam et al., 2014). Several researches with large datasets from different populations reveal an increased risk of vascular events in IPF patients (Hubbard et al., 2008; Sode et al., 2010; Sprunger et al., 2012; Schulman and Crowther, 2012). Also, coagulant and plasminergic proteases are likely to have fibrotic actions, which involve cell-mediated responses via receptors (e.g., PARs and uPAR) and coreceptors (e.g., integrins) (Schuliga, et al., 2018). Based on the above studies, it is thought that there may be a potential benefit to the use of anticoagulants in patients with IPF. There is increasing awareness that the broader pharmacologic properties of statins, ACEI, ARB, and anticoagulants encompass the abilities to modulate local fibroproliferative pathways in a variety of organ systems or prolong the survival of IPF patients.

Existing studies have reported divergent findings on the link between medications used for cardiovascular diseases and fibrotic disease processes. The potential effect of these medications in interstitial fibrosis remains unclear. IPF remains a progressive disease, and new antifibrotic therapies do not reverse existing fibrosis. To address this knowledge gap, we conducted a systematic review and meta-analysis of all medications used in cardiovascular diseases to evaluate their relative efficacy and safety for IPF. Therefore, evaluating the effect of the potential adjuvant therapy may offer new approaches in the management of IPF.

METHODS

Our systematic review and meta-analysis was conducted under the Cochrane Handbook (Higgins et al., 2020). Reporting was consistent with the Preferred Reporting Items for Systematic Reviews and Meta-Analyses (PRISMA) (Guise et al., 2017).

Search Strategy

We systematically searched PubMed, Embase, Web of Science, Cochrane Library (Cochrane Central Register of Controlled Trials), and two Chinese databases (China National Knowledge Infrastructure database and China Wanfang database) to identify non-randomized studies of cardiovascular medications for IPF published from January 2000 to July 2021, with no language restriction. The full search strategy was employed using combinations of MeSH terms and text words around "statin," "hydroxymethylglutaryl-CoA reductase inhibitors," "ACEI," "angiotensin-converting enzyme inhibitors," "angiotensin converting enzyme inhibitors," "ARB," "angiotensin receptor antagonists," "angiotensin receptor blockers," "anticoagulants," "anticoagulant drugs," "idiopathic pulmonary fibrosis," "IPF," "pulmonary fibroses," "non-randomised studies," "retrospective studies," "prospective studies," "cohort studies," "case-control studies," and "clinical trial." Additional studies were derived from screening the reference lists of included non-randomized studies and previous systematic reviews.

Eligibility Criteria

We included the studies with the following criteria: 1) they included participants with diagnosis of IPF; 2) intervention involving any form of statins, ACEI, ARB, and anticoagulants; 3) controls including placebo or other IPF therapy; and 4) reporting disease-related outcomes including mortality and pulmonary function.

Data Extraction

Two independent authors (W-TZ and B-CZ) assessed all studies for eligibility, extracted the data, and assessed study quality. Disagreements were resolved by consensus-based discussion. The full-text articles were downloaded, and the same inclusion criteria were used to decide whether to include or exclude articles. Each reviewer carried out the quality assessment of each selected article, assessed the

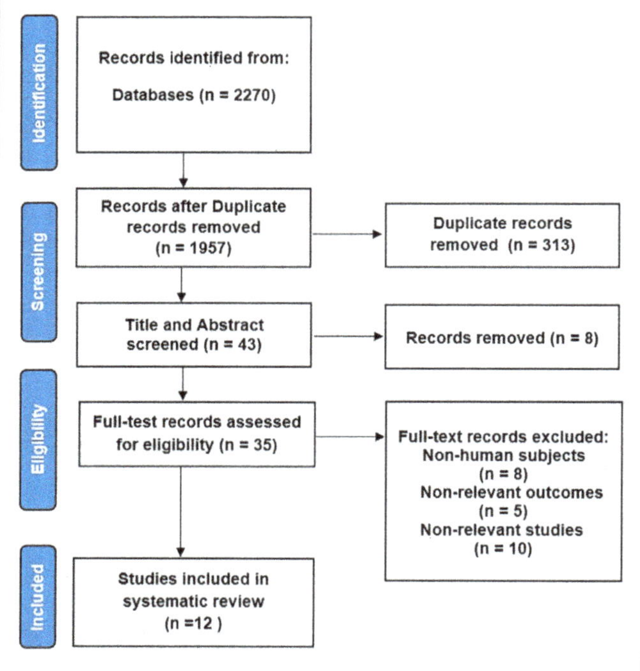

FIGURE 1 | Flowchart.

completeness of the data extraction, and confirmed the quality rating to reduce bias independently.

Quality Assessment

Three authors (W-TZ, B-CZ, and X-JW) evaluated all the included studies. Any disagreement was solved through discussion and rechecking of the article. For the included studies, the Cochrane risk of bias tool ROBINS-I was used to assess the risk of bias (Sterne et al., 2016), including 1) confounding, 2) selection of participants into the study, 3) classification of interventions, 4) intended intervention, 5) missing data, 6) measurement of outcomes, and 7) selection of the reported results and other possible sources of bias. In this way, all articles selected for inclusion in the review were graded under the categories of low, moderate, serious, critical, or no information risk of bias.

Data Synthesis

Primary outcome measurements of survival data were performed. Since survival data include survival outcomes such as survival rate, mortality, censoring, and survival time, we merged the survival data in the meta-analysis. Secondary outcomes were forced vital capacity (FVC) decline and IPF-related mortality. Where more than one study reported the same outcome measured in similar way, a meta-analysis was undertaken. Alternatively, a narrative synthesis of the findings was conducted. For meta-analysis, we calculated a hazard ratio (HR) and 95% CIs using a fixed-effects model. Heterogeneity of included studies was quantified using the chi-squared test (Q test) and I^2 statistic. We used RevMan software for statistical analysis.

RESULTS

Study Selection and Characteristics of the Included Studies

We initially identified 2,270 potentially relevant publications through database searches and other sources. After deleting 313 duplicate articles, we screened the titles and abstracts of 43 related articles. Thirty-five articles were selected for full-text review. Ultimately, 12 studies met our inclusion criteria and were included for the final analysis (**Figure 1**). The characteristics of studies included in the systematic review and meta-analysis are shown in **Table 1**.

Risk of Bias

A total of 12 non-randomized studies were included in this study, of which seven were retrospective studies and five were prospective studies. The above studies were reasonable for non-randomized studies, but none of them could achieve the quality of well-implemented randomized trials. Therefore, the overall bias was assessed as moderate-to-serious risk (**Figure 2**). The lack of diagnostic criteria for IPF in a prospective cohort study (Ekström and Bornefalk-Hermansson, 2016) based on the National Swedevox Register, where approximately 80% of the patients had IPF, assessed the bias in selection of participants as high risk. One retrospective cohort study (Durheim Michael T, 2020) had data from 740 hospitals in the United States, but the data registration information was not stated in the article, so the bias due to missing data was assessed as moderate risk. Although five studies (Nadrous Hassan F, 2004; Durheim Michael T, 2020; M Lambert Eline, 2021; Kubo et al., 2005; Tomassetti S, 2013) had no indications for selective reporting, they lacked evidence support such as prior registration information or data analysis plan, so their bias in selection of the reported result was assessed as a moderate risk of bias.

Meta-Analysis Result of Statin

Of seven included statin studies, six studies reported the survival data. In the fixed-effects meta-analysis, statin use was associated with a reduction in mortality (HR, 0.89; 95% CI 0.83–0.97) (**Figure 3A**).

Two studies involving 1,685 patients reported on a composite measure of FVC decline of >10% or death. The meta-analysis did not demonstrate any significant relationship between statin use and the composite outcome (HR, 0.86; 95% CI 0.73–1.02) (**Figure 3B**).

Meta-Analysis Result of Angiotensin-Converting Enzyme Inhibitor/ Angiotensin Receptor Blocker

Four studies involving 1,955 patients reported a relationship between ACEI/ARB use and survival data. The meta-analysis did not demonstrate any significant relationship between ACEI/ ARB use and survival data (HR, 0.92; 95% CI 0.73–1.15) (**Figure 4**).

Meta-Analysis Result of Anticoagulants

Six studies involving 2,172 patients reported a relationship between anticoagulant use and survival data. Although the

TABLE 1 | Characteristics of the included studies.

Type	Author, year	Country	Study design	Intervention	Control	Outcome	Conclusion
Statin	Nadrous et al. (2004)	United States	Retrospective	Statin $n = 35$	No statin $N = 442$	Mean survival HR 0.97; 95% CI 0.62–1.52 (p = 0.985)	These data do not suggest a beneficial effect of statins on survival in patients with IPF.
	Vedel-Krogh et al. (2015)	Denmark	Retrospective	Statin $n = 261$	No statin $N = 522$	All-cause Mortality HR 0.76; 95% CI 0.62–0.93 (p = 0.05)	Among patients with interstitial lung disease, statin use was associated with reduced all-cause mortality.
	Ekström and Bornefalk-Hermansson (2016)	Sweden	Prospective cohort study	Statin $n = 122$	No statin $N = 340$	All-cause mortality HR 1.13; 95% CI 0.81–1.57	There was no association between statin treatment and survival.
	Kreuter et al. (2017)	United States	Prospective population-based study	Statin $n = 276$	No statin	All-cause mortality HR 0.54; 95% CI 0.24–1.21 (p = 0.1369)	This study indicated that statins may have a beneficial effect on clinical outcomes in IPF.
					$N = 348$	IPF-related mortality HR 0.36; 95% CI 0.14–0.95 (p = 0.0393)	
					—	FVC decline or death HR 0.71; 95% CI 0.48–1.07 (p = 0.1032)	
—	Kreuter et al. (2018)	INPULSIS	Retrospective	Statin $n = 312$	No statin	Annual rate of decline in FVC mean	It showed a numerically lower FVC decline in placebo-treated patients who were receiving statins at baseline.
					$N = 749$	Difference 50.8 ml/year; 95% CI 10.9–112.5 (p = 0.1065)	
					—	FVC decline or death HR 1.01; 95% CI 0.72–1.41 (p = 0.9700)	
—	Durheim et al. (2020)	United States	Retrospective cohort study	Statin $n = 4,775$	No statin $N = 4,892$	In-hospital mortality OR 0.76; 95% CI 0.67–0.87 (p < 0.001)	Statins significantly associated with a lower risk of in-hospital mortality.
—	Lambert et al. (2021)	Belgium	Retrospective	Statin $n = 171$	No statin	Survival HR 0.82; 95% CI 0.50–1.35 (p = 0.428)	This study demonstrated a significant beneficial effect of statin therapy on IPF evolution, particularly on FVC and DLCO decline, but not significantly affecting survival.
					$N = 152$	Annual FVC% difference 2.9%, CI 1.6–4.4 (p < 0.001)	
					—	DLCO% decline difference 1.3%, CI 0.24–2.3 (p = 0.013)	
Anticoagulants	Kubo et al. (2005)	Japan	Prospective study	Warfarin $n = 23$	No warfarin $n = 33$	Survival HR 2.9; 95% CI 1.0–8.0 (p = 0.04)	Anticoagulant therapy has a beneficial effect on survival in patients with IPF.
—	Tomassetti et al. (2013)	Italy	Retrospective cohort study	Warfarin $n = 25$	None $n = 25$	Survival HR 4.8; 95% CI 1.8–12.8 (p = 0.002) Interval to disease progression HR 2.7; 95% CI 1.2–6.5 (p = 0.023)	In this retrospective study, patients treated with anticoagulants had a worse survival and a shorter interval to disease progression.
—	Kreuter et al. (2017)	United States	Prospective study	Anticoagulants $n = 32$	No anticoagulants $n = 592$	All-cause mortality HR 2.6; 95% CI 0.7–8.8 (p = 0.136) IPF-related mortality HR 4.7; 95% CI 1.1–19.3 (p = 0.034)	This post-hoc analysis suggests that anticoagulants used for non-IPF indications may have unfavorable effects in IPF patients

(Continued on following page)

TABLE 1 | (*Continued*) Characteristics of the included studies.

Type	Author, year	Country	Study design	Intervention	Control	Outcome	Conclusion
—	King et al. (2021)	United States	Retrospective cohort study	Direct oral anticoagulants (DOACs) n = 57	No anticoagulants n = 1,070	All-cause mortality or transplant HR 1.368; 95% CI 0.500–3.737 Transplant-free survival HR 1.510; 95% CI 0.709–3.215	In patients with IPF, DOACs were not associated with increase in risk of death or transplant and reduction in transplant-free survival.
—	King et al. (2021)	United States	Retrospective cohort study	Warfarin n = 49	No anticoagulants n = 1,070	All-cause mortality or transplant HR 2.566; 95% CI 1.095–6.0165 Transplant-free survival HR 2.101; 95% CI 1.025–4.307	In patients with IPF, warfarin was associated with increase in risk of death or transplant and reduction in transplant-free survival.
—	Lambert et al. (2021)	Belgium	Retrospective review	Anticoagulants n = 49	No anticoagulants 274	Survival HR 1.25; 95% CI 0.71–2.21 (p = 0.444) DLCO decline (difference −1.3%, CI 2.6–0.02 (p = 0.055)	This study suggests that anticoagulant use showed a trend towards worse DLCO decline in IPF patients, but no effect on survival.
ACEI/ARB	Nadrous et al. (2004)	United States	Retrospective	ACEI n = 52	No ACEI/ARB N = 425	Mean survival HR 1.05; 95% CI 0.73–1.52 (p = 0.776)	These data do not suggest a beneficial effect of ACEI on survival in patients with IPF.
—	Ekström and Bornefalk-Hermansson (2016)	Sweden	Perspective cohort study	ACEI/ARB n = 161	No ACEI/ARB N = 301	All-cause mortality HR 0.63; 95% CI 0.47–0.85	ACEI/ARB treatment is related to improving the survival of IPF patients.
—	Kreuter et al. (2019)	United States	Prospective population-based study	ACEI n = 111	No ACEI/ARB N = 392	All-cause mortality HR 1.2; 95% CI 0.5–2.8 (p = 0.737) Disease progression HR 0.6; 95% CI 0.4–0.9 (p = 0.026)	This analysis suggests that ACEI treatment may potentially be associated with slightly better outcomes in patients with IPF.
—	Kreuter et al. (2019)	United States	Prospective population-based study	ARB n = 121	No ACEI/ARB N = 392	All-cause mortality HR 2.2; 95% CI 1.2–4.3 (p = 0.017)	ARB treatment may potentially be associated with greater risk of all-cause.

Note. The INPULSIS studies were performed at 205 sites in 24 countries in the Americas, Europe, Asia, and Australia.
HR, hazard ratio; IPF, idiopathic pulmonary fibrosis; FVC, forced vital capacity; DLCO, diffusing capacity of the lungs for carbon monoxide; DOACs, direct oral anticoagulants; ACEI, angiotensin-converting enzyme inhibitor; ARB, angiotensin receptor blocker.

meta-analysis did not demonstrate any significant relationship between anticoagulant use and survival data (HR, 1.16; 95% CI 0.62–2.19) (**Figure 5**), five of six studies included in the meta-analysis showed that patients given anticoagulant medication remained at increased risk of mortality.

DISCUSSION

IPF is defined as a chronic, progressive, fibrosing ILD of unknown etiology. Multiple studies have revealed associated pulmonary as well as extra-pulmonary comorbidities (Buendía-Rold´an et al., 2017). Likewise, patients are more at risk for cardiovascular disorders such as ischemic heart disease, atrial fibrillation, and thrombotic vascular events. To reduce their cardiovascular risk, many IPF patients receive cardiovascular medications like statins, ACEI, ARB, and anticoagulants (Hubbard, et al., 2008). Existing studies have reported divergent findings on the link between medications used for cardiovascular diseases and fibrotic disease processes. Given the increasing awareness that pharmacologic properties of statins, ACEI, ARB, and anticoagulants encompass the abilities to modulate fibroproliferative pathways, therefore,

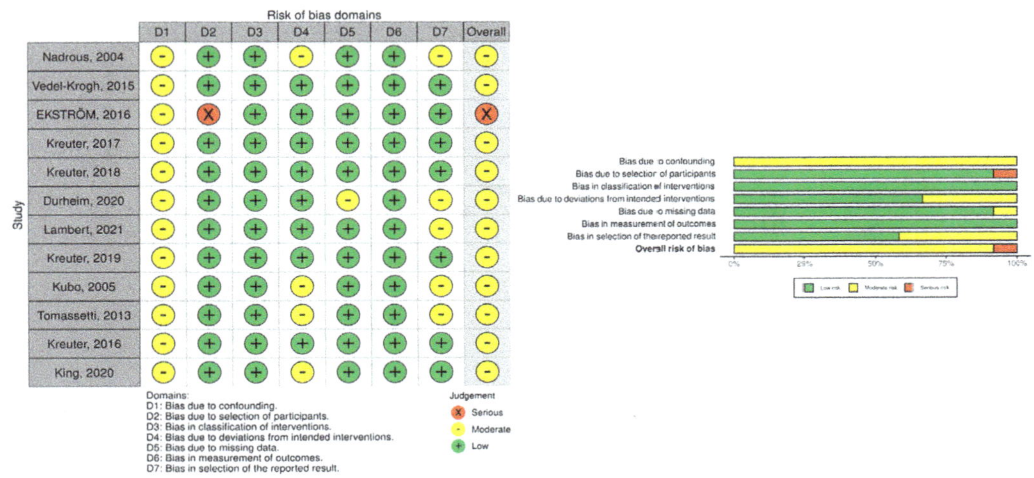

FIGURE 2 | Risk of bias graph.

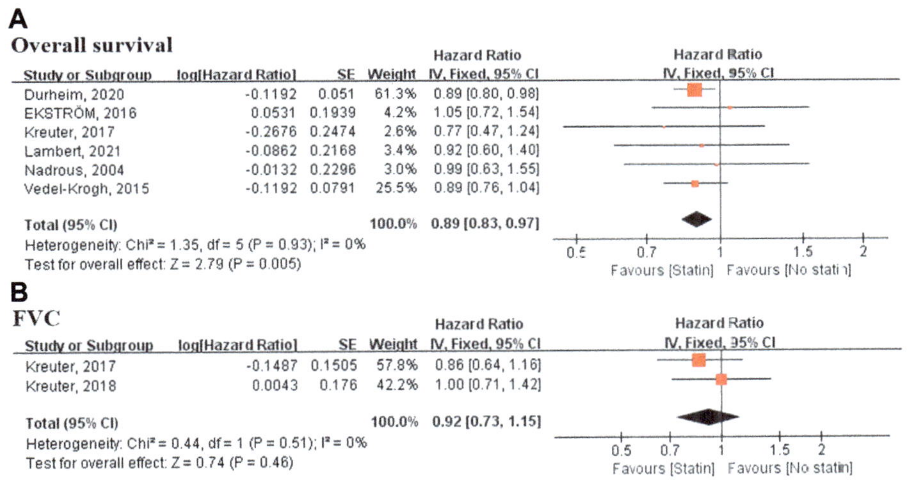

FIGURE 3 | Meta-analyses of the included studies examining overall survival and FVC for statin vs. no statin. The marker size indicates the relative weight of the study, as it contributes to the results of the overall comparison. IV indicates inverse-variance random-effects analysis; HR, hazard ratio; FVC, forced vital capacity.

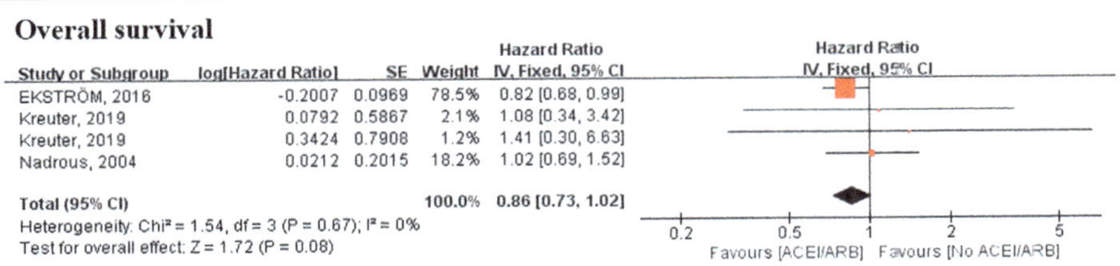

FIGURE 4 | Meta-analyses of the included studies examining overall survival for ACEI/ARB vs. no ACEI/ARB. The marker size indicates the relative weight of the study, as it contributes to the results of the overall comparison. IV indicates inverse-variance random-effects analysis; HR, hazard ratio; ACEI, angiotensin-converting enzyme inhibitor; ARB, angiotensin receptor blocker.

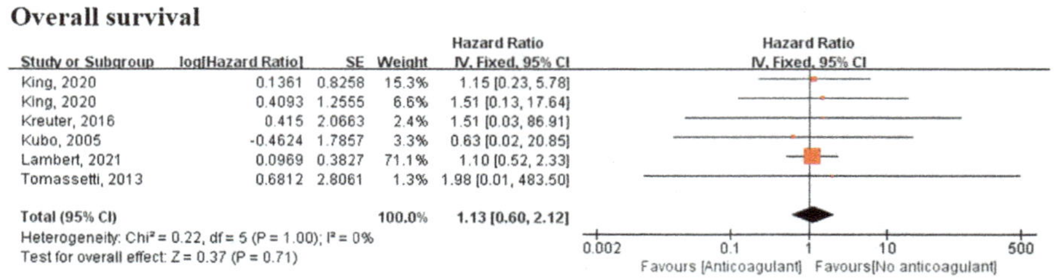

FIGURE 5 | Meta-analyses of the included studies examining overall survival for anticoagulant vs. no anticoagulant. The marker size indicates the relative weight of the study, as it contributes to the results of the overall comparison. IV indicates inverse-variance random-effects analysis; HR, hazard ratio.

identifying the treatment with the best safety and efficacy is important. This systematic review and meta-analysis including 12 non-randomized studies, covering four types of cardiovascular medications, aimed to evaluate the relationship between cardiovascular medications and IPF. To the best of our knowledge, this is currently the first systematic review and meta-analysis investigating different types of cardiovascular medications for IPF. Our study suggested a consistent relationship between statin therapy and all-cause mortality in IPF population. There was no statistically significant association between ACEI/ARB use and decline in FVC. Meanwhile, although the meta-analysis did not demonstrate any significant relationship between anticoagulant use and survival data, we found that all the six studies related to survival data showed the result that patients given anticoagulant medication remained at increased risk of mortality.

Regarding the statin use in IPF patients, of seven included studies, five studies reported survival analysis, through which three studies suggested a beneficial effect of statins on survival. One study reported IPF-related mortality, which suggested that statin use at baseline significantly reduced chance of IPF-related death. Two studies reported on a composite measure of FVC decline of >10% or death with no statistically difference. Regarding the ACEI/ARB use in IPF patients, of four included studies, only one study suggested that ACEI/ARB treatment is related to improving the survival of IPF patients, same with the result of meta-analysis. Regarding the anticoagulant use in IPF patients, of six included studies, only one study suggested that warfarin has a beneficial effect on survival in patients with IPF. Interestingly, others all indicated that patients treated with anticoagulants had a worse survival. Above all, we found that among the cardiovascular medications, only statin was beneficial to survival data of IPF patients. However, since only one study reported IPF-related death, we could not specify the true pharmacological action on IPF clearly. More studies focused on the outcome of IPF-related death should be conducted in the future.

This study has some limitations. Firstly, we concentrated our research on published literatures and did not screen gray literature. This is because the use of the risk of bias tools ROBINS-I requires very explicit and comprehensive reporting of the primary research study. Secondly, most studies used all-cause mortality and survival rate but not IPF-related death as their primary outcomes. So the causes of death were missing in the majority of studies. Thirdly, all studies included are non-randomized, and half of the studies are retrospective. Therefore, there exists some bias due to missing data and confounding that cannot be avoided. Given these challenges, larger-scale samples and higher-quality studies are needed in the future to draw conclusions about the exact causal relationship between survival data of IPF and cardiovascular medications.

Nevertheless, a crucial strength of the present study lies in the large number of included patients and full analysis of the relationship between different types of cardiovascular medications and survival data. Lastly, we would like to propose two suggestions for future clinical trials especially randomized controlled trials (RCTs) of cardiovascular medications for IPF. The combination, especially with antifibrotic drugs, could maximize the treatment effects of cardiovascular medications, but the majority of included trials were not clarified. If the included patients are grouped according to different antifibrotic treatments or non-antifibrotic treatments, then we can then classify and synthesize the outcome data as different types of syndromes in the systematic review, and the analyzed results can provide more pointed guidance for clinical practice. On the other hand, the quality of life of patients was not reported in most of the included studies. As IPF is defined as a chronic, progressive ILD, the multidimensional quality of life is an indispensable indicator and evaluation tool to show the trend of treatment effectiveness. We suggested that future prospective trials should be improved in related fields.

CONCLUSION

Our study suggested a consistent relationship between statin therapy and survival data in IPF population. However, there is currently insufficient evidence to conclude the effect of ACEI, ARB, and anticoagulant therapy on IPF population especially to the disease-related outcomes in IPF. Considering the limitations of available literature, we would recommend a prospective RCT or cohort study that captures IPF-related outcomes of cardiovascular medications and use of concurrent antifibrotic treatment.

AUTHOR CONTRIBUTIONS

All authors were involved in the review, interpretation of the results, and manuscript preparation. W-TZ, Q-YL, and

C-MX conceived and designed the study. W-TZ and X-JW drafted the report. X-JW and B-CZ did the data analysis. W-TZ, X-JW, C-MX, X-YJ, LP, W-LW, Q-YL, G-DH, and B-CZ revised the report and approved the final version before submission.

REFERENCES

Bjoraker, J. A., Ryu, J. H., Edwin, M. K., Myers, J. L., Tazelaar, H. D., Schroeder, D. R., et al. (1998). Prognostic Significance of Histopathologic Subsets in Idiopathic Pulmonary Fibrosis. *Am. J. Respir. Crit. Care Med.* 157 (1), 199–203. doi:10.1164/ajrccm.157.1.9704130

Buendía-Roldán, I., Mejía, M., Navarro, C., and Selman, M. (2017). Idiopathic Pulmonary Fibrosis: Clinical Behavior and Aging Associated Comorbidities. *Respir. Med.* 129, 46–52. doi:10.1016/j.rmed.2017.06.001

Chobanian, A. V., Bakris, G. L., Black, H. R., Cushman, W. C., Green, L. A., Izzo, J. L., et al. (2003). The Seventh Report of the Joint National Committee on Prevention, Detection, Evaluation, and Treatment of High Blood Pressure: the JNC 7 Report. *JAMA* 289 (19), 2560–2572. doi:10.1001/jama.289.19.2560

Durheim, M. T., Judy, J., Bender, S., Neely, M. L., Baumer, D., Robinson, S. B., et al. (2020). A Retrospective Study of In-Hospital Mortality in Patients with Idiopathic Pulmonary Fibrosis between 2015 and 2018. *Medicine (Baltimore)* 99 (47), e23143. doi:10.1097/MD.0000000000023143

Ekström, M., and Bornefalk-Hermansson, A. (2016). Cardiovascular and Antacid Treatment and Mortality in Oxygen-dependent Pulmonary Fibrosis: A Population-Based Longitudinal Study. *Respirology* 21 (4), 705–711. doi:10.1111/resp.12781

Gao, F., Fish, B. L., Moulder, J. E., Jacobs, E. R., and Medhora, M. (2013). Enalapril Mitigates Radiation-Induced Pneumonitis and Pulmonary Fibrosis if Started 35 Days after Whole-Thorax Irradiation. *Radiat. Res.* 180 (5), 546–552. doi:10.1667/RR13350.1

Guise, J. M., Butler, M. E., Chang, C., Viswanathan, M., Pigott, T., Tugwell, P., et al. (2017). AHRQ Series on Complex Intervention Systematic Reviews-Paper 6: PRISMA-CI Extension Statement and Checklist. *J. Clin. Epidemiol.* 90 (undefined), 43–50. doi:10.1016/j.jclinepi.2017.06.016

Hubbard, R. B., Smith, C., Le Jeune, I., Gribbin, J., and Fogarty, A. W. (2008). The Association between Idiopathic Pulmonary Fibrosis and Vascular Disease: a Population-Based Study. *Am. J. Respir. Crit. Care Med.* 178 (12), 1257–1261. doi:10.1164/rccm.200805-725OC

Hyldgaard, C., Hilberg, O., and Bendstrup, E. (2014). How Does Comorbidity Influence Survival in Idiopathic Pulmonary Fibrosis? *Respir. Med.* 108 (4), 647–653. doi:10.1016/j.rmed.2014.01.008

version 6.1 (updated September 2020) J. P. T. Higgins, J. Thomas, J. Chandler, M. Cumpston, T. Li, M. J. Page, et al. (Editors) (2020). *Cochrane Handbook for Systematic Reviews of Interventions* (Cochrane. Available from www.training.cochrane.org/handbook.

King, C. S., Freiheit, E., Brown, A. W., Shlobin, O. A., Aryal, S., Ahmad, K., et al. (2021). Association between Anticoagulation and Survival in Interstitial Lung Disease: An Analysis of the Pulmonary Fibrosis Foundation Patient Registry. *Chest* 159 (4), 1507–1516. doi:10.1016/j.chest.2020.10.019

Kreuter, M., Bonella, F., Maher, T. M., Costabel, U., Spagnolo, P., Weycker, D., et al. (2017). Effect of Statins on Disease-Related Outcomes in Patients with Idiopathic Pulmonary Fibrosis. *Thorax* 72 (2), 148–153. doi:10.1136/thoraxjnl-2016-208819

Kreuter, M., Costabel, U., Richeldi, L., Cottin, V., Wijsenbeek, M., Bonella, F., et al. (2018). Statin Therapy and Outcomes in Trials of Nintedanib in Idiopathic Pulmonary Fibrosis. *Respiration* 95 (5), 317–326. doi:10.1159/000486286

Kreuter, M., Lederer, D. J., Molina-Molina, M., Noth, I., Valenzuela, C., Frankenstein, L., et al. (2019). Association of Angiotensin Modulators with the Course of Idiopathic Pulmonary Fibrosis. *Chest* 156 (4), 706–714. doi:10.1016/j.chest.2019.04.015

Kruzliak, P., Hare, D. L., Zvonicek, V., Klimas, J., and Zulli, A. (2015). Simvastatin Impairs the Induction of Pulmonary Fibrosis Caused by a Western Style Diet: a Preliminary Study. *J. Cel Mol Med* 19 (11), 2647–2654. doi:10.1111/jcmm.12637

Kubo, H., Nakayama, K., Yanai, M., Suzuki, T., Yamaya, M., Watanabe, M., et al. (2005). Anticoagulant Therapy for Idiopathic Pulmonary Fibrosis. *Chest* 128 (3), 1475–1482. doi:10.1378/chest.128.3.1475

Lambert, M. E., Wuyts, W. A., Yserbyt, J., and De Sadeleer, L. J. (2021). Statins: Cause of Fibrosis or the Opposite? Effect of Cardiovascular Drugs in Idiopathic Pulmonary Fibrosis. *Respir. Med.* 176 (undefined), 106259. doi:10.1016/j.rmed.2020.106259

LaRosa, J. C., He, J., and Vupputuri, S. (1999). Effect of Statins on Risk of Coronary Disease: a Meta-Analysis of Randomized Controlled Trials. *JAMA* 282 (24), 2340–2346. doi:10.1001/jama.282.24.2340

Molteni, A., Wolfe, L. F., Ward, W. F., Ts'ao, C. H., Molteni, L. B., Veno, P., et al. (2007). Effect of an Angiotensin II Receptor Blocker and Two Angiotensin Converting Enzyme Inhibitors on Transforming Growth Factor-Beta (TGF-Beta) and Alpha-Actomyosin (Alpha SMA), Important Mediators of Radiation-Induced Pneumopathy and Lung Fibrosis. *Curr. Pharm. Des.* 13 (13), 1307–1316. doi:10.2174/138161207780618777

Nadrous, H. F., Ryu, J. H., Douglas, W. W., Decker, P. A., and Olson, E. J. (2004). Impact of Angiotensin-Converting Enzyme Inhibitors and Statins on Survival in Idiopathic Pulmonary Fibrosis. *Chest* 126 (2), 438–446. doi:10.1378/chest.126.2.438

Navaratnam, V., Fogarty, A. W., McKeever, T., Thompson, N., Jenkins, G., Johnson, S. R., et al. (2014). Presence of a Prothrombotic State in People with Idiopathic Pulmonary Fibrosis: a Population-Based Case-Control Study. *Thorax* 69 (3), 207–215. doi:10.1136/thoraxjnl-2013-203740

Oka, H., Ishii, H., Iwata, A., Kushima, H., Toba, S., Hashinaga, K., et al. (2013). Inhibitory Effects of Pitavastatin on Fibrogenic Mediator Production by Human Lung Fibroblasts. *Life Sci.* 93 (null), 968–974. doi:10.1016/j.lfs.2013.10.026

Piepho, R. W. (2000). Overview of the Angiotensin-Converting-Enzyme Inhibitors. *Am. J. Health Syst. Pharm.* 57 Suppl 1 (57 Suppl. 1), S3–S7. doi:10.1093/ajhp/57.suppl_1.S3

Raghu, G., Collard, H. R., Egan, J. J., Martinez, F. J., Behr, J., Brown, K. K., et al. (2011). An Official ATS/ERS/JRS/ALAT Statement: Idiopathic Pulmonary Fibrosis: Evidence-Based Guidelines for Diagnosis and Management. *Am. J. Respir. Crit. Care Med.* 183 (6), 788–824. doi:10.1164/rccm.2009-040GL

Schuliga, M., Grainge, C., Westall, G., and Knight, D. (2018). Westall Glen., and Knight DarrylThe Fibrogenic Actions of the Coagulant and Plasminogen Activation Systems in Pulmonary Fibrosis. *Int. J. Biochem. Cel Biol.* 97 (undefined), 108–117. doi:10.1016/j.biocel.2018.02.016

Schulman, S., and Crowther, M. A. (2012). How I Treat with Anticoagulants in 2012: New and Old Anticoagulants, and when and How to Switch. *Blood* 119 (13), 3016–3023. doi:10.1182/blood-2011-10-378950

Sode, B. F., Dahl, M., Nielsen, S. F., and Nordestgaard, B. G. (2010). Venous Thromboembolism and Risk of Idiopathic Interstitial Pneumonia: a Nationwide Study. *Am. J. Respir. Crit. Care Med.* 181 (10), 1085–1092. doi:10.1164/rccm.200912-1951OC

Sprunger, D. B., Olson, A. L., Huie, T. J., Fernandez-Perez, E. R., Fischer, A., Solomon, J. J., et al. (2012) Pulmonary Fibrosis Is Associated with an Elevated Risk of Thromboembolic Disease. *Eur. Respir. J.* 39 (1), 125–132. doi:10.1183/09031936.00041411

Sterne, J. A., Hernán, M. A., Reeves, B. C., Savović, J., Berkman, N. D., Viswanathan, M., et al. (2016). ROBINS-I: a Tool for Assessing Risk of Bias in Non-randomised Studies of Interventions. *BMJ* 355 (undefined), i4919. doi:10.1136/bmj.i4919

Tomassetti, S., Ruy, J. H., Gurioli, C., Ravaglia, C., Buccioli, M., Tantalocco, P., et al. (2013). The Effect of Anticoagulant Therapy for Idiopathic Pulmonary Fibrosis in Real Life Practice. *Sarcoidosis Vasc. Diffuse Lung Dis.* 30 (2), 121–127.

Turner, J. M., and Kodali, R. (2020). Should Angiotensin-Converting Enzyme Inhibitors Ever Be Used for the Management of Hypertension? *Curr. Cardiol. Rep.* 22 (9), 95. doi:10.1007/s11886-020-01352-8

Uhal, B. D., Gidea, C., Bargout, R., Bifero, A., Ibarra-Sunga, O., Papp, M., et al. (1998). Captopril Inhibits Apoptosis in Human Lung Epithelial Cells: a Potential Antifibrotic Mechanism. *Am. J. Physiol.* 275 (5), L1013–L1017. doi:10.1152/ajplung.1998.275.5.L1013

Vedel-Krogh, S., Nielsen, S. F., and Nordestgaard, B. G. (2015). Statin Use Is Associated with Reduced Mortality in Patients with Interstitial Lung Disease. *PLoS One* 10 (10), e0140571. doi:10.1371/journal.pone.0140571

7

Latent Transforming Growth Factor-β Binding Protein-2 Regulates Lung Fibroblast-to-Myofibroblast Differentiation in Pulmonary Fibrosis *via* NF-κB Signaling

Menglin Zou[1†], Jingfeng Zou[2†], Xingxing Hu[1†], Weishuai Zheng[1], Mingyang Zhang[1] and Zhenshun Cheng[1]*

[1]*Department of Respiratory and Critical Care Medicine, Zhongnan Hospital of Wuhan University, Wuhan, China,* [2]*Department of Respiratory and Critical Care Medicine, Jiangxi Provincial People's Hospital, Nanchang, China*

Correspondence:
Zhenshun Cheng
zhenshun_cheng@126.com

[†]*These authors have contributed equally to this work and share first authorship*

Despite past extensive studies, the mechanisms underlying pulmonary fibrosis (PF) still remain poorly understood. The aberrantly activated lung myofibroblasts, predominantly emerging through fibroblast-to-myofibroblast differentiation, are considered to be the key cells in PF, resulting in excessive accumulation of extracellular matrix (ECM). Latent transforming growth factor-β (TGFβ) binding protein-2 (LTBP2) has been suggested as playing a critical role in modulating the structural integrity of the ECM. However, its function in PF remains unclear. Here, we demonstrated that lungs originating from different types of patients with PF, including idiopathic PF and rheumatoid arthritis-associated interstitial lung disease, and from mice following bleomycin (BLM)-induced PF were characterized by increased LTBP2 expression in activated lung fibroblasts/myofibroblasts. Moreover, serum LTBP2 was also elevated in patients with COVID-19-related PF. LTBP2 silencing by lentiviral shRNA transfection protected against BLM-induced PF and suppressed fibroblast-to-myofibroblast differentiation *in vivo* and *in vitro*. More importantly, LTBP2 overexpression was able to induce differentiation of lung fibroblasts to myofibroblasts *in vitro*, even in the absence of TGFβ1. By further mechanistic analysis, we demonstrated that LTBP2 silencing prevented fibroblast-to-myofibroblast differentiation and subsequent PF by suppressing the phosphorylation and nuclear translocation of NF-κB signaling. LTBP2 overexpression-induced fibroblast-to-myofibroblast differentiation depended on the activation of NF-κB signaling *in vitro*. Therefore, our data indicate that intervention to silence LTBP2 may represent a promising therapy for PF.

Keywords: pulmonary fibrosis, latent transforming growth factor-β binding protein-2, fibroblast-to-myofibroblast differentiation, extracellular matrix, NF-κB signaling

---

Abbreviations: BLM, bleomycin; ECM, extracellular matrix; HRCT, high-resolution computed tomography; IPF, idiopathic pulmonary fibrosis; LTBP2, latent transforming growth factor-β binding protein-2; MAPK, mitogen-activated protein kinase; NF-κB, nuclear factor kappa B; PF, pulmonary fibrosis; RA-ILD, rheumatoid arthritis-associated interstitial lung disease; α-SMA, α-smooth muscle actin; TGFβ, transforming growth factor-β; UIP, usual interstitial pneumonia.

INTRODUCTION

Pulmonary fibrosis (PF) is a type of chronic and progressive lung interstitial disease, characterized by the irreversible scarring and remodeling of the lung (Kolahian et al., 2016). The fibrogenic triggers remain controversial, but identifiable triggers probably include cigarette smoke (Wilson and Wynn, 2009), respiratory infections such as the 2019 novel coronavirus disease (COVID-19) (George et al., 2020), and connective tissue diseases/autoimmune disorders such as rheumatoid arthritis (RA) and scleroderma (Wilson and Wynn, 2009; Spagnolo et al., 2018). However, PF can also manifest without any known etiology, which is termed "idiopathic" (IPF) (Lederer and Martinez, 2018). To date, the mechanisms underlying PF remain poorly understood, so there are limited therapeutic options and poor prognosis. Therefore, novel agents targeted against the fibrotic process are urgently needed.

The currently accepted pathogenic theories suggest that formation of fibrotic foci and excessive deposition of extracellular matrix (ECM) proteins, such as hyaluronan, fibronectin, and interstitial collagens, are principal events in PF (Kolahian et al., 2016). Following lung injury, quiescent fibroblasts become activated and transform into α-smooth muscle actin (α-SMA)-expressing myofibroblasts, resulting in excess accumulation of ECM components (Wynn, 2011). Thus, targeting the fibroblast-to-myofibroblast differentiation process and ECM synthesis would provide a potential therapeutic strategy for PF.

Latent transforming growth factor-β (TGFβ) binding protein-2 (LTBP2) is a member of the fibrillin/LTBP ECM proteins family, which includes LTBP-1, -2, -3, and -4 (Gibson et al., 1995; Robertson et al., 2015). LTBPs play a critical role in modulating the structural integrity of the ECM, and in the assembly and secretion of the latent TGF-β (Miyazono et al., 1991). Unlike the other LTBPs, LTBP2 is unable to bind to latent TGFβ (Anderson et al., 2008; Robertson et al., 2015). Thus, the function of LTBP2 has not been fully clarified. Previous studies have demonstrated that high expression of LTBP2 was associated with poor outcome and tumor progression in thyroid and gastric cancer. Moreover, knockdown of LTBP2 inhibited the proliferation and invasion in thyroid carcinoma and gastric cancer cells (Wan et al., 2017; Wang et al., 2018). Enomoto et al. (2018) found that LTBP2 was secreted from lung myofibroblasts and was potentially a novel prognostic blood biomarker reflecting the level of differentiation of lung fibroblasts into myofibroblasts in IPF patients. However, there has been very little research using LTBP2-knockout mice to assess lung fibrosis, and the exact function of LTBP2 in lung (myo) fibroblasts and PF remains unknown.

Nuclear factor kappa B (NF-κB), a well-characterized transcription factor, regulates many genes responsible for the generation of proinflammatory molecules and profibrogenic cytokines, which promote inflammatory response and fibrosis (Christman et al., 2000; Wilson and Wynn, 2009; Meng et al., 2014). The activation of the NF-κB signaling pathway resulted in the apoptotic resistance of lung fibroblasts (Golan-Gerstl et al., 2012), but blocking NF-κB signaling attenuated bleomycin (BLM)-induced lung fibrosis *via* suppressing myofibroblast differentiation (Hou et al., 2018). A previous study showed that LTBP2 knockdown by siRNA reduced the degree of myocardial fibrosis by suppressing activation of the NF-κB signaling pathway (Pang et al., 2020). However, research regarding whether the NF-κB signaling is related to LTBP2 in PF has rarely been reported.

In the current study, we characterized the expression pattern of LTBP2 and investigated for the first time its role in lung fibroblasts' differentiation to myofibroblasts and lung fibrosis. We showed that LTBP2 silencing by lentiviral shRNA transfection attenuated PF by suppressing lung fibroblast-to-myofibroblast differentiation and ECM deposition *via* blocking NF-κB signaling.

MATERIALS AND METHODS

Human Samples

Lung tissues from patients with IPF (n = 3) and rheumatoid arthritis-associated interstitial lung disease (RA-ILD) (n = 3) were collected in the Zhongnan Hospital of Wuhan University. Three normal lung biopsies from resection of cancer were used as controls. IPF patients fulfilled the American Thoracic Society (ATS)/European Respiratory Society (ERS) consensus diagnostic criteria (Raghu et al., 2018). RA was classified according to the 1987 American College of Rheumatology (ACR) classification criteria (Arnett et al., 1988) and a definitive diagnosis of ILD was evident by clinical features, chest high-resolution computed tomography (HRCT), laboratory findings, and/or surgical lung biopsy. The pattern in RA-ILD patients was usual interstitial pneumonia (UIP) based on HRCT and/or histopathological pattern in this study. COVID-19 diagnosis was made according to the nucleic acid test, and PF in COVID-19 survivors was diagnosed by chest CT images. Six patients with COVID-19-related PF and 13 age-, and male sex-matched COVID-19 survivors without PF were included in the present study. As healthy controls, serum samples were also collected from 11 healthy volunteers who worked or had worked at Zhongnan Hospital of Wuhan University.

BLM-Induced Lung Fibrosis Model

We used 8- to 10-week-old male C57BL/6 mice housed in a specific pathogen-free environment with sterilized food and water. For BLM-induced fibrosis studies, mice under pentobarbital anesthesia received a single intratracheal injection of 3 mg/kg BLM (Hisun, Zhejiang, China) dissolved in 50 μl of saline. Control mice were intratracheally injected with 50 μl saline. At 28 days later, mice were euthanized. Parts of the lung lobes were fixed in 4% paraformaldehyde (PFA) for histopathologic analyses, and parts were frozen for further analysis.

Lentivirus Production and Transfection

Three different mouse LTBP2 shRNAs and scrambled shRNA were designed and synthesized by GeneChem (Shanghai, P.R. China). The target sequences of shRNAs are shown in

Supplementary Table S1. The shRNA1 with the best silencing efficiency was chosen for further animal experiments. C57BL/6 mice under anesthesia were intratracheally administrated with scrambled shRNA or LTBP2 shRNA at a dose of 3.5×10^7 transduction units per mouse. Five days later, mice were challenged with BLM for lung fibrosis experiments.

Lung Histological Analysis

The lower lung tissues were fixed in 4% PFA for 24 h, sliced mid-sagittally, and embedded in paraffin. Then 4 μm sections were stained with hematoxylin-eosin (H&E) for structured observation, or with Masson's trichrome staining for detection of collagen deposition. In H&E staining, the severity of fibrosis was estimated from 0 to 8 by the Ashcroft score (Ashcroft et al., 1988).

Immunohistochemistry Staining

Tissue sections were deparaffinized and heated in EDTA buffer, followed by treatment with 3% H_2O_2 in methanol for 10 min and blocking with 5% normal serum. Tissue sections were incubated with primary antibody overnight at 4°C, and then incubated with secondary antibody for 50 min at room temperature, visualized with DAB chromogen, and counterstained with hematoxylin.

FACS Protocol

Mouse lung cells from the BLM 28 days group were incubated with antibodies against the following lineage-specific cell surface markers: CD45, CD31, viability dye, CD11b, and CD11c. When isolating lung fibroblasts from mice, anti-PDGFRα antibody was added. We defined fibroblasts as lineage-negative and PDGFRα-positive cells. Then we further analyzed the transcription of key profibrotic genes in LTBP2-expressing and LTBP2-negative lung fibroblasts.

Hydroxyproline Assay

Total hydroxyproline content of lung tissues were analyzed with the Hydroxyproline Assay Kit (Cat. No: A030-2, Jiancheng, Nanjing, China) according to the manufacturer's protocol. In brief, the lung tissue homogenates were centrifuged and the supernatant was collected. Subsequently, hydroxyproline content in lung tissues was evaluated by the absorbance at 550 nm. The results were expressed as μg hydroxyproline/mg wet lung.

Culture and Lentiviral Infection of HFL1 Cells

HFL1 cells, the human pulmonary fibroblast cell line, were purchased from iCell Bioscience (Shanghai, China). HFL1 cells were cultured in complete medium containing Kaighn's modification of Ham's F-12 (F12K) medium (Hyclone, Logan, UT, United States) supplemented with 10% fetal bovine serum (FBS, Gibco; Thermo Fisher Scientific, Inc., Waltham, MA, United States) and 1% antibiotics (100 μg/ml streptomycin and 100μ/ml penicillin) in a humidified atmosphere of 5% CO_2 at 37°C. Three different human LTBP2 shRNAs and scrambled shRNA were designed and synthesized by GeneChem (Shanghai, P.R. China). The target sequences of shRNAs are shown in **Supplementary Table S2**. The shRNA3 with the best silencing efficiency was chosen for further experiments. For functional studies, HFL1 cells were plated in 6-well plates (1×10^5 cells/well), and infected with scrambled shRNA or LTBP2 shRNA at the multiplicity of infection (MOI = 40). After 8 h, the medium was replaced with fresh complete medium and the cells were incubated with 4 μg/ml puromycin for 72 h when the cells reached 70–80% confluence. Then the cells were stimulated with PBS or 10 ng/ml TGF-β1 (PeproTech, Rocky Hill, NJ, United States) for 48 h.

LTBP2 Plasmids Construction and Transfection

Human LTBP2 cDNA was synthesized and cloned into GV230 vector (GeneChem, Shanghai, P.R. China). Transfection was carried out using the Lipo8000™ Transfection Reagent (Beyotime, Shanghai, China) according to the manufacturer's instructions. HFL1 cells were pretreated with BAY 11-7082 (MedChem Express, NJ, United States) for 1 h followed by transfection with LTBP2 plasmids.

Immunofluorescence

HFL1 cells or tissue sections were fixed in 4% PFA, then permeabilized with 0.2% Triton X-100 for 10 min, and blocked in 5% bovine serum albumin for 60 min. The cells or tissue sections were incubated with primary antibody overnight at 4°C, and subsequently incubated with appropriate secondary antibody for 1 h at room temperature. Nuclei were stained with DAPI for 3 min.

Quantitative RT-PCR

Total RNAs were extracted from tissues and cells using TRIzol reagent (Invitrogen, Carlsbad, CA, United States). Total RNAs were reversely transcribed to cDNAs using the Prime Script RT Reagent Kit (TaKaRa, Dalian, China) according to the manufacturer's instructions. For quantitative analysis of mRNA expression, the SYBR Green PCR kit (Toyobo, Osaka, Japan) was used to amplify the target gene using the manufacturer's protocol. Relative mRNA levels of the target gene were normalized to GAPDH mRNA expression by using the $2^{-\Delta\Delta CT}$ method.

The Mouse Primer Sequences Used in the Study Were Listed as Follows

LTBP2: forward, 5′-ACACTTGCGACTGCTTTGAGG-3′, reverse, 5′-CAGTGGCAGCGATAGGAACC-3`; α-SMA: forward, 5′-GATAGAACACGGCATCATCACC-3′, reverse, 5′-CATAATCTGGGTCATTTTCTCCC-3`; Fibronectin: forward, 5′-GCAAGGAAACAAGCAAATGC-3′, reverse, 5′-GTTGTAGGTGAACGGGAGGAC-3`; Col1α1: forward, 5′-CTGACTGGAAGAGCGGAGAG-3′, reverse, 5′-CGG

CTGAGTAGGGAACACAC-3`; Col2α1: forward, 5′-GAC GCCATGAAAGTTTTCTGC-3′, reverse, 5′-CCCTCAGTG GACAGTAGACGG-3`; IL-1β: forward, 5′-GAAATGCCA CCTTTTGACAGTG-3′, reverse, 5′-TGGATGCTCTCA TCAGGACAG-3`; IL-6: forward, 5′-CTGCAAGAGACT TCCATCCAG-3′, reverse, 5′-AGTGGTATAGACAGGTCT GTTGG-3`; TNFα: forward, 5′-TTCTCATTCCTGCTTGTG G-3′, reverse, 5′-ACTTGGTGGTTTGCTACG-3`; GAPDH: forward, 5′-TGAAGGGTGGAGCCAAAAG-3′, reverse, 5′-AGTCTTCTGGGTGGCAGTGAT-3`.

The Human Primer Sequences Used in the Study Were Listed as Follows

LTBP2: forward, 5′-ACAGCAAACAGCACCAACCAC-3′, reverse, 5′-CTCATCGGGAATGACCTCCTC-3`; α-SMA: forward, 5′-CTTGAGAAGAGTTACGAGTTGC-3′, reverse, 5′-GATGCTGTTGTAGGTGGTTTC-3`; Fibronectin: forward, 5′-GTGGCAGAAGGAATATCTCGG-3′, reverse, 5′-TCTAAAGGCATGAAGCACTCAA-3`; Col1α1: forward, 5′-GCCAAGACGAAGACATCCCA-3′, reverse, 5′-CGTCAT CGCACAACACCTTG-3`; GAPDH: forward, 5′-CATCAT CCCTGCCTCTACTGG-3′, reverse, 5′-GTGGGTGTCGCT GTTGAAGTC-3`.

Western Blot Analysis

The protein concentration was measured using bicinchoninic acid assay kit (Aspen, Wuhan, China). Nuclear extracts were prepared with a nuclear and cytoplasmic protein extraction kit (Beyotime, Shanghai, China) according to the manufacturer's instructions for the detection of NF-κB p65 and phospho-NF-κB p65 (phospho s536) protein expression. Protein samples were separated by SDS-PAGE and transferred to PVDF membranes (Millipore, Bedford, MA, United States). The membranes were then blocked with 5% non-fat milk in TBST buffer for 2 h, and subsequently incubated with the appropriate primary antibodies at appropriate dilutions overnight at 4°C. After washing, the membranes were incubated with horseradish peroxidase (HRP)-conjugated secondary antibodies at room temperature for 2 h. The bands were visualized using the electrochemiluminescence (ECL) system (Tanon, Shanghai, China). The primary antibody against antibodies to α-SMA, collagen I, fibronectin, and Glyceraldehyde-3-phosphate dehydrogenase (GAPDH) were purchased from Abcam (Cambridge, MA, United States). Antibodies for total NF-κB p65, phospho-NF-κB p65 (phospho s536) and Lamin B were purchased from Cell Signaling Technology (Danvers, MA). Antibody against LTBP2 was purchased from Santa Cruz Biotechnology (Santa Cruz, CA, United States). Goat anti-rabbit and anti-mouse horseradish peroxidase (HRP)-conjugated secondary antibodies were acquired from Aspen (Wuhan, China).

Enzyme-Linked Immunosorbent Assay

LTBP2 protein levels in serum, bronchoalveolar lavage fluid (BALF), and cell culture media were detected using the Mouse LTBP2 ELISA Kit (ELK Biotechnology, Wuhan, China) and the Human LTBP2 ELISA Kit (ELK Biotechnology, Wuhan, China) following the manufacturers' instructions.

Statistical Analysis

All data were analyzed using the Statistical Package for the Social Sciences software (SPSS 21.0, Chicago, IL, United States) and presented as mean ± standard deviation (SD). Significant differences were determined by one-way ANOVA for multiple comparisons and Student's *t*-test for pairwise comparisons between two groups. *p* values less than 0.05 were considered significant.

RESULTS

LTBP2 Is Overexpressed in IPF Patients and BLM-Injured Mice

To verify LTBP2 as a candidate gene in PF, we first assessed LTBP2 expression in lung tissues of IPF patients. LTBP2 was almost undetectable in normal lung tissues, but it was highly expressed in the lungs from patients with IPF (**Figure 1A**). To address the above assumption, we further investigated LTBP2 expression in the PF murine model with a single intratracheal administration of BLM. We also observed considerably increased LTBP2 immunohistochemical staining in active fibrotic areas (**Figure 1B**). Furthermore, BLM upregulated LTBP2 levels in serum and BALF of mice with PF, and LTBP2 levels in BLM 28 days group were higher than those in BLM 7 days group (**Figures 1C,D**). Collectively, these findings support that IPF patients and BLM-induced mice are characterized by LTBP2 overexpression.

LTBP2 Is Co-localized in Activated Lung Fibroblasts/Myofibroblasts

Next, we stained LTBP2 and the marker proteins of lung fibroblast activation in fibrotic lungs with IPF patients and mice. The increased expression of LTBP2 was detected in α-SMA -positive or collagen-I-positive cells, suggesting that LTBP2 was co-localized in activated fibroblasts/myofibroblasts of IPF lungs (**Figures 2A,B**). Murine models of PF showed that LTBP2 expression was detected in vimentin-positive fibroblasts, and the increased expression of LTBP2 was co-localized with α-SMA and collagen-I in lung fibrotic regions (**Figures 2C–E**). To further investigate the role of LTBP2 in lung fibroblast activation, we sorted LTBP2-expressing and LTBP2-negative fibroblasts from BLM-induced mice lungs (**Supplementary Figure S1A**) and analyzed the transcription of key profibrotic genes. As shown in **Figure 2F**, LTBP2-expressing fibroblasts expressed higher mRNA levels for Acta2, Col1α1, Col2α1, and fibronectin compared to LTBP2-negative fibroblasts. Taken together, our data indicate that LTBP2 is highly expressed in activated lung fibroblasts/myofibroblasts and positively related with lung fibroblast activation.

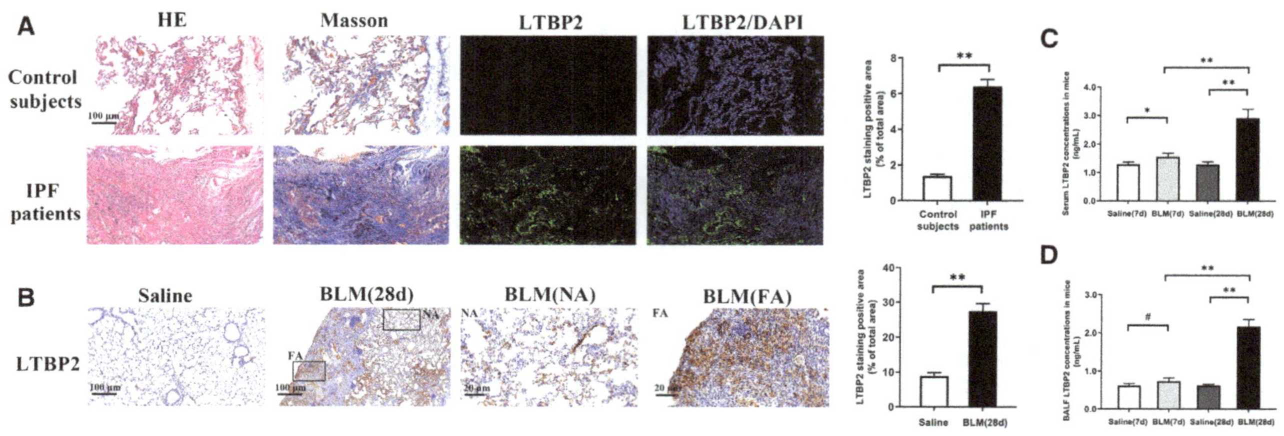

FIGURE 1 | LTBP2 is overexpressed in IPF patients and mice with BLM induction. **(A)** Representative Hematoxylin-eosin staining, Masson's trichrome staining, and immunofluorescence staining of LTBP2 (green) in the lung sections from normal people and IPF patients. Nuclei are stained with DAPI (blue); Scale bar = 100 μm. Quantification of positive staining area was measured and statistically analyzed. n = 3, $^{**}p < 0.01$. **(B)** Immunohistochemistry for LTBP2 expression in the lungs of mice. Scale bar = 100 μm. NA stands for normal area; FA stands for fibrotic area; Scale bar = 20 μm. Quantification of positive staining area was measured and statistically analyzed. n = 3, $^{**}p < 0.01$ **(C)** LTBP2 levels in serum of mice. n = 6, $^{*}p < 0.05$, $^{**}p < 0.01$ **(D)** LTBP2 levels in BALF of mice. n = 6, $^{\#}p > 0.05$, $^{**}p < 0.01$. Data are represented as means ± SD. Statistical analysis was performed by one-way ANOVA or *t*-test.

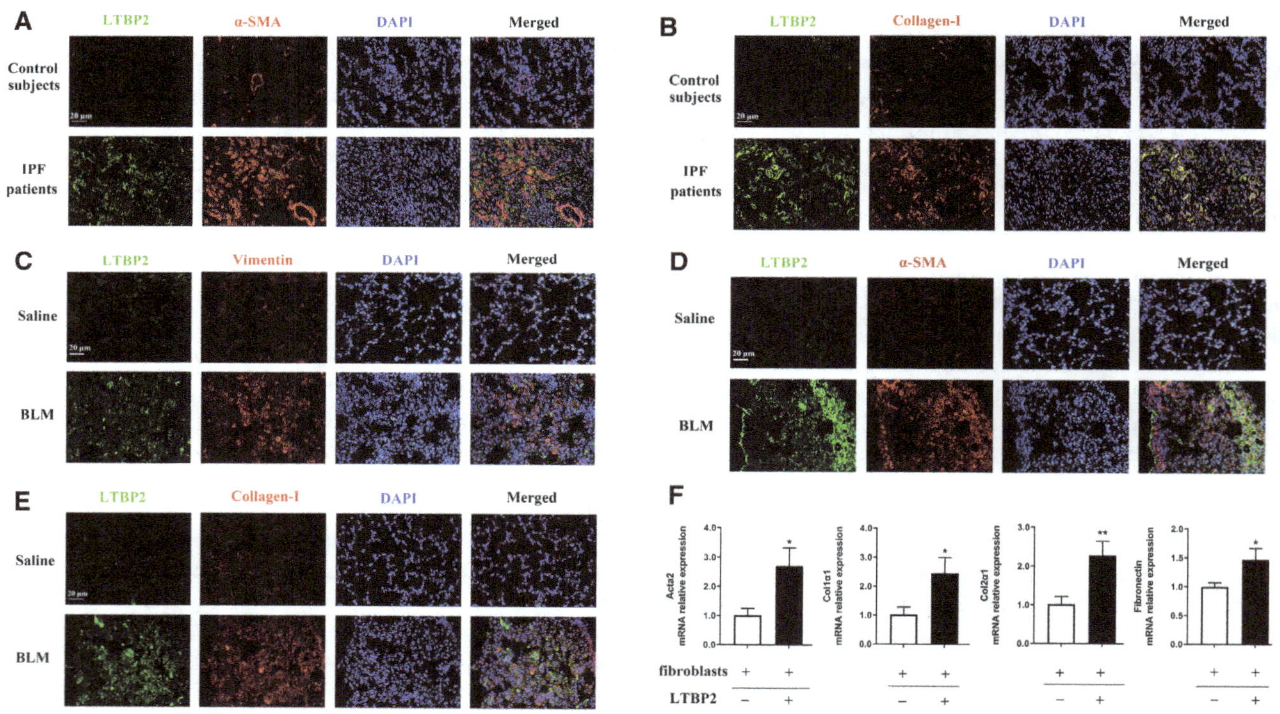

FIGURE 2 | LTBP2 is co-localized in activated lung fibroblasts/myofibroblasts. **(A)** Representative results for co-immunostaining of LTBP2 (green) and α-SMA (red) in the lung sections from patients with IPF (n = 3). Scale bar = 20 μm. **(B)** Representative results for co-immunostaining of LTBP2 (green) and collagen-I (red) in the lung sections from patients with IPF (n = 3). Scale bar = 20 μm. **(C)** Results for co-immunostaining of LTBP2 (green) and vimentin (red) in mice lungs (n = 3). Scale bar = 20 μm. **(D)** Representative results for co-immunostaining of LTBP2 (green) and α-SMA (red) in mice lungs (n = 3). Scale bar = 20 μm. **(E)** Results for co-immunostaining of LTBP2 (green) and collagen-I (red) in mice lungs (n = 3). Scale bar = 20 μm. **(F)** qRT-PCR analysis of Acta2, Col1α1, Col2α1, and Fibronectin in LTBP2-expressing and LTBP2-negative lung fibroblasts (n = 3 per group). $^{*}p < 0.05$, $^{**}p < 0.01$. Nuclei are stained with DAPI (blue). Data are represented as means ± SD. Statistical significance was analyzed using *t*-test.

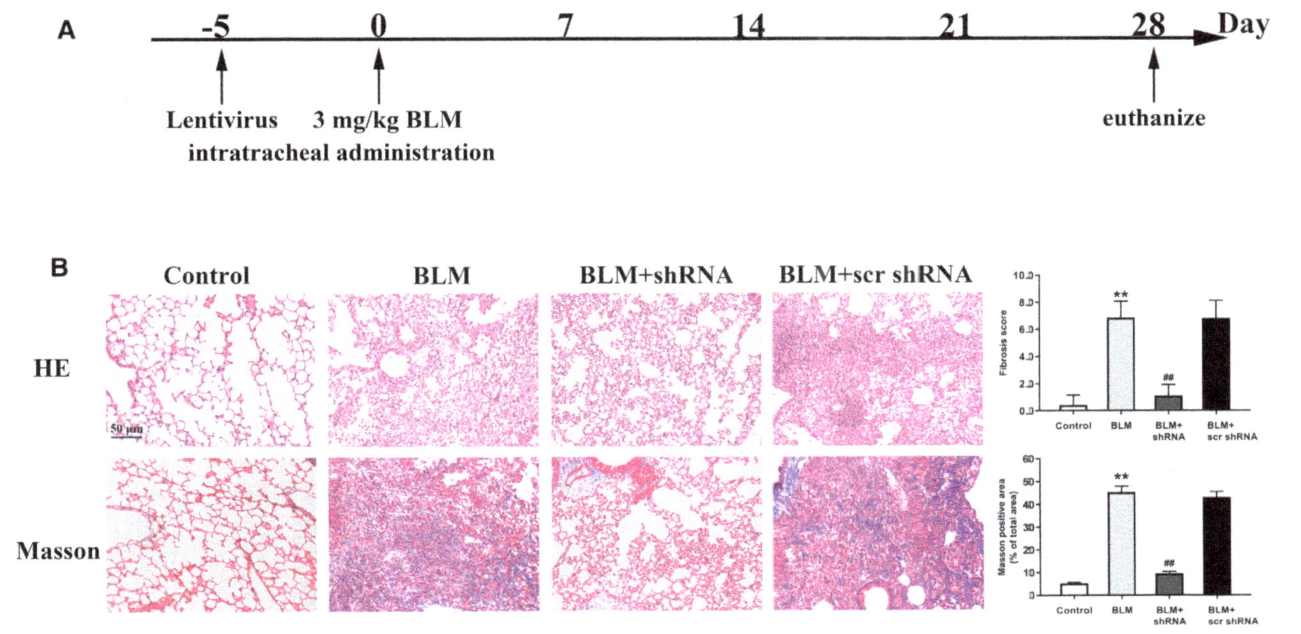

FIGURE 3 | LTBP2 silencing attenuates BLM-induced pulmonary fibrosis in mice. **(A)** Strategy for knockdown LTBP2 in BLM-induced lung fibrosis mouse model. Mice were received an intratracheal injection of LTBP2 shRNA, scrambled shRNA (scr shRNA), or left untreated. Five days later, mice were received a single intratracheal administration of BLM or saline **(B)** Representative histopathological sections of lung tissues by Hematoxylin-eosin staining and Masson's trichrome staining in mice. Scale bar = 50 μm. Fibrotic score was measured using the Ashcroft method. Quantification of postive Masson's staining area was measured and statistically analyzed. n = 6, $^{**}p < 0.01$ vs. control, $^{\#\#}p < 0.01$ vs. BLM + scr shRNA. Data are represented as means ± SD. Statistical analysis was performed by one-way ANOVA.

LTBP2 Silencing Attenuates BLM-Induced PF in Mice

To reveal the role of LTBP2 in PF, we designed three lentivirus shRNAs for LTBP2 silencing. We chose shRNA1 for further *in vivo* experiments because of its silencing efficiency (**Supplementary Figures S1B, S1C**). BLM-induced increase of LTBP2 protein was dramatically reduced in mice lungs after LTBP2 shRNA administration (~59% decrease; **Supplementary Figure S1D**). LTBP2 silencing attenuated the extent and intensity of the lung injury, fibrosis regions formation, and collagen deposition, as demonstrated by H&E staining, Masson's Trichome staining, and Ashcroft scores assessment (**Figure 3B**). These results suggest that LTBP2 silencing protects against BLM-induced PF in mice.

Next, we analyzed the inflammatory response of LTBP2 silencing in mice 7 days after BLM treatment. In BLM-challenged mice, a significant increase in the alveolar wall thickness and serious inflammatory cell infiltration were observed. LTBP2 shRNA administration tended to reduce lung inflammation in BLM-treated mice, but this was not significant. Consistently, similar levels of cytokines IL-1β, IL-6, and TNFα were detected in BLM + LTBP2 scr shRNA-treated and BLM + LTBP2 shRNA-treated mice (**Supplementary Figure S1E**). These data suggest that LTBP2 silencing attenuates BLM-induced lung fibrosis without affecting the inflammatory response in response to lung injury.

LTBP2 Silencing Inhibits Fibroblast-to-Myofibroblast Differentiation and ECM Accumulation in Fibrotic Lungs of BLM-Stimulated Mice

The differentiation of fibroblasts to α-SMA expressing myofibroblasts is a pivotal event in the process of PF, resulting in excess accumulation of ECM components (Wynn, 2011). Abnormal ECM proteins deposition, including α-SMA, fibronectin, and collagen I, also drives PF progression (Herrera et al., 2018). Therefore, we investigated whether LTBP2 silencing attenuated PF by suppressing fibroblasts' differentiation to myofibroblasts and decreasing the deposition of ECM proteins.

Desmin, an intermediate filament protein, can identify stromal cells with fibroblastic morphology. Our results for co-immunostaining suggested that LTBP2 expression was detected in desmin-positive fibroblasts from the BLM + scr shRNA group. However, LTBP2 expression was decreased in those from the BLM + shRNA group (**Supplementary Figure S1F**). These data suggested that LTBP2 shRNA administration decreased LTBP2 expression in lung fibroblasts. As shown in **Figure 4A**, desmin-positive lung fibroblasts had a myofibroblast marker (α-SMA) in the BLM-stimulated mice, which verified the involvement of fibroblasts' differentiation to myofibroblasts in the fibrotic process. Notably, LTBP2 silencing prevented this differentiation. We also found that α-SMA and fibronectin expressions were significantly increased in the BLM-challenged mice. However, LTBP2 silencing significantly blunted

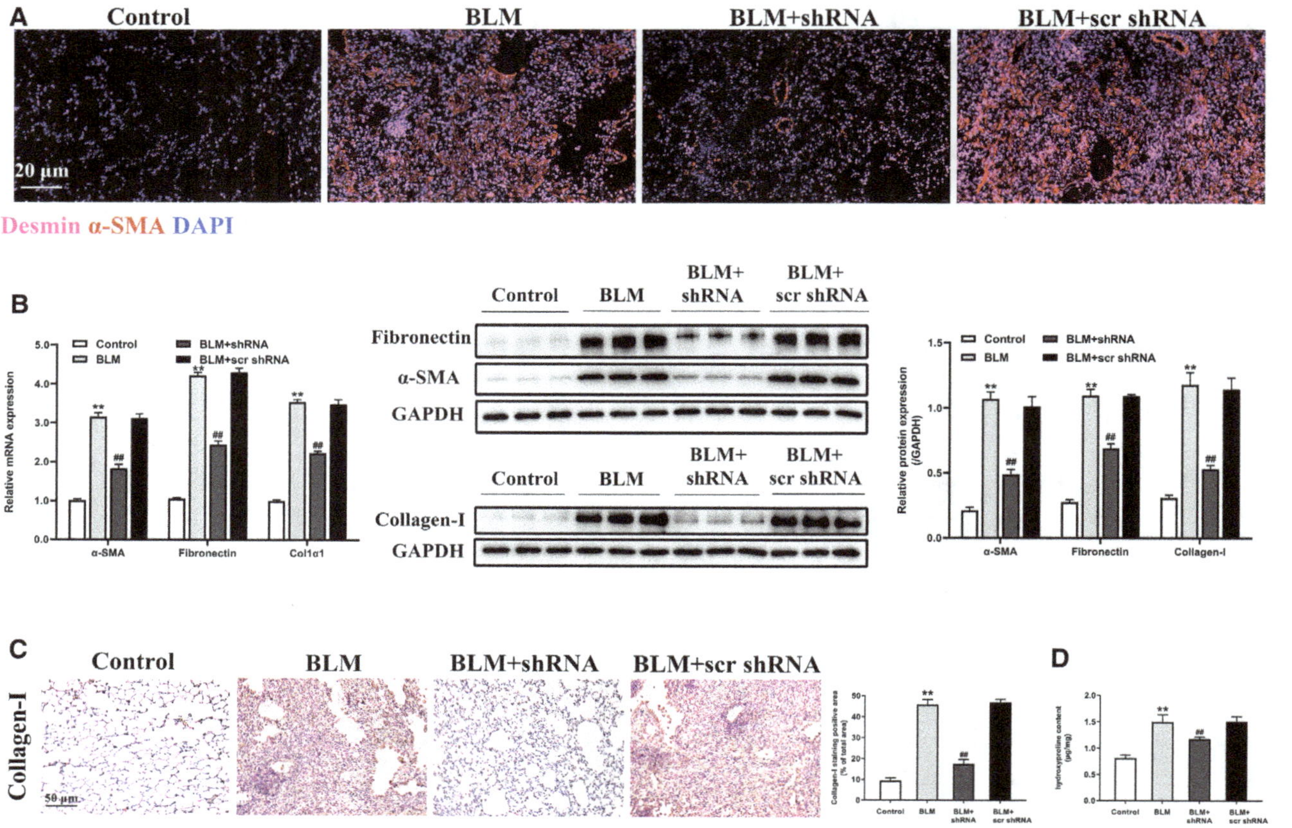

FIGURE 4 | LTBP2 silencing inhibits fibroblast-to-myofibroblast differentiation and ECM accumulation in fibrotic lungs of BLM-stimulated mice. **(A)** Immunofluorescence analysis of desmin (pink) and α-SMA (red) were performed to assess the lung fibroblast-to-myofibroblast differentiation. Nuclei are stained with DAPI (blue). Scale bar = 20 μm. **(B)** Quantitative RT-PCR and western blot analysis of α-SMA, fibronectin, and collagen I in the lungs of mice. GAPDH was detected as the internal control **(C)** Immunohistochemistry for collagen I expression in the lungs of mice. Scale bar = 50 μm. Quantification of positive staining area was measured and statistically analyzed **(D)** The levels of hydroxyproline in the lungs of mice. n = 6, $^{**}p < 0.01$ vs. control, $^{\#\#}p < 0.01$ vs. BLM + scr shRNA. Data are represented as means ± SD. Statistical analysis was performed by one-way ANOVA.

upregulation in α-SMA and fibronectin expression levels in mice lungs (**Figure 4B**). Moreover, LTBP2 silencing significantly reduced lung collagen accumulation, indicated by Western blot, immunohistochemical staining, and the lung hydroxyproline levels (**Figures 4B–D**). Taken together, these results suggest that LTBP2 silencing is protective against fibrogenesis, possibly *via* limiting the BLM-induced fibroblast-to-myofibroblast differentiation and ECM deposition.

LTBP2 Silencing Inhibits TGFβ1-Induced Differentiation of Fibroblasts *in Vitro*

TGFβ1 is a key profibrotic cytokine known to mediate the process of PF by lung fibroblasts accumulation and differentiation (Györfi et al., 2018). To determine whether the results in mice were reproducible in human cells, we analyzed the LTBP2 expression in HFL1 cells with or without stimulation by TGFβ1. TGFβ1 increased LTBP2 mRNA level and protein expression in HFL1 cells during fibroblasts' differentiation to myofibroblasts, which was characterized by the increased expression of the marker gene α-SMA (**Supplementary Figure S1G**).

We next evaluated the effect of LTBP2 silencing on lung fibroblast differentiation by transfecting HFL1 cells with scrambled shRNA or LTBP2 shRNA combined with subsequent TGF-β1 stimulation. We designed three lentivirus shRNAs for human LTBP2 silencing and chose shRNA3 for further experiments because of its silencing efficiency (**Supplementary Figure S1H**). A significant reduction in the protein expressions of α-SMA, fibronectin, and collagen I was observed in HFL1 cells transfected with LTBP2 shRNA alone compared with scrambled shRNA (**Figure 5A** and **Supplementary Figure S1I**). Moreover, LTBP2 silencing abrogated TGFβ1-induced increases in α-SMA, fibronectin, and collagen I in HFL1 cells (**Figure 5A**). Consistently, immunofluorescence staining showed a lower number of α-SMA-positive cells and less collagen expression in HFL1 cells transfected with LTBP2 shRNA (**Figures 5B,C**). Collectively, these results suggest that LTBP2 silencing

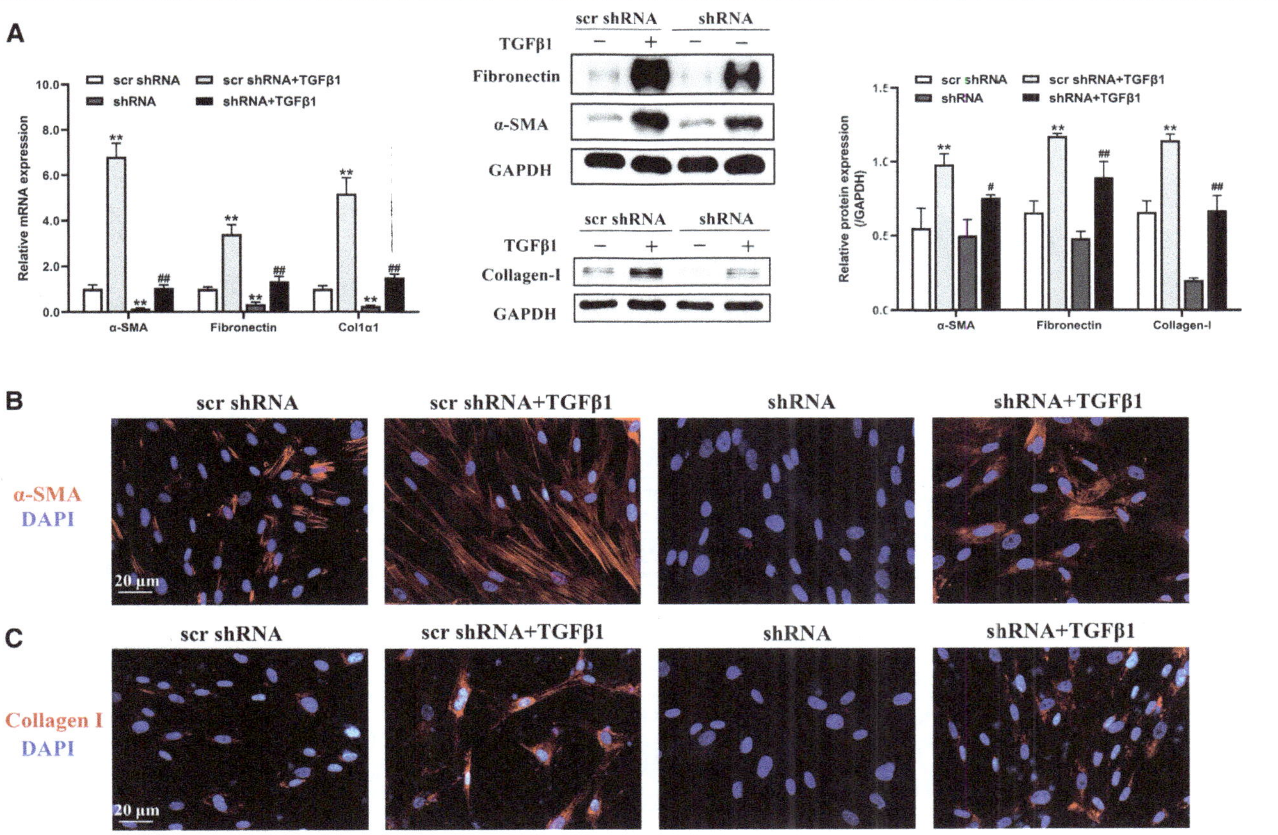

FIGURE 5 | LTBP2 silencing inhibits TGFβ1-induced differentiation of fibroblasts *in vitro*. **(A)** Quantitative RT-PCR and western blot analysis of α-SMA, fibronectin, and collagen I in HFL1 cells transfected with scrambled shRNA or LTBP2 shRNA followed by PBS or TGF-β1 stimulation. GAPDH was detected as the internal control. $^{**}p < 0.01$ vs. scr shRNA, $^{\#}p < 0.05$, $^{\#\#}p < 0.01$ vs. scr shRNA + TGFβ1 **(B)** Representative immunofluorescence staining of α-SMA (red) in HFL1 cells. Nuclei are stained with DAPI (blue). Scale bar = 20 μm. **(C)** Representative immunofluorescence staining of collagen I (red) in HFL1 cells. Nuclei are stained with DAPI (blue). Scale bar = 20 μm. Data are represented as means ± SD, n = 3. Statistical analysis was performed by one-way ANOVA.

suppresses TGFβ1-induced fibroblasts' differentiation to myofibroblasts in HFL1 cells.

LTBP2 Silencing Suppresses the Activation of NF-κB Signaling After BLM Treatment

Increased nuclear translocation of activated NF-κB initiates a cascade of responses, including abundant expression of proinflammatory molecules and profibrogenic cytokines that have been shown to be involved in the pathogenesis of PF (Christman et al., 2000; Meng et al., 2014). To elucidate the underlying mechanism of LTBP2 on lung fibroblasts differentiation and ECM deposition, we analyzed the effect of administering LTBP2 shRNA on NF-κB signaling in mice lungs. The results revealed that BLM administration induced phosphorylated NF-κB p65 subunit translocation from cytoplasm into nucleus (**Figure 6A**). Western blot further confirmed that BLM significantly increased both p65 nuclear translocation and phosphorylated p65 levels, confirming the activation of NF-κB signaling (**Figure 6B**). However, LTBP2 silencing inhibited the BLM-induced phosphorylation and nuclear translocation of the NF-κB p65 subunit (**Figures 6A,B**). These results suggest that LTBP2 silencing represses the activation of NF-κB signaling in the BLM-induced lung fibrosis murine model.

LTBP2 Silencing Suppresses the Activation of NF-κB Signaling Induced by TGFβ1

As demonstrated previously here, LTBP2 silencing inhibited the phosphorylation and nuclear translocation of NF-κB signaling in mice lungs. The effect of LTBP2 silencing on TGF-β1 -induced NF-κB signaling activation in HFL1 cells was subsequently evaluated by immunofluorescence assay and Western blot. As shown in **Figure 7**, TGFβ1 stimulated phosphorylated NF-κB p65 subunit translocation from cytoplasm into nucleus. However, TGFβ1-induced phosphorylation and nuclear translocation of NF-κB p65 subunit in HFL1 cells were blunted by LTBP2 shRNA transfection. These results suggest that LTBP2 silencing suppresses the activation of NF-κB signaling during TGF-β1 stimulation.

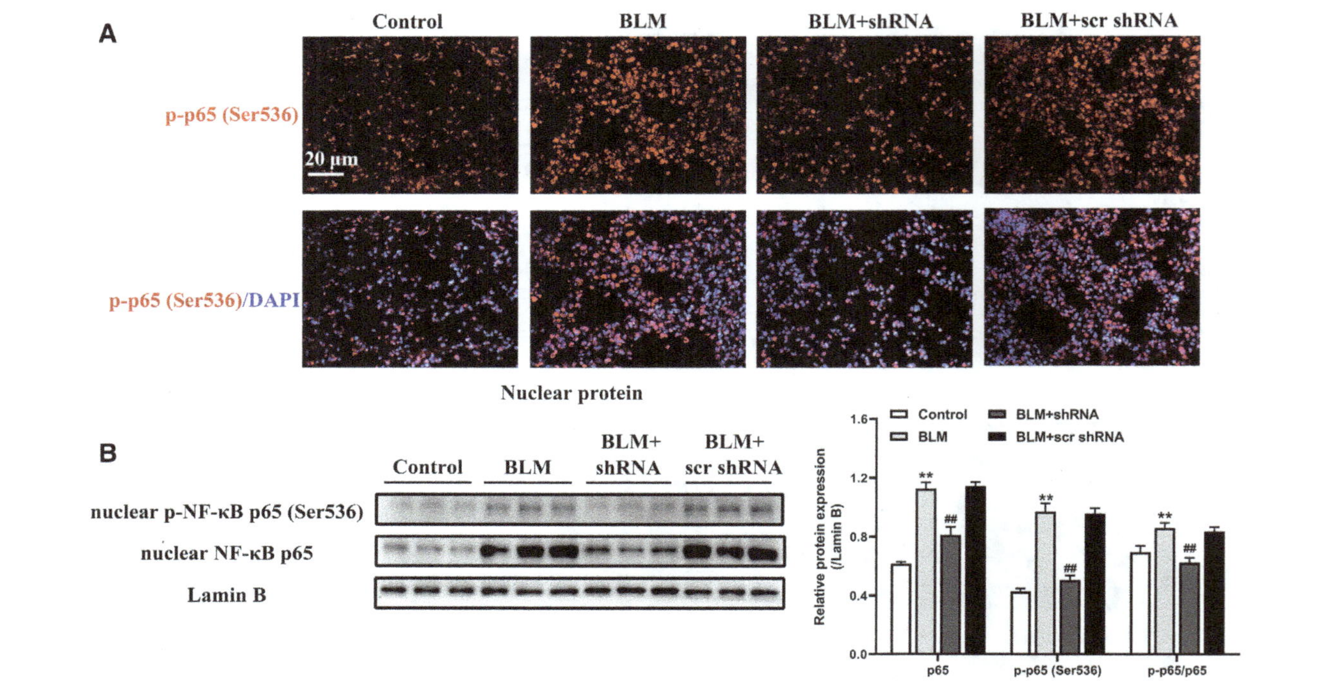

FIGURE 6 | LTBP2 silencing suppresses the activation of NF-κB signaling after BLM treatment. **(A)** Representative immunofluorescence staining of phospho-NF-κB p65 (ser536) (red) in mice lungs. Nuclei are stained with DAPI (blue). Scale bar = 20 μm. **(B)** Western blot analysis of nuclear NF-κB p65 and nuclear phospho-NF-κB p65 (ser536) in the lungs of mice. Lamin B was detected as the internal control. n = 6, $^{**}p < 0.01$ vs. control, $^{\#\#}p < 0.01$ vs. BLM + scr shRNA. Data are represented as means ± SD. Statistical analysis was performed by one-way ANOVA.

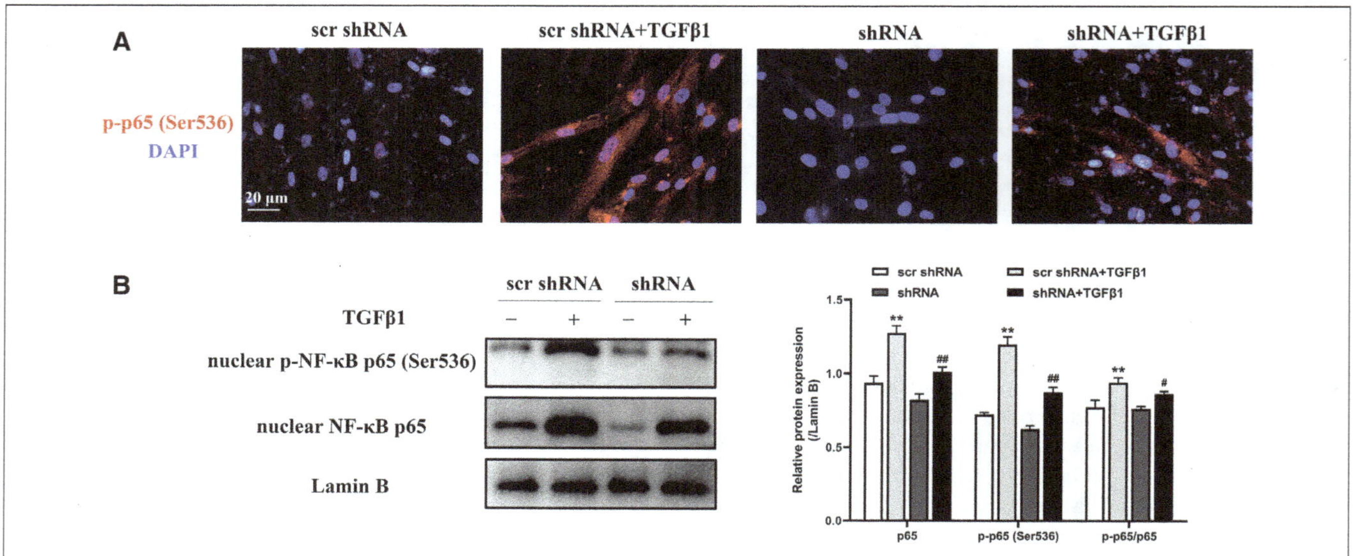

FIGURE 7 | LTBP2 silencing suppresses the activation of NF-κB signaling induced by TGFβ1. **(A)** Representative immunofluorescence staining of phospho-NF-κB p65 (ser536) (red) in HFL1 cells transfected with scrambled shRNA or LTBP2 shRNA followed by PBS or TGF-β1 stimulation. Nuclei are stained with DAPI (blue). Scale bar = 20 μm. **(B)** Western blot analysis of nuclear NF-κB p65 and nuclear phospho-NF-κB p65 (ser536) in HFL1 cells. Lamin B was detected as the internal control. $^{**}p < 0.01$ vs. scr shRNA, $^{\#}p < 0.05$, $^{\#\#}p < 0.01$ vs. scr shRNA + TGFβ1. Data are represented as means ± SD, n = 3. Statistical analysis was performed by one-way ANOVA.

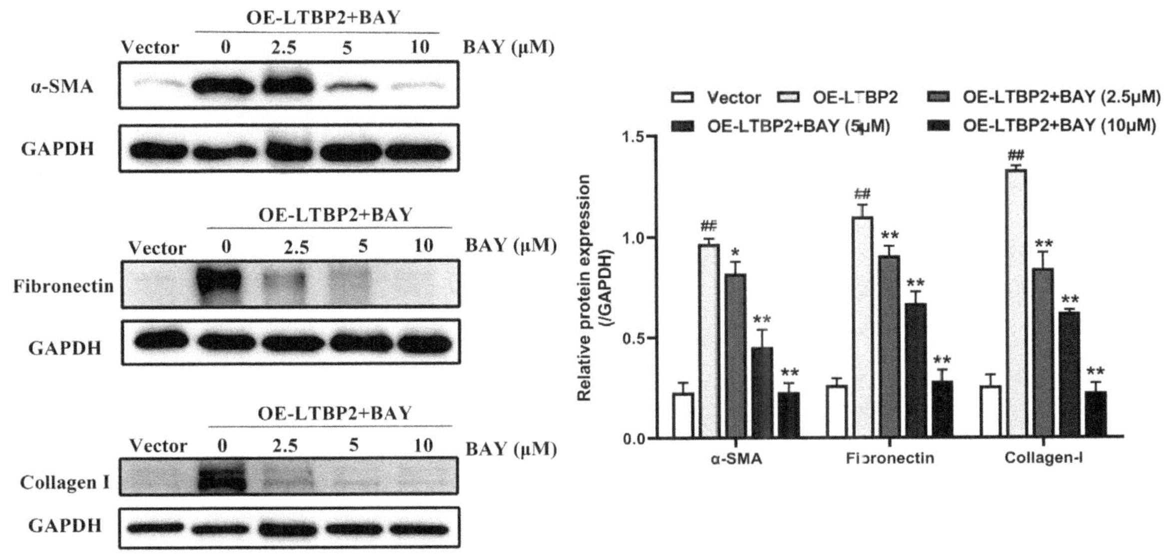

FIGURE 8 | LTBP2 overexpression-induced lung fibroblast-to-myofibroblast differentiation depends on NF-κB phosphorylation and nuclear translocation *in vitro*. Western blot analysis of α-SMA, fibronectin, and collagen I in HFL1 cells transfected with LTBP2 cDNA and/or BAY 11-7082 or vector. GAPDH was detected as the internal control. $^{\#\#}p < 0.01$ vs. vector. $^{*}p < 0.05$, $^{**}p < 0.01$ vs. OE-LTBP2. Data are represented as means ± SD, n = 3. Statistical analysis was performed by one-way ANOVA.

LTBP2 Overexpression-Induced Lung Fibroblast-To-Myofibroblast Differentiation Depends on NF-κB Phosphorylation and Nuclear Translocation *in Vitro*

We further examined whether LTBP2 is sufficient alone to regulate lung fibroblast differentiation by conducting a gain-of-function experiment. Interestingly, LTBP2 overexpression induced significant changes in the protein levels of α-SMA, fibronectin, and collagen I (**Figure 8** and **Supplementary Figure S1J**). These results suggest that LTBP2 overexpression is able to induce lung fibroblasts' differentiation to myofibroblasts in HFL1 cells, even in the absence of TGFβ1.

BAY is a compound in widespread use as an anti-inflammatory agent, and acts as an inhibitor of the activation of the transcription factor NF-κB (Pierce et al., 1997; Hou et al., 2018). Therefore, we next used BAY to investigate the effect of NF-κB signaling on lung fibroblast differentiation induced by LTBP2 overexpression. Our results demonstrated that BAY alone did not affect cell viability, and BAY significantly inhibited LTBP2 overexpression-induced nuclear translocation of the NF-κB p65 subunit (**Supplementary Figures S1K, S1L**). LTBP2 overexpression induced increases in α-SMA, fibronectin, and collagen I expressions, which was also suppressed by BAY in a dose-dependent manner, with concentrations ranging from 2.5 to 10 μM (**Figure 8**).

LTBP2 Expression Is Up-Regulated in RA-ILD Patients and COVID-19-Related PF

We further investigated LTBP2 expression in PF with other different pathological origins. Compared with control group, lung samples originating from RA-ILD patients exhibited increased LTBP2 expression, while co-immunostaining of α-SMA suggested that LTBP2 was co-localized in activated fibroblasts/myofibroblasts (**Figure 9A**). As LTBP2 was a secreted protein, we measured serum LTBP2 concentrations in patients with PF secondary to COVID-19. Baseline characteristics are summarized in **Supplementary Table S3**. Serum levels of LTBP2 were similar between healthy controls and COVID-19 patients without PF (mean: 7.45 ng/ml (median: 6.53) compared with 7.04 ng/ml (median: 7.06), $p > 0.05$; **Figure 9B**). However, serum LTBP2 concentrations in patients with COVID-19-related PF were significantly higher than those in COVID-19 patients without developing PF (mean: 18.51 ng/ml (median: 17.51) compared with 7.04 ng/ml (median: 7.06), $p < 0.01$; **Figure 9B**).

DISCUSSION

In the present study, we identified that LTBP2 is upregulated in different types of patients with PF, including IPF, RA-ILD, and COVID-19-related PF, and in mice following BLM-induced PF. Specifically, LTBP2 is overexpressed in activated fibroblasts/myofibroblasts in fibrotic lung tissues. Our data show that LTBP2 silencing protects against BLM-induced PF and suppresses fibroblast-to-myofibroblast differentiation *via* blocking NF-κB signaling *in vivo* and *in vitro*. Interestingly, LTBP2 overexpression promotes lung fibroblast-to-myofibroblast differentiation *in vitro*, even in the absence of TGFβ1, which depends on the activation of NF-κB signaling. Taken together, our results support that strategy aimed at silencing LTBP2 may provide a viable therapy against PF.

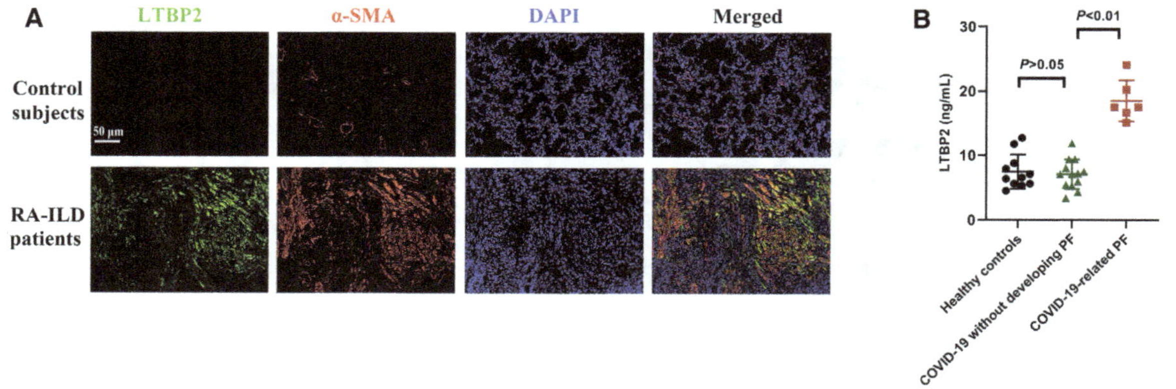

FIGURE 9 | LTBP2 expression is up-regulated in RA-ILD patients and COVID-19-related PF. **(A)** Representative results for co-immunostaining of LTBP2 (green) and α-SMA (red) in the lung sections from patients with RA-ILD (n = 3). Scale bar = 50 μm. **(B)** Serum LTBP2 concentrations in healthy controls (n = 11), COVID-19 patients without PF (n = 13), and patients with PF secondary to COVID-19 (n = 6). Data are represented as means ± SD. Statistical analysis was performed by one-way ANOVA.

LTBP2 has a broad tissue distribution and plays a structural role within elastic fibers in most cases (Shipley et al., 2000). LTBP2 may be associated with organ fibrosis, including the heart (Pang et al., 2020) and skin (Sideek et al., 2016). A previous study showed that serum LTBP2 concentrations in IPF patients were significantly higher than those in healthy controls, but the exact role of LTBP2 in PF had not been well understood (Enomoto et al., 2018). The BLM-induced lung fibrosis model, is able to reproduce many aspects of human IPF and other fibrotic ILDs, and is the best-characterized and most extensively used animal model (Liu et al., 2017). Here, we observed that lung tissues originating from different types of patients with PF, including IPF and RA-ILD, and from mice following BLM-induced PF were characterized by increased LTBP2 expression. Moreover, serum LTBP2 was also elevated in patients with COVID-19-related PF. Consistently, Li et al. (Li et al., 2021) demonstrated that LTBP2 was highly expressed in lungs of mice with PF. More importantly, we found that LTBP2 silencing by lentiviral transfection attenuated BLM-induced PF in mice. Therefore, our results provide evidence of the profibrotic role of LTBP2 in PF.

Fibrotic diseases are typically characterized by a progressive, vicious cycle of abnormally high myofibroblast accumulation. The activated myofibroblast is thought to be the main source of pathological ECM in fibrosis (El Agha et al., 2017; Philp et al., 2018). It has been reported that myofibroblasts in PF could originate from multiple cellular sources, including resident fibroblasts, circulating fibrocytes, epithelial cells, pericytes, and endothelial cells (El Agha et al., 2017; Walsh et al., 2018). Of these, resident fibroblasts make a major contribution to the myofibroblast population in PF (Hoyles et al., 2011) and the differentiation of fibroblasts to myofibroblasts is the primary feature during the progression of PF (Wynn, 2011). Consistent with these findings, we found that fibrotic mice lungs and lung samples originating from IPF and RA-ILD patients exhibited increases in the activated fibroblasts/myofibroblasts marker, and this pathological change was accompanied by increased LTBP2 expression. More importantly, we demonstrated that silencing LTBP2 inhibited fibroblast-to-myofibroblast differentiation and ECM deposition in BLM-treated mice lungs. This is in line with several studies that LTBP2 knockdown decreased collagen expression in myocardial fibrosis (Pang et al., 2020) and ECM gene expression in trabecular meshwork cells (Suri et al., 2018). Moreover, the above *in vivo* findings were further verified by *in vitro* observations that LTBP2 silencing inhibited TGF-β1-mediated fibroblast-to-myofibroblast differentiation in HFL1 cells. Through gain- and loss-of-function assays, we validated LTBP2 was essential and sufficient for TGF-β1-induced lung fibroblast differentiation *in vitro*. It was worth noting that in our study, the differences using the shRNA *in vitro* were less robust than data *in vivo*. We speculated that the results might be related to the difference in the best silencing efficiency of mouse LTBP2 shRNA and human LTBP2 shRNA, and besides fibroblasts, LTBP2 in other types of cells from mouse lungs might play a role in the phenotype through other different mechanisms. Collectively, these findings suggest that LTBP2 is a key regulator of fibroblast differentiation to myofibroblast in PF.

We then further investigated the molecular mechanism by which LTBP2 regulated fibroblast-to-myofibroblast differentiation in PF. As an important transcription factor, NF-κB transcription complexes consists of various homo- and heterodimers, including the subunits p50, p52, c-Rel, RelA (p65), and RelB (Sun, 2017). Previous studies have highlighted the significance of NF-κB signaling in the progression of PF (Inayama et al., 2006; Sun et al., 2015; Hou et al., 2018). Consistent with these reports, we found that the NF-κB signaling was activated by BLM or TGFβ1 *in vivo* or *in vitro*, respectively. Previous data have shown that LTBP2 knockdown inactivated the NF-κB signaling pathway, subsequently decelerating the progression of myocardial fibrosis (Pang et al., 2020). Our results suggested that LTBP2 silencing suppressed the activation of NF-κB signaling *in vivo* and *in vitro*. More importantly, we demonstrated that LTBP2 overexpression directly activated the NF-κB signaling and that LTBP2 overexpression-induced fibroblast-to-myofibroblast differentiation depended on the activation of NF-κB signaling *in vitro*. Contrary to our and others' results, Kan et al. (Kan et al., 2015) reported that LTBP2 negatively regulated NF-κB p65 by decreasing phosphorylation of p65 at serine 536, inhibiting active phosphorylated p65 nuclear localization and weakening the p65 DNA-binding ability in nasopharyngeal carcinoma. We speculate LTBP2 may have a specific molecular function in each tissue type. NF-κB can be activated by mitogen-activated protein kinases (MAPKs) (Luo et al., 2010). A previous study has already showed that inhibiting MAPKs suppressed the angiotensin II-stimulated NF-κB cascade in HFL1 cells (Meng et al., 2014). Ren et al. (2015) found that upon a transcriptional analysis and interrogation of the KEGG database, LTBP2 knockdown affected the MAPK signaling pathway in HeLa cells. In human MSU-1.1 fibroblasts, a central bioactive region of LTBP-2 stimulated the expression of inactively TGF-β1 *via* p38 MAPK signaling pathways (Sideek et al., 2017). Therefore, in the future, it is necessary to further study the relationship between LTBP2 and MAPKs signaling in PF. While NF-κB is a key signaling pathway targeted by LTBP2 in PF, we cannot rule out the involvement of other signaling pathways which would be very interesting to explore in future studies. In addition, although LTBP2 has not been reported to have transcription factor-like functions, a previous study showed that LTBP2 was one of the super-enhancer-driven pathogenic genes in lung fibrosis and Myc was one of the transcription factors binding to the LTBP2 super-enhancer (Li et al., 2021). Therefore, it's not ruled out that LTBP2 may directly regulate promoter activity of α-SMA, fibronectin and Col1α, and it would be necessary to explore in the future.

PF is not a single disease. Instead, it is the result of various processes that cause widespread scarring in the lungs. In this study, we investigated LTBP2 expression in three PF with different pathological origins: IPF, RA-ILD and COVID-19-related PF. IPF is defined as UIP based on HRCT and/or histopathological pattern after exclusion of other known causes of ILD (Raghu et al., 2018). IPF patients demonstrate large heterogeneity in their pulmonary manifestation of fibrosis, and it is generally not regarded as an inflammatory disease (Strieter and Mehrad, 2009). RA is a systemic inflammatory autoimmune disorder that can be associated with extra-articular manifestations in up to 50% of patients (Turesson, 2013). Among those with multiple extra-articular manifestations, ILD is the most frequent and worsens the disease prognosis (Bongartz et al., 2010). Contrary to ILD associated with other connective tissue diseases, the most prevalent pattern in RA-ILD is UIP followed by nonspecific interstitial pneumonia (Wu et al., 2019). Compared to RA patients with a non-UIP pattern, a proportion of those with UIP have similar phenotype and mortality as IPF (Song et al., 2013; Samara et al., 2017). The pattern in RA-ILD patients included in the current study is UIP. Moreover, IPF and RA-ILD share some phenotypic characteristics, autoimmune features, and a genetic background (Juge et al., 2020). The hallmarks of IPF and RA-ILD are both fibroblast/myofibroblast hyperproliferation, fibroblast foci formation, and ECM protein deposition. PF has been recognized as a potential sequela among COVID-19 survivors. Virus-induced lung injury, immune response, and attempts at healing are central to the process of fibrogenesis (Ojo et al., 2020). Features of COVID-19 presents some common points with IPF and RA-ILD, typically characterized by a chronic progression over time and possibly complicated by acute exacerbation (Manfredi et al., 2020). Our data showed that LTBP2 expression was up-regulated in patients with IPF, RA-ILD and COVID-19-related PF. However, our study has limitations in BLM-induced PF murine model and it would be necessary to use different animal models to further evaluate the exact role of LTBP2 in RA-ILD and COVID-19-related PF in future studies.

CONCLUSION

In summary, our study demonstrates that LTBP2 serves as a pro-fibrotic regulator in pulmonary fibrogenesis and that LTBP2 regulates fibroblasts' differentiation to myofibroblasts *via* NF-κB signaling. Therefore, LTBP2 may be a potential therapeutic target for the treatment of PF.

AUTHOR CONTRIBUTIONS

ZC designed the study. MeZ, JZ, and XH performed the *in vivo* and *in vitro* experiments. MeZ, WZ and MiZ analyzed the experimental data. MeZ and XH wrote the manuscript with input from all co-authors. MeZ, JZ, and XH have contributed equally to this work and share first authorship.

SUPPLEMENTARY MATERIAL

Supplementary Figure S1 | **(A)** Gating strategy for sorting of LTBP2-positive and LTBP2-negative murine lung fibroblasts **(B)** L929 cells were co-transfected with scrambled shRNA, LTBP2 shRNA1, LTBP2 shRNA2, LTBP2 shRNA3. Silencing efficiency was detected by qRT-PCR ($n = 3$, $^{*}P < 0.05$, $^{**}P < 0.01$ vs. scr shRNA). **(C)** Mice were received an intratracheal injection of LTBP2 shRNA1-GFP, and mice lung sections were viewed under a fluorescent microscope to assess the transduction efficiency ($n = 6$). Scale bar = 20 μm. **(D)** Western blot analysis of LTBP2 expression in mice lungs. $n = 3$, $^{**}P < 0.01$ vs. control, $^{\#\#}P < 0.01$ vs. BLM + scr shRNA. **(E)** Mice were treated as indicated and samples were collected on day 7 after intratracheal administration of BLM. Representative Hematoxylin-eosin staining in mice lungs. Scale bar = 100 μm; Total protein concentration in the BALF; The numbers of total cells, macrophages, neutrophils, and lymphocytes counted in the BALF; Quantitative RT-PCR analysis of IL-1β, IL-6, and TNFα in mice lungs. $n = 6$, $^{**}P < 0.01$ vs. control, $^{\#}P > 0.05$ vs. BLM + scr shRNA. **(F)** Immunofluorescence analysis of desmin (red) and LTBP2 (pink) were performed in mice lungs. Nuclei are stained with DAPI (blue). Scale bar = 20 μm, $n = 3$. **(G)** HFL1 cells were treated with TGF-β1 or PBS. Representative immunofluorescence staining, quantitative RT-PCR, and western blot analysis of α-SMA in HFL1 cells. Red, α-SMA; blue, nuclei; Scale bar = 20 μm. $n = 3$, $^{**}P < 0.01$ vs. control; LTBP2 expression in HFL1 cells was assessed using immunofluorescence staining, quantitative RT-PCR, and western blot. Green, LTBP2; blue, nuclei; Scale bar = 20 μm. LTBP2 levels in culture supernatant were measured by ELISA. $n = 3$, $^{**}P < 0.01$ vs. control. **(H)** HFL1 cells were co-transfected with scrambled shRNA, LTBP2 shRNA1, LTBP2 shRNA2, LTBP2 shRNA3. Silencing efficiency was detected by qRT-PCR and western blot ($n = 3$, $^{*}P < 0.05$, $^{**}P < 0.01$ vs. scr shRNA). **(I)** Western blot analysis of α-SMA, fibronectin, and collagen I in HFL1 cells transfected with scrambled shRNA or LTBP2 shRNA. $n = 3$, $^{**}P < 0.01$ vs. scr shRNA. **(J)** Western blot analysis of LTBP2 expression in HFL1 cells transfected with LTBP2 cDNA or vector. $n = 3$, $^{**}P < 0.01$ vs. vector. **(K)** HFL1 cells were treated with BAY 11-7082 for 48h. The cell viability was detected by CCK-8 assay kit. $n = 9$, $^{\#}P > 0.05$ vs. control. **(L)** Western blot analysis of nuclear NF-κB p65 expression in HFL1 cells transfected with LTBP2 cDNA and/or BAY 11-7082 or vector. $n = 3$, $^{\#\#}P < 0.01$ vs. vector. $^{**}P < 0.01$ vs. OE-LTBP2. Data are represented as means ± SD. Statistical analysis was performed by one-way ANOVA or *t*-test.

REFERENCES

Anderson, S. B., Goldberg, A. L., and Whitman, M. (2008). Identification of a Novel Pool of Extracellular Pro-myostatin in Skeletal Muscle. *J. Biol. Chem.* 283, 7027–7035. doi:10.1074/jbc.M706678200

Arnett, F. C., Edworthy, S. M., Bloch, D. A., McShane, D. J., Fries, J. F., Cooper, N. S., et al. (1988). The American Rheumatism Association 1987 Revised Criteria for the Classification of Rheumatoid Arthritis. *Arthritis Rheum.* 31, 315–324. doi:10.1002/art.1780310302

Ashcroft, T., Simpson, J. M., and Timbrell, V. (1988). Simple Method of Estimating Severity of Pulmonary Fibrosis on a Numerical Scale. *J. Clin. Pathol.* 41, 467–470. doi:10.1136/jcp.41.4.467

Bongartz, T., Nannini, C., Medina-Velasquez, Y. F., Achenbach, S. J., Crowson, C. S., Ryu, J. H., et al. (2010). Incidence and Mortality of Interstitial Lung Disease in Rheumatoid Arthritis: a Population-Based Study. *Arthritis Rheum.* 62 (6), 1583–1591. doi:10.1002/art.27405

Christman, J. W., Sadikot, R. T., and Blackwell, T. S. (2000). The Role of Nuclear Factor-Kappa B in Pulmonary Diseases. *Chest* 117, 1482–1487. doi:10.1378/chest.117.5.1482

El Agha, E., Kramann, R., Schneider, R. K., Li, X., Seeger, W., Humphreys, B. D., et al. (2017). Mesenchymal Stem Cells in Fibrotic Disease. *Cell Stem Cell* 21, 166–177. doi:10.1016/j.stem.2017.07.011

Enomoto, Y., Matsushima, S., Shibata, K., Aoshima, Y., Yagi, H., Meguro, S., et al. (2018). LTBP2 Is Secreted from Lung Myofibroblasts and Is a Potential Biomarker for Idiopathic Pulmonary Fibrosis. *Clin. Sci. (Lond)* 132, 1565–1580. doi:10.1042/CS20180435

George, P. M., Wells, A. U., and Jenkins, R. G. (2020). Pulmonary Fibrosis and COVID-19: The Potential Role for Antifibrotic Therapy. *Lancet Respir. Med.* 8, 807–815. doi:10.1016/S2213-2600(20)30225-3

Gibson, M. A., Hatzinikolas, G., Davis, E. C., Baker, E., Sutherland, G. R., and Mecham, R. P. (1995). Bovine Latent Transforming Growth Factor Beta 1-Binding Protein 2: Molecular Cloning, Identification of Tissue Isoforms, and Immunolocalization to Elastin-Associated Microfibrils. *Mol. Cel. Biol.* 15, 6932–6942. doi:10.1128/mcb.15.12.6932

Golan-Gerstl, R., Wallach-Dayan, S. B., Zisman, P., Cardoso, W. V., Goldstein, R. H., and Breuer, R. (2012). Cellular FLICE-like Inhibitory Protein Deviates Myofibroblast Fas-Induced Apoptosis toward Proliferation during Lung Fibrosis. *Am. J. Respir. Cel. Mol. Biol.* 47, 271–279. doi:10.1165/rcmb.2010-0284RC

Györfi, A. H., Matei, A.-E., and Distler, J. H. W. (2018). Targeting TGF-β Signaling for the Treatment of Fibrosis. *Matrix Biol.* 68-69, 8–27. doi:10.1016/j.matbio.2017.12.016

Herrera, J., Henke, C. A., and Bitterman, P. B. (2018). Extracellular Matrix as a Driver of Progressive Fibrosis. *J. Clin. Invest.* 128, 45–53. doi:10.1172/JCI93557

Hou, J., Ma, T., Cao, H., Chen, Y., Wang, C., Chen, X., et al. (2018). TNF-α-induced NF-Kb Activation Promotes Myofibroblast Differentiation of LR-MSCs and Exacerbates Bleomycin-Induced Pulmonary Fibrosis. *J. Cel. Physiol.* 233, 2409–2419. doi:10.1002/jcp.26112

Hoyles, R. K., Derrett-Smith, E. C., Khan, K., Shiwen, X., Howat, S. L., Wells, A. U., et al. (2011). An Essential Role for Resident Fibroblasts in Experimental Lung Fibrosis Is Defined by Lineage-specific Deletion of High-Affinity Type II Transforming Growth Factor β Receptor. *Am. J. Respir. Crit. Care Med.* 183, 249–261. doi:10.1164/rccm.201002-0279OC

Inayama, M., Nishioka, Y., Azuma, M., Muto, S., Aono, Y., Makino, H., et al. (2006). A Novel IkappaB Kinase-Beta Inhibitor Ameliorates Bleomycin-Induced Pulmonary Fibrosis in Mice. *Am. J. Respir. Crit. Care Med.* 173, 1016–1022. doi:10.1164/rccm.200506-947OC

Juge, P. A., Crestani, B., and Dieudé, P. (2020). Recent Advances in Rheumatoid Arthritis-Associated Interstitial Lung Disease. *Curr. Opin. Pulm. Med.* 26 (5), 477–486. doi:10.1097/MCP.0000000000000710

Kan, R., Shuen, W. H., Lung, H. L., Cheung, A. K., Dai, W., Kwong, D. L., et al. (2015). NF-κB P65 Subunit Is Modulated by Latent Transforming Growth Factor-β Binding Protein 2 (LTBP2) in Nasopharyngeal Carcinoma HONE1 and HK1 Cells. *PLoS One* 10, e0127239. doi:10.1371/journal.pone.0127239

Kolahian, S., Fernandez, I. E., Eickelberg, O., and Hartl, D. (2016). Immune Mechanisms in Pulmonary Fibrosis. *Am. J. Respir. Cel. Mol. Biol.* 55, 309–322. doi:10.1165/rcmb.2016-0121TR

Lederer, D. J., and Martinez, F. J. (2018). Idiopathic Pulmonary Fibrosis. *N. Engl. J. Med.* 378, 1811–1823. doi:10.1056/NEJMra1705751

Li, H., Zhao, C., Li, Z., Yao, K., Zhang, J., Si, W., et al. (2021). Identification of Potential Pathogenic Super-enhancers-driven Genes in Pulmonary Fibrosis. *Front. Genet.* 12, 644143. doi:10.3389/fgene.2021.644143

Liu, T., De Los Santos, F. G., and Phan, S. H. (2017). The Bleomycin Model of Pulmonary Fibrosis. *Methods Mol. Biol.* 1627, 27–42. doi:10.1007/978-1-4939-7113-8_2

Luo, S. F., Fang, R. Y., Hsieh, H. L., Chi, P. L., Lin, C. C., Hsiao, L. D., et al. (2010). Involvement of MAPKs and NF-kappaB in Tumor Necrosis Factor Alpha-Induced Vascular Cell Adhesion Molecule 1 Expression in Human Rheumatoid Arthritis Synovial Fibroblasts. *Arthritis Rheum.* 62, 105–116. doi:10.1002/art.25060

Manfredi, A., Luppi, F., Cassone, G., Vacchi, C., Salvarani, C., and Sebastiani, M. (2020). Pathogenesis and Treatment of Idiopathic and Rheumatoid Arthritis-Related Interstitial Pneumonia. The Possible Lesson from COVID-19 Pneumonia. *Expert Rev. Clin. Immunol.* 16 (8), 751–770. doi:10.1080/1744666X.2020.1803064

Meng, Y., Yu, C. H., Li, W., Li, T., Luo, W., Huang, S., et al. (2014). Angiotensin-converting Enzyme 2/angiotensin-(1-7)/Mas axis Protects against Lung Fibrosis by Inhibiting the MAPK/NF-κB Pathway. *Am. J. Respir. Cel. Mol. Biol.* 50, 723–736. doi:10.1165/rcmb.2012-0451OC

Miyazono, K., Olofsson, A., Colosetti, P., and Heldin, C. H. (1991). A Role of the Latent TGF-Beta 1-Binding Protein in the Assembly and Secretion of TGF-Beta 1. *EMBO J.* 10, 1091–1101. doi:10.1002/j.1460-2075.1991.tb08049.x

Ojo, A. S., Balogun, S. A., Williams, O. T., and Ojo, O. S. (2020). Pulmonary Fibrosis in COVID-19 Survivors: Predictive Factors and Risk Reduction Strategies. *Pulm. Med.* 2020, 6175964. doi:10.1155/2020/6175964

Pang, X. F., Lin, X., Du, J. J., and Zeng, D. Y. (2020). LTBP2 Knockdown by siRNA Reverses Myocardial Oxidative Stress Injury, Fibrosis and Remodelling during Dilated Cardiomyopathy. *Acta Physiol. (Oxf.)* 228, e13377. doi:10.1111/apha.13377

Philp, C. J., Siebeke, I., Clements, D., Miller, S., Habgood, A., John, A. E., et al. (2018). Extracellular Matrix Cross-Linking Enhances Fibroblast Growth and Protects against Matrix Proteolysis in Lung Fibrosis. *Am. J. Respir. Cel. Mol. Biol.* 58, 594–603. doi:10.1165/rcmb.2016-0379OC

Pierce, J. W., Schoenleber, R., Jesmok, G., Best, J., Moore, S. A., Collins, T., et al. (1997). Novel Inhibitors of Cytokine-Induced IkappaBalpha Phosphorylation and Endothelial Cell Adhesion Molecule Expression Show Anti-inflammatory Effects *In Vivo*. *J. Biol. Chem.* 272, 21096–21103. doi:10.1074/jbc.272.34.21096

Raghu, G., Remy-Jardin, M., Myers, J. L., Richeldi, L., Ryerson, C. J., Lederer, D. J., et al. (2018). Diagnosis of Idiopathic Pulmonary Fibrosis. An Official ATS/ERS/JRS/ALAT Clinical Practice Guideline. *Am. J. Respir. Crit. Care Med.* 198, e44–e68. doi:10.1164/rccm.201807-1255ST

Ren, Y., Lu, H., Zhao, D., Ou, Y., Yu, K., Gu, J., et al. (2015). LTPB2 Acts as A Prognostic Factor and Promotes Progression of Cervical Adenocarcinoma. *Am. J. Transl. Res.* 7 (6), 1095–1105.

Robertson, I. B., Horiguchi, M., Zilberberg, L., Dabovic, B., Hadjiolova, K., and Rifkin, D. B. (2015). Latent TGF-β-Binding Proteins. *Matrix Biol.* 47, 44–53. doi:10.1016/j.matbio.2015.05.005

Samara, K. D., Trachalaki, A., Tsitoura, E., Koutsopoulos, A. V., Lagoudaki, E. D., Lasithiotaki, I., et al. (2017). Upregulation of Citrullination Pathway: From Autoimmune to Idiopathic Lung Fibrosis. *Respir. Res.* 18 (1), 218. doi:10.1186/s12931-017-0692-9

Shipley, J. M., Mecham, R. P., Maus, E., Bonadio, J., Rosenbloom, J., McCarthy, R. T., et al. (2000). Developmental Expression of Latent Transforming Growth Factor Beta Binding Protein 2 and its Requirement Early in Mouse Development. *Mol. Cel. Biol.* 20, 4879–4887. doi:10.1128/MCB.20.13.4879-4887.2000

Sideek, M. A., Smith, J., Menz, C., Adams, J. R. J., Cowin, A. J., and Gibson, M. A. (2017). A Central Bioactive Region of LTBP-2 Stimulates the Expression of TGF-B1 in Fibroblasts via Akt and P38 Signalling Pathways. *Int. J. Mol. Sci.* 18 (10), 2114. doi:10.3390/ijms18102114

Sideek, M. A., Teia, A., Kopecki, Z., Cowin, A. J., and Gibson, M. A. (2016). Co-localization of LTBP-2 with FGF-2 in Fibrotic Human Keloid and Hypertrophic Scar. *J. Mol. Histol.* 47, 35–45. doi:10.1007/s10735-015-9645-0

Song, J. W., Lee, H. K., Lee, C. K., Chae, E. J., Jang, S. J., Colby, T. V., et al. (2013). Clinical Course and Outcome of Rheumatoid Arthritis-Related

Usual Interstitial Pneumonia. *Sarcoidosis. Vasc. Diffuse. Lung Dis.* 30 (2), 103–112.

Spagnolo, P., Lee, J. S., Sverzellati, N., Rossi, G., and Cottin, V. (2018). The Lung in Rheumatoid Arthritis: Focus on Interstitial Lung Disease. *Arthritis Rheumatol.* 70, 1544–1554. doi:10.1002/art.40574

Strieter, R. M., and Mehrad, B. (2009). New Mechanisms of Pulmonary Fibrosis. *Chest* 136 (5), 1364–1370. doi:10.1378/chest.09-0510

Sun, S. C. (2017). The Non-canonical NF-Kb Pathway in Immunity and Inflammation. *Nat. Rev. Immunol.* 17, 545–558. doi:10.1038/nri.2017.52

Sun, X., Chen, E., Dong, R., Chen, W., and Hu, Y. (2015). Nuclear Factor (NF)-κB P65 Regulates Differentiation of Human and Mouse Lung Fibroblasts Mediated by TGF-β. *Life Sci.* 122, 8–14. doi:10.1016/j.lfs.2014.11.033

Suri, F., Yazdani, S., and Elahi, E. (2018). LTBP2 Knockdown and Oxidative Stress Affect Glaucoma Features Including TGFβ Pathways, ECM Genes Expression and Apoptosis in Trabecular Meshwork Cells. *Gene* 673, 70–81. doi:10.1016/j.gene.2018.06.038

Turesson, C. (2013). Extra-articular Rheumatoid Arthritis. *Curr. Opin. Rheumatol.* 25 (3), 360–366. doi:10.1097/BOR.0b013e32835f693f

Walsh, S. M., Worrell, J. C., Fabre, A., Hinz, B., Kane, R., and Keane, M. P. (2018). Novel Differences in Gene Expression and Functional Capabilities of Myofibroblast Populations in Idiopathic Pulmonary Fibrosis. *Am. J. Physiol. Lung Cel. Mol. Physiol.* 315, L697–L710. doi:10.1152/ajplung.00543.2017

Wan, F., Peng, L., Zhu, C., Zhang, X., Chen, F., and Liu, T. (2017). Knockdown of Latent Transforming Growth Factor-β (TGF-B)-Binding Protein 2 (LTBP2) Inhibits Invasion and Tumorigenesis in Thyroid Carcinoma Cells. *Oncol. Res.* 25, 503–510. doi:10.3727/096504016X14755368915591

Wang, J., Liang, W. J., Min, G. T., Wang, H. P., Chen, W., and Yao, N. (2018). LTBP2 Promotes the Migration and Invasion of Gastric Cancer Cells and Predicts Poor Outcome of Patients with Gastric Cancer. *Int. J. Oncol.* 52, 1886–1898. doi:10.3892/ijo.2018.4356

Wilson, M. S., and Wynn, T. A. (2009). Pulmonary Fibrosis: Pathogenesis, Etiology and Regulation. *Mucosal Immunol.* 2, 103–121. doi:10.1038/mi.2008.85

Wu, E. K., Ambrosini, R. D., Kottmann, R. M., Ritchlin, C. T., Schwarz, E. M., and Rahimi, H. (2019). Reinterpreting Evidence of Rheumatoid Arthritis-Associated Interstitial Lung Disease to Understand Etiology. *Curr. Rheumatol. Rev.* 15 (4), 277–289. doi:10.2174/1573397115666190116102451

Wynn, T. A. (2011). Integrating Mechanisms of Pulmonary Fibrosis. *J. Exp. Med.* 208, 1339–1350. doi:10.1084/jem.20110551

8

Challenges for Clinical Drug Development in Pulmonary Fibrosis

Eric S. White[1], *Matthew Thomas*[2], *Susanne Stowasser*[3] *and Kay Tetzlaff*[3,4]*

[1]Boehringer Ingelheim Pharmaceuticals, Inc., Ridgefield, CT, United States, [2]Boehringer Ingelheim Pharma GmbH & Co. KG, Biberach, Germany, [3]Boehringer Ingelheim International GmbH, Ingelheim am Rhein, Germany, [4]Department of Sports Medicine, University of Tübingen, Tübingen, Germany

***Correspondence:**
Kay Tetzlaff
kay.tetzlaff@boehringer-ingelheim.com*

Pulmonary fibrosis is a pathologic process associated with scarring of the lung interstitium. Interstitial lung diseases (ILDs) encompass a large and heterogenous group of disorders, a number of which are characterized by progressive pulmonary fibrosis that leads to respiratory failure and death. Idiopathic pulmonary fibrosis (IPF) has been described as an archetype of progressive fibrosing ILD, and the development of pirfenidone and nintedanib has been a major breakthrough in the treatment of patients with this deadly disease. Both drugs principally target scar-forming fibroblasts and have been shown to significantly slow down the accelerated decline of lung function by approximately 50%. In addition, nintedanib has been approved for patients with other progressive fibrosing ILDs and systemic sclerosis-associated ILD. However, there is still no cure for pulmonary fibrosis and no meaningful improvement of symptoms or quality of life has been shown. Advancement in research, such as the advent of single cell sequencing technology, has identified additional pathologic cell populations beyond the fibroblast which could be targeted for therapeutic purposes. The preclinical and clinical development of novel drug candidates is hampered by profound challenges such as a lack of sensitive clinical outcomes or suitable biomarkers that would provide an early indication of patient benefit. With the availability of these anti-fibrotic treatments, it has become even more difficult to demonstrate added efficacy, in particular in short-term clinical studies. Patient heterogeneity and the paucity of biomarkers of disease activity further complicate clinical development. It is conceivable that future treatment of pulmonary fibrosis will need to embrace more precision in treating the right patient at the right time, explore novel measures of efficacy, and likely combine treatment options.

Keywords: lung disease, interstitial, clinical trial, drugs, fibroblast, pharmaceutical research, pharmacology

INTRODUCTION

The last decade has been a game changer for idiopathic pulmonary fibrosis (IPF) from a research as well as from a clinical perspective. A shift of understanding of the pathogenesis from a chronic inflammatory to an epithelial driven disorder resulting from repetitive alveolar epithelial injury and aberrant repair (Selman et al., 2001; King et al., 2011) as well as a refinement of diagnostic criteria for IPF (Raghu et al., 2012) finally enabled a breakthrough in the treatment of patients with this devastating disease with the approval of nintedanib and pirfenidone (Richeldi et al., 2011; Raghu et al., 2012; King et al., 2014).

IPF is the most common form of idiopathic interstitial pneumonia within a large and heterogenous group of disorders referred to as interstitial lung diseases (ILD) (Travis et al., 2013). IPF is, by definition, a chronic progressive fibrosing ILD characterized by inexorable worsening of symptoms, lung function and early mortality (Raghu et al., 2018) and is considered the prototypical progressive fibrotic ILD. However, such longitudinal disease behaviour (termed "progressive fibrotic phenotype") is not restricted to IPF but applies to other ILDs with even greater heterogeneity compared to IPF (Travis et al., 2013; Wells et al., 2018). It is postulated that progressive fibrosing ILDs also share similarities in pathogenic mechanisms implicated in fibrotic remodeling (Wollin et al., 2019). Consequently, pirfenidone and nintedanib were separately investigated in a basket approach, similar to oncology, including non-IPF patients with differing underlying etiologies but a common progressive fibrotic clinical disease course (Flaherty et al., 2019; Behr et al., 2021), further supporting the concept of the progressive fibrotic phenotype and leading to the approval of nintedanib in patients with progressive fibrosing interstitial lung disease (Brown et al., 2020).

Undoubtedly these advances and, specifically, the approvals of antifibrotic drugs for the treatment of (idiopathic) pulmonary fibrosis have fuelled basic, translational and clinical research and drug development in this field. However, key challenges will have to be tackled across disciplines in the next decade to ultimately embark on a path of patient-centricity and precision medicine in drug development and to provide benefit to patients beyond "just" slowing lung function decline. These include identification of patients earlier in their disease course to ultimately prevent development of or even reverse fibrosis, validation of prognostic and predictive biomarkers to enable the right treatment for the right patient at the right time, developing better disease models, clinical outcome parameters and, ultimately, targeting the mechanisms involved in lung repair and regeneration.

This review aims to shed light on some of these key challenges from an industry research and development perspective.

EVOLVING MECHANISMS OF PULMONARY FIBROSIS

Both pirfenidone and nintedanib—the current standard of care for medications for idiopathic and other forms of pulmonary fibrosis—were borne of the desire to inhibit aberrant fibroblast activity. Fibroblast populations are responsible for providing structure to organs, so are thus an essential part of the repair process following damage. Fibroblast proliferation, migration and transition toward myofibroblasts, which preferentially deposit collagen to form scar tissue, are healthy processes when controlled to be transient (Ushakumary et al., 2021). However, the dysregulation of these processes leads to uncontrolled fibrogenesis—a fundamental driver or "master mechanism" of pulmonary fibrosis. Anti-fibrotic therapies address elements of these pathologic pathways through inhibition of fibroblast-centric growth factors (Conte et al., 2014; Wollin et al., 2014)

The advent of single cell seq technologies have greatly expanded our view of pathologic processes to reach beyond the fibroblast (Habermann et al., 2019; Reyfman et al., 2019; Adams et al., 2020). We now recognize profound changes in epithelial stem cell populations which drive perturbed barrier repair and impaired lung function. Disease-specific "aberrant basaloid" cells may be derived from dysregulated secretory cell phenotypes or dysfunctional/transitional alveolar type 2 populations (Adams et al., 2020; Jaeger et al., 2020; Strunz et al., 2020). Signaling thought to drive the perturbed epithelial repair include oxidative and endoplasmic reticulum stress (Burman et al., 2018; Otoupalova et al., 2020). An additional "master mechanism" for consideration is the phenotypic alteration to macrophage populations driving a loss of homeostatic control within a fibrotic lung. Although long associated with progressive pulmonary fibrosis (Keogh and Crystal, 1982), early attempts to modulate macrophage migration into the lung failed (Raghu et al., 2015)—likely due to the translational limitations of previously dominant murine M1/M2 hypothesis of macrophage pathobiology. Triggered, again, by SCseq studies, we have now expanded our knowledge of macrophages and fibrosis to reveal a key role for efferocytosis in the effective (anti-fibrotic) repair of the lung (Morse et al., 2019; Gerlach et al., 2021). Furthermore, biomarker evidence of senescence in pulmonary fibrosis (Ryu et al., 2017) is being unraveled across "master mechanisms"—linked to dysregulated fibroblasts, aberrant epithelial stem cell populations and as drivers of a pro-fibrotic macrophage phenotype (Álvarez et al., 2017; DePianto et al., 2021). Furthermore, we are now understanding more than ever that to consider any cell population in isolation is to miss the (mis-) communication between different populations—cell types which collude to drive fibrosis relentlessly forward (Raredon, Systems Biol 2020; Le et al., 2021). Preclinical research into the "immunofibrotic niche" (summarized in **Figure 1**) has opened new avenues for drug discovery.

We now look to promote a homeostatic balance of macrophages, rejuvenate small airway and alveolar epithelial progenitor populations and correct the mutual dysfunctional crosstalk between epithelium and underlying fibroblasts. Yet the ambition to explore novel targets within the immune fibrotic niche preclinically will bring even greater challenges as they are translated to the clinic—requiring an ever greater degree of therapeutic precision.

CHALLENGES IN PRECLINICAL RESEARCH OF EMERGING THERAPEUTICS

Anti-fibrotic therapeutics were validated with *in vitro* and *in vivo* systems focused upon fibroblast biology. Fibroblasts stimulated with platelet-derived growth factor (PDGF) will proliferate, or with transforming growth factor (TGF)ß transition to scar-forming myofibroblasts. Bleomycin-induced fibrosis in mice/rats model inflammatory, then fibrotic, changes followed by resolution waves of pathobiology—yet have shown limited

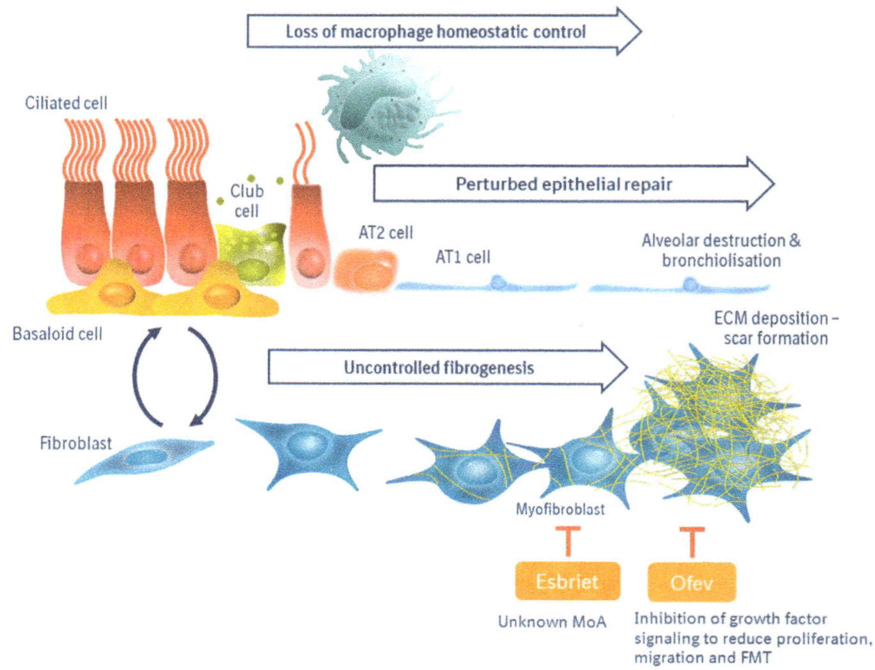

FIGURE 1 | Master Mechanisms of the immunofibrotic niche. Pathologic drivers in pulmonary fibrosis can be viewed as three "master mechanisms": Uncontrolled fibrogenesis, driven by pro-fibrotic growth factors and tissue stiffness, is the current point of intervention for standards of care "anti-fibrotics." Perturbed epithelial repair is due to dysregulated/transitional small airway and/or alveolar progenitor populations, leading to senescence, impaired barrier function and poor gas exchange. Loss of macrophage homeostatic control is characterized by an imbalance of pro-fibrotic vs. pro-repair macrophage phenotypes to resulting in less efferocytosis and heighted inflammation within the lung. The immunofibrotic niche is interconnected, where macrophage activity and phenotype can be influenced by senescent fibroblasts; aberrant signals from epithelium promote fibrosis and scar-forming fibroblasts hinder effective epithelial repair.

translational value (Moeller et al., 2008). It is interesting to note that although fibroblasts remain the principal target cell population of both nintedanib and pirfenidone, this does not preclude some effects on other cell populations—either directly or as a consequence of altering the dynamics within the immune-fibrotic niche (Huang et al., 2017).

The next generation of novel therapeutics need innovative *in vitro* and *in vivo* systems. By enriching the environment in which primary co-cultured cells act and react *in vitro*, including stimuli which are more representative of the pathophysiologic situation, we increase the likelihood of observing a difference between healthy and diseased cells. Once observed, this 'differential patient biology' can form the basis of novel therapeutic discovery. For example, we can observe a reciprocal influence of primary small airway epithelial cells (SAECs), grown at air-liquid interface, together with fibroblasts (see **Figure 2**). When derived from healthy donors, epithelial cells exert a protective effect on fibroblasts challenged with a fibrosis-driving growth factor (TGFß). However, if derived from pulmonary fibrosis patient donors or conditioned with stimuli from fibrosis patients, SAECs can drive fibrotic transition in fibroblasts in the absence of stimulation (Le et al., 2020).

In vivo models, although no longer the source of novel targets, are nevertheless fundamental to understanding pharmacokinetic (PK) vs target engagement (TE) vs pharmacodynamic (PD) relationships of drug candidates. Yet, we strive to enhance the translational relevance of PD measures—functional measures or biomarkers—to capture more elements of the immune-fibrotic niche. Bleomycin models can be enhanced by using older mice, thus partially negating the transient nature of the fibrosis observed, or by using a model of repetitive instillation to create a more durable fibrotic response (Redente et al., 2021). Furthermore, microCT measures have been developed to better mimic diagnostic measures from the clinic (Ruscitti et al., 2017). Alternative models have been developed which better reveal the perturbed epithelial elements of pulmonary fibrosis, such as the model of SPC mutation, which creates an alveolar type 2 cell-driven fibrotic response (Nureki et al., 2018). Few rodent models have come closer to patient biology than that which uses a combination of humanized mice, low-dose bleomycin and adoptively transferred patient epithelial cells reproduce the lung reticulation patterns so characteristic of usual interstitial pneumonia (UIP) seen in IPF (Jaeger et al., 2020).

Novel *in vitro* and *in vivo* systems can now be assessed for greater translational relevance by the comparative computational analysis of gene expression changes in an assay vs patient material. Thus, individual pathways/processes, and the impact of test compounds upon them, can be effectively matched to the appropriate assay. It is with preclinical systems such as these that we can create first evidence in support of either combination or differentiation for a next generation therapeutic with standard of

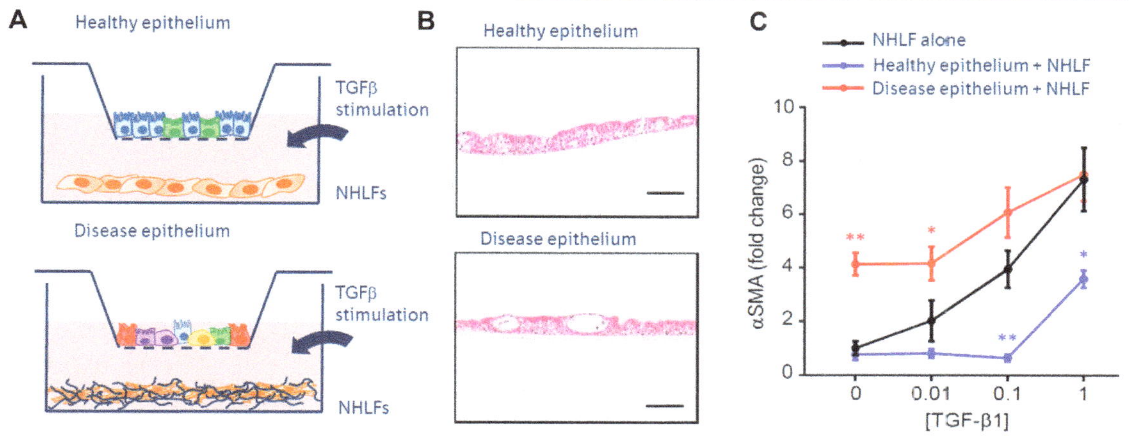

FIGURE 2 | Next generation co-culture assays of epithelial:fibroblast crosstalk. **(A)** Schematics of epithelial cells, cultured in inserts at air-liquid interface from primary basal epithelium isolated from healthy or fibrosis patient lungs. Normal healthy lung fibroblasts (NHLFs) co-cultured in the below wells—stimulated with increasing concentrations of TGFβ. **(B)** H&E images of healthy vs diseased (fibrotic) epithelium, showing fewer ciliated cells and more secretory populations. **(C)** Mono-culture NHLF response to TGFβ dose response (black), showing increased a-smooth muscle actin—an indicator of fibroblast to myofibroblast transition. Fibrotic epithelium promotes fibroblast transition in the absence of TGFβ (red). Healthy epithelial co-culture protects fibroblasts from pro-fibrotic effects of TGFβ.

care anti-fibrotics. Through these technological breakthroughs, it is now possible to employ precision pharmacology, and thus set the stage for clinical assessment of precision therapies.

CHALLENGES IN CLINICAL DEVELOPMENT OF EMERGING THERAPEUTICS

Enrichment Strategies and Efficacy Endpoints

The widespread regulatory approval of nintedanib and pirfenidone to reduce the rate of decline in a key measure of lung function, forced vital capacity (FVC), is seen as a major advance for the treatment of patients with IPF (and, in the case of nintedanib, for patients with systemic sclerosis-associated ILD and with chronic fibrosing ILDs with a progressive phenotype). However, this success is also accompanied by new challenges for drug developers. In the ideal clinical trial, all patients enrolled in the trial would experience the event the study drug is designed to prevent/treat, such that patients receiving active drug will demonstrate clear efficacy as compared to placebo. This is especially important in conditions which take a long time to manifest or in which relatively few patients experience the event. Indeed, fibrotic ILDs often progress slowly; thus, in some patients it may take years to see significant declines in lung physiology or increased fibrosis on high-resolution computed tomography (HRCT) scans, and clinical trials often require primary endpoints to be measured after a minimum of 12 months to allow sufficient patients to demonstrate progression. Yet even in such circumstances, a proportion of patients will not demonstrate significant loss of lung function. As an example, in the pivotal INPULSIS trials of nintedanib in patients with IPF, 15% of placebo-treated patients demonstrated either no decline or an improvement in FVC over the 52-week trial period (Brown et al., 2019). Similar findings were observed in the INBUILD trial of nintedanib in patients with progressive fibrotic ILDs (Maher et al., 2021).

For fibrotic ILDs, a current challenge is identifying which patients will develop progression over a relatively short period of time or are at increased risk for exacerbations or death. This is critical not only for planning of clinical trials but also for clinical care; patients likely to experience faster progression or at risk for adverse outcomes might be prioritized on transplant lists or followed more closely in the clinic. Efforts to develop prognostic information in patients with fibrotic ILDs have intensified greatly over the recent past, with numerous investigators evaluating a panoply of potential biomarkers. Such biomarkers may be genetic (Fingerlin et al., 2013; Stuart et al., 2015; Herazo-Maya et al., 2017), metabolomic (Zhao et al., 2017; Nambiar et al., 2021), circulating soluble factors in plasma or serum (Rosas et al., 2008; Makiguchi et al., 2016; Maher et al., 2017; Organ et al., 2019), cell-based (Morse et al., 2019; Karampitsakos et al., 2021), image-based (Justet et al., 2017; Salisbury et al., 2017; Win et al., 2018; Derlin et al., 2021), or based on clinical characteristics (Ley et al., 2012; Ryerson et al., 2014; Morisset et al., 2017). While these efforts are laudable and show promise, none is yet sufficiently validated to be used in clinical practice. For clinical trial planning, enrichment strategies based on biomarkers are similarly not well validated, yet are desperately needed. One possible exception to the current lack of enrichment biomarkers is the imaging pattern of usual interstitial pneumonia (UIP) seen on HRCT scanning. UIP is the radiologic and histopathologic pattern associated with IPF, as well as other ILDs that may demonstrate more rapid progression in a similar fashion. Indeed, in the INBUILD trial of nintedanib for treatment of patients with non-IPF progressive fibrotic ILDs of varying causes, patients with an HRCT pattern of UIP demonstrated similar declines in FVC over 52 weeks as has been seen in prior IPF trials (Flaherty et al., 2019).

But for which outcome should we be trying to enrich? Historically, registrational trials for both nintedanib and pirfenidone in patients with IPF were predicated on a primary endpoint of annualized rate of decline of FVC (ml/year) or change in FVC from baseline (ml), supported by additional secondary outcomes such as a trend for reduced mortality, further strengthening FVC as a valid surrogate endpoint. Subsequent studies in IPF, as well asother fibrosing ILDs, have similarly focused on the rate of FVC decline given the precedent set by nintedanib and pirfenidone. Certainly, slowing the rate of decline in lung function for patients with IPF and other progressive ILDs is a worthy goal; data suggest that rate of decline of lung function, both FVC and diffusing capacity for carbon monoxide (DLCO), correlates with time to mortality (Collard et al., 2003; Latsi et al., 2003). This correlation between lung function decline and mortality bolstered active discussions with authorities, in particular the US FDA, which finally accepted FVC as a surrogate outcome marker for mortality in IPF; the acceptance of FVC decline was also based on review of study data from both the nintedanib and pirfenidone clinical development programs (Karimi-Shah and Chowdhury, 2015). Now, evolving real-world data suggest that patients with IPF receiving antifibrotic medication demonstrate better survival than those not treated (Guenther et al., 2018; Behr et al., 2020), lending credence to the concept that FVC decline is an appropriate surrogate for mortality (Karimi-Shah and Chowdhury, 2015). However, the relationship between lung function decline and mortality is indirect and doesn't capture the impact of progressive ILDs on patients' quality of life, symptoms and/or disability. Further, clinical experience tells us that the rate of decline of lung function in IPF and other ILDs is not necessarily linear over time; therefore, careful thought must be given to identifying, validating, and qualifying novel endpoints to determine the impact of new therapeutics for these patients.

Trial Design Challenges

Both nintedanib and pirfenidone utilized classical drug development approaches with large and long phase II dose-ranging studies. For example, the trial providing proof of clinical concept for nintedanib was a dose-ranging study exploring four doses of nintedanib versus placebo that randomized 432 patients with IPF to treatment over 1 year (Richeldi et al., 2011). This study was followed by two large placebo-controlled confirmatory phase III studies comprising a total of 1,066 patients with IPF randomized to 52 weeks of treatment with nintedanib or placebo to establish pivotal efficacy and safety data for submission (Richeldi et al., 2014).

However, newer drug candidates will be required to utilize different clinical development approaches, for a variety of reasons. First, IPF (and the majority of other progressive fibrosing ILDs) are rare-to-uncommon diseases and, thus, the patient pool available for inclusion in clinical studies in these indications is limited. Coupled with increased drug development efforts in pulmonary fibrosis by numerous companies, several drug candidates are currently being investigated in phase II and phase III studies (Spagnolo et al., 2020) which leadsto competition for patients among potential trials. One potential solution to this problem was recently demonstrated by the successful conduct of the INBUILD trial, in which patients with various fibrosing ILDs (excluding IPF) who all shared a common phenotype of progressive disease were randomized to receive placebo or nintedanib (Flaherty et al., 2017). This "basket" study showed that in patients with a UIP-like pattern on HRCT but an underlying diagnosis other than IPF, nintedanib has a similar effect on slowing the rate of decline in FVC compared to what was seen in prior IPF trials (Flaherty et al., 2019). Moreover, patients with fibrosing ILD with other radiologic fibrotic patterns, but still with a prior history of disease progression, equally benefitted from nintedanib (Flaherty et al., 2019). This suggests that pooling patients who have different disease etiologies a but similar longitudinal clinical behavior may be an appropriate enrichment strategy, although this concept remains a source of debate (Wells et al., 2018; Wolters et al., 2018).

Second, accelerated new drug development timelines are necessary due to pragmatic considerations for our patients as well as costs: a long phase II study with endpoints measured 1 year after study initiation is no longer sustainable for patients or sponsors. However, the ability to demonstrate a statistically significant treatment difference in rate of FVC decline at a timepoint earlier than 52 weeks is dependent upon the degree of patient heterogeneity within a cohort and the variability inherent in lung function testing. As a result, increased sample sizes are required to achieve the power needed to detect significant differences in rate of FVC decline. Interestingly, retrospective analyses of nintedanib and pirfenidone clinical development programs suggest that a separation in the rate of decline of FVC with antifibrotic treatment may be apparent after 26 weeks. Some sponsors have recently reported results demonstrating treatment effects in phase II trials of patients with IPF after only 12 weeks (Maher et al., 2018; Palmer et al., 2018). Ziritaxestat, for example, an autotaxin (an enzyme catalyzing lysophosphatidylcholine into lysophosphatidic acid [LPA]) inhibitor demonstrated favorable effects on mean change from baseline in FVC after 12 weeks, with an increase of 8 ml in the active group versus a reduction of 87 ml on placebo (Maher et al., 2018). Similarly, treatment of antifibrotic-naïve patients with IPF with the LPA receptor antagonist BMS-986020 also resulted in a slowing of the rate of decline in FVC compared to placebo-treated patients, although the results were not statistically significant until 26 weeks (Palmer et al., 2018).

Finally, new drug candidates for patients with IPF or other progressive fibrosing ILDs can no longer ethically be compared to true placebo, as standard of care therapies (with their associated adverse effects) now exist for these patients. This adds further complexity and challenges on clinical trial design: any treatment (or adverse) effects seen for newer therapeutics could be attributed to the investigational compound or the standard background therapy; the room for improvement in lung function on top of standard of care is variable and limited and affecting sample size; patient populations will be heterogenous including all-comers, i.e., patients without background antifibrotic standard of care (either naïve to antifibrotic treatment or having stopped previous standard of care for tolerability or effectiveness reasons) and patients with concomitant approved antifibrotic treatments. Moreover, in the future, newer therapeutics may be designed to improve the lives of patients with IPF and other fibrosing ILDs as measured by different endpoints (e.g. quality of life, imaging, or other biomarkers of disease activity), which may be difficult to interpret in the face of combination therapy.

Approaches to Increase Trial Efficiency

Given the challenge of recruiting enough patients in a timely fashion to identify drug efficacy in pulmonary fibrotic diseases, drug developers may seek to take advantage of a number of methods to speed development program efficiency. Such methods may involve innovative statistical modeling, novel trial design approaches, biomarker enrichment strategies, or some combination thereof. One example of innovative statistical modeling, called Bayesian dynamic borrowing (Dron et al., 2019), utilizes data from historical control cohorts to decrease the required number of control subjects, in some cases by up to 80%, without compromising statistical results (Dron et al., 2019). Similarly, efficiency in clinical development programs may be realized through the use of "master protocol" designs, such as confirmatory basket, umbrella and platform trials (Angus et al., 2019; Collignon et al., 2020). For example, adaptive platform trials (APTs) are perhaps least similar to the gold-standard randomized control trial, in that they study multiple interventions in a single disease (or condition) in a perpetual manner, with interventions allowed to enter or leave the platform on the basis of a decision algorithm' (Woodcock and LaVange, 2017) rather than compare a single intervention with a control group. This approach allows for multiple treatment comparators to enter or leave a trial without having to halt the study or pause other investigative arms. Moreover, as the name implies, APTs may utilize within-trial adaptations such as response-adaptive randomization that allow for arms of a trial that are showing promise to preferentially recruit subsequent subjects, or rules that allow for transitioning from one phase to the next during the course of a trial (Angus et al., 2019). Finally, utilization of various biomarkers to allow early read-out of efficacy signals or to enrich trials for patients who will demonstrate progression over the course of a trial could also potentially improve study efficiency. While there are no universally agreed-upon biomarkers to achieve this goal, there has been substantial progress recently to detect blood biomarkers predictive of disease progression in IPF, such as markers of epithelial cell dysfunction and extracellular matrix remodeling: serum levels of surfactant protein A (SP-A) and D (SP-D) have been found correlated with reduced survival (Greene et al., 2002; Maher et al., 2017), and serum levels of Krebs von den Lungen 6 (KL-6) have been shown to be associated with acute exacerbations of IPF and mortality (Ishikawa et al., 2012; Maher et al., 2017). Cancer antigens CA 19-9 and CA-125 have been shown to be elevated in patients with progressive disease (Maher et al., 2017). Genetic variants of MUC5B and TOLLIP have been associated with disease progression (Oldham et al., 2015). Thus, opportunities are emerging to allow for enriching clinical trials for patients at higher risk of IPF progression; however, none of the molecular biomarkers have yet been validated in larger clinical trials. Also, it is likely that not a single biomarker, but a biomarker signature will most reliably predict disease progression. Fewer data are available on possible therapeutic biomarkers; recent studies have demonstrated a short-term dynamic change in various putative biomarker analytes in response to therapeutics that might be predictive of a subsequent response to therapy (Nanthakumar et al., 2019; Jenkins et al., 2020; Luo et al., 2020). Further studies of such biomarker effects will be necessary but suggest the feasibility of biomarker-driven studies to improve clinical trial efficiency. In conclusion, biomarkers are not ready for prime time yet. They are increasingly being used to indicate target engagement or proof of clinical principle, but no biomarkers are available to substitute FVC as an endpoint in pivotal clinical studies in fibrosing interstitial lung diseases.

Regulatory Requirements

The regulatory hurdles for registration of new drug candidates for IPF or fibrotic ILDs have been high in the past, requiring at least two replicate pivotal trials meeting their primary efficacy endpoint (i.e., decline in FVC) and providing acceptable safety over 1 year treatment duration. However, some light at the end of the tunnel can be seen that authorities may be increasingly willing to deviate from these classical rigid requirements, given the remaining high unmet need in pulmonary fibrosis and the challenges with existing clinical endpoints. An example is the recent approval byUS FDA of tocilizumab, an IL-6 inhibitor, to slow the rate of FVC decline in systemic sclerosis-associated ILD. This FDA approval is based on data from a single phase III randomized controlled clinical trial in 210 SSc-ILD patients with supportive evidence coming from a similar preceding (phase II) trial. The phase III trial did not meet its primary endpoint change from baseline to week 48 in the modified Rodnan Skin Score, a standard outcome measure for skin fibrosis in systemic sclerosis (Khanna et al., 2020), but showed stabilization of lung function in participants who received tocilizumab (mean change −14 vs. −255 ml; mean difference 241 ml), similar to the effect observed in the phase II trial which also missed its primary endpoint (Khanna et al., 2016). This recent approval indicates acknowledgement by the FDA of shortcomings and difficulties of available clinical endpoints for SSc-ILD, and that robust evidence may even by proven by consistent and substantial treatment differences in secondary outcomes such as FVC used in these studies.

CONCLUSION

Pulmonary fibrosis is believed to result from aberrant repair of repeated epithelial injury. Application of new technologies has shifted our research focus beyond fibroblast biology into the immune-fibrotic niche and its complex dysregulated interplay of diverse cell populations. Differential patient biology using cell systems and tissue directly from patients and patient-relevant stimuli, as well as enhanced *in vivo* animal models reflecting the fibrotic niche, has become the starting point for precision drug discovery. Clinical development of new therapeutics for the treatment of rare fibrotic lung conditions is hampered by e.g., patient heterogeneity and the lack of appropriate biomarkers to predict the disease trajectory for the individual patient to enable enrichment strategies. This imposes major challenges on clinical trial design and project development timelines. These will hopefully be overcome by improved and efficient trial designs which are accepted by regulatory authorities and ultimately pave the way to precision medicine approaches to provide the right treatment at the right time to the right patient suffering from pulmonary fibrosis.

AUTHOR CONTRIBUTIONS

All authors listed have equally contributed to the conceptualization of this manuscript and have made a substantial, direct, and intellectual contribution to the work and approved it for publication.

REFERENCES

Adams, T. S., Schupp, J. C., Poli, S., Ayaub, E. A., Neumark, N., Ahangari, F., et al. (2020). Single-Cell RNA-Seq Reveals Ectopic and Aberrant Lung-Resident Cell Populations in Idiopathic Pulmonary Fibrosis. *Sci. Adv.* 6, eaba1983. doi:10.1126/sciadv.aba1983

Álvarez, D., Cárdenes, N., Sellarés, J., Bueno, M., Corey, C., Hanumanthu, V. S., et al. (2017). IPF Lung Fibroblasts Have a Senescent Phenotype. *Am. J. Physiol.-Lung Cell Mol. Physiol.* 313, L1164–L1173. doi:10.1152/ajplung.00220.2017

Angus, D. C., Alexander, B. M., Berry, S., Buxton, M., Lewis, R., Paoloni, M., et al. (2019). Adaptive Platform Trials: Definition, Design, Conduct and Reporting Considerations. *Nat. Rev. Drug Discov.* 18, 797–807. doi:10.1038/s41573-019-0034-3

Behr, J., Prasse, A., Kreuter, M., Johow, J., Rabe, K. F., Bonella, F., et al. (2021). Pirfenidone in Patients with Progressive Fibrotic Interstitial Lung Diseases Other Than Idiopathic Pulmonary Fibrosis (RELIEF): A Double-Blind, Randomised, Placebo-Controlled, Phase 2b Trial. *Lancet Respir. Med.* 9, 476–486. doi:10.1016/s2213-2600(20)30554-3

Behr, J., Prasse, A., Wirtz, H., Koschel, D., Pittrow, D., Held, M., et al. (2020). Survival and Course of Lung Function in the Presence or Absence of Antifibrotic Treatment in Patients with Idiopathic Pulmonary Fibrosis: Long-Term Results of the INSIGHTS-IPF Registry. *Eur. Respir. J.* 56, 1902279. doi:10.1183/13993003.02279-2019

Brown, K. K., Flaherty, K. R., Cottin, V., Raghu, G., Inoue, Y., Azuma, A., et al. (2019). Lung Function Outcomes in the INPULSIS® Trials of Nintedanib in Idiopathic Pulmonary Fibrosis. *Respir. Med.* 146, 42–48. doi:10.1016/j.rmed.2018.11.012

Brown, K. K., Martinez, F. J., Walsh, S. L. F., Thannickal, V. J., Prasse, A., Schlenker-Herceg, R., et al. (2020). The Natural History of Progressive Fibrosing Interstitial Lung Diseases. *Eur. Respir. J.* 55, 2000085. doi:10.1183/13993003.00085-2020

Burman, A., Tanjore, H., and Blackwell, T. S. (2018). Endoplasmic Reticulum Stress in Pulmonary Fibrosis. *Matrix Biol.* 68-69, 355–365. doi:10.1016/j.matbio.2018.03.015

Collard, H. R. T. E. K., Jr., King, T. E., Bartelson, B. B., Vourlekis, J. S., Schwarz, M. I., and Brown, K. K. (2003). Changes in Clinical and Physiologic Variables Predict Survival in Idiopathic Pulmonary Fibrosis. *Am. J. Respir. Crit. Care Med.* 168, 538–542. doi:10.1164/rccm.200211-1311oc

Collignon, O., Gartner, C., Haidich, A-B., Hemmings, R. J., Hofner, B., Petavy, F., et al. (2020). Current Statistical Considerations and Regulatory Perspectives on the Planning of Confirmatory Basket, Umbrella, and Platform Trials. *Clin. Pharm. Therap.* 107 (5), 1059–1067. doi:10.1002/cpt.1804

Conte, E., Gili, E., Fagone, E., Fruciano, M., Iemmolo, M., and Vancheri, C. (2014). Effect of Pirfenidone on Proliferation, TGF-β-Induced Myofibroblast Differentiation and Fibrogenic Activity of Primary Human Lung Fibroblasts. *Eur. J. Pharm. Sci.* 58, 13–19. doi:10.1016/j.ejps.2014.02.014

DePianto, D. J., Heiden, J. A. V., Morshead, K. B., Sun, K. H., Modrusan, Z., Teng, G., et al. (2021). Molecular Mapping of Interstitial Lung Disease Reveals a Phenotypically Distinct Senescent Basal Epithelial Cell Population. *JCI Insight* 6, e143626. doi:10.1172/jci.insight.143626

Derlin, T., Jaeger, B., Jonigk, D., Apel, R. M., Freise, J., Shin, H. O., et al. (2021). Clinical Molecular Imaging of Pulmonary CXCR4 Expression to Predict Outcome of Pirfenidone Treatment in Idiopathic Pulmonary Fibrosis. *Chest* 159, 1094–1106. doi:10.1016/j.chest.2020.08.2043

Dron, L., Golchi, S., Hsu, G., and Thorlund, K. (2019). Minimizing Control Group Allocation in Randomized Trials Using Dynamic Borrowing of External Control Data - an Application to Second Line Therapy for Non-small Cell Lung Cancer. *Contemp. Clin. Trials Commun.* 16, 100446. doi:10.1016/j.conctc.2019.100446

Fingerlin, T. E., Murphy, E., Zhang, W., Peljto, A. L., Brown, K. K., Steele, M. P., et al. (2013). Genome-Wide Association Study Identifies Multiple Susceptibility Loci for Pulmonary Fibrosis. *Nat. Genet.* 45, 613–620. doi:10.1038/ng.2609

Flaherty, K. R., Brown, K. K., Wells, A. U., Clerisme-Beaty, E., Collard, H. R., Cottin, V., et al. (2017). Design of the PF-ILD Trial: A Double-Blind, Randomised, Placebo-Controlled Phase III Trial of Nintedanib in Patients with Progressive Fibrosing Interstitial Lung Disease. *BMJ Open Respir. Res.* 4, e000212. doi:10.1136/bmjresp-2017-000212

Flaherty, K. R., Wells, A. U., Cottin, V., Devaraj, A., Walsh, S. L. F., Inoue, Y., et al. (2019). Nintedanib in Progressive Fibrosing Interstitial Lung Diseases. *N. Engl. J. Med.* 381, 1718–1727. doi:10.1056/nejmoa1908681

Gerlach, B. D., Ampomah, P. B., Yurdagul, A., Liu, C., Lauring, M. C., Wang, X., et al. (2021). Efferocytosis Induces Macrophage Proliferation to Help Resolve Tissue Injury. *Cell Metab* 33, 2445–2463.e8. doi:10.1016/j.cmet.2021.10.015

Greene, K. E., King, T. E., Kuroki, Y., Bucher-Bartelson, B., Hunninghake, G. W., Newman, L. S., et al. (2002). Serum Surfactant Proteins-A and -D as Biomarkers in Idiopathic Pulmonary Fibrosis. *Eur. Respir. J.* 19, 439–446. doi:10.1183/09031936.02.00081102

Guenther, A., Krauss, E., Tello, S., Wagner, J., Paul, B., Kuhn, S., et al. (2018). The European IPF Registry (eurIPFreg): Baseline Characteristics and Survival of Patients with Idiopathic Pulmonary Fibrosis. *Respir. Res.* 19, 141. doi:10.1186/s12931-018-0845-5

Habermann, A. C., Gutierrez, A. J., Bui, L. T., Yahn, S. L., Winters, N. I., Calvi, C. L., et al. (2019). Single-Cell RNA-Sequencing Reveals Profibrotic Roles of Distinct Epithelial and Mesenchymal Lineages in Pulmonary Fibrosis. *Biorxiv* 6, 753806. doi:10.1101/7538068

Herazo-Maya, J. D., Sun, J., Molyneaux, P. L., Li, Q., Villalba, J. A., Tzouvelekis, A., et al. (2017). Validation of a 52-gene Risk Profile for Outcome Prediction in Patients with Idiopathic Pulmonary Fibrosis: an International, Multicentre, Cohort Study. *Lancet Respir. Med.* 5, 857–868. doi:10.1016/s2213-2600(17)30349-1

Huang, J., Maier, C., Zhang, Y., Soare, A., Dees, C., Beyer, C., et al. (2017). Nintedanib Inhibits Macrophage Activation and Ameliorates Vascular and Fibrotic Manifestations in the Fra2 Mouse Model of Systemic Sclerosis. *Ann. Rheum. Dis.* 76, 1941–1948. doi:10.1136/annrheumdis-2016-210823

Ishikawa, N., Hattori, N., Yokoyama, A., and Kohno, N. (2012). Utility of KL-6/MUC1 in the Clinical Management of Interstitial Lung Diseases. *Respir. Investig.* 50, 3–13. doi:10.1016/j.resinv.2012.02.001

Jaeger, B., Schupp, J. C., Plappert, L., Terwolbeck, O., Kayser, G., Engelhard, P., et al. (2020). Airway Basal Cells Show a Dedifferentiated KRT17highPhenotype and Promote Fibrosis in Idiopathic Pulmonary Fibrosis. *bioRxiv.* doi:10.1101/2020.09.04.283408

Jenkins, G., Noth, I., Selman, M., Cottin, V., Nishioka, Y., Song, J. W., et al. (2020). Effects of Nintedanib on Markers of Epithelial Damage in Subjects with IPF: Data from the INMARK Trial. *Eur. Respir. J.*, 5187. doi:10.1183/13993003.congress-2020.5187

Justet, A., Laurent-Bellue, A., Thabut, G., Dieudonné, A., Debray, M. P., Borie, R., et al. (2017). [18F]FDG PET/CT Predicts Progression-free Survival in Patients with Idiopathic Pulmonary Fibrosis. *Respir. Res.* 18, 74. doi:10.1186/s12931-017-0556-3

Karampitsakos, T., Torrisi, S., Antoniou, K., Manali, E., Korbila, I., Papaioannou, O., et al. (2021). Increased Monocyte Count and Red Cell Distribution Width as Prognostic Biomarkers in Patients with Idiopathic Pulmonary Fibrosis. *Respir. Res.* 22, 140. doi:10.1186/s12931-021-01725-9

Karimi-Shah, B. A., and Chowdhury, B. A. (2015). Forced Vital Capacity in Idiopathic Pulmonary Fibrosis--FDA Review of Pirfenidone and Nintedanib. *N. Engl. J. Med.* 372, 1189–1191. doi:10.1056/nejmp1500526

Keogh, B. A., and Crystal, R. G. (1982). Alveolitis: the Key to the Interstitial Lung Disorders. *Thorax* 37, 1–10. doi:10.1136/thx.37.1.1

Khanna, D., Denton, C. P., Jahreis, A., van Laar, J. M., Frech, T. M., Anderson, M. E., et al. (2016). Safety and Efficacy of Subcutaneous Tocilizumab in Adults with Systemic Sclerosis (faSScinate): A Phase 2, Randomised, Controlled Trial. *Lancet* 387, 2630–2640. doi:10.1016/s0140-6736(16)00232-4

Khanna, D., Lin, C. J. F., Furst, D. E., Goldin, J., Kim, G., Kuwana, M., et al. (2020). Tocilizumab in Systemic Sclerosis: A Randomised, Double-Blind, Placebo-Controlled, Phase 3 Trial. *Lancet Respir. Med.* 8, 963–974. doi:10.1016/s2213-2600(20)30318-0

King, T. E., Bradford, W. Z., Castro-Bernardini, S., Fagan, E. A., Glaspole, I., Glassberg, M. K., et al. (2014). A Phase 3 Trial of Pirfenidone in Patients with Idiopathic Pulmonary Fibrosis. *N. Engl. J. Med.* 370, 2083–2092. doi:10.1056/nejmoa1402582

King, T. E., Pardo, A., and Selman, M. (2011). Idiopathic Pulmonary Fibrosis. *Lancet* 378, 1949–1961. doi:10.1016/s0140-6736(11)60052-4

Latsi, P. I., du Boisdu, Nicholson, R. M. A. G., Nicholson, A. G., Colby, T. V., Bisirtzoglou, D., Nikolakopoulou, A., et al. (2003). Fibrotic Idiopathic Interstitial Pneumonia: the Prognostic Value of Longitudinal Functional Trends. *Am. J. Respir. Crit. Care Med.* 168, 531–537. doi:10.1164/rccm.200210-1245oc

Le, H. Q., Hill, M. A., Kollak, I., Keck, M., Schroeder, V., Wirth, J., et al. (2021). An EZH2-Dependent Transcriptional Complex Promotes Aberrant Epithelial Remodelling after Injury. *Embo Rep.* 22, e52785. doi:10.15252/embr.202152785

Le, H. Q., Hill, M. A., Kollak, I., Skronska-Wasek, W., Schroeder, V., Wirth, J., et al. (20202020). A Polycomb-Independent Role of EZH2 in TGFβ1-Damaged Epithelium Triggers a Fibrotic cascade with Mesenchymal Cells. *Biorxiv* 0729, 225300. doi:10.1101/2020.07.29.225300

Ley, B., Ryerson, C. J., Vittinghoff, E., Ryu, J. H., Tomassetti, S., Lee, J. S., et al. (2012). A Multidimensional Index and Staging System for Idiopathic Pulmonary Fibrosis. *Ann. Intern. Med.* 156, 684–691. doi:10.7326/0003-4819-156-10-201205150-00004

Luo, Y., Decato, B., Palmer, S. M., Du, S., Charles, E. D., Sand, J. M. B., et al. (2020). Evaluation of Collagen Neoepitope Biomarkers in a Phase 2 Trial of BMS-986020, a Lysophosphatidic Acid Receptor Antagonist, for the Treatment of Idiopathic Pulmonary Fibrosis. *Am. J. Respir. Crit. Care Med.* 201, A2751. doi:10.1164/ajrccm-conference.2020.201.1_meetingabstracts.a2751

Maher, T. M., Oballa, E., Simpson, J. K., Porte, J., Habgood, A., Fahy, W. A., et al. (2017). An Epithelial Biomarker Signature for Idiopathic Pulmonary Fibrosis: An Analysis from the Multicentre PROFILE Cohort Study. *Lancet Respir. Med.* 5, 946–955. doi:10.1016/s2213-2600(17)30430-7

Maher, T. M., van der Aar, E. M., Van de Steen, O., Allamassey, L., Desrivot, J., Dupont, S., et al. (2018). Safety, Tolerability, Pharmacokinetics, and Pharmacodynamics of GLPG1690, a Novel Autotaxin Inhibitor, to Treat Idiopathic Pulmonary Fibrosis (FLORA): A Phase 2a Randomised Placebo-Controlled Trial. *Lancet Respir. Med.* 6, 627–635. doi:10.1016/s2213-2600(18)30181-4

Maher, T. M., Cerri, S., Hallowell, R. W., Koschel, D., Pope, J., Tolle, L., et al. (2021). Effect of Nintedanib on Categorical Changes in Fvc in Patients with Progressive Fibrosing Ilds: Further Analyses of the INBUILD Trial. Available at: https://acrabstracts.org/abstract/effect-of-nintedanib-on-categorical-changes-in-fvc-in-patients-with-progressive-fibrosing-ilds-further-analyses-of-the-inbuild-trial/.

Makiguchi, T., Yamada, M., Yoshioka, Y., Sugiura, H., Koarai, A., Chiba, S., et al. (2016). Serum Extracellular Vesicular miR-21-5p is a Predictor of the Prognosis in Idiopathic Pulmonary Fibrosis. *Respir. Res.* 17, 110. doi:10.1186/s12931-016-0427-3

Moeller, A., Ask, K., Warburton, D., Gauldie, J., and Kolb, M. (2008). The Bleomycin Animal Model: A Useful Tool to Investigate Treatment Options for Idiopathic Pulmonary Fibrosis. *Int. J. Biochem. Cell Biol.* 40, 362–382. doi:10.1016/j.biocel.2007.08.011

Morisset, J., Vittinghoff, E., Lee, B. Y., Tonelli, R., Hu, X., Elicker, B. M., et al. (2017). The Performance of the GAP Model in Patients with Rheumatoid Arthritis Associated Interstitial Lung Disease. *Respir. Med.* 127, 51–56. doi:10.1016/j.rmed.2017.04.012

Morse, C., Tabib, T., Sembrat, J., Buschur, K. L., Bittar, H. T., Valenzi, E., et al. (2019). Proliferating SPP1/MERTK-Expressing Macrophages in Idiopathic Pulmonary Fibrosis. *Eur. Respir. J.* 54, 1802441. doi:10.1183/13993003.02441-2018

Nambiar, S., Tan, D. B. A., Clynick, B., Bong, S. H., Rawlinson, C., Gummer, J., et al. (2021). Untargeted Metabolomics of Human Plasma Reveal Lipid Markers Unique to Chronic Obstructive Pulmonary Disease and Idiopathic Pulmonary Fibrosis. *Prot. Clin. Appl.* 15, 2000039. doi:10.1002/prca.202000039

Nanthakumar, C. B., Eley, J., Man, Y., Gudmann, N. S., Chambers, R. C., Blanchard, A., et al. (2019). Omipalisib Modulates Extracellular Matrix Turnover in IPF Patients: Exploratory Biomarker Analysis from a Phase I Proof of Mechanism Study. *Am. J. Respir. Crit. Care Med.* 199, A7301. doi:10.1164/ajrccm-conference.2019.199.1_meetingabstracts.a7301

Nureki, S. I., Tomer, Y., Venosa, A., Katzen, J., Russo, S. J., Jamil, S., et al. (2018). Expression of Mutant Sftpc in Murine Alveolar Epithelia Drives Spontaneous Lung Fibrosis. *J. Clin. Invest.* 128, 4008–4024. doi:10.1172/jci99287

Oldham, J. M., Ma, S. F., Martinez, F. J., Anstrom, K. J., Raghu, G., Schwartz, D. A., et al. (2015). TOLLIP, MUC5B, and the Response to N-Acetylcysteine Among Individuals with Idiopathic Pulmonary Fibrosis. *Am. J. Respir. Crit. Care Med.* 192, 1475–1482. doi:10.1164/rccm.201505-1010oc

Organ, L. A., Duggan, A. R., Oballa, E., Taggart, S. C., Simpson, J. K., Kang'ombe, A. R., et al. (2019). Biomarkers of Collagen Synthesis Predict Progression in the PROFILE Idiopathic Pulmonary Fibrosis Cohort. *Respir. Res.* 20, 148. doi:10.1186/s12931-019-1118-7

Otoupalova, E., Smith, S., Cheng, G., and Thannickal, V. J. (2020). Oxidative Stress in Pulmonary Fibrosis. *Compr. Physiol.* 10, 509–547. doi:10.1002/cphy.c190017

Palmer, S. M., Snyder, L., Todd, J. L., Soule, B., Christian, R., Anstrom, K., et al. (2018). Randomized, Double-Blind, Placebo-Controlled, Phase 2 Trial of BMS-986020, a Lysophosphatidic Acid Receptor Antagonist for the Treatment of Idiopathic Pulmonary Fibrosis. *Chest* 154, 1061–1069. doi:10.1016/j.chest.2018.08.1058

Raghu, G., Collard, H. R., Egan, J. J., Martinez, F. J., Behr, J., Brown, K. K., et al. (2012). An Official ATS/ERS/JRS/ALAT Statement: Idiopathic Pulmonary Fibrosis: Evidence-Based Guidelines for Diagnosis and Management. *Am. J. Respir. Crit. Care Med.* 183, 788–824. doi:10.1164/rccm.2009-040gl

Raghu, G., Martinez, F. J., Brown, K. K., Costabel, U., Cottin, V., Wells, A. U., et al. (2015). CC-chemokine Ligand 2 Inhibition in Idiopathic Pulmonary Fibrosis: a Phase 2 Trial of Carlumab. *Eur. Respir. J.* 46, 1740–1750. doi:10.1183/13993003.01558-2014

Raghu, G., Remy-Jardin, M., Myers, J. L., Richeldi, L., Ryerson, C. J., Lederer, D. J., et al. (2018). Diagnosis of Idiopathic Pulmonary Fibrosis. An Official ATS/ERS/JRS/ALAT Clinical Practice Guideline. *Am. J. Respir. Crit. Care Med.* 198, e44–e68. doi:10.1164/rccm.201807-1255st

Redente, E. F., Black, B. P., Backos, D. S., Bahadur, A. N., Humphries, S. M., Lynch, D. A., et al. (2021). Persistent, Progressive Pulmonary Fibrosis and Epithelial Remodeling in Mice. *Am. J. Respir. Cell Mol. Biol.* 64, 669–676. doi:10.1165/rcmb.2020-0542ma

Reyfman, P. A., Walter, J. M., Joshi, N., Anekalla, K. R., McQuattie-Pimentel, A. C., Chiu, S., et al. (2019). Single-cell Transcriptomic Analysis of Human Lung Provides Insights into the Pathobiology of Pulmonary Fibrosis. *Am. J. Respir. Crit. Care Med.* 199, 1517–1536. doi:10.1164/rccm.201712-2410oc

Richeldi, L., Costabel, U., Selman, M., Kim, D. S., Hansell, D. M., Nicholson, A. G., et al. (2011). Efficacy of a Tyrosine Kinase Inhibitor in Idiopathic Pulmonary Fibrosis. *N. Engl. J. Med.* 365, 1079–1087. doi:10.1056/nejmoa1103690

Richeldi, L., du Bois, R. M., Raghu, G., Azuma, A., Brown, K. K., Costabel, U., et al. (2014). Efficacy and Safety of Nintedanib in Idiopathic Pulmonary Fibrosis. *N. Engl. J. Med.* 370, 2071–2082. doi:10.1056/nejmoa1402584

Rosas, I. O., Richards, T. J., Konishi, K., Zhang, Y., Gibson, K., Lokshin, A. E., et al. (2008). MMP1 and MMP7 as Potential Peripheral Blood Biomarkers in

Idiopathic Pulmonary Fibrosis. *PLoS Med.* 5, e93. doi:10.1371/journal.pmed.0050093

Ruscitti, F., Ravanetti, F., Essers, J., Ridwan, Y., Belenkov, S., Vos, W., et al. (2017). Longitudinal Assessment of Bleomycin-Induced Lung Fibrosis by Micro-CT Correlates with Histological Evaluation in Mice. *Multidiscip Respir. Med.* 12, 8. doi:10.1186/s40248-017-0089-0

Ryerson, C. J., Vittinghoff, E., Ley, B., Lee, J. S., Mooney, J. J., Jones, K. D., et al. (2014). Predicting Survival across Chronic Interstitial Lung Disease: the ILD-GAP Model. *Chest* 145, 723–728. doi:10.1378/chest.13-1474

Ryu, C., Sun, H., Gulati, M., Herazo-Maya, J. D., Chen, Y., Osafo-Addo, A., et al. (2017). Extracellular Mitochondrial DNA is Generated by Fibroblasts and Predicts Death in Idiopathic Pulmonary Fibrosis. *Am. J. Respir. Crit. Care Med.* 196, 1571–1581. doi:10.1164/rccm.201612-2480oc

Salisbury, M. L., Tolle, L. B., Xia, M., Murray, S., Tayob, N., Nambiar, A. M., et al. (2017). Possible UIP Pattern on High-Resolution Computed Tomography is Associated with Better Survival Than Definite UIP in IPF Patients. *Respir. Med.* 131, 229–235. doi:10.1016/j.rmed.2017.08.025

Selman, M., King, T. E., and Pardo, A. (2001). American Thoracic Society, European Respiratory Society, American College of Chest PhysiciansIdiopathic Pulmonary Fibrosis: Prevailing and Evolving Hypotheses about its Pathogenesis and Implications for Therapy. *Ann. Intern. Med.* 134, 136. doi:10.7326/0003-4819-134-2-200101160-00015

Spagnolo, P., Kropski, J. A., Jones, M. G., Lee, J. S., Rossi, G., Karampitsakos, T., et al. (2021). Idiopathic Pulmonary Fibrosis: Disease Mechanisms and Drug Development. *Pharmacol. Ther.* 222, 107798. doi:10.1016/j.pharmthera.2020.107798

Strunz, M., Simon, L. M., Ansari, M., Kathiriya, J. J., Angelidis, I., Mayr, C. H., et al. (2020). Alveolar Regeneration through a Krt8+ Transitional Stem Cell State that Persists in Human Lung Fibrosis. *Nat. Commun.* 11, 3559. doi:10.1038/s41467-020-17358-3

Stuart, B. D., Choi, J., Zaidi, S., Xing, C., Holohan, B., Chen, R., et al. (2015). Exome Sequencing Links Mutations in PARN and RTEL1 with Familial Pulmonary Fibrosis and Telomere Shortening. *Nat. Genet.* 47, 512–517. doi:10.1038/ng.3278

Travis, W. D., Costabel, U., Hansell, D. M., King, T. E., Lynch, D. A., Nicholson, A. G., et al. (2013). An Official American Thoracic Society/European Respiratory Society Statement: Update of the International Multidisciplinary Classification of the Idiopathic Interstitial Pneumonias. *Am. J. Respir. Crit. Care Med.* 188, 733–748. doi:10.1164/rccm.201308-1483st

Ushakumary, M. G., Riccetti, M., and Perl, A. T. (2021). Resident Interstitial Lung Fibroblasts and Their Role in Alveolar Stem Cell Niche Development, Homeostasis, Injury, and Regeneration. *Stem Cells Transl. Med.* 10, 1021–1032. doi:10.1002/sctm.20-0526

Wells, A. U., Brown, K. K., Flaherty, K. R., Kolb, M., and Thannickal, V. J. (2018). What's in a Name? That Which we Call IPF, by Any Other Name Would Act the same. *Eur. Respir. J.* 51, 1800692. doi:10.1183/13993003.00692-2018

Win, T., Screaton, N. J., Porter, J. C., Ganeshan, B., Maher, T. M., Fraioli, F., et al. (2018). Pulmonary 18F-FDG Uptake Helps Refine Current Risk Stratification in Idiopathic Pulmonary Fibrosis (IPF). *Eur. J. Nucl. Med. Mol. Imaging* 45, 806–815. doi:10.1007/s00259-017-3917-8

Wollin, L., Distler, J. H. W., Redente, E. F., Riches, D. W. H., Stowasser, S., Schlenker-Herceg, R., et al. (2019). Potential of Nintedanib in Treatment of Progressive Fibrosing Interstitial Lung Diseases. *Eur. Respir. J.* 54, 1900161. doi:10.1183/13993003.00161-2019

Wollin, L., Maillet, I., Quesniaux, V., Holweg, A., and Ryffel, B. (2014). Antifibrotic and Anti-Inflammatory Activity of the Tyrosine Kinase Inhibitor Nintedanib in Experimental Models of Lung Fibrosis. *J. Pharmacol. Exp. Ther.* 349, 209–220. doi:10.1124/jpet.113.208223

Wolters, P. J., Blackwell, T. S., Eickelberg, O., Loyd, J. E., Kaminski, N., Jenkins, G., et al. (2018). Time for a Change: Is Idiopathic Pulmonary Fibrosis Still Idiopathic and Only Fibrotic. *Lancet Respir. Med.* 6, 154–160. doi:10.1016/s2213-2600(18)30007-9

Woodcock, J., and LaVange, L. M. (2017). Master Protocols to Study Multiple Therapies, Multiple Diseases, or Both. *N. Engl. J. Med.* 377, 62–70. doi:10.1056/nejmra1510062

Zhao, Y. D., Yin, L., Archer, S., Lu, C., Zhao, G., Yao, Y., et al. (2017). Metabolic Heterogeneity of Idiopathic Pulmonary Fibrosis: a Metabolomic Study. *BMJ Open Respir. Res.* 4, e000183. doi:10.1136/bmjresp-2017-000183

9

Common Molecular Pathways between Post-COVID-19 Syndrome and Lung Fibrosis

*Laura Bergantini *, Alessandro Mainardi, Miriana d'Alessandro, Paolo Cameli, David Bennett, Elena Bargagli and Piersante Sestini*

Department of Medical Sciences, Surgery and Neurosciences, Respiratory Disease and Lung Transplant Unit, Respiratory Diseases and Transplant Unit, Siena University, Siena, Italy

***Correspondence:**
Laura Bergantini
laurabergantini@gmail.com*

The pathogenetic mechanism of post-Covid-19 pulmonary fibrosis is currently a topic of intense research interest, but still largely unexplored. The aim of this work was to carry out a systematic exploratory search of the literature (Scoping review) to identify and systematize the main pathogenetic mechanisms that are believed to be involved in this phenomenon, in order to highlight the same molecular aspect of the lung. These aims could be essential in the future for therapeutic management. We identified all primary studies involving in post COVID19 syndrome with pulmonary fibrosis as a primary endpoint by performing data searches in various systematic review databases. Two reviewers independently reviewed all abstracts (398) and full text data. The quality of study has been assess through SANRA protocol. A total of 32 studies involving were included, included the possible involvement of inflammatory cytokines, concerned the renin-angiotensin system, the potential role of galectin-3, epithelial injuries in fibrosis, alveolar type 2 involvement, Neutrophil extracellular traps (NETs) and the others implied other specific aspects (relationship with clinical and mechanical factors, epithelial transition mesenchymal, TGF-β signaling pathway, midkine, caspase and macrophages, genetics). In most cases, these were narrative reviews or letters to the editor, except for 10 articles, which presented original data, albeit sometimes in experimental models. From the development of these researches, progress in the knowledge of the phenomenon and hopefully in its prevention and therapy may originate.

Keywords: lung fibrosis, post covid19 syndrome, molecular aspects, pathogenetic mechanisms, literature review

INTRODUCTION

Severe acute respiratory syndrome coronavirus-2 (SARS-CoV-2) infection can generate a systemic disease named coronavirus disease-2019 (COVID-19) (Cameli et al., 2021a).

Since the start of the outbreak, one of the first observations has been the impressive heterogeneity of phenotypic response to SARS-CoV-2 infection among individuals (Benetti et al., 2020). The suitability of antiviral defenses, genetic predisposition together with immunologic defenses is known to influence the severity of the disease and to contribute to the development of COVID-19 associated cytokine storm (Liu et al., 1996; Maltezou et al., 2021; Shakaib et al., 2021). Moreover, sequelae of

Abbreviations: HRCT, High Resolution Computed Tomography; IL-, interleukin; IPF, Idiopathic pulmonary fibrosis; LFT, Lung Function Tests; PFT, Pulmonary Functional Test; TGF-β, Tumor Growth Factor-β.

disease as well as the risk of irreversible organ damage due to COVID-19 are still far from being properly assessed.

Post-COVID syndrome was described for the first time in spring 2020, characterized by persistent symptoms for many weeks after acute infection resolution (Daga et al., 2021; Fallerini et al., 2021; Maltezou et al., 2021). Patients who do not require hospitalization develop post-COVID syndrome in 10–35% cases, while hospitalized patients showed symptoms for up to 80% (Carvalho-Schneider et al., 2021; Cameli et al., 2021b). Even though they are still poorly understood, the immunological dysregulations are probably associated with post-COVID syndrome: in particular, patients with prolonged symptoms duration maintained antigen-specific T-cell response magnitudes to the virus in $CD4^+$ and increased T follicular helper cells (Tfh) populations throughout late convalescence while those experiencing a full recover demonstrated an decline of these cellular population (d'Alessandro et al., 2020a; Bergantini et al., 2021a; Files et al., 2021; d'Alessandro et al., 2021b). Different common proteins have been proposed as markers of diagnosis, prognosis or severity for COVID-19 development (d'Alessandro et al., 2021a; Pavli et al., 2021; Billoir et al., 2021), although Post-Acute Sequalae of COVID-19 immune signatures associated with these syndromes are very poorly investigated.

Although review papers are available on post-COVID syndrome (Gianola et al., 2020), to the best of our knowledge, there is no specific evidence concerning the similar molecular aspects between COVID-19 syndrome and chronic, irreversible pulmonary sequelae, such as lung fibrosis. Of note, SARS-CoV2-infection induces direct cytopathic effects against type II pneumocytes, that is considered a key event in the pathogenesis of idiopathic pulmonary fibrosis (IPF) (d'Alessandro et al., 2021a).

The aim of this work was to carry out a systematic exploratory search of the literature (Scoping review) to identify and systematize the main pathogenetic mechanisms that are believed to be involved in this phenomenon, in order to highlight the same molecular aspect of the lung. These aims could be essential in the future for therapeutic management.

METHODS

A scoping review methodology was used, following the methods called scoping review protocol (Tricco et al., 2018). In this paper, descriptive thematic analysis, later detailed, is used to understand any molecular and/or pathways protein involvement present in both IPF and as a consequences of a COVID-19. This article conforms to the Scale for Assessment of Narrative Review Articles (SANRA) guidelines (Baethge et al., 2019).

Eligibility Criteria

The inclusion criteria were peer-reviewed empirical or perspective papers (including editorials or commentaries) with 1) relevance to the study topic: Covid-19 disease or pandemic, fibrogenetic pathways, underlying pathogenetic mechanism, reciprocal influence between SARS-COV-2 and fibrotic lung disease; 2) type of journal: preferences for journals relating to the pneumology area with full text or abstract; 3) type of study: review, case report, case series, original article, letter to the editor. Studies were excluded if 1) did not satisfy the relevance to the topic of study; 2) did not adequately report objectives and conclusions; 3) did not carry full text.

Information Sources and Search

A systematic literature search was conducted from 19 March 2020 to 15 May 2021 in the PubMed, European Centre for Disease Prevention and Control, World Health organization (WHO) Global research on coronavirus disease (COVID-19) (https://www.who.int/emergencies/diseases/novel-coronavirus-2019/global-research-on-novel-coronavirus-2019-ncov), Cochrane Libraryonline database. The search term, which has been included in our Boolean search syntax, is as follows: COVID-19 AND ("lung fibrosis" OR "pulmonary fibrosis" OR "interstitial lung disease", "pulmonary fibrosis and post-COVID19" OR "pulmonary fibrosis, post- COVID syndrome"). The search was limited to the English language and the availability of the full text and abstracts.

We included elements of the grey literature (e.g., official reports from international organizations), bioXiv, medXiv, arXiv online database. During the initial searches, we have found a living repository of that literature, hosted by the United Nations. That freely accessible repository (https://www.un.org/development/desa/disabilities/covid-19.html (Accessed date: 15 December 2020)) provides key grey literature resources from the United Nations, their specialty agencies, and from partner institutions (e.g., Disabled Person's Organizations) alike (Management of post-acute, 2021). With this new information, and to produce timely results as intended, we opted to include the grey literature and narrow the review coverage to the peer-reviewed literature and preprint studies. An iterative development process is common in scoping reviews, with some decisions—as long as justified and reported—taken as new information comes by, since scoping reviews usually explore and map out initially unchartered territories (Colquhoun et al., 2020; Jesus et al., 2020; Updated methodological guidance for the conduct of scoping reviews - PubMed, 2021).

Selection Process

The abstract and titles screenings and the full-text assessments were made against the eligibility criteria and were conducted by two independent reviewers (M.d, E.B.), after pilot screenings with over 80% agreements, overseen by the leading review author (L.B.). Any discrepancies were resolved through consensus or the leading author's input.

Data Charting and Items

Following a coding structure elaborated by members of the research team, one author (D.B.) extracted formal data elements (publication type, sources, geographies addressed, objectives and main findings) with a random 5% verified by another (P.C). Regarding the content of the literature included, three independent reviewers (LB, A.M and P.S.) extracted text quotations on 1) consequences of a COVID-19 infection on people 2) or common molecular pattern with lung fibrosis. These independent extractions were later paired for the

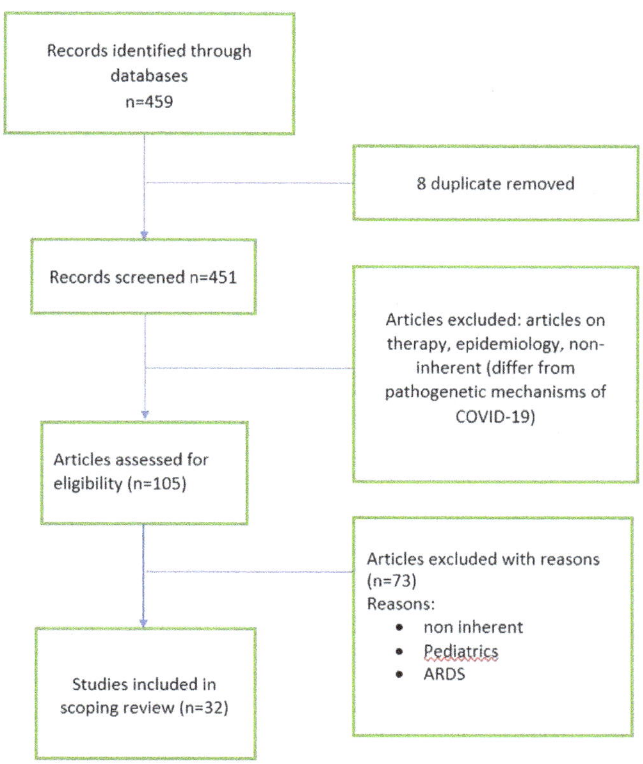

FIGURE 1 | Flowchart of selected manuscript.

qualitative data synthesis, which was also informed by a brief synthesis of each paper developed by two reviewers independently. Then, the content of these extractions after being merged (i.e., presented as the combined extractions of all reviewers), as well as reviewers' combined synthesis of each paper. Flowchart of selected articles were reported in **Figure 1**.

RESULTS

Synthesis of the Results Simple Descriptive Data

The literature search yielded the entire text. Therefore, we selected 32 studies included the possible involvement of inflammatory cytokines, concerned the renin-angiotensin system, the potential role of galectin-3, epithelial injuries in fibrosis, alveolar type 2 involvement, Neutrophil extracellular traps (NETs) and the others implied other specific aspects (relationship with clinical and mechanical factors, epithelial transition mesenchymal, TGF-β signaling pathway, midkine, caspase and macrophages, genetics). These were reviews or letters to the editor, 10 were original article, which presented original data, albeit sometimes in experimental models. The principal extracellular and intracellular mechanisms were reported in **Figures 2**, **3**, while **Figure 4** summerized the main pathological processes that lead to fibrosis.

Quality Assessment Following SANRA Assessment

The results of SANRA were reported in **Table 1**. All 96 ratings (3 raters × 32 manuscripts) were used for statistical analysis. The mean sum score across all 32 manuscripts was 8.9 out of 12 possible points (SD 2.6, range 7.75–11, median 9). Highest scores were rated for item 4 (referencing) (mean 1.78), item 6 (Appropriate presentation of data) (mean 1.75) and item 1 (Justification of the article's importance for the readership)

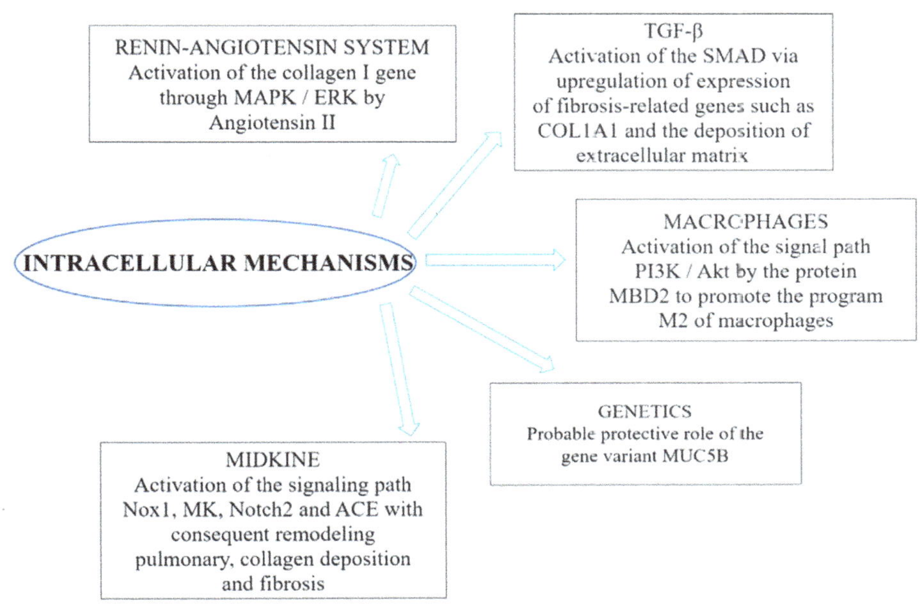

FIGURE 2 | Intracellular mechanisms involved in post COVID-19 syndrome.

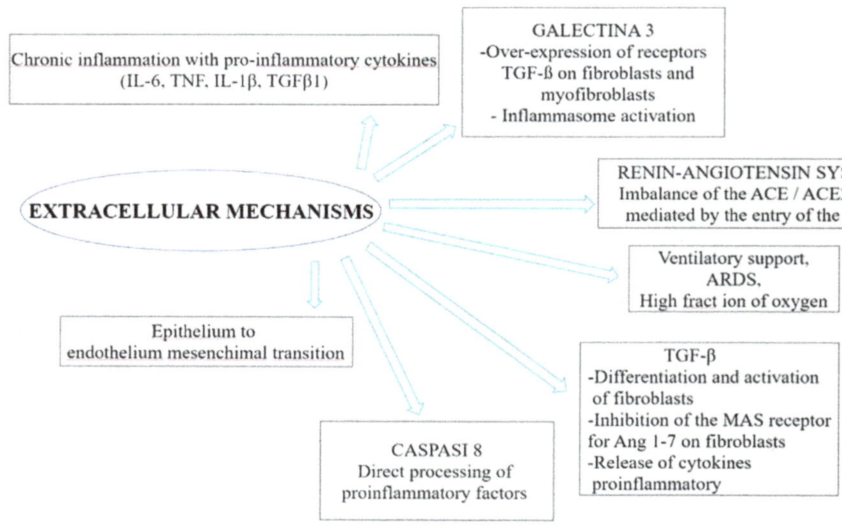

FIGURE 3 | Extracellular mechanisms involved in post COVID-19 syndrome.

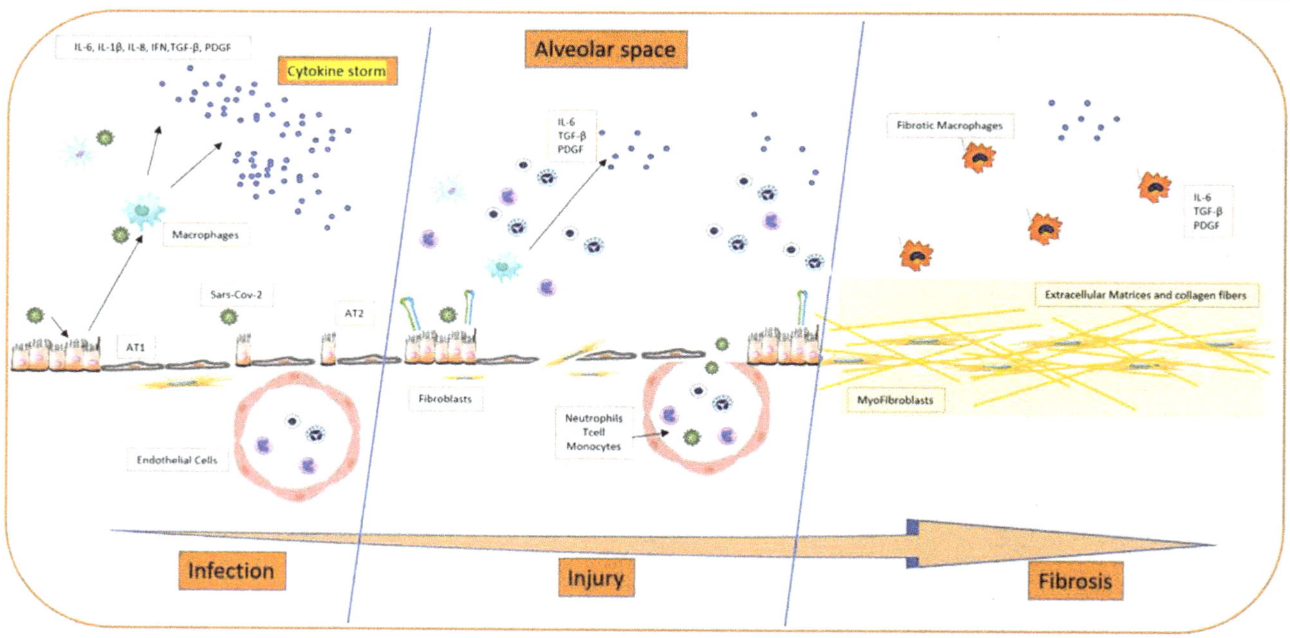

FIGURE 4 | Process of development of fibrosis on Sars COV-2 patients.

(mean 1.65) whereas items 2, 3, 5 had the lowest scores (means of 1.5, 0.84 and 1.43, respectively).

Cytokine Pathways and Development of Fibrosis

Most of the studies identified "cytokine storm" as the pathogenetic mechanism leading to fibrosis, based on the release of proinflammatory cytokines. In fact, aberrant inflammation associated with dysregulated repair mechanisms and fibrogenesis can lead to fibrogenesis (Bergantini et al., 2021b; Bergantini et al., 2022). Changes in the cellular and molecular environment in lung tissue secondary to viral infection, as found in COVID-19, were the key factors behind fibrosis development. Ongoing damage occurs in tissues secondary to inflammation, leading to overexpression of inflammatory cytokines, including

TABLE 1 | SANRA Score for quality assessment.

No.	Title and authors	Justification of the article's importance for the readership	Statement of concrete aims or formulation of questions	Description of the literature search	Referencing	Scientific reasoning	Appropriate presentation of data	Total score
1	Post-COVID lung fibrosis: The tsunami that will follow the earthquake Udwadia ZF, Koul PA, Richeldi L. 2021	1	1	0	2	1	1	6
2	Physiology of Midkine and Its Potential Pathophysiological Role in COVID-19. Sanino G, Bosco M, Terrazzano 2020	1	1	0	2	2	2	8
3	Healing after COVID-19: are survivors at risk for pulmonary fibrosis? McDonald LT. 2021	1	1	0	2	1	2	7
4	A Dangerous Consequence of the Recent Pandemic: Early Lung Fibrosis Following COVID-19 Pneumonia—Case Reports. Scelfo C, Fontana M, Casalini E, et al., 2020	2	2	1	2	2	2	11
5	The second wave of desaturation in coronavirus disease 2019 Alghizzawi MI, Ata F, Yousaf Z, et al., 2021	2	2	1	2	1	2	10
6	Investigation into molecular mechanisms and high-frequency core TCM for pulmonary fibrosis secondary to COVID-19 based on network pharmacology and data mining Yu MX, Song X, Ma XQ, Hao CX, Huang JJ, Yang WH 2021	2	2	2	2	2	2	12
7	Discharge may not be the end of treatment: Pay attention to pulmonary fibrosis caused by severe COVID-19 Zhang C, Wu Z, Li JW, et al., 2021	1	1	0	2	1	2	7
8	MBD2 serves as a viable target against pulmonary fibrosis by inhibiting macrophage M2 program Wang Y, Zhang L, Wu GR, et al., 2021	2	2	2	2	2	2	12
9	Novel insight from the first lung transplant of a COVID-19 patient Chen XJ, Li K, Xu L, et al., 2021	2	2	2	2	1	2	11
10	Post-COVID-19 pneumonia pulmonary fibrosis Tale S, Ghosh S, Meitei SP, Kolli M, Garbhapu AK, Pudi S. 2020	1	0	0	0	1	0	2
11	Persistent viral activity, cytokine storm, and lung fibrosis in a case of severe COVID-19 Xu G, Liu Y, Liao M, et al., 2020	2	2	1	2	1	2	10
12	Lung transplantation for pulmonary fibrosis secondary to severe COVID-19 Bharat A, Querrey M, Markov NS, et al., 2020	2	2	1	2	2	2	11
13	SARS-CoV-2 triggers inflammatory responses and cell death through caspase-8 activation Li S, Zhang Y, Guan Z, et al., 2020	2	1	2	2	2	2	11
14	Endothelial to mesenchymal transition: a precursor to post-COVID-19 interstitial pulmonary fibrosis and vascular obliteration? Eapen MS, Lu W, Gaikwad AV, et al., 2020	1	1	0	2	1	2	7
15	Hyperinflammation and Fibrosis in Severe COVID-19 Patients: Galectin-3, a Target Molecule to Consider Garcia-Revilla J, Deierborg T, Venero JL, Boza-Serrano A. 2020	2	2	0	2	2	2	10
16	SARS-CoV-2 Pathogenesis: Imbalance in the Renin-Angiotensin System Favors Lung Fibrosis Delpino MV, Quarleri J 2020	1	2	0	2	1	2	8
17	Immunopathology of galectin-3: an increasingly promising target in COVID-19 Caniglia JL, Asuthkar S, Tsung AJ, Guda MR, Velpula KK. 2020	2	1	1	2	2	2	10
18	Converging pathways in pulmonary fibrosis and Covid-19 - The fibrotic link to disease severity Wigén J, Löfdahl A, Bjermer L, Elowsson-Rendin L, Westergren-Thorsson G. 2020	1	1	0	2	1	2	7
19	Alveolar cells under mechanical stressed niche: critical contributors to pulmonary fibrosis. Yang J, Pan X, Wang L, Yu G. 2020	2	2	0	2	1	2	9

(Continued on following page)

TABLE 1 | (*Continued*) SANRA Score for quality assessment.

No.	Title and authors	Justification of the article's importance for the readership	Statement of concrete aims or formulation of questions	Description of the literature search	Referencing	Scientific reasoning	Appropriate presentation of data	Total score
20	SARS-CoV-2 induces transcriptional signatures in human lung epithelial cells that promote lung fibrosis. Xu J, Xu X, Jiang L, Dua K, Hansbro PM, Liu G. 2020	2	2	2	2	2	2	12
21	Post-COVID-19 Pulmonary Fibrosis: A Lifesaving Challenge Prakash J, Bhattacharya PK, Priye S, Kumar N. 2021	1	1	0	2	1	1	6
22	Long-Term Respiratory and Neurological Sequelae of COVID-19. Wang F, Kream RM, Stefano GB. 2020	2	1	0	2	1	1	7
23	COVID-19: The Potential Treatment of Pulmonary Fibrosis Associated with SARS-CoV-2 Infection Lechowicz K, Drożdżal S, Machaj F, et al., 2020	2	1	0	2	1	2	8
24	Michalski JE, Kurche JS, Schwartz DA. From ARDS to pulmonary fibrosis: the next phase of the COVID-19 pandemic? Transl Res. 2021 September 20:S1931-5244 (21)00243–7. 10.1016/j.trsl.2021.09.001. Epub ahead of print. PMID: 34547499; PMCID: PMC8452088	2	2	1	2	1	1	9
25	Shen H, Zhang N, Liu Y, Yang X, He Y, Li Q, Shen X, Zhu Y, Yang Y. The Interaction Between Pulmonary Fibrosis and COVID-19 and the Application of Related Anti-Fibrotic Drugs. Front Pharmacol. 2022 January 5; 12:805535. 10.3389/fphar.2021.805535. PMID: 35069217; PMCID: PMC8766975	2	1	1	1	2	1	8
26	Stoyanov GS, Yanulova N, Stoev L, Zgurova N, Mihaylova V, Dzhenkov DL, Stoeva M, Stefanova N, Kalchev K, Petkova L. Temporal Patterns of COVID-19-Associated Pulmonary Pathology: An Autopsy Study. Cureus. 2021 December 19; 13 (12):e20522. 10.7759/cureus.20522. PMID: 35103119; PMCID: PMC8769076	1	1	1	1	2	2	8
27	Colarusso C, Maglio A, Terlizzi M, Vitale C, Molino A, Pinto A, Vatrella A, Sorrentino R. Post-COVID-19 Patients Who Develop Lung Fibrotic-like Changes Have Lower Circulating Levels of IFN-β but Higher Levels of IL-1α and TGF-β. Biomedicines. 2021 December 17; 9 (12):1931. 10.3390/biomedicines9121931. PMID: 34944747; PMCID: PMC8698335	2	2	2	2	2	2	12
28	Sinha S, Castillo V, Espinoza CR, Tindle C, Fonseca AG, Dan JM, Katkar GD, Das S, Sahoo D, Ghosh P. COVID-19 lung disease shares driver AT2 cytopathic features with Idiopathic pulmonary fibrosis. bioRxiv (Preprint). 2021 December 26:2021.11.28.470269. 10.1101/2021.11.28.470269. PMID: 34873597; PMCID: PMC8647648	2	2	1	1	2	2	10
29	Giacomelli C, Piccarducci R, Marchetti L, Romei C, Martini C. Pulmonary fibrosis from molecular mechanisms to therapeutic interventions: lessons from post-COVID-19 patients. Biochem Pharmacol. 2021 November; 193:114812. 10.1016/j.bcp.2021.114812. Epub 2021 October 21. PMID: 34687672; PMCID: PMC8546906	2	2	1	1	1	2	9
30	Middleton EA, He XY, Denorme F, Campbell RA, Ng D, Salvatore SP, Mostyka M, Baxter-Stoltzfus A, Borczuk AC, Loda M, Cody MJ, Manne BK, Portier I, Harris ES, Petrey AC, Beswick EJ, Caulin AF, Iovino A, Abegglen LM, Weyrich AS, Rondina MT, Egeblad M, Schiffman JD, Yost CC. Neutrophil extracellular traps contribute to immunothrombosis in COVID-19 acute respiratory distress syndrome. Blood. 2020 September 3; 136 (10):1169–1179. 10.1182/blood.2020007008. PMID: 32597954; PMCID: PMC7472714	2	2	1	1	1	2	9

(Continued on following page)

TABLE 1 | (*Continued*) SANRA Score for quality assessment.

No.	Title and authors	Justification of the article's importance for the readership	Statement of concrete aims or formulation of questions	Description of the literature search	Referencing	Scientific reasoning	Appropriate presentation of data	Total score
31	Pandolfi L, Bozzini S, Frangipane V, Percivalle E, De Luigi A, Violatto MB, Lopez G, Gabanti E, Carsana L, D'Amato M, Morosini M, De Amici M, Nebuloni M, Fossali T, Colombo R, Saracino L, Codullo V, Gnecchi M, Bigini P, Baldanti F, Lilleri D, Meloni F. Neutrophil Extracellular Traps Induce the Epithelial-Mesenchymal Transition: Implications in Post-COVID-19 Fibrosis. Front Immunol. 2021 June 14; 12:663303. 10.3389/fimmu.2021.663303. PMID: 34194429; PMCID: PMC8236949	2	2	2	2	2	2	12
32	Mongelli A, Barbi V, Gottardi Zamperla M, Atlante S, Forleo L, Nesta M, Massetti M, Pontecorvi A, Nanni S, Farsetti A, Catalano O, Bussotti M, Dalla Vecchia LA, Bachetti T, Martelli F, La Rovere MT, Gaetano C. Evidence for Biological Age Acceleration and Telomere Shortening in COVID-19 Survivors. Int J Mol Sci. 2021 June 7; 22 (11):6151. 10.3390/ijms22116151. PMID: 34200325; PMCID: PMC8201243	1	1	2	2	1	1	8

transforming growth factor-β1 (TGF-β), tumor necrosis factor-α (TNF-α), interleukin-1 (IL-1) and interleukin-6 (IL-6). These mediators, in turn, stimulates the proliferation of type 2 alveolar cells and increases the recruitment of fibroblasts. Eventually, the cascade can lead to an increased production and storage of extracellular matrix (ECM), compromising the architecture of alveolar-capillary membrane leading to impaired gas exchange and hypoxemia (Vietri et al., 2019; Alghizzawi et al., 2021). These assumptions are confirmed by Yu MX, et al., that, by exploiting data mining and network pharmacology, showed that the molecular mechanisms of PF secondary to COVID-19 are mainly related to the TNF signaling pathway, the cytokine-cytokine receptor interaction pathway and the NF-κB signaling pathway. Among cytokines, interleukin 6 (IL-6), TNF and IL-1β have been identified as key targets associated with PF secondary to COVID-19 (Yu et al., 2021).

A recent paper by Colarusso C et al. demonstrated that Post Covid patients with lung fibrosis-like symptoms had higher levels of IL-1α and TGF-β, but lower levels of IFN-β (Colarusso et al., 2021). Interestingly it is well known that IL-1α and TGF-β were highly released by peripheral blood mononuclear cells (PBMCs) obtained by patients with IPF, sharing the same immunological alteration (Terlizzi et al., 2022).

Furthermore, as pointed out by Lechowicz K, et al., there are similar cytokine profiles in IPF and COVID-19, suggesting similar pathological mechanisms underlying fibrosis development between these two diseases. Vesicular-type endothelial cells II are a major source of fibrogenic factors: they stimulate the hyperproliferation of type II follicular cells, recruit fibroblasts in fibrotic loci and induce differentiation and activation of fibroblasts in myofibroblasts. Myofibroblasts are responsible for the excessive accumulation of ECM basement membranes and interstitial tissues, which ultimately leads to the loss of alveolar-capillary barrier function (Lechowicz et al., 2020).

Sinha S. and colleagues with the help of artificial intelligence, demonstrating that COVID-19 resembles idiopathic pulmonary fibrosis (IPF) by sharing prognostic signatures. In particular the pathognomonic Alveolar type 2 (AT2) cytopathic changes, associated with DNA damage induced by oxidative stress that culminates into progenitor state arrest, senescence-associated secretory phenotype (SASP) and an IL15-centric cytokine storm faithfully recapitulate the host immune induced by SARS-CoV-2 and IPF (Sinha et al., 2021). From pathogenetic point of view, in IPF patients AT2 cells was shown to release fibrogenic factors and cytokine (including monocyte chemoattractant protein-1 (MCP-1), TGF-β1, TNF-α, IL-1β, and IL-6). Subsequently, a feedback mechanism stimulates hyperproliferation of AT2 cells, followed by the recruitment of fibroblasts into the fibroblastic foci, and induce the latter to begin myofibroblasts, leading to alveolar function loss (Razzaque and Taguchi, 2003; Satija and Lal, 2007).

The Entrance of the Virus Into the Cells: ACE2 and the Role of Integrins

The renin-angiotensin system (RAS) plays a key role in maintaining blood pressure but is also often involved in lung disease. RAS dysregulation has been implicated in pulmonary fibrosis onset, in particular due to the downstream actions of angiotensin I (Ang I), which is cleaved by ACE into angiotensin II (Ang II); Ang II promotes inflammatory and fibrotic responses through the receptor (AT1R). The other arm in the RAS involves the cleavage of Ang I into Ang (1–9) by (ACE2) and counteracts the ACE arm. Events downstream of Ang (1–9) result in a reduction in inflammation and fibrosis (Gheblawi et al., 2020). In addition, ACE2 also acts on Ang II by converting it into Ang (1–7), which further attenuates inflammation (Wigén et al., 2020). Thus, ACE2 acts as a negative regulator of the renin-angiotensin system. SARS-COV-2 infection is associated with a downregulation ofACE2 expression leading to a ACE/ACE2 ratio imbalance in favor of ACE, thus accelerating the production of angiotensin II (Dalan et al., 2020). The latter, in addition to being a powerful vasoconstrictor, induces the activation of IL-6, TNFα and an increase recruitment of neutrophils and macrophages in alveolar spaces, as well as the direct damage of endothelium. Ang II has also been shown to promote the activation of the collagen I gene via MAPK/ERK in order to generate a fibrotic response (Chang et al., 2021; Giacomelli et al., 2021).

Furthermore, pulmonary fibrosis tissue from IPF patients have shown an increased expression of ACE2 in fibroblasts, make fibrotic patients more susceptible to virus entrance (Shen et al., 2022).

Moreover, SARS-CoV-2 contributes to the activation of the host's proinflammatory and profibrotic pathways, including those associated with RAS (McDonald, 2021). In support of these hypotheses, the study by Delpino MVet al. points out that higher viral load in respiratory secretions were accompanied by significantly increased serum AngII levels in patients with COVID-19 pneumonia compared to healthy individuals (Delpino and Quarleri, 2020).

Regarding the role of adhesion molecules, it was demonstrated that SARS-CoV-2 virus is able to bind integrins with the consequances of increase viral entry into cells. Avβ6 Integrin appears to have high affinity for the SARS-CoV-2 virus andit has been directly implicated in IPF pathogenesis, suggesting a link between these seemingly distinct processes (Michalski et al., 2022). In IPF αvβ6 integrin is upregulated and it is able to promote TGFβ1 pro-fibrotic functions. The level of expression correlates with prognosis, making this integrin not only a potential biomarker of disease progression, but also an therapeutic target (John et al., 2020).

Galectin-3 and Pulmonary Fibrosis

The role of Gal-3 as a mediator of pulmonary fibrosis has long been investigated: higher levels of Gal-3 have now been widely associated with the development of interstitial lung diseases. Following cellular stress, the secretion of Gal-3 by macrophages upregulates TGF-ß receptors on fibroblasts and myofibroblasts. This in turn activates these cells, initiating the formation of granulation tissue (*via* collagen deposition) which is eventually remodeled into a fibrous scar. This Gal-3 mediated pathway is widespread throughout the body, not just in the lungs, and is critical for the development of fibrotic change in the liver, kidneys and even the heart (Caniglia et al., 2020). Recently, RNAseq analysis performed on several immune cells in the lungs of COVID-19 patients has provided valuable insights in this setting. Indeed, the study by Garcia-Revilla J, Deierborg T et al. (Garcia-Revilla et al., 2020) points out how Gal3 appears to be elevated in proliferative T lymphocytes associated with severe COVID-19 and that in a subset of pro-fibrogenic macrophages, Gal3 was one of the most upregulated genes in association with TREM2 and SPP1, both of which are involved in the disease and in pulmonary fibrosis. Furthermore, it has also been reported that SARS-CoV-2, like the H5N1 influenza virus, can activate the NLRP3 inflammasome by exploiting the action of Gal3 which in turn governs the release of proinflammatory cytokines such as: IL-1, IL-6, TNFα and IL-1β (d'Alessandro et al., 2020b; Garcia-Revilla et al., 2020; d'Alessandro et al., 2021c).

Other Specific Factors Related to the Development of Lung Fibrosis

3.6.1 Mechanical and Clinical Factors

As mentioned above, it is recognized that the disease caused by SARS-CoV-2 induces the activation of a complex pathway of cytokines that could cause various manifestations lung damage, including a pro-fibrotic pathway (Marchioni et al., 2018). So much so that a similar pro-fibrotic pathway is also involved in the development of some types of pulmonary fibrosis, such as IPF. It should be noted that, in many cases, the clinical syndrome associated with this pathogen is comparable to acute distress syndrome (ARDS), in which fibrotic damage is a possible and well-known consequence.

However there is also significant controversy within the pulmonary community as to the "uniqueness" of COVID-19 ARDS induced pulmonary fibrosis (Bos, 2020).

Mechanical ventilation may also play a role in worsening lung damage and easing the development of fibrosis, and some patients have shown the presence of fibrosis, even after different types of support and varying disease severity. Furthermore, the potential pro-fibrotic role represented by oxygen free radicals (ROS) produced by the prolonged and intensive use of a high-flow oxygen therapy must also be considered (Scelfo et al., 2020).

ENDOTHELIUM-MESENCHIMAL AND EPITHELIUM-MESENCHIMAL TRANSITION

Endothelium-mesenchymal transition occurs when endothelial cells respond to an external insult or internal pathological condition, transforming into a more aggressive mesenchymal state, causing irreversible vascular damage or fibrosis (Yang et al., 2020). Like the endothelium-mesenchymal transition, the epithelium-mesenchymal transition (EMT) is also known to play a crucial role in organ fibrosis. In this process, epithelial cells transform into a mesenchymal phenotype accompanied by basement membrane degradation, epithelial loss and mesenchymal protein gain (Yang et al., 2020). It would appears that this insidious viral infection leads to increased activation of epithelial and endothelial cells through endothelium-epithelial mesenchymal transitions, thus again potentially contributing to post-COVID-19 pulmonary fibrosis (Eapen et al., 2020).

The shared origin of epithelial injury between COVID-19-related ARDS and diseases such as IPF likely represents another unifying aspect of pulmonary fibrosis. Given the connection between the degree of epithelial injury and subsequent fibrosis, these associations could be indicative of a more severe manifestation of post-ARDS fibrosis than other virally-mediated etiologies.

This may also explain why others have described COVID-19-related ARDS as distinct from other types of ARDS (Sisson et al., 2010; Evidence of typepneum, 2022).

Another important mechanisms that highlight similarity between pulmonary fibrosis and COVID-19 regards the role of surfactant proteins. Surfactant is able to form a layer on the alveolar epithelium. At this level, surfactant reduce surface tension that allow the expansion of alveoli and gas exchange (Agassandian and Mallampalli, 2013). Surfactant also participate in host defense against infections and inflammation (Wang et al., 2021a). Alveolar type 2 cells is able to synthesize, secrete, andrecycle pulmonary surfactant, fundamental factor for alveolar stability and host immunity (Calkovska et al., 2021). Moreover it is important to evidence that AT2 produce cytokines and grow factors that affect immunity of the lungs (Calkovska et al., 2021). Surfactant proteins- A, B, C, and D are the main protein of surfanctant.

Several author reported the depletion of surfactant through virus-induced lysis of Type II pneumocytes with associated hyaline membrane formation in COVID-19 ARDS patients (Xu et al., 2020a).

It is also known that polymorphisms of Surfactant Protein (SP)-A, B and D showed association with idiopathic pulmonary fibrosis and various other pulmonary diseases (Wang et al., 2021a).

For these reasons the treatment with surfactant has been proposed for COVID-19 patients (Piva et al., 2021).

THE ROLES OF TGF-Β

TGF-β is a highly expressed key player in nearly all fibrotic processes.

This cytokine promotes redox imbalance by increasing the level of ROS and suppressing antioxidant enzymes. In viral infection-induced pulmonary fibrosis (including SARS-COV-2), oxidative stress increases in epithelial cells, thereby stimulating the production and release of TGF-β, leading to excessive migration, proliferation, activation and differentiation of fibroblasts into myofibroblasts. The latter cells are an important producer of collagenous and non-collagenous matrix molecules. Furthermore, TGF-β regulates AngII-induced collagen expression with subsequent accumulation and inflammation of ECM. In this scenario, activated fibroblasts induce further injury and death in alveolar epithelial cells, thus creating a vicious circle of interactions between profibrotic epithelial cells and fibroblasts that leads to the formation of non-functional scar tissue. Furthermore, TGF-β could also be responsible for inhibiting the expression of the Mas receptor for Ang1-7 in fibroblasts, thus antagonizing the antifibrotic capabilities of the hepatopeptide. In this microenvironment, TGF-β will be able to act on alveolar macrophages by stimulating the secretion of IL-4, IL-6 and IL-13, thus favoring the development of fibrosis (Delpino and Quarleri, 2020). As proof of this, TGF-β messenger RNA transcripts have been observed significantly in alveolar epithelial cells after SARS-CoV-2 infection (Xu et al., 2020b). Furthermore, under stimulation of repeated lesions or inflammation, TGF-β can recruit the type I receptor (TGFB1), thus activating intracellular signaling pathways, in particular the SMAD pathway, with upregulation of the expression of fibrosis-related genes (COL1A1, COL3A1, TIMP1, etc.,) and to the deposition of the extracellular matrix (Vaz de Paula et al., 2021; Zhang et al., 2021). Another interesting thing is that the SARS-CoV-1 nucleocapsid protein can directly promote the upregulation of TGF-β expression. Considering that the similarity of the nucleocapsid protein between SARS-CoV-2 and SARS-CoV-1 is up to 90%, it is possible to hypothesize that SARS-CoV-2 will also have a similar molecular mechanism (Wang et al., 2020). Very recently a study on the autopsy of COVID-19 patients analyzing the morphological and dynamics changes in the pulmonary parenchyma. Type II pneumocyte hyperplasia, alveolar cell multinucleation, and endothelitis resulted the most common alteration observed in this cohort, but without specificity. However the onset of these changes correlates to the onset of clinically established complications and also with the early detection of the development of severe post-COVID syndrome complications (Stoyanov et al., 2021).

ROLE OF MACROPHAGES

Macrophages are deeply involved in the "dialogue" between innate and adaptive immunity. The function and polarization of macrophages vary greatly depending on their anatomical location and the physical environment in which they are found. Pulmonary macrophages are divided into two subgroups based on their location: alveolar macrophages and interstitial macrophages. In addition to classification by location, macrophages can dynamically move between two activated forms: classically activated (M1) and alternately activated (M2), in response to ever-changing environmental factors. M1 macrophages act primarily as a host defense system to eliminate pathogens by generating pro-inflammatory chemokines and cytokines such as TNF-α, while M2 macrophages exhibit anti-inflammatory properties and engage in remodeling of the extracellular matrix. M2 macrophages are actively involved in the pathogenesis of pulmonary fibrosis (Wang et al., 2020). Furthermore, there is compelling evidence that DNA methylation, one of the main epigenetic mechanisms, is also involved in the pathogenesis of pulmonary fibrosis (Sanders et al., 2012; McErlean et al., 2021). In this regard, there are proteins called MBD, in particular MBD2, which by binding to these methylated areas mediate their activation or repression. Going into more detail, MBD2 improves PI3K/Akt signaling to promote the M2 program of macrophages and consequently the fibrogenesis process. All this is extremely important because MBD2 was found to be highly expressed in pulmonary macrophages of patients with COVID19 and that the loss of MBD2 leads to a marked reduction in the accumulation of M2 macrophages in the lung, with a reduction in fibrotic commitment (Wang et al., 2021b; McErlean et al., 2021).

Role of Caspasi 8

Caspase 8 is the main regulator of several cell death pathways, including apoptosis, necroptosis and pyroptosis. Its role in regulating inflammatory responses has recently been reported in the context of fungal infection (Gringhuis et al., 2012). It would appear that SARS-CoV-2 induces activation of caspase-8 to trigger cell apoptosis and to directly process inflammatory factors such as pro-IL-1β, which are essential later to trigger the pulmonary fibrotic process. Consistent with this notion, massive infiltrations of inflammatory cells, necrotic cell debris, and interstitial fibrosis have been observed in the post-mortem lungs of COVID-19 patients. Overall, these mechanisms could lead to severe lung damage and immune pathogenesis during SARS-CoV-2 infection. Thus, this suggests that caspase-8 activation may play a central role in SARS-CoV-2-induced apoptosis and inflammatory and fibrotic responses (Li et al., 2020).

Role of Midkine and NETosis

Midkine is a heparin-binding growth factor and shows a physiological role in embryonic development (Kadomatsu et al., 1988). It is also poorly expressed in the cells of the adult organism, while it is strongly increased in tumor cells and correlated with a less favorable prognosis in cancer patients (Maeda et al., 2007). As demonstrated by the study by Weckbach et al. it should be noted that midkine is significantly involved in causing inflammation and in the production of proinflammatory cytokines (Weckbach et al., 2011). This growth factor is also an important physiological mediator of RAS and has been found to be significantly increased in patients with ARDS (Kadomatsu, 2010; Zhang and Baker, 2017). Furthermore, midkine, in viral infections, including COVID-19, may promote the infiltration of neutrophils, the formation of NETs and be involved in lung remodeling and fibrosis, through the deposition of collagen through Nox1, MK, Notch2 signaling pathway.

Different factors inducing NETs resulted increased in autopsies of COVID-19 patients (Middleton et al., 2020). In fact NETs promoting cytokine storm through NFκB pathway activation in alveolar epithelial cells that triggers ROS production. Furthermore, NETs can induce the EMT in lung epithelial cells, thus further supporting NET role in fibrosis pathogenesis (Middleton et al., 2020; Pandolfi et al., 2021; d'Alessandro et al., 2022). So much so that anti-midkine monoclonal antibodies have been proposed as a new potential therapeutic strategies in COVID-19 (Sanino et al., 2020).

Genetic Aspects

From a genetic point of view, not much evidence is available in the literature: most studies try to investigate the genetic correlations between IPF and severe COVID-19. In this regard, in one of these studies, it was observed that the most important genetic risk factor for IPF, the variant MUC5B, seems to confer protection against COVID-19. However, it should be noted that the observed effect could be due to the protective effects of mucin overproduction on the airways or be a consequence of the selection bias. Therefore, further investigation is needed to address this apparent paradox (Fadista et al., 2021). Furthermore, in another study based on experimental models, it was found that SARS-CoV-2 infection increases the messenger RNA transcripts of ACE2, TGFB1, CTGF and FN1 in alveolar epithelial cells. These same changes were also found in the lung tissues of patients with pulmonary fibrosis (Xu et al., 2020b).

The epigenetic alteration has also been suggested in the pathogenesis of post-Covid patients developed pulmonary fibrosis. In COVID-19, patients bearing shorter telomeres in their peripheral leukocytes have been proposed to be at risk of worse prognoses. Telomere length is a marker of aging: progressive telomere shortening is a well-characterized phenomenon observed in older adults and attributed to the so-called telomere attrition (Mongelli et al., 2021). Telomere shortening is a strong predictive factor of poor prognosis in patients with IPF and short telomeres have more rapid disease progression (Molina-Molina, 2019; Mongelli et al., 2021).

CONCLUSION

In general, fibrosis is a normal repair process and is almost inevitably preceded by other tissue changes and inflammatory reactions. In the case of repeated or chronic lung damage, fibrosis becomes aberrant wound healing due to the dysregulation of the fibroblasts and the extensive deposition of collagen and elastin. While pulmonary fibrosis development and progression is the main actor of IPF, fibrogenic processes are also present in the evolution of COVID-19.

The topic of the pathogenetic mechanism of post-Covid-19 pulmonary fibrosis is currently a topic of intense research interest, but still largely at a speculative level. From the development of these researches, progress in the knowledge of the phenomenon and hopefully in its prevention and therapy may originate.

AUTHOR CONTRIBUTIONS

LB AM, and PS contributed to conception and design of the study. MD'A organized the database. PC and PS performed the statistical analysis. DB wrote the first draft of the manuscript. EB and LB wrote sections of the manuscript. All authors contributed to manuscript revision, read, and approved the submitted version.

REFERENCES

Agassandian, M., and Mallampalli, R. K. (2013). Surfactant Phospholipid Metabolism. *Biochim. Biophys. Acta* 1831, 612–625. doi:10.1016/j.bbalip.2012.09.010

Alghizzawi, M. I., Ata, F., Yousaf, Z., Alhiyari, M. A. A., Bint I Bilal, A., Elhiday, A., et al. (2021). The Second Wave of Desaturation in Coronavirus Disease 2019. *New Microbes New Infect.* 41, 100866. doi:10.1016/j.nmni.2021.100866

Baethge, C., Goldbeck-Wood, S., and Mertens, S. (2019). SANRA-a Scale for the Quality Assessment of Narrative Review Articles. *Res. Integr. Peer Rev.* 4, 5. doi:10.1186/s41073-019-0064-8

Benetti, E., Giliberti, A., Emiliozzi, A., Valentino, F., Bergantini, L., Fallerini, C., et al. (2020). Clinical and Molecular Characterization of COVID-19 Hospitalized Patients. *PLoS One* 15, e0242534. doi:10.1371/journal.pone.0242534

Bergantini, L., Bargagli, E. M., d'Alessandro, M., Refini, R. M., Cameli, P., Galasso, L., et al. (2021a). Prognostic Bioindicators in Severe COVID-19 Patients. *Cytokine* 141, 155455. doi:10.1016/j.cyto.2021.155455

Bergantini, L., d'Alessandro, M., Cameli, P., Cavallaro, D., Gangi, S., Cekorja, B., et al. (2021b). NK and T Cell Immunological Signatures in Hospitalized Patients with COVID-19. *Cells* 10 (11), 3182. doi:10.3390/cells10113182

Bergantini, L., d'Alessandro, M., Cameli, P., Otranto, A., Luzzi, S., Bianchi, F., et al. (2022). Cytokine Profiles in the Detection of Severe Lung Involvement in Hospitalized Patients With COVID-19: The IL-8/IL-32 Axis. *Cytokine* 151, 155804. doi:10.1016/j.cyto.2022.155804

Billoir, P., Alexandre, K., Duflot, T., Roger, M., Miranda, S., Goria, O., et al. (2021). Investigation of Coagulation Biomarkers to Assess Clinical Deterioration in SARS-CoV-2 Infection. *Front. Med. (Lausanne)* 8, 670694. doi:10.3389/fmed.2021.670694

Bos, L. D. J. (2020). COVID-19-related Acute Respiratory Distress Syndrome: Not So Atypical. *Am. J. Respir. Crit. Care Med.* 202, 622–624. doi:10.1164/rccm.202004-1423LE

Calkovska, A., Kolomaznik, M., and Calkovsky, V. (2021). Alveolar Type II Cells and Pulmonary Surfactant in COVID-19 Era. *Physiol. Res.* 70, S195–S208. doi:10.33549/physiolres.934763

Cameli, P., Bergantini, L. M., and d'Alessandro, E. B. (2021a). High-dose Steroids for the Treatment of Severe COVID-19: a New Therapeutic Tool?, *Intern. Emerg. Med.* 16(5):1329–1330. doi:10.1007/s11739-021-02722-y

Cameli, P., Bargagli, E., Bergantini, L., d'Alessandro, M., Giugno, B., Gentili, F., et al. (2021b). Alveolar Nitric Oxide as a Biomarker of COVID-19 Lung Sequelae: A Pivotal Study. *Antioxidants (Basel)* 10 (9), 1350. doi:10.3390/antiox10091350

Caniglia, J. L., Guda, M. R., Asuthkar, S., Tsung, A. J., and Velpula, K. K. (2020). A Potential Role for Galectin-3 Inhibitors in the Treatment of COVID-19. *PeerJ* 8, e9392. doi:10.7717/peerj.9392

Carvalho-Schneider, C., Laurent, E., Lemaignen, A., Beaufils, E., Bourbao-Tournois, C., Laribi, S., et al. (2021). Follow-up of Adults with Noncritical COVID-19 Two Months after Symptom Onset. *Clin. Microbiol. Infect.* 27, 258–263. doi:10.1016/j.cmi.2020.09.052

Chang, R., Mamun, A., Dominic, A., and Le, N.-T. (2021). SARS-CoV-2 Mediated Endothelial Dysfunction: The Potential Role of Chronic Oxidative Stress, Front. *Physiol* 0. doi:10.3389/fphys.2020.605908

Colarusso, C., Maglio, A., Terlizzi, M., Vitale, C., Molino, A., Pinto, A., et al. (2021). Post-COVID-19 Patients Who Develop Lung Fibrotic-like Changes Have Lower Circulating Levels of IFN-β but Higher Levels of IL-1α and TGF-β. *Biomedicines* 9, 1931. doi:10.3390/biomedicines9121931

Colquhoun, H. L., Jesus, T. S., O'Brien, K. K., Tricco, A. C., Chui, A., Zarin, W., et al. (2020). Scoping Review on Rehabilitation Scoping Reviews. *Arch. Phys. Med. Rehabil.* 101, 1462–1469. doi:10.1016/j.apmr.2020.03.015

Dalan, R., Bornstein, S. R., El-Armouche, A., Rodionov, R. N., Markov, A., Wielockx, B., et al. (2020). The ACE-2 in COVID-19: Foe or Friend? *Horm. Metab. Res.* 52, 257–263. doi:10.1055/a-1155-0501

d'Alessandro, M., Bergantini, L., Cameli, P., Curatola, G., Remediani, L., Bennett, D., et al. (2021a). Siena COVID, Serial KL-6 Measurements in COVID-19 Patients. *Intern. Emerg. Med.* 16 (6), 1541–1545. doi:10.1007/s11739-020-02614-7

d'Alessandro, M., Bergantini, L., Cameli, P., Curatola, G., Remediani, L., Sestini, P., et al. (2021b). Peripheral Biomarkers' Panel for Severe COVID-19 Patients. *J. Med. Virol.* 93 (3), 1230–1232. doi:10.1002/jmv.26577

d'Alessandro, M., Bergantini, L., Fossi, A., De Vita, E., Perillo, F., Luzzi, L., et al. (2021c). The Role of Galectins in Chronic Lung Allograft Dysfunction. *Lung* 199 (3), 281–288. doi:10.1007/s00408-021-00449-3

d'Alessandro, M., Cameli, P., Refini, R. M., Bergantini, L., Alonzi, V., Lanzarone, N., et al. (2020a). Serum KL-6 concentrations as a Novel Biomarker of Severe COVID-19. *J. Med. Virol.* 92 (10), 2216–2220. doi:10.1002/jmv.26087

d'Alessandro, M., De Vita, E., Bergantini, L., Mazzei, M. A., di Valvasone, S., Bonizzoli, M., et al. (2020b). Galactin-1, 3 and 9: Potential Biomarkers in Idiopathic Pulmonary Fibrosis and Other Interstitial Lung Diseases. *Respir. Physiol. Neurobiol.* 282, 103546. doi:10.1016/j.resp.2020.103546

d'Alessandro, M., Conticini, E., Bergantini, L., Cameli, P., Cantarini, L., Frediani, B., et al. (2022). Neutrophil Extracellular Traps in ANCA-Associated Vasculitis and Interstitial Lung Disease: A Scoping Review. *Life* 12 (2), 317. doi:10.3390/life12020317

Daga, S., Fallerini, C., Baldassarri, M., Fava, F., Valentino, F., Doddato, G., et al. (2021). Employing a Systematic Approach to Biobanking and Analyzing Clinical and Genetic Data for Advancing COVID-19 Research. *Eur. J. Hum. Genet.* 29 (5), 745–759. doi:10.1038/s41431-020-00793-7

Delpino, M. V., and Quarleri, J (2020). SARS-CoV-2 Pathogenesis: Imbalance in the Renin-Angiotensin System Favors Lung Fibrosis. *Front. Cel. Infect. Microbiol.* 0. doi:10.3389/fcimb.2020.00340

Eapen, M. S., Lu, W., Gaikwad, A. V., Bhattarai, P., Chia, C., Hardikar, A., et al. (2020). Endothelial to Mesenchymal Transition: a Precursor to post-COVID-19 Interstitial Pulmonary Fibrosis and Vascular Obliteration? *Eur. Respir. J.* 56, 2003167. doi:10.1183/13993003.03167-2020

Evidence of type II pneumocyte apoptosis in the pathogenesis of idiopathic pulmonary fibrosis (IFP)/usual interstitial pneumonia (UIP) - PubMed (2022). Available at: https://pubmed.ncbi.nlm.nih.gov/11215282/(accessed February 5, 2022).

Fadista, J., Kraven, L. M., Karjalainen, J., Andrews, S. J., Geller, F., au, fnm., et al. (2021). Shared Genetic Etiology between Idiopathic Pulmonary Fibrosis and COVID-19 Severity. *EBioMedicine* 65, 103277. doi:10.1016/j.ebiom.2021.103277

Fallerini, C., Daga, S., Mantovani, S., Benetti, E., Picchiotti, N., Francisci, D., et al. (2021). Association of Toll-Like Receptor 7 Variants With Life-Threatening COVID-19 Disease in Males: Findings From a Nested Case-Control Study. *Elife* 10, e67569. doi:10.7554/eLife.67569

Files, J. K., Sarkar, S., Fram, T. R., Boppana, S., Sterrett, S., Qin, K., et al. (2021). Duration of post-COVID-19 Symptoms Is Associated with Sustained SARS-CoV-2-specific Immune Responses. *JCI Insight* 6, 151544. doi:10.1172/jci.insight.151544

Garcia-Revilla, J., Deierborg, T., Venero, J L., and Boza-Serrano, A. (2020). Hyperinflammation and Fibrosis in Severe COVID-19 Patients: Galectin-3, a Target Molecule to Consider, Front. *Immunol* 0. doi:10.3389/fimmu.2020.02069

Gheblawi, M , Wang, K., Viveiros, A., Nguyen, Q., Zhong, J. C., Turner, A. J., et al. (2020). Angiotensin-Converting Enzyme 2: SARS-CoV-2 Receptor and Regulator of the Renin-Angiotensin System: Celebrating the 20th Anniversary of the Discovery of ACE2. *Circ. Res.* 126, 1456–1474. doi:10.1161/CIRCRESAHA.120.317015

Giacomelli, C., Piccarducci, R., Marchetti, L., Romei, C., and Martini, C. (2021). Pulmonary Fibrosis from Molecular Mechanisms to Therapeutic Interventions: Lessons from post-COVID-19 Patients. *Biochem. Pharmacol.* 193, 114812. doi:10.1016/j.bcp.2021.114812

Gianola, S., Jesus, T. S., Bargeri, S., and Castellini, G. (2020). Characteristics of Academic Publications, Preprints, and Registered Clinical Trials on the COVID-19 Pandemic. *PLoS ONE* 15, e0240123. doi:10.1371/journal.pone.0240123

Gringhuis, S I., Kaptein, T. M., Wevers, B. A., Theelen, B., van der Vlist, M., Boekhout, T., et al. (2012). Dectin-1 Is an Extracellular Pathogen Sensor for the Induction and Processing of IL-1β via a Noncanonical Caspase-8 Inflammasome. *Nat. Immunol.* 13, 246–254. doi:10.1038/ni.2222

Jesus, T. S., Kamalakannan, S., Bhattacharjya, S., Bogdanova, Y., Arango-Lasprilla, J. C., Bentley, J., et al. (2020). People with Disabilities and Other Forms of Vulnerability to the COVID-19 Pandemic: Study Protocol for a Scoping Review and Thematic Analysis. *Arch. Rehabil. Res. Clin. Transl* 2, 100079. doi:10.1016/j.arrct.2020.100079

John, A. E., Graves, R. H., Pun, K. T., Vitulli, G., Forty, E. J., Mercer, P. F., et al. (2020). Translational Pharmacology of an Inhaled Small Molecule αvβ6 Integrin Inhibitor for Idiopathic Pulmonary Fibrosis. *Nat. Commun.* 11, 4659. doi:10.1038/s41467-020-18397-6

Kadomatsu, K. (2010). Midkine Regulation of the Renin-Angiotensin System. *Curr. Hypertens. Rep.* 12, 74–79. doi:10.1007/s11906-010-0092-8

Kadomatsu, K., Tomomura, M., and Muramatsu, T. (1988). cDNA Cloning and Sequencing of a New Gene Intensely Expressed in Early Differentiation Stages of Embryonal Carcinoma Cells and in Mid-gestation Period of Mouse Embryogenesis. *Biochem. Biophys. Res. Commun.* 151, 1312–1318. doi:10.1016/S0006-291X(88)80505-9

Lechowicz, K., Drożdżal, S., Machaj, F., Rosik, J., Szostak, B., Zegan-Barańska, M., et al. (2020). COVID-19: The Potential Treatment of Pulmonary Fibrosis Associated with SARS-CoV-2 Infection. *J. Clin. Med.* 9, E1917. doi:10.3390/jcm9061917

Li, S., Zhang, Y., Guan, Z., Li, H., Ye, M., Chen, X., et al. (2020). SARS-CoV-2 Triggers Inflammatory Responses and Cell Death through Caspase-8 Activation. *Signal. Transduct Target. Ther.* 5, 235–310. doi:10.1038/s41392-020-00334-0

Liu, R., Paxton, W. A., Choe, S., Ceradini, D., Martin, S. R., Horuk, R., et al. (1996). Homozygous Defect in HIV-1 Coreceptor Accounts for Resistance of Some Multiply-Exposed Individuals to HIV-1 Infection. *Cell.* 86, 367–377. doi:10.1016/s0092-8674(00)80110-5

Maeda, S., Shinchi, H., Kurahara, H., Mataki, Y., Noma, H., Maemura, K., et al. (2007). Clinical Significance of Midkine Expression in Pancreatic Head Carcinoma. *Br. J. Cancer* 97, 405–411. doi:10.1038/sj.bjc.6603879

Maltezou, H. C., Pavli, A., and Tsakris, A. (2021). Post-COVID Syndrome: An Insight on its Pathogenesis. *Vaccines (Basel)* 9, 497. doi:10.3390/vaccines9050497

Management of post-acute covid-19 in primary care | The BMJ. Available at: https://www.bmj.com/content/370/bmj.m3026 (accessed June 21, 2021).

Marchioni, A., Tonelli, R., Ball, L., Fantini, R., Castaniere, I., Cerri, S., et al. (2018). Acute Exacerbation of Idiopathic Pulmonary Fibrosis: Lessons Learned from Acute Respiratory Distress Syndrome? *Crit. Care* 22, 80. doi:10.1186/s13054-018-2002-4

McDonald, L. T. (2021). Healing after COVID-19: Are Survivors at Risk for Pulmonary Fibrosis? *Am. J. Physiol. Lung Cel Mol Physiol* 320, L257–L265. doi:10.1152/ajplung.00238.2020

McErlean, P., Bell, C. G., Hewitt, R. J., Busharat, Z., Ogger, P. P., Ghai, P., et al. (2021). DNA Methylome Alterations Are Associated with Airway Macrophage Differentiation and Phenotype during Lung Fibrosis, Am J Respir Crit Care Med. 204(8):954–966. doi:10.1164/rccm.202101-0004OC

Michalski, J. E., Kurche, J. S., and Schwartz, D. A. (2022). From ARDS to Pulmonary Fibrosis: the Next Phase of the COVID-19 Pandemic? *Transl Res.* 241, 13–24. doi:10.1016/j.trsl.2021.09.001

Middleton, E. A., He, X. Y., Denorme, F., Campbell, R. A., Ng, D., Salvatore, S. P., et al. (2020). Neutrophil Extracellular Traps Contribute to Immunothrombosis in COVID-19 Acute Respiratory Distress Syndrome. *Blood* 136, 1169–1179. doi:10.1182/blood.2020007008

Molina-Molina, M. (2019). Telomere Shortening Is behind the Harm of Immunosuppressive Therapy in Idiopathic Pulmonary Fibrosis. *Am. J. Respir. Crit. Care Med.* 200, 274–275. doi:10.1164/rccm.201812-2330ED

Mongelli, A., Barbi, V., Gottardi Zamperla, M., Atlante, S., Forleo, L., Nesta, M., et al. (2021). Evidence for Biological Age Acceleration and Telomere Shortening in COVID-19 Survivors. *Int. J. Mol. Sci.* 22, 6151. doi:10.3390/ijms22116151

Pandolfi, L., Bozzini, S., Frangipane, V., Percivalle, E., De Luigi, A., Violatto, M. B., et al. (2021). Neutrophil Extracellular Traps Induce the Epithelial-Mesenchymal Transition: Implications in Post-COVID-19 Fibrosis. *Front. Immunol.* 12, 663303. doi:10.3389/fimmu.2021.663303

Pavli, A., Theodoridou, M., and Maltezou, H. C. (2021). Post-COVID Syndrome: Incidence, Clinical Spectrum, and Challenges for Primary Healthcare Professionals. *Arch. Med. Res.* 52, 575–581. doi:10.1016/j.arcmed.2021.03.010

Piva, S., DiBlasi, R. M., Slee, A. E., Jobe, A. H., Roccaro, A. M., Filippini, M., et al. (2021). Surfactant Therapy for COVID-19 Related ARDS: a Retrospective Case-Control Pilot Study. *Respir. Res.* 22, 20. doi:10.1186/s12931-020-01603-w

Razzaque, M. S., and Taguchi, T. (2003). Pulmonary Fibrosis: Cellular and Molecular Events. *Pathol. Int.* 53, 133–145. doi:10.1046/j.1440-1827.2003.01446.x

Sanders, Y. Y., Ambalavanan, N., Halloran, B., Zhang, X., Liu, H., Crossman, D. K., et al. (2012). Altered DNA Methylation Profile in Idiopathic Pulmonary Fibrosis. *Am. J. Respir. Crit. Care Med.* 186, 525–535. doi:10.1164/rccm.201201-0077OC

Sanino, G., Bosco, M., and Terrazzano, G. (2020). Physiology of Midkine and its Potential Pathophysiological Role in COVID-19. *Front. Physiol.* 0. doi:10.3389/fphys.2020.616552

Satija, N., and Lal, S. K. (2007). The Molecular Biology of SARS Coronavirus. *Ann. N. Y Acad. Sci.* 1102, 26–38. doi:10.1196/annals.1408.002

Scelfo, C., Fontana, M., Casalini, E., Menzella, F., Piro, R., Zerbini, A., et al. (2020). A Dangerous Consequence of the Recent Pandemic: Early Lung Fibrosis Following COVID-19 Pneumonia - Case Reports. *TCRM* Vol 16, 1039–1046. doi:10.2147/TCRM.S275779

Shakaib, B., Zohra, T., Ikram, A., Shakaib, M. B., Ali, A., Bashir, A., et al. (2021). A Comprehensive Review on Clinical and Mechanistic Pathophysiological Aspects of COVID-19 Malady: How Far Have We Come? *Virol. J.* 18, 120. doi:10.1186/s12985-021-01578-0

Shen, H., Zhang, N., Liu, Y., Yang, X., He, Y., Li, Q., et al. (2022). The Interaction between Pulmonary Fibrosis and COVID-19 and the Application of Related Anti-fibrotic Drugs. *Front. Pharmacol.* 12, 805535. doi:10.3389/fphar.2021.805535

Sinha, S., Castillo, V., Espinoza, C. R., Tindle, C., Fonseca, A. G., Dan, J. M., et al. (2021). COVID-19 Lung Disease Shares Driver AT2 Cytopathic Features with Idiopathic Pulmonary Fibrosis. *BioRxiv*, 470269. doi:10.1101/2021.11.28.470269

Sisson, T. H., Mendez, M., Choi, K., Subbotina, N., Courey, A., Cunningham, A., et al. (2010). Targeted Injury of Type II Alveolar Epithelial Cells Induces Pulmonary Fibrosis. *Am. J. Respir. Crit. Care Med.* 181, 254–263. doi:10.1164/rccm.200810-1615OC

Stoyanov, G. S., Yanulova, N., Stoev, L., Zgurova, N., Mihaylova, V., Dzhenkov, D. L., et al. (2021). Temporal Patterns of COVID-19-Associated Pulmonary Pathology: An Autopsy Study, *Cureus.* 13 (12) e20522. doi:10.7759/cureus.20522

Terlizzi, M., Molino, A., Colarusso, C., Donovan, C., Imitazione, P., Somma, P., et al. (2022). Activation of the Absent in Melanoma 2 Inflammasome in Peripheral Blood Mononuclear Cells from Idiopathic Pulmonary Fibrosis Patients Leads to the Release of Pro-fibrotic Mediators. *Front. Immunol.* 9 (2018), 670. doi:10.3389/fimmu.2018.00670

Tricco, A. C., Lillie, E., Zarin, W., O'Brien, K. K., Colquhoun, H., Levac, D., et al. (2018). PRISMA Extension for Scoping Reviews (PRISMA-ScR): Checklist and Explanation. *Ann. Intern. Med.* 169, 467–473. doi:10.7326/M18-0850

Updated methodological guidance for the conduct of scoping reviews - PubMed. Available at: https://pubmed.ncbi.nlm.nih.gov/33038124/(accessed July 28, 2021).

Vaz de Paula, C. B., Nagashima, S., Liberalesso, V., Collete, M., da Silva, F. P. G., Oricil, A. G. G., et al. (2021). COVID-19: Immunohistochemical Analysis of TGF-β Signaling Pathways in Pulmonary Fibrosis. *Int. J. Mol. Sci.* 23, 168. doi:10.3390/ijms23010168

Vietri, L., Bennett, D., Cameli, P., Bergantini, L., Cillis, G., Sestini, P., et al. (2019). Serum Amyloid A in Patients With Idiopathic Pulmonary Fibrosis. *Respir. Investig.* 57 (5), 430–434. doi:10.1016/j.resinv.2019.03.010

Wang, F., Kream, R. M., Stefano, G. B., Respiratory, Long-Term., and Sequelae, Neurological. (2020). Long-Term Respiratory and Neurological Sequelae of COVID-19. *Med. Sci. Monit.* 26, e928996. doi:10.12659/MSM.928996

Wang, S., Li, Z., Wang, X., Zhang, S., Gao, P., and Shi, Z. (2021). The Role of Pulmonary Surfactants in the Treatment of Acute Respiratory Distress Syndrome in COVID-19. *Front. Pharmacol.* 12, 698905. doi:10.3389/fphar.2021.698905accessed February 7, 2022)

Wang, Y., Zhang, L., Wu, G.-R., Zhou, Q., Yue, H., Rao, L.-Z., et al. (2021). MBD2 Serves as a Viable Target against Pulmonary Fibrosis by Inhibiting Macrophage M2 Program. *Sci. Adv.* 7, eabb6075. doi:10.1126/sciadv.abb6075

Weckbach, L. T., Muramatsu, T., and Walzog, B. (2011). Midkine in Inflammation. *ScientificWorldJournal* 11, 2491–2505. doi:10.1100/2011/517152

Wigén, J., Löfdahl, A., Bjermer, L., Elowsson Rendin, L., and Westergren-Thorsson, G. (2020). Converging Pathways in Pulmonary Fibrosis and Covid-19 - the Fibrotic Link to Disease Severity. *Respir. Med. X* 2, 100023. doi:10.1016/j.yrmex.2020.100023

Xu, J., Xu, X., Jiang, L., Dua, K., Hansbro, P. M., and Liu, G. (2020). SARS-CoV-2 Induces Transcriptional Signatures in Human Lung Epithelial Cells that Promote Lung Fibrosis. *Respir. Res.* 21, 182. doi:10.1186/s12931-020-01445-6

Xu, Z., Shi, L., Wang, Y., Zhang, J., Huang, L., Zhang, C., et al. (2020). Pathological Findings of COVID-19 Associated with Acute Respiratory Distress Syndrome. *Lancet Respir. Med.* 8, 420–422. doi:10.1016/S2213-2600(20)30076-X

Yang, J., Pan, X., Wang, L., and Yu, G. (2020). Alveolar Cells under Mechanical Stressed Niche: Critical Contributors to Pulmonary Fibrosis. *Mol. Med.* 26, 95. doi:10.1186/s10020-020-00223-w

Yu, M. X., Song, X., Ma, X. Q., Hao, C. X., Huang, J. J., and Yang, W. H. (2021). Investigation into Molecular Mechanisms and High-Frequency Core TCM for Pulmonary Fibrosis Secondary to COVID-19 Based on Network Pharmacology and Data Mining. *Ann. Palliat. Med.* 10, 3960–3975. doi:10.21037/apm-20-1384

Zhang, C., Wu, Z., Li, J. W., Tan, K., Yang, W., Zhao, H., et al. (2021). Discharge May Not Be the End of Treatment: Pay Attention to Pulmonary Fibrosis Caused by Severe COVID-19. *J. Med. Virol.* 93, 1378–1386. doi:10.1002/jmv.26634

Zhang, H., and Baker, A. (2017). Recombinant Human ACE2: Acing Out Angiotensin II in ARDS Therapy. *Crit. Care* 21, 305. doi:10.1186/s13054-017-1882-z

10

An Herbal Product Alleviates Bleomycin-Induced Pulmonary Fibrosis in Mice *via* Regulating NF-κB/TNF-α Signaling in Macrophages

Fei Jing[1], Xi Chen[2], Jingbo Xue[1], Kai Huang[2], Feng Xing[1], Xudong Hu[3], Yuan Peng[1] and Chenghai Liu[1,2,4]**

[1]Institute of Liver Diseases, Shuguang Hospital Affiliated to Shanghai University of Traditional Chinese Medicine, Shanghai, China, [2]Shanghai Key Laboratory of Traditional Chinese Clinical Medicine, Shanghai, China, [3]School of Basic Medical Sciences, Shanghai University of Traditional Chinese Medicine, Shanghai, China, [4]Key Laboratory of Liver and Kidney Diseases, Ministry of Education, Shanghai, China

***Correspondence:**
Chenghai Liu
chenghai.liu@outlook.com
Yuan Peng
pengyuan1026@shutcm.edu.cn

Background and aim: Pro-inflammatory macrophages aggravated progress of pulmonary fibrosis (PF) both in patients and animal models. Fuzheng Huayu (FZHY) formula, a Chinese herbal product, is effective in treating pulmonary fibrosis in our previous study. But its action mechanism against PF relating to macrophage activation was unclear. This study was designed to evaluate the anti-fibrotic and anti-inflammatory roles of FZHY in pulmonary fibrosis and to elucidate the potential mechanisms.

Methods: Network pharmacology was employed to identify the interrelationships among compounds of FZHY, potential targets and putative pathways on anti-pulmonary fibrosis. According to the data of bioinformatics analysis, the key pharmacological target for FZHY against PF was screened. The network pharmacological prediction was validated by a series of experimental assays, including CCK8, western blot and immunofluorescence staining. Then molecular mechanism of FZHY on relating to the predictive target were studied in bleomycin induced pulmonary fibrosis in mice with methylprednisolone as a positive control, and in lipopolysaccharide (LPS) stimulated cultured macrophages in culture, respectively.

Results: The network pharmacology analysis reveal that a total of 12 FZHY–PF crossover proteins were filtered into a protein-protein interaction network complex and designated as the potential targets of FZHY against pulmonary fibrosis, while TNF-α signal pathway ranked at the top. FZHY and methylprednisolone could attenuate the lung fibrosis and decrease pulmonary TNF-α expression in bleomycin induced fibrotic mice, without

---

Abbreviations: PF, pulmonary fibrosis; TCM, Traditional Chinese Medicine; FZHY, Fuzheng Huayu; BMDM, bone marrow-derived macrophages; LPS, lipopolysaccharide; RCT, randomized controlled trial; NMPA, National Medical Products Administration; COPD, chronic obstructive pulmonary disease; TCMSP, Traditional Chinese Medicine Systems Pharmacology database and Analysis Platform; BATMAN-TCM, Bioinformatics Analysis Tool for Molecular Mechanism of Traditional Chinese Medicine; GEO, Gene Expression Omnibus; OMIM, Online Mendelian Inheritance in Man; GO, Gene Ontology; KEGG, Kyoto Encyclopedia of Genes and Genomes; PVDF, polyvinylidene fluoride; PPI, protein–protein interaction; PBS, phosphate-buffered saline; NC, nitrocellulose; SDS-PAGE, SDS-polyacrylamide gel electrophoresis; DEGs, differentially expressed genes.

difference between two treatments. While TNF-α was mainly originated from macrophages identified by double fluorescent staining of TNF-α and F4/80. LPS stimulated cultured macrophage polarization and activation demonstrated by the enhance contents of TNF-α and iNOS but decreased level of Arg-1. FZHY could alleviate the LPS stimulated macrophage polarization and activation demonstrated by decreasing TNF-α and iNOS and increasing Arg-1. In particular, FZHY could significantly reduce the production of p65 and the nuclear translocation of phosphorylated p65.

Conclusion: Fuzheng Huayu formula has a good effect against pulmonary fibrosis induced by bleomycin in mice, whose action mechanism was associated with down-regulation of NF-κB/TNF-α signaling pathway in pro-inflammatory macrophages. These findings provided an important strategy for developing new agents against lung fibrosis and accelerated FZHY product application on patients with lung fibrosis.

Keywords: fuzheng huayu formula, pulmonary fibrosis, network pharmacology, macrophages, TNF-α signal pathway, NF-κB, lipopolysaccharide, methylprednisolone

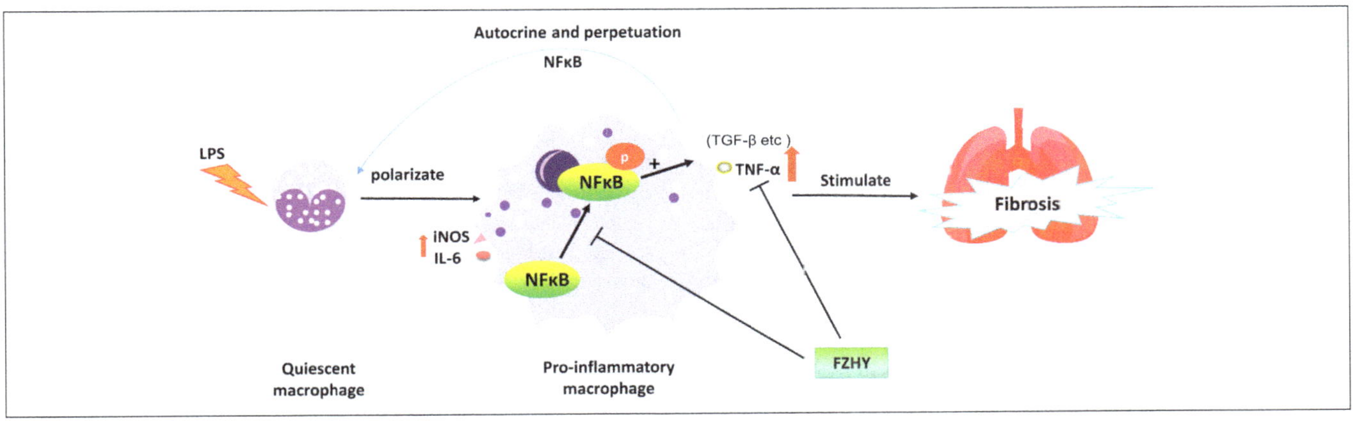

INTRODUCTION

Pulmonary fibrosis (PF) is a chronic interstitial lung disease caused by various insults including chemical materials, smoke, microbial infection, etc (Noble et al., 2012). As a highly heterogeneous and lethal pathological process, pulmonary fibrosis is characteristic of collage deposition and architecture destruction in lung that ultimately induce organ malfunction, disruption of gas exchange, and death from respiratory failure (Wynn, 2011). There are very limited therapeutic options for PF, except lung transplantation, two antifibrotic drugs, Pirfenidone and nintedanib have been approved by FDA for PF treatment (King et al., 2014; Karimi-Shah and Chowdhury, 2015). But the therapeutic effects of these two agents were not completely satisfactory in clinic (Ahluwalia et al., 2014; Kingwell, 2014). In fact, pulmonary fibrosis has complicated processes involving multiple targets, refractory to be treated or cured with single targeted agent. Traditional Chinese Medicine (TCM) is characterized by multiple components and multiple targets, as well as rich experiences of treating chronic lung diseases. Therefore, the efforts to develop the anti-lung fibrotic agents from TCM could be a practical approach to meet the clinic emerging needs.

Fuzheng Huayu (FZHY) formula is a botanic product composed of six herbs (**Table 1**). The randomized controlled trial (RCT) studies in multi centers had approved that FZHY could regress liver fibrosis due to hepatitis B (Wang et al., 2018). It was approved as an herbal product for liver fibrosis treatment by China National Medical Products Administration (NMPA) since 2002, and clinic trails in US for liver fibrosis due to HCV has been carried out. The action mechanism of FZHY against liver fibrosis was integrative, involving in protection of hepatocyte inflammation, inhibition of stellate cell activation via TGF-β/Smads pathway, and regulating hepatic matrix metabolism etc. (Liu et al., 2009). And recently, we found that FZHY could regulate immunity in diseased liver (Zhang et al., 2020). In particular, FZHY was found to have favorable effects on pulmonary interstitial inflammation and fibrosis in Bleomycin induced rats in our previous study (Dai et al., 2006; Tan et al., 2007), and helpful in improving lung function for Chronic obstructive pulmonary disease (COPD) patients as well [Published in Chinese]. However, little is known about the mechanism of action for FZHY against lung fibrosis.

TABLE 1 | Components of Fuzheng Huayu formula.

Chinese name	Plant sources	Medicinal parts	Preparation amount (g)
Danshen	Salvia Miltiorrhizae Bge (Labiatae)	radix	8
Chongcao	artificial fermentation cordyceps	mycelia	4
Taoren	Prunus persica (L.) Batsch (Rosaceae)	fruit	2
Jiaogulan	Gynostemma pentaphyllum (Thunb)	whole herb	6
Songhuafen	Pinus massoniana Lamb (Pinaceae)	pollen	2
Wuweizi	Schisandrae Chinensis (Turcz.)Baill	fruit	2

Pulmonary fibrosis is associated with inflammation characterized by the recruitment of macrophages, neutrophils and lymphocytes in the airways (Ward and Hunninghake, 1998). Among these, macrophage infiltration was the most crucial for regulating the progression of lung fibrosis (Wynn and Vannella, 2016; Yao et al., 2016).

Activation of macrophages could accelerate the recruitment and activation of other immune cells, thus further amplify the pulmonary inflammation, initiate and develop lung fibrosis. During this period, inflammatory mediators (eg. TNF-α) and pro-fibro-genic factors (eg. TGF-β1) were released, which accelerated the deterioration of the lung tissue, stimulated fibroblast activation. As a result, overproduction and deposition of ECM were accumulated in the lung tissue, and eventually fibrosis occurred. Could FZHY play its action against-lung fibrosis via anti-inflammation as it acted against liver fibrosis via protecting hepatocyte from injury and inflammation? Or are there any other mechanisms, through which FZHY plays a comprehensive role in preventing or regressing lung fibrosis?

By focusing on the above questions, we applied a network pharmacology approach with online database to search for probable target genes of FZHY related to pulmonary fibrosis treatment. Then a series of experimental assays were performed *in vivo* and *in vitro* to validate the effects of FZHY on pulmonary fibrosis and their underlying mechanism (**Figure 1**). With the above works, we predicted that TNF-α was the main target of FZHY against pulmonary fibrosis, which had been validated in Bleomycin induced lung fibrosis model in mice. Moreover, macrophage was the main resource of TNF-α in diseased lung, and we elucidated that FZHY could inhibit pro-inflammatory macrophage activation via NF-κB/TNF-α signaling pathway, which was closely associated with its efficacy on lung fibrosis. These results might represent a breakthrough in the potential use of FZHY for pulmonary fibrosis treatment.

MATERIALS AND METHODS

Ethics

All experimental procedures complied with the Guidelines for Experimentation of Shuguang Hospital, affiliated with Shanghai University of Traditional Chinese Medicine. The protocols were reviewed and approved by the Ethics Committee of the institution.

Databases

Data on the canonical name and molecular weight of the compounds in FZHY were obtained from the Traditional Chinese Medicine Systems Pharmacology database and Analysis Platform (TCMSP; http://tcmspw.com/tcmsp.php, version 2.3, updated on april 30, 2021 (Ru et al., 2014), the Bioinformatics Analysis Tool for Molecular Mechanism of Traditional Chinese Medicine (BATMAN-TCM; http://bionet.ncpsb.org/batman-tcm/, updated on april 30, 2021) (Liu et al., 2016), and PubChem (https://pubchem.ncbi.nlm.nih.gov, updated on april 1, 2021; (Kim et al., 2019). To identify the compounds with high levels of oral absorption, usability, and biological activity for further study, candidate components were screened and selected based on the following two parameters: 1) oral bioavailability (OB) of ≥30% and 2) drug-likeness (DL) of ≥0.18.

Prediction of Drug-Related Targets of Bioactive Components

Predicted target genes of FZHY ingredients were screened in two online databases, TCMSP and BATMAN-TCM (Ru et al., 2014; Liu et al., 2016). The known therapeutic targets of these ingredients were confirmed by referring to DrugBank database (www.drugbank.ca, updated on 28 February 2020) and designated as the putative targets of FZHY. The putative targets were designated as the drug-related genes.

Prediction of PF-Related Genes From Gene Expression Omnibus Profiles

Gene expression microarray data (GSE76808) on the gene expression profiles of PF in patients with and without systemic sclerosis-related interstitial lung disease were obtained from Gene Expression Omnibus (GEO) database of the National Center for Biotechnology Information (https://www.ncbi.nlm.nih.gov/geo), a public functional genomics data repository. Data of 18 lung samples were obtained, four of which from individuals without PF (GSM2038281, GSM2038282, GSM2038283 and GSM2038284) and 14 of which from patients with PF (GSM2038267, GSM2038268, GSM2038269, GSM2038270, GSM2038271, GSM2038272, GSM2038273, GSM2038274,

GSM2038275, GSM2038276, GSM2038277, GSM2038278, GSM2038279 and GSM2038280). By using the data from the whole human genome microarray, we analyzed the potential therapeutic targets for patients with and without PF by employing the LIMMA package in the R language. An adjusted p value of <0.05 and a fold change (FC) of >1.2 were selected as the cutoff criteria. The potential genes were considered PF-related target genes and processed by using Strawberry Perl (version 5.30.0.1) and R (version 4.0.2) with the Bioconductor packages.

Prediction of PF-Related Targets From Online Databases

Information regarding the various genes associated with PF were obtained from the GeneCards database (http://www.genecards.org) and Online Mendelian Inheritance in Man (OMIM) database (http://omim.org/), which are knowledge bases of human genes and genetic disorders (Hamosh et al., 2005; Stelzer et al., 2016). The key search terms used in two databases were "lung fibrosis" and "Pulmonary fibrosis" and the results were exported online.

Processing of Data on Potential Hub Genes Involved in Effects of FZHY on PF

The predictions of PF-related genes and putative drug-related genes were verified by VennDiagram R package. Overlapping genes were considered as potential hub genes related to the preventative effects of FZHY against PF.

Network Construction and Analysis

On the basis of the potential hub genes identified through the aforementioned process, a protein–protein interaction (PPI) network was established by public Search Tool for the Retrieval of Interacting Genes/Proteins database (https://string-db.org, updated 21 May 2021) (Szklarczyk et al., 2015). The minimum required interaction score was set to 0.7 to improve the accuracy of results. For further observations of biological functions of the hub genes, the cluster Profiler package was used to explore and visualize the data used in the pathway and functional enrichment analysis. Cytoscape (version 3.7.1) was used to construct and visualize a network of the compound–target protein-differential genes, which can be used to identify the target proteins that connect between compounds and differential genes in PF.

Gene Ontology and Kyoto Encyclopedia of Genes and Genomes Pathway Analysis

To identify the functional annotation and pathway enrichment associated with the potential genes, a pathway enrichment analysis was performed by Gene Ontology (GO) annotation database (http://www.geneontology.org) and Kyoto Encyclopedia of Genes and Genomes (KEGG) (http://www.genome.jp/kegg) using cluster Profiler R package (Ashburner et al., 2000; Kanehisa et al., 2019). The enrich plot and DOSE Bioconductor packages were used to visualize the enrichment results and facilitate the interpretation process (Yu et al., 2015). Biological process (BP), molecular function (MF), and cellular component (CC) were used to visualize the functional annotation and pathway of potential genes. Enrichment with a p value of <0.05 was considered statistically significant, and an adjusted p value of <0.05 was set as the threshold value.

Drug Preparation and Identification

FZHY formula was purchased from Shanghai Sundise Traditional Chinese Medicine Co., Ltd, and was prepared as previously described (Liu et al., 2019; Wu et al., 2019) **Table 2**.

Mouse Models

Male C57BL/6 mice (24 ± 2 g) were supplied by Zhejiang Vital River Laboratory Animal Technology Co., Ltd. (License No: SCXK (Zhe)2019–0001). The mice were fed in the Experimental Animal Center of Shanghai University of Traditional Chinese Medicine and were acclimatized to the animal center conditions for 3 days before experiments. The mice were given Rodent Laboratory Chow and water ad libitum and maintained under controlled conditions with a temperature of 22–25°C, relative humidity of 46–52%, and a 12/12-h light/dark cycle (lights on at 7a.m.). Our experiments were conducted in accordance with the Animal Ethics Committee of Shanghai University of Traditional Chinese Medicine (License No: PZSHUTCM200821006).

Bleomycin-Induced Murine Pulmonary Fibrosis Model

We utilized a modified model of bleomycin-induced pulmonary fibrosis according to our previous work (Tan et al., 2007). Briefly, Bleomycin (CSN10472, Csnpharm, USA) dissolved in saline was administrated via trachea route at a single dose of 2 mg/kg at day 0. The sham-treated mice were treated with the identical volume of normal saline.

Animal Groups and Experimental Design

To evaluate the effect of FZHY on PF, 46 C57BL/6 mice were randomly divided into four treatment groups: normal control (n = 10), model control (n = 12), FZHY treatment (n = 12) and positive control (n = 12). Mice in model control, FZHY treatment and positive control groups were received bleomycin via trachea route to induce pulmonary fibrosis model at Day 0. In addition, for FZHY treatment groups, FZHY was administered daily through oral gavage at doses of 5.6 g/kg body weight once a day for 20 consecutive days. The daily amount of FZHY was equivalent to 10 times of the clinical dose of 60 kg/day body weight in adults. Mice in positive control group was intragastrically administered methylprednisolone (Pfizer Italia Srl, H20150245) at a daily dose of 10 mg/kg body weight. For the normal control and model control groups, the mice were treated with saline through gavage. All mice were sacrificed with pentobarbital sodium and killed 24 h after the last administration.

Pulmonary Histopathology

Morphological evaluation was performed on formalin-fixed, paraffin-embedded lung tissue sections and stained with hematoxylin and eosin (HE) to investigate levels of lung inflammation in accordance with manufacturer's procedures. For estimating the lung collagen deposition, Masson's trichrome staining (collagen stains blue) and picrosirius red staining (collagen stains red) were performed. The images were analyzed using a light microscope (Olympus BX40, Japan).

Immunohistochemical Analysis

Immunohistochemical analysis was performed to detect TNF-α and F4/80 expressions in lung tissues. In brief, paraffin-embedded sections were deparaffinized in xylene twice for 10 min and rehydrated in graded concentrations of ethanol (100%, 95%, 90%, 80% and 70%) and then submerged to water. For antigen retrieval, the whole sections were submerged in antigenic retrieval buffer and microwaved. They were then treated with 3% hydrogen peroxide in methanol to inactivate the endogenous enzymes. Sequentially, the sections were incubated with 5% bovine serum albumin (BSA) for 20 min in room temperature to block nonspecific binding. Sections were incubated with anti-TNFα (Absin, abs131997, China) or F4/80 (CST, 70076T, USA) overnight at 4°C, respectively. After washing with phosphate-buffered saline (PBS), tissue sections were treated with secondary antibodies, followed by incubation with conjugated horseradish peroxidase–streptavidin. Tissue sections were then counter-stained with hematoxylin, dehydrated and mounted.

Immunofluorescence Staining

The lung tissue sections or cells were fixed with cold acetone for 30 min and treated with 0.5% TritonX-100 for 2 min. Then they were blocked with 1% bovine serum albumin for 40 min, and stained with primary antibody. After washing, they were incubated with fluorescent secondary antibody. Nuclei were stained with 4′, 6-diamidino-2-phenylindole (DAPI; ab228549, abcam, USA). Images and photographs were obtained by Olympus confocal microscope.

Isolation of Murine Bone Marrow-Derived Macrophages

10–12 weeks old male C57BL/6 mice were euthanized. Subsequently, the knee joint was cut and both ends of tibia and femur were removed one by one. The bones were washed with sterile PBS. The ends of the bones were removed to flush out the bone marrow with DMEM containing penicillin-streptomycin. Next, the bone marrow was resuspended and passed through a 70 μm nylon filter to remove debris and unwanted tissue. Cells were centrifuged for 10 min at 1,500 rpm. The cell pellet was resuspended in 3 ml red blood cell (RBC) lysis buffer. RBCs were lysed for 2 min at room temperature (RT). Cells were separated by centrifugation (10 min, RT, 1,500 rpm). RBC-free cell pellets were resuspended in DMEM containing of 10% FBS without penicillin-streptomycin, and cells were enumerated by using a TC-20 cell counter (Biorad, USA). Cells were adjusted to 3.0×10^5 cells/ml in BMDM medium and seeded into T150 flask (NEST, China). Medium was changed 4 days later. After 7 days of culture, 99% of the attached cells were BMDMs.

Cell Viability Assay

CCK8 cell viability kit (HY-K0301, MCE, China) was used to detect cell viability. Briefly, BMDMs were seeded in 96-well plates (3×10^4 cells/well) and 100 μl of 10% CCK8 solution were added into each well, followed by incubation in a humidified incubator for 2 h at 37°C, 5% CO_2. After the incubation, absorbance was measured at 450 nm and 630 nm using a microplate reader (BioTEK, MQX200R, USA).

Cytokine Quantification

TNF-α (227846-011, Thermofisher, Austria) and IL-6 (234277-008, Thermofisher, Austria) released in supernatants were quantified by ELISA according to manufacturer's protocol.

Western Blot Analysis

Cell pellets or lung tissues were lysed with RIPA buffer containing a complete cocktail of protease inhibitors in western blot analysis (53153900, Roche, Germany). Proteins were quantified by BCA Protein Assay (WA322434, Thermofisher, USA) and equal amounts (20 μg) of total protein lysates from each sample were separated by SDS-polyacrylamide gel electrophoresis (SDS-PAGE). Separated proteins were then transferred onto polyvinylidene fluoride (PVDF) or nitrocellulose (NC) membranes. Membranes were blocked with blocking buffer (WB315798, Thermofisher,USA) and then incubated with the following primary antibodies respectively: anti-TNF-α (1/1,000; 11948T, CST,USA), anti-Arg1 (1/1,000; 93668S, CST, USA), anti-iNos(1/1,000; 13120S, CST, USA), anti- NF-κB (1/1,000; 8242S, CST, USA), anti-p-NF-κB (1/1,000; 3033S, CST, USA), and anti-GAPDH (1/5000; 60004-1-Ig, Proteintech, China). Membranes were then thoroughly rinsed and incubated with species-matched HRP-conjugated secondary antibodies. Protein bands were visualized by ECL Western blot detection reagents (4600SF, Tanon, China) in accordance with manufacturer's protocol or defined by scanning (Odyssey, USA) and quantified by computer-assisted image analysis system.

Real-Time Fluorescence Quantitative Polymerase Chain Reaction

Total RNA was extracted using TRIzol Reagent (Sangon Biotech, Shanghai, China) in accordance with manufacturer's protocol. After the concentration of RNA was determined, 500 ng of total RNA was used as the template for reverse transcription into single-stranded cDNA by Reverse Transcription Reagent Kit with gDNA Eraser (Takara, Dalian, China). Real-time fluorescence quantitative polymerase chain reaction was performed using SYBR Premix Ex Taq (Tli RNaseH Plus; Takara) and ViiA seven Real-Time PCR System (ABI, Carlsbad, CA, USA). The β-actin gene was amplified as an internal control, and the primer sequences are listed in **Table 3**. The relative gene quantities compared with β-actin were calculated through the $2^{-\Delta\Delta CT}$ method.

Statistical Analysis

All data were analyzed using PASW Statistics software (version 20). Differences between groups were assessed through a nonparametric one-way analysis of variance. Values were presented as mean ± standard deviation. $p < 0.05$ was considered statistically significant.

TABLE 2 | The chemical components of FZHY for FZHY quality control.

Compounds (marker)	Quality criterion
Salvianolic acid B (from Danshen)	Should be no less than 15.6 mg in 24 g of FZHY raw materials (daily dose)
Sodium Danshensu (from Danshen)	Should be no less than 13.2 mg in 24 g of FZHY raw materials (daily dose)
Adenosine (from Chongcao)	Should be no less than 4.8 mg in 24 g of FZHY raw materials (daily dose)
Schisandrin B (from Wuweizi)	Should be no less than 2.28 mg in 24 g of FZHY raw materials (daily dose)

TABLE 3 | Real-time quantitative PCR primers used in this study.

Gene	Forward (5'→3')	Reverse (5'→3')
TNF-α	TAG CCA GGA GGG AGA ACA GA	CCA GTG AGT GAA AGG GAC AGA
β-actin	TGA CGA GGC CCA GAG CAA GA	ATG GGC ACA GTG TGG GTG AC

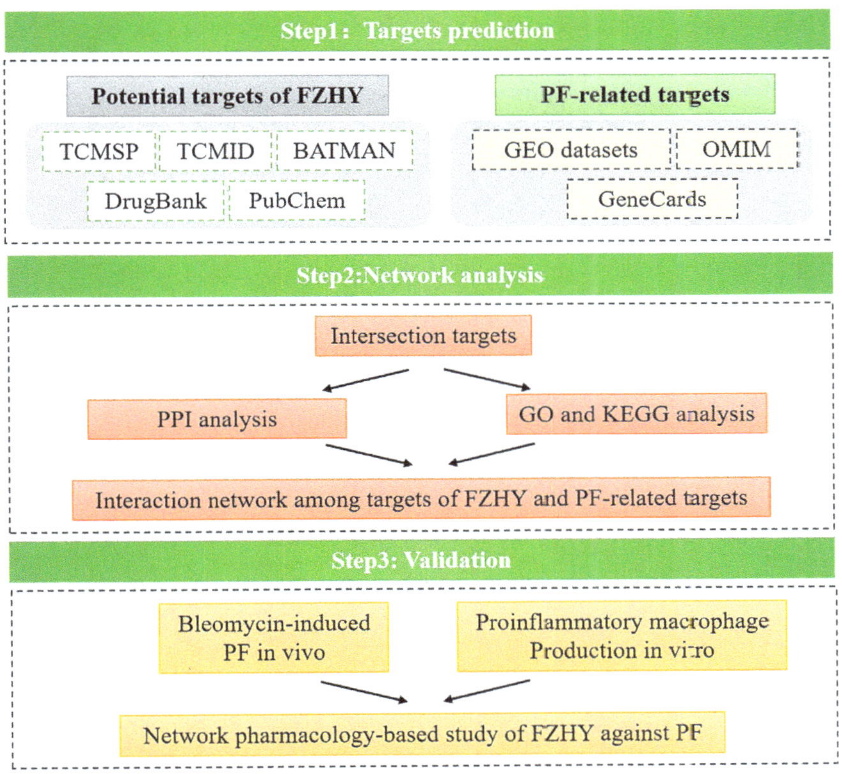

FIGURE 1 | Flow chart.

RESULTS

Putative Ingredients and Targets for FZHY

We selected a total of 141 ingredients based on the following criteria for the absorption, distribution, metabolism, and excretion (ADME) properties of drugs with potential biological effects at a systematic level: OB ≥ 30% and DL ≥ 0.18 (**Supplementary Table S1**). The potential targets of FZHY were predicted by referring to the TCMSP, BATMAN-TCM and DrugBank databases, as described in the Materials and Methods section. A total of 197 potential target genes for FZHY were identified (**Supplementary Table S2**) after the redundant data were removed.

Differentially Expressed mRNAs in Patients With and Without PF

By using the raw data from the GSE76808 dataset, we analyzed mRNA expression profiles in the lung samples from patients with and without PF. **Figure 2A** presents a heatmap of the

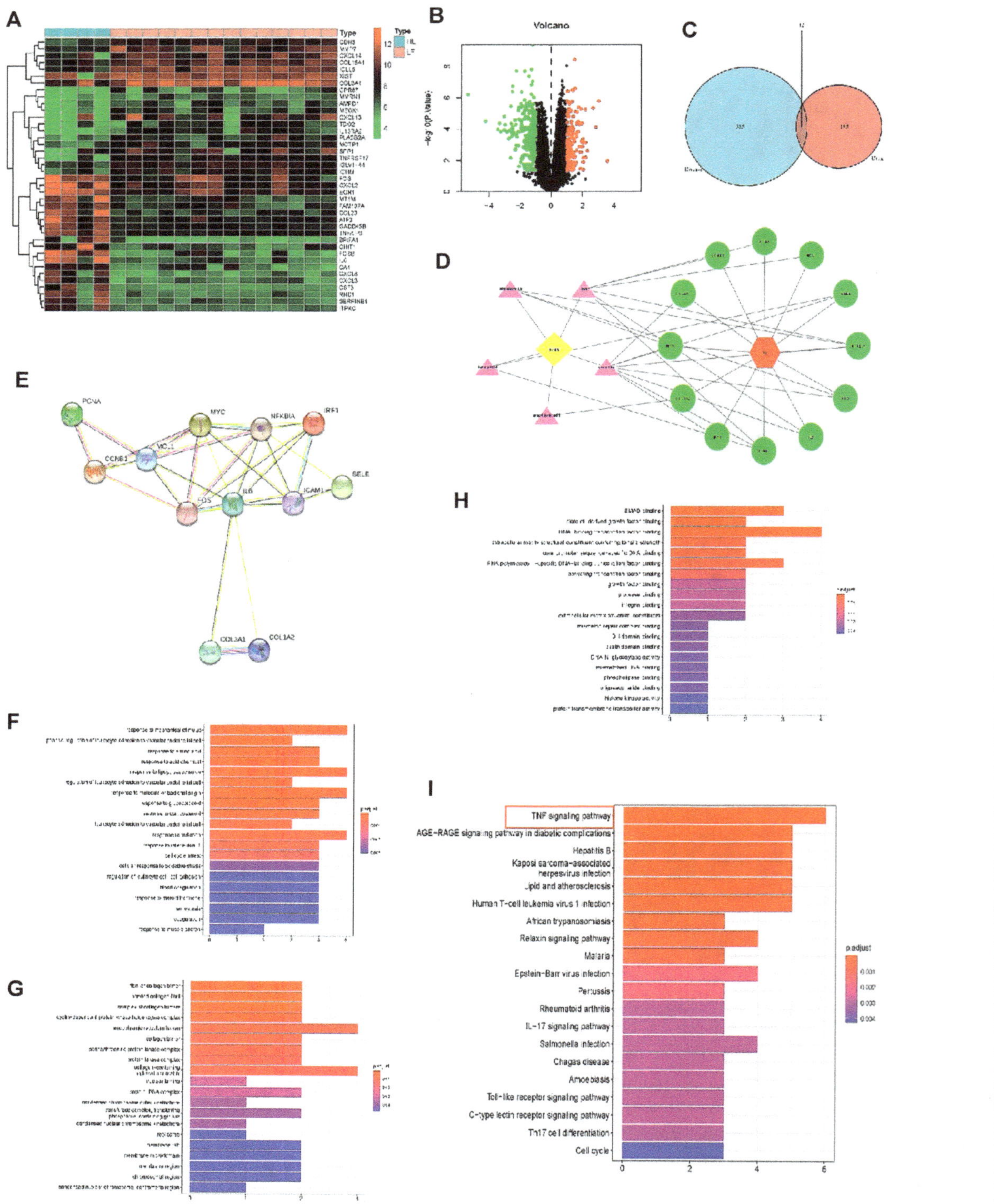

FIGURE 2 | Analyses of the different potential therapeutic targets between PF and healthy lung tissues. **(A)** The heatmap comparing the different gene expressions between PF and healthy lung tissues was shown. **(B)** The volcano plot of *p* values as a function of weighted fold change for mRNAs in PF and healthy lung tissues. The vertical dotted line delimits up- and down-regulation. Red and green plots represent significant up-regulated and down-regulated mRNAs with>1.2-fold change and corrected $p < 0.05$, respectively. **(C)** Venn diagram of FZHY- and PF-related proteins. The overlapped genes were considered as the potential hub genes of FZHY against PF. **(D)** The Component-Target protein network. The violet triangles represent the candidate active compounds in FZHY. The green circles represent the gene names of target proteins of PF. **(E)** Cluster analysis of the PPI network. 12 FZHY-PF crossover proteins were filtered into the PPI network complex. **(F–H)** Bioinformatic analyses of drug-disease intersection proteins. Gene ontology annotations, including BP **(F)**, CC **(G)** and MF **(H)** analysis. **(I)** KEGG pathway enrichment analysis of 12 putative targets. **(I)** PF-related KEGG pathway enrichment was presented.

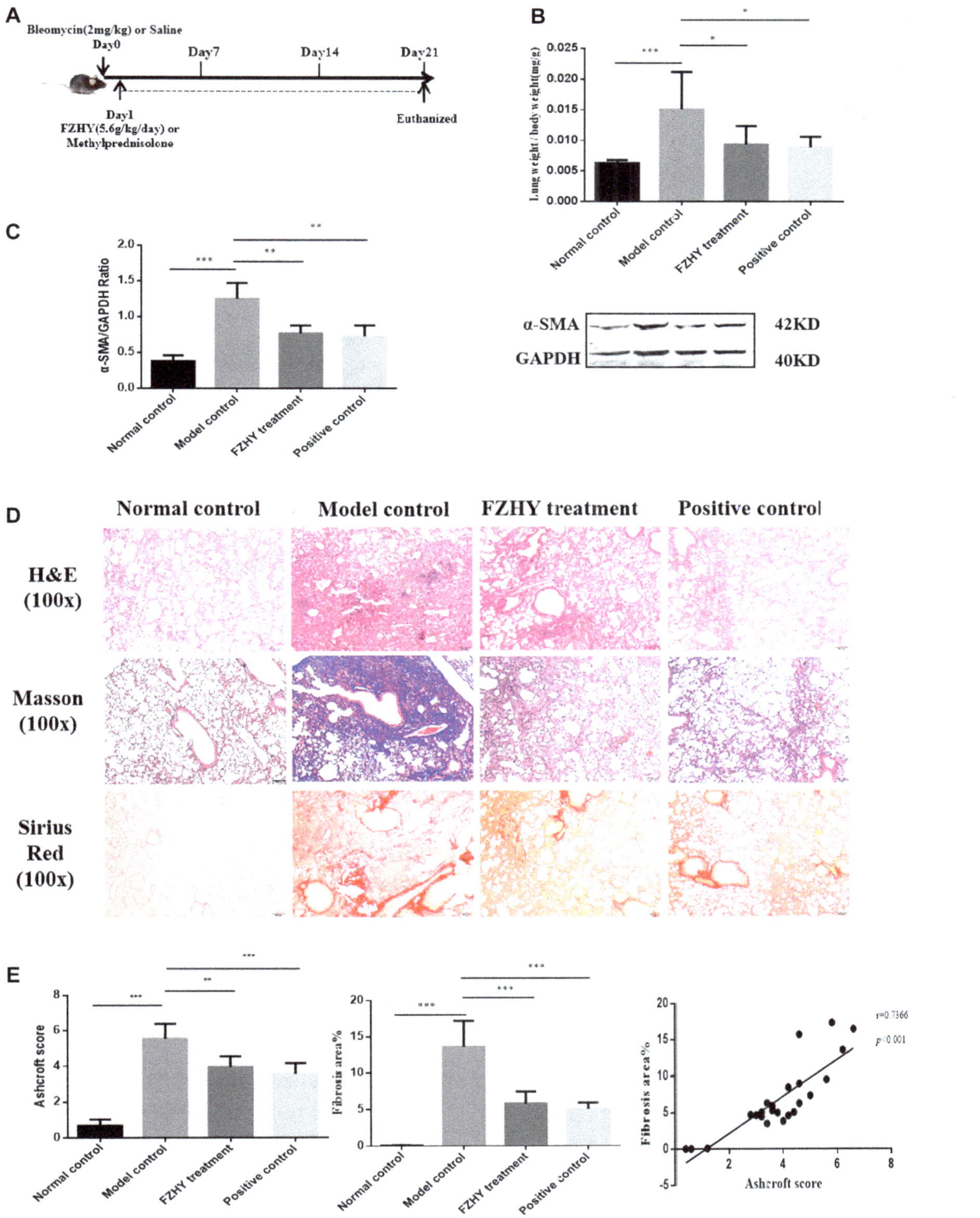

FIGURE 3 | FZHY treatment attenuates bleomycin-induced lung fibrosis *in vivo*. **(A)** Lung fibrosis was induced by bleomycin at day 0. Then mice were administered with FZHY or methylprednisolone once a day for 20 consecutive days. 24 h after FZHY administration, all mice were sacrificed. **(B)** Ratio of lung weight to body weight in each group. **(C)** α-SMA protein expression in each group. **(D)** Pathological analysis including H&E, Masson, Sirius red stains at ×100 magnification in each tissue specimen. **(E)** Semi-quantitative analysis for collagen deposition. $^{*}p < 0.05$; $^{**}p < 0.01$; $^{***}p < 0.001$.

TABLE 4 | The potential hub genes of FZHY against PF.

Gene	Full name
ICAM1	Intercellular Adhesion Molecule 1
IL6	Interleukin 6
FOS	Fos Proto-Oncogene
NFKBIA	Nuclear factor Kappa B inhibitor alpha
SELE	Selectin E
MCL1	Myeloid cell leukemia 1 protein
PCNA	Proliferating Cell Nuclear Antigen
CCNB1	cyclin B1
COL3A1	Collagen Type III Alpha 1 Chain
MYC	MYC proto-oncogene, bHLH transcription factor
COL1A2	Collagen Type I Alpha 2 Chain
IRF1	Interferon Regulatory Factor 1

expression of the top 40 genes in the lung samples from the patients with PF and the controls. Volcano plot filtering identified 397 differentially expressed mRNAs ($p < 0.05$, $|FC| > 1.2$, **Figure 2B**). Among them, 158 mRNAs were upregulated, and 239 mRNAs were downregulated. **Supplementary Table S3** presented the detailed information regarding these therapeutic targets used in the data analysis. In addition, the PF-related targets were predicted using the GeneCards and OMIM online databases (**Supplementary Tables S4, S5**).

Construction of FZHY Target-PF Network

Based on the identified FZHY- and PF-related target genes, a Venn diagram of the FZHY- and PF-related proteins was created. The overlapping genes were considered differentially expressed genes (DEGs) and designated as potential hub genes for the effects of FZHY on PF (**Figure 2C**). A total of 12 DEGs were filtered into the PPI network complex and presumed to be related to the effects of FZHY on PF (**Figure 2D**; **Table 4**). In addition, a PPI network of the 12 DEGs was constructed (**Figure 2E**).

To identify the relevant gene functions, the GO annotation, consisting of the BP, CC, and MF categories, displayed in **Figures 2F–H**, was assayed for the 12 DEGs by using R software. After KEGG analysis, DEGs were mapped to 53 KEGG pathways (**Figure 2I** and **Supplementary Table S6**). Notably, the top one ranked KEGG pathway was TNF signal pathway.

FZHY Ameliorated Bleomycin-Induced Lung Fibrosis

The pulmonary fibrotic mice were intervened with FZHY and methylprednisolone as positive drug respectively (**Figure 3A**). Since the intratracheal instillation of bleomycin in mice results in lung injury, which peaks 3–5 days later, and was followed by pulmonary fibrosis at 21 days (Chua et al., 2005; Budinger et al., 2006), the efficacy of FZHY and methylprednisolone on bleomycin-induced lung fibrosis in mice was evaluated 21 days after the administration. Compared with the normal mice, the lung weight was increased in model control (**Figure 3B**). FZHY and methylprednisolone treatment significantly decreased the lung weight compared to the model control (**Figure 3B**). The collagen deposition in lungs evaluated by Masson and Sirius red staining, and fibroblast activation measured as α-SMA expression with western blot (**Figure 3C**), was significantly increased in model control mice, but were decreased in FZHY and methylprednisolone groups compared to the model control. Also pulmonary inflammation appeared to also be more severe after bleomycin challenge, while FZHY treatment alleviated the inflammatory response in lung tissues (**Figure 3D**). Besides, the semi-quantitation for lung fibrosis with a numerical fibrotic scale was conducted (*Ashcroft score*) (**Figure 3E**). In, similar tendency in effects of FZHY against bleomycin-induced pulmonary fibrosis was observed, and there is no difference for the lung weight, fibrotic areas and α-SMA expression between FZHY and methylprednisolone. The results revealed that bleomycin-treated mice exhibited the increase of inflammation and collagen deposition, while FZHY treatment could suppress the changes caused by bleomycin.

FZHY Reduced Expression of TNF-α in Macrophages in Mice Pulmonary Fibrosis *in vivo*

TNF-α expression in lung tissue was measured by immunohistochemical staining and western-blot assay. As shown in **Figures 4A–E**, positive staining, protein and gene (mRNA) expression of TNF-α were markedly increased in model control group than that in the normal mice. In particular, most of the positive staining of TNF-α located in lung interstitial area. Compared with the model group, TNF-α expression was remarkably decreased after FZHY or methylprednisolone as positive drug, but there is no significant difference between two treatment groups. To confirm whether expression of TNF-α was contributed by the inflammatory macrophages, we conducted double stains with antibodies of F4/80 [a mouse macrophage surface marker, (Austyn and Gordon, 1981; Lee et al., 1985)]. As **Figures 4F-G** showed that there were obvious increased positive stains for the single F4/80, and both F4/80 and TNF-α, i.e. inflammatory macrophages in model control group, compared to the normal mice, but those positive stains were decreased in FZHY or methylprednisolone treatment without difference between two treatments. These data revealed that FZHY treatment could significantly inhibited the aggregation of inflammatory macrophages in the lung.

FZHY Downregulated TNF-α Expression via NF-κB Pathway in LPS-Stimulated BMDMs

To elucidate the regulatory mechanism of FZHY on TNF-α expression in macrophages, we investigated the anti-inflammatory effects of FZHY on LPS-stimulated BMDMs. Firstly, BMDMs were incubated with 25–200 μg/ml of FZHY for 24 h, and there was no obvious cell toxicity during this dose scope. Secondly, BMDMs were exposed with 100 ng/ml and 200 ng/ml of LPS to induce proinflammatory polarization *in vitro, respectively.* Subsequently, cells were incubated with 25–100 μg/ml of FZHY for 24 h, the contents of TNF-α and IL-6 in cell supernatant were significantly inhibited by FZHY with

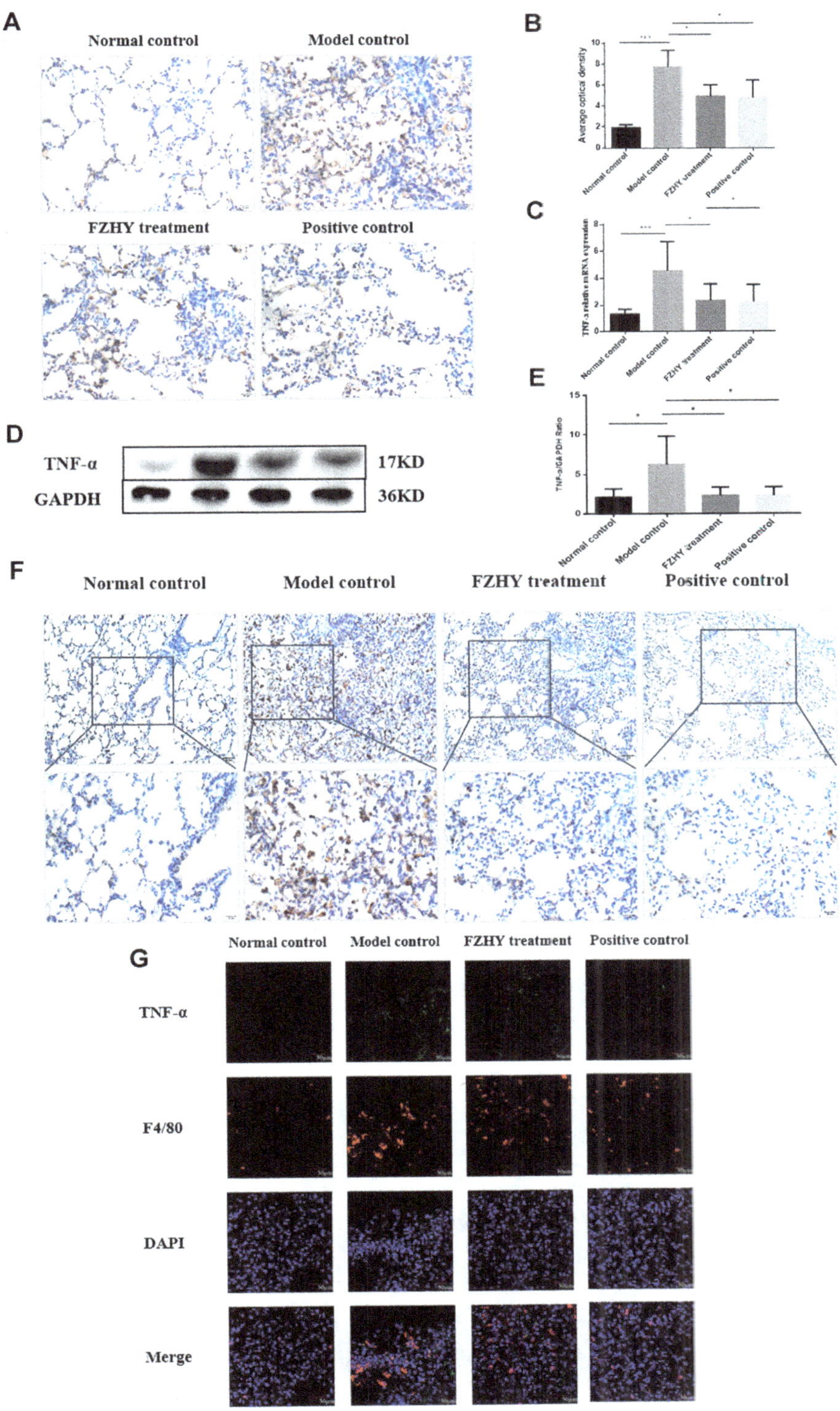

FIGURE 4 | FZHY reduced expression of TNF-α in macrophages in mice Pulmonary Fibrosis *in vivo* **(A–B)** Immunohistochemistry for expression of TNF-α in the lung tissue (A; magnification, ×400) and semi-quantitative analysis for the positive-stain of TNF-α **(B)**. **(C)** mRNA expression of TNF-α in the lung tissue. **(D–E)** Western blot for TNF-α of the lung tissue **(D)** and histograms for Western blot results **(E)**. **(F)** Immunohistochemistry for expression of F4/80 in the lung tissue. **(G)** Representative immunofluorescence confocal microscopy images of F4/80 and TNF-α; red transfected into F4/80; green transfected into TNF-α. $^{*}p < 0.05$; $^{**}p < 0.01$; $^{***}p < 0.001$.

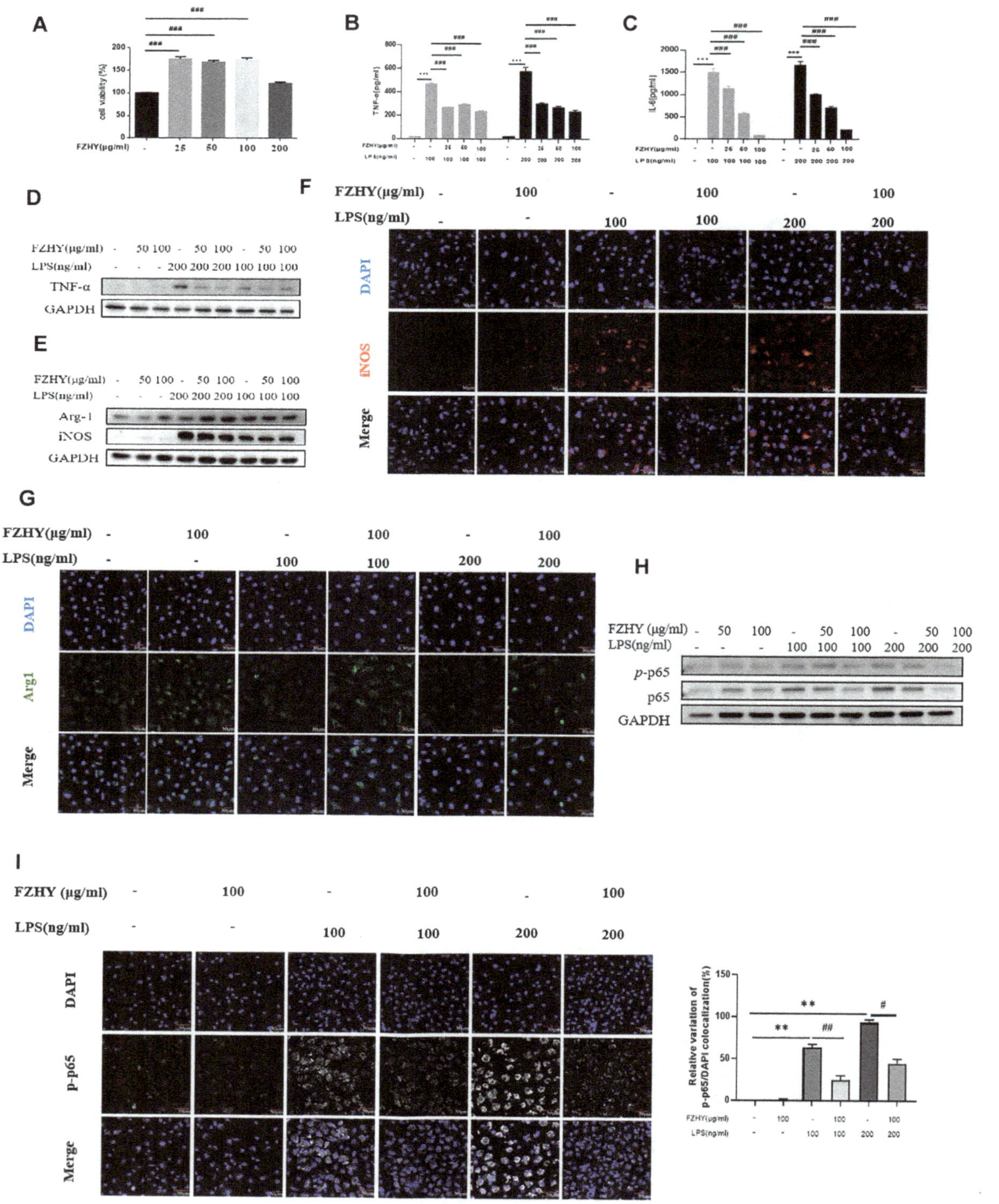

FIGURE 5 | FZHY reduced the expression of TNF-α in LPS-inducedmacrophages in vitro. (A) Viability ofBMDMsat 24 h incubatedwith different concentrations of FZHY assessed byCCK8assay.BMDMswere treated withLPS (100 or 200 ng/ml) with or without FZHY(25 μg/ml, 50 μg/ml, 100 μg/ml) for 24 h (B–C) Levels of TNF-α and IL-6 in supernatant after 24 h incubated with different concentrations of FZHY observed by Elisa kits. (D) Western blot analysis for TNF-α, (E) Arg1 and iNos of the LPS-stimulated BMDMs. Representative immunofluorescence microscopy images of iNos (F) and Arg1 (G). (H) Western blot analysis for p65 and p-p65 production in the LPS-stimulated BMDMs.(I) Representative images of immunofluorescence staining of p-p65 NF-κB (white) nuclear translocation. Cell nuclei are detected by 4′,6-diamidino-2-phenylindole (DAPI) (blue). Scale bars, 50 μm. Semi-quantitative evaluation of p-p65NF-κB nuclear translocation, as evidenced by the colocalization experiments.Results are expressed asmeans ± SDof the relative percentage of p-p65 nuclei-positively stained cells to the total number of cells. Ten fields per condition were analyzed. *$p < 0.05$, **$p < 0.01$, ***$p < 0.001$; #$p < 0.05$, ##$p < 0.01$, ###$p < 0.001$.

a dose dependent manner (**Figures 5B,C**), which revealed that FZHY might be able to act a vital role in resisting inflammation by M1 macrophage polarization *in vitro*.

To confirm the anti-inflammatory effect of FZHY *in vitro*, we checked TNF-α expression with by western blot, the results showed that FZHY incubation for 24 h decreased TNF-α expression in LPS stimulated BMDM (**Figure 5D; Supplementary Figure S5D**). Besides, FZHY decreased the levels of iNos and enhanced Arg-1 (**Figure 5E; Supplementary Figure S5E**), respectively. In addition, compared with those in the LPS-simulated BMDMs (**Figures 5F,G**), immunofluorescence stains of Arg-1 and iNos were exhibited with the same tendency after FZHY incubation.

In further analysis, expression of component (p65) of NF-κB, the key transcription factor of TNF-α signal pathway, was significantly increased after LPS stimulation at a dose dependent manner. In contrast, levels of NF-κB components in pro-inflammatory BMDMs were effectively down-regulated in **Figures 5H,I; Supplementary Figure S5H**. The NF-κB nuclear translocation was moderately blocked after incubation of FZHY, which was demonstrated by the positive nuclear immunostaining (**Figures 5H,I; Supplementary Figure S5H**). Taken together, these results implicated that FZHY could inhibit activation of proinflammatory macrophages through NF-κB/TNF-α pathway.

DISCUSSION

Pulmonary fibrosis is characterized by an excess accumulation of collagen deposition in the lung tissue, accompanied by progressive dyspnea and worsening of pulmonary function with a high mortality rate. It has highly heterogeneous etiologies and complicated pathologic mechanisms. Although fibroblasts activation and differentiation played a pivot role in lung fibrogenesis, inflammatory mediators such as TNF and IL-1β have an important effect on the initiation and development of lung fibrosis. Macrophages and many other cells produce TNF after exposure to silica and bleomycin etc. While, methylprednisolone, the most used drug to inhibit inflammatory diseases in clinic, was effective for some type of lung fibrosis (Wynn, 2011). In current study, we firstly found that TNF-α related pathway could be the target of FZHY against lung fibrosis with informatic analysis, then FZHY was confirmed to inhibit the development of lung fibrosis in bleomycin-induced mice model, whereas methylprednisolone used as a positive control. Lastly, it revealed that the action mechanism of FZHY against lung fibrosis was associated with NF-κB/TNF-α signaling in LPS-stimulated macrophage.

Lung fibrosis is an orchestra process involving integrating mechanisms. TCM or herbal medicines comprise various active components, which could produce synergistic or antagonistic interactions among components through its multicomponent and multitarget principles (Wang et al., 2014). It is difficult to understand and uncover the main action mechanism of TCM due to its complexity. While a network pharmacology approach has the characteristic of integration and entirety, which is a very suitable tool to predict the target profiles and pharmacological mechanisms of active substances in TCM (Li and Zhang, 2013). FZHY formula, a traditional Chinese medicine formula, is used to treat liver fibrosis and cirrhosis in China. FZHY has been shown to have no serious adverse reactions and exerts antifibrotic effects through targeting multiple molecules (Chen et al., 2019). In our previous studies, FZHY could protect lung injury and fibrosis induced by bleomycin in rats, and improve pulmonary function in patients with COPD [Published in Chinese]. Herein, we applied the network pharmacology method to predict the mechanism of FZHY on lung fibrosis development. Given FZHY and other TCM products were taken orally, OB (Xu et al., 2012) and DL (Walters and Murcko, 2002), two ADME-related models, are the main factors affecting the absorption of drugs in gastrointestinal tract. Thus, we screened the bioactive components of FZHY by using two parameters: OB ≥ 30% and DL ≥ 0.18. A total of 197 active components were identified as FZHY-related genes, and 12 Differentially Expressed Genes (DEGs) were identified by bioinformatical analysis. To understand the relevant gene functions and the possible pathways of 12 DEGs, GO and KEGG pathway enrichment was analyzed through R software. The results revealed that TNF signaling pathway was markedly ranked first for FZHY action mechanism against lung fibrosis.

Studies have shown that TNF was a prerequisite for the development of pulmonary fibrosis, and $TNF^{-/-}$ mice were completely unaffected by inflammation and fibrosis. The expression of TNF could not only trigger the initial acute inflammatory response to bleomycin-induced lung tissue injury, but also provide chronic inflammatory signals and lead to the progress of pulmonary fibrosis (Oikonomou et al., 2006). Therefore, the treatment strategy of inhibiting TNF production is of great significance in the treatment of pulmonary fibrosis. Based on the analysis results of network pharmacology, we further verified the anti-pulmonary fibrosis mechanism of FZHY by inhibiting TNF pathway *in vivo* and *in vitro*. Inflammatory macrophages are the main source of TNF(Shapouri-Moghaddam et al., 2018). In our animal experiment, the histological results showed that inflammation and coagulative necrosis were pronounced in the bleomycin-treated mice, while FZHY and methylprednisolone reduced lung inflammation and collagen deposition *in vivo*. Given inflammation is closely associated with the infiltration of macrophages in the lung, expressions of TNF-α and F4/80, a gold marker for macrophage, were observed to locate the origin of cells that mainly expressed TNF-α. The double staining result showed that macrophage is the main resource of TNF-α and increased in bleomycin-induced pulmonary fibrosis in mice. Meanwhile, FZHY and methylprednisolone decreased $TNF\text{-}\alpha^{+}F4/80^{+}$ cell staining. It indicated that FZHY might inhibit experimental pulmonary fibrosis via down-regulate the activation of pro-inflammatory macrophages expressing TNF-α. In the *in-vitro* study, we revealed that FZHY inhibited pro-inflammatory macrophages activation, demonstrated by a decrease in release of TNF-α, IL-6 and iNOS, but increase of Arg1 in LPS-induced BMDMs. These above results suggested that FZHY might play an anti-pulmonary fibrosis role by inhibiting the inflammatory polarization of macrophages and reducing the production of TNF.

The most potent stimulus for eliciting TNF production by macrophage is LPS(Shapouri-Moghaddam et al., 2018), which could promote TNF production via NF-kB pathway (Tang et al.,

2021). Therefore, blockade of NF-kB pathway is crucial step to inhibit macrophage activation and improve inflammation. NF-κB phosphorylation is a hallmark of NF-κB function to activate NF-κB-dependent transcription (Chen and Ivashkiv, 2010). p65 is one of the important subunits of NF-κB. Inhibiting p65 activation, that is, inhibiting the production of p-p65, can reduce LPS-induced acute lung injury and reduce the production of TNF(Yang et al., 2021). In the study, we observed NF-κB nuclear translocation in LPS-stimulated activation of pro-inflammatory macrophages with confocal immunofluorescence, and found that FZHY could significantly reduce the production and nuclear translocation of p65, indicating that FZHY could inhibit macrophage activation and inflammation via NF-κB/TNF-α pathway.

Our work indicates that macrophage is the important target cell for the therapy of pulmonary fibrosis, which was also proposed in liver fibrosis (Tacke, 2017). However, whether FZHY could influence lung fibroblasts directly via NF-κB/TNF-α pathway? What is the anti-pulmonary fibrosis molecular target in NF-κB/TNF-α pathway for the active components of FZHY? The answers to these questions would be our next research topic.

CONCLUSION

FZHY was effective in alleviating pulmonary fibrosis, whose action mechanism was associated with regulation of NF-κB/TNF-α signaling pathway in pro-inflammatory macrophages. These findings provided an important strategy for developing new agents against lung fibrosis and accelerated FZHY product application on patients with lung fibrosis.

AUTHOR CONTRIBUTIONS

CL and FX conceived and designed the project; FJ, XC, YP, JX, and KH conducted the experiments; YP and FJ analyzed the data and wrote the manuscript; YP and XH revised the manuscript; CL made the final critical revision to the manuscript.

REFERENCES

Ahluwalia, N., Shea, B. S., and Tager, A. M. (2014). New Therapeutic Targets in Idiopathic Pulmonary Fibrosis. Aiming to Rein in Runaway Wound-Healing Responses. *Am. J. Respir. Crit. Care Med.* 190, 867–878. doi:10.1164/rccm.201403-0509PP

Ashburner, M., Ball, C. A., Blake, J. A., Botstein, D., Butler, H., Cherry, J. M., et al. (2000). Gene Ontology: Tool for the Unification of Biology. The Gene Ontology Consortium. *Nat. Genet.* 25, 25–29. doi:10.1038/75556

Austyn, J. M., and Gordon, S. (1981). F4/80, a Monoclonal Antibody Directed Specifically against the Mouse Macrophage. *Eur. J. Immunol.* 11, 805–815. doi:10.1002/eji.1830111013

Budinger, G. R., Mutlu, G. M., Eisenbart, J., Fuller, A. C., Bellmeyer, A. A., Baker, C. M., et al. (2006). Proapoptotic Bid Is Required for Pulmonary Fibrosis. *Proc. Natl. Acad. Sci. U S A.* 103, 4604–4609. doi:10.1073/pnas.0507604103

Chen, J., Hu, Y., Chen, L., Liu, W., Mu, Y., and Liu, P. (2019). The Effect and Mechanisms of Fuzheng Huayu Formula against Chronic Liver Diseases. *Biomed. Pharmacother.* 114, 108846. doi:10.1016/j.biopha.2019.108846

Chen, J., and Ivashkiv, L. B. (2010). IFN-γ Abrogates Endotoxin Tolerance by Facilitating Toll-like Receptor-Induced Chromatin Remodeling. *Proc. Natl. Acad. Sci. U S A.* 107, 19438–19443. doi:10.1073/pnas.1007816107

Chua, F., Gauldie, J., and Laurent, G. J. (2005). Pulmonary Fibrosis: Searching for Model Answers. *Am. J. Respir. Cell Mol Biol* 33, 9–13. doi:10.1165/rcmb.2005-0062TR

Dai, G. Z., Chen, R. X., and Wei, H. C. (2006). Effect of Dahuang Zhechong Pill on Content of Amino Acids in Hippocampal Tissue of Ischemic Cerebral Hemorrhagic Rats. *Zhongguo Zhong Xi Yi Jie He Za Zhi* 26, 538–540.

Hamosh, A., Scott, A. F., Amberger, J. S., Bocchini, C. A., and Mckusick, V. A. (2005). Online Mendelian Inheritance in Man (OMIM), a Knowledgebase of Human Genes and Genetic Disorders. *Nucleic Acids Res.* 33, D514–D517. doi:10.1093/nar/gki033

Kanehisa, M., Sato, Y., Furumichi, M., Morishima, K., and Tanabe, M. (2019). New Approach for Understanding Genome Variations in KEGG. *Nucleic Acids Res.* 47, D590–D595. doi:10.1093/nar/gky962

Karimi-Shah, B. A., and Chowdhury, B. A. (2015). Forced Vital Capacity in Idiopathic Pulmonary Fibrosis-FDA Review of Pirfenidone and Nintedanib. *N. Engl. J. Med.* 372, 1189–1191. doi:10.1056/NEJMp1500526

Kim, S., Chen, J., Cheng, T., Gindulyte, A., He, J., He, S., et al. (2019). PubChem 2019 Update: Improved Access to Chemical Data. *Nucleic Acids Res.* 47, D1102–D1109. doi:10.1093/nar/gky1033

King, T. E., Jr., Bradford, W. Z., Castro-Bernardini, S., Fagan, E. A., Glaspole, I., Glassberg, M. K., et al. (2014). A Phase 3 Trial of Pirfenidone in Patients with Idiopathic Pulmonary Fibrosis. *N. Engl. J. Med.* 370, 2083–2092. doi:10.1056/NEJMoa1402582

Kingwell, K. (2014). InterMune and Boehringer Blaze Trails for Idiopathic Pulmonary Fibrosis Drugs. *Nat. Rev. Drug Discov.* 13, 483–484. doi:10.1038/nrd4382

Lee, S. H., Starkey, P. M., and Gordon, S. (1985). Quantitative Analysis of Total Macrophage Content in Adult Mouse Tissues. Immunochemical Studies with Monoclonal Antibody F4/80. *J. Exp. Med.* 161, 475–489. doi:10.1084/jem.161.3.475

Li, S., and Zhang, B. (2013). Traditional Chinese Medicine Network Pharmacology: Theory, Methodology and Application. *Chin. J. Nat. Med.* 11, 110–120. doi:10.1016/S1875-5364(13)60037-0

Liu, C., Hu, Y., Xu, L., Liu, C., and Liu, P. (2009). Effect of Fuzheng Huayu Formula and its Actions against Liver Fibrosis. *Chin. Med.* 4, 12. doi:10.1186/1749-8546-4-12

Liu, H. L., Lv, J., Zhao, Z. M., Xiong, A. M., Tan, Y., Glenn, J. S., et al. (2019). Fuzhenghuayu Decoction Ameliorates Hepatic Fibrosis by Attenuating Experimental Sinusoidal Capillarization and Liver Angiogenesis. *Sci. Rep.* 9, 18719. doi:10.1038/s41598-019-54663-4

Liu, Z., Guo, F., Wang, Y., Li, C., Zhang, X., Li, H., et al. (2016). BATMAN-TCM: a Bioinformatics Analysis Tool for Molecular mechANism of Traditional Chinese Medicine. *Sci. Rep.* 6, 21146. doi:10.1038/srep21146

Noble, P. W., Barkauskas, C. E., and Jiang, D. (2012). Pulmonary Fibrosis: Patterns and Perpetrators. *J. Clin. Invest.* 122, 2756–2762. doi:10.1172/JCI60323

Oikonomou, N., Harokopos, V., Zalevsky, J., Valavanis, C., Kotanidou, A., Szymkowski, D. E., et al. (2006). Soluble TNF Mediates the Transition from Pulmonary Inflammation to Fibrosis. *PLoS One* 1, e108. doi:10.1371/journal.pone.0000108

Ru, J., Li, P., Wang, J., Zhou, W., Li, B., Huang, C., et al. (2014). TCMSP: a Database of Systems Pharmacology for Drug Discovery from Herbal Medicines. *J. Cheminform* 6, 13. doi:10.1186/1758-2946-6-13

Shapouri-Moghaddam, A., Mohammadian, S., Vazini, H., Taghadosi, M., Esmaeili, S. A., Mardani, F., et al. (2018). Macrophage Plasticity, Polarization, and Function in Health and Disease. *J. Cell Physiol* 233, 6425–6440. doi:10.1002/jcp.26429

Stelzer, G., Rosen, N., Plaschkes, I., Zimmerman, S., Twik, M., Fishilevich, S., et al. (2016). The GeneCards Suite: From Gene Data Mining to Disease Genome Sequence Analyses. *Curr. Protoc. Bioinformatics* 54, 1.30.1–1.30.33. doi:10.1002/cpbi.5

Szklarczyk, D., Franceschini, A., Wyder, S., Forslund, K., Heller, D., Huerta-Cepas, J., et al. (2015). STRING V10: Protein-Protein Interaction Networks, Integrated over the Tree of Life. *Nucleic Acids Res.* 43, D447–D452. doi:10.1093/nar/gku1003

Tacke, F. (2017). Targeting Hepatic Macrophages to Treat Liver Diseases. *J. Hepatol.* 66, 1300–1312. doi:10.1016/j.jhep.2017.02.026

Tan, S. Z., Liu, C. H., Zhang, W., Lu, X., Ye, W. C., Cai, Z. Z., et al. (2007). Effects of Fuzheng Huayu Recipe on MMP-2 Activity and Type IV Collagen Expression at Fibrotic Lung. *Zhongguo Zhong Yao Za Zhi* 32, 835–839.

Tang, J., Xu, L., Zeng, Y., and Gong, F. (2021). Effect of Gut Microbiota on LPS-Induced Acute Lung Injury by Regulating the TLR4/NF-kB Signaling Pathway. *Int. Immunopharmacol* 91, 107272. doi:10.1016/j.intimp.2020.107272

Walters, W. P., and Murcko, M. A. (2002). Prediction of 'drug-Likeness'. *Adv. Drug Deliv. Rev.* 54, 255–271. doi:10.1016/s0169-409x(02)00003-0

Wang, C. Y., Bai, X. Y., and Wang, C. H. (2014). Traditional Chinese Medicine: a Treasured Natural Resource of Anticancer Drug Research and Development. *Am. J. Chin. Med.* 42, 543–559. doi:10.1142/S0192415X14500359

Wang, T., Zhou, X., Liu, H., Wang, J., Zhang, P., Zhu, Y., et al. (2018). Fuzheng Huayu Capsule as an Adjuvant Treatment for HBV-Related Cirrhosis: A Systematic Review and Meta-Analysis. *Phytother Res.* 32, 757–768. doi:10.1002/ptr.6009

Ward, P. A., and Hunninghake, G. W. (1998). Lung Inflammation and Fibrosis. *Am. J. Respir. Crit. Care Med.* 157, S123–S129. doi:10.1164/ajrccm.157.4.nhlbi-10

Wu, R., Dong, S., Cai, F. F., Chen, X. L., Yang, M. D., Liu, P., et al. (2019). Active Compounds Derived from Fuzheng Huayu Formula Protect Hepatic Parenchymal Cells from Apoptosis Based on Network Pharmacology and Transcriptomic Analysis. *Mol.*24, 338. doi:10.3390/molecules24020338

Wynn, T. A. (2011). Integrating Mechanisms of Pulmonary Fibrosis. *J. Exp. Med.* 208, 1339–1350. doi:10.1084/jem.20110551

Wynn, T. A., and Vannella, K. M. (2016). Macrophages in Tissue Repair, Regeneration, and Fibrosis *Immunity* 44, 450–462. doi:10.1016/j.immuni.2016.02.015

Xu, X., Zhang, W., Huang, C., Li, Y., Yu, H., Wang, Y., et al. (2012). A Novel Chemometric Method for the Prediction of Human Oral Bioavailability. *Int. J. Mol. Sci.* 13, 6964–6982. doi:10.3390/ijms13066964

Yang, K., Li, B., and Chen, J. (2021). Knockdown of Phosphoinositide-dependent Kinase 1 (PDK1) Inhibits Fibrosis and Inflammation in Lipopolysaccharide-Induced Acute Lung Injury Rat Model by Attenuating NF-κB/p65 Pathway Activation. *Ann. Transl Med.* 9, 1671 doi:10.21037/atm-21-5476

Yao, Y., Wang, Y., Zhang, Z., He, L., Zhu, J., Zhang, M., et al. (2016). Chop Deficiency Protects Mice against Bleomycin-Induced Pulmonary Fibrosis by Attenuating M2 Macrophage Production. *Mol. Ther.* 24, 915–925. doi:10.1038/mt.2016.36

Yu, G., Wang, L. G., Yan, G. R., and He, Q. Y. (2015). DOSE: an R/Bioconductor Package for Disease Ontology Semantic and Enrichment Analysis. *Bioinformatics* 31, 608–609. doi:10.1093/bioinformatics/btu684

Zhang, M., Liu, H. L., Huang, K., Peng, Y., Tao, Y. Y., Zhao, C. Q., et al. (2020). Fuzheng Huayu Recipe Prevented and Treated CCl4-Induced Mice Liver Fibrosis through Regulating Polarization and Chemotaxis of Intrahepatic Macrophages via CCL2 and CX3CL1. *Evid. Based Complement. Alternat Med.* 2020, 8591892. doi:10.1155/2020/8591892

11

Electronic Cigarette Exposure Enhances Lung Inflammatory and Fibrotic Responses in COPD Mice

*Hongwei Han[1,2], Guangda Peng[1], Maureen Meister[3], Hongwei Yao[4], Jenny J. Yang[5], Ming-Hui Zou[6], Zhi-Ren Liu[1] and Xiangming Ji[3]**

[1]Department of Biology, Georgia State University, Atlanta, GA, United States, [2]Division of Pulmonary and Critical Care, Department of Medicine, Massachusetts General Hospital, Harvard Medical School, Boston, MA, United States, [3]Department of Nutrition, Georgia State University, Atlanta, GA, United States, [4]Division of Biology and Medicine, Department of Molecular Biology, Cell Biology and Biochemistry, Brown University, Providence, RI, United States, [5]Department of Chemistry, Georgia State University, Atlanta, GA, United States, [6]Center for Molecular and Translational Medicine, Georgia State University, Atlanta, GA, United States

***Correspondence:**
Xiangming Ji
xji4@gsu.edu

Although a few studies show that the use of electronic nicotine delivery systems (ENDS) may ameliorate objective and subjective outcomes in COPD smokers who switched to electronic cigarettes, it is unclear whether e-cigarette exposure alters lung pathological features and inflammatory response in COPD. Here, we employed βENaC-overexpressing mice bearing COPD-like pulmonary abnormality, and exposed them to ENDS. We found that ENDS exposure aggravated airspace enlargement and mucus production in βENaC-overexpressing mice, which was associated with increased MMP12 and Muc5ac, respectively. ENDS exposure to mice significantly increased the numbers of macrophages, particularly in M2 macrophages in bronchoalveolar lavage (BAL) fluid, despite ENDS did not induce M2 macrophage polarization in a cultured murine macrophage cell line (RAW264.7). There were no changes in neutrophils in BAL fluid by ENDS exposure. Multiple cytokine productions were increased including M-CSF, IL-1rα, IL-10, and TGF-β1, in BAL fluid from mice when exposed to ENDS. The Sirius Red staining and hydroxyproline assay showed ENDS-exposed mice displayed enhanced fibrotic phenotypes compared to control mice. In conclusion, ENDS exposure enhances airspace enlargement, mucus secretion, and fibrogenesis in COPD mice. This is associated with increased MMP12, inflammatory responses, and M2 macrophage phenotype. This study provides pre-clinical data implicating that electronic cigarette exposure is not safe in COPD patients who want to replace traditional cigarettes with ENDS.

Keywords: ENDS, COPD, M2 macrophage, lung fibrosis, inflammation

INTRODUCTION

Electronic nicotine delivery systems (ENDS), also referred to as e-cigarettes, are electronic devices that produce an aerosol by heating a liquid that contains nicotine predominantly (Breland et al., 2017). ENDS is generated for stopping traditional cigarette smoking that is a major risk factor for chronic obstructive pulmonary disease (COPD). Some studies show that ENDS use may ameliorate objective and subjective outcomes in COPD smokers who switched to e-cigarettes, which is associated with abstinence and conventional smoking reduction (Polosa et al., 2016;

Polosa et al., 2020). However, ENDS is not safe. Emerging evidence shows that ENDS trigger severe lung injuries and lead to the development of various lung diseases (Shields et al., 2017; Gilpin, 2019; Bhatt et al., 2020; Bhatta and Glantz, 2020; Mcalinden et al., 2020; Traboulsi et al., 2020). In 2019, an epidemic of E-cigarette-associated lung injury affected 49 states of the United States with over 2,600 cases and 60 deaths reported (Belok et al., 2020; Cherian et al., 2020). Moreover, growing evidence reveals that ENDS use is directly associated with the diagnosis of COPD in humans in recent years, and the exposure to ENDS is reported to induce COPD-like phenotype in mice (Garcia-Arcos et al., 2016; Bowler et al., 2017; Perez et al., 2019; Xie et al., 2020). However, the mechanisms have not been fully uncovered yet.

COPD is a primary leading cause of death affecting an estimated 328 million worldwide (Eisner et al., 2010; Quaderi and Hurst, 2018). It is characterized by progressive and irreversible airflow obstruction caused by chronic lung inflammation, in which innate immune cells play a pivotal role (Rovina et al., 2013; Barnes, 2016). Especially, macrophages are key effector cells in COPD which orchestrate immune responses (Kapellos et al., 2018). Macrophages are observed remarkedly increased in lung tissues and bronchoalveolar lavage (BAL) fluid of COPD patients and are associated with COPD severity (Hiemstra, 2013). In general, macrophages consist of two major phenotypes (Mosser and Edwards, 2008). M1 macrophages, referred to as classically activated macrophages, have been described as cytotoxic and pro-inflammatory, and are characterized by secretion of pro-inflammatory cytokines such as interferon (IFN)-γ, IL-6, and IL-12 (Mantovani et al., 2004; Mantovani et al., 2013). M2 macrophages, referred to as alternatively activated macrophages, are considered anti-inflammatory and are related to tissue repair and fibrosis, producing majorly anti-inflammatory cytokines including transforming growth factor β1 (TGF-β1), IL-4, IL-10, M-CSF (Gordon and Martinez, 2010; Martinez and Gordon, 2014; Chávez-Galán et al., 2015). Two phenotypes can switch between each other by different stimuli (Das et al., 2015; Funes et al., 2018). Multiply research groups have reported an alteration of immunophenotypes of macrophages towards M2 phenotype in COPD subjects, with cytokine production skew towards an M2 profile in blood and BAL samples from patients, suggesting M2 macrophages phenotype is a critical player in COPD disease progression (Eapen et al., 2017a; Eapen et al., 2017b; Da Silva et al., 2020). However, it is unclear whether macrophages undergo phenotype alterations after ENDS exposure in COPD, understanding of which would be of great importance to uncover the impact of ENDS on COPD.

It has been shown that βENaC-overexpressing mice have COPD-like pulmonary abnormalities, including mucous hypersecretion, inflammatory and emphysematous phenotypes and pulmonary dysfunction (Johannesson et al., 2012; Seys et al., 2015; Shuto et al., 2016). In this study, we employed βENaC-overexpressing mice and exposed them to ENDS to determine whether ENDS aggravate or exacerbate COPD-like pathological changes. We also measured macrophage immunophenotype and lung fibrogenesis in these mice exposed to ENDS. We observed a significant exacerbation of COPD features in these mice, along with a remarkable change in multiple cytokine production in COPD mice after exposure to ENDS. Further investigations elucidated that the ENDS challenge increased the total macrophage population but did not change neutrophil numbers. Macrophage phenotype was altered with an increase in M2 phenotype after ENDS exposure. In addition, fibrotic phenotypes were enhanced in ENDS-exposed mice, evidenced by a dramatic increase in the level of pro-fibrotic cytokine TGF-β1 and an augment in collagen production. For the first time, our study shows that the ENDS affect macrophage phenotype alteration during COPD development in mice, which leads to an enhancement of lung fibrosis.

MATERIALS AND METHODS

Animal Model

βENaC mice with C57BL/6J background were obtained from the Jackson Laboratory. All animal procedures described were approved by the Institutional Animal Care and Use Committee (IACUC) at Georgia State University. βENaC mice were bred with wild-type C57BL/6J mice to produce hemizygous βENaC for our studies. Animals were genotyped to determine the genetic overexpression of *Scnn1b*. Briefly, tail snips were harvested and lysed in Proteinase K at 56°C water bath overnight. DNA was extracted by Dneasy Blood and Tissue kit (Qiagen, Foster City, CA). The overexpression of the mouse *Scnn1b* gene was identified by PCR (Forward: CCTCCAAGA GTTCAACTACCG; Reverse: TCTACCAGCTCAGCCACA GTG) (Mall et al., 2004). After PCR, samples were run on a 4% agarose gel containing ethidium bromide. Mice carrying *Scnn1b* overexpression were tagged as βENaC mice for future studies.

Electronic Nicotine Delivery Systems Exposure to βENaC Mice

At 12-week of age, mice (n = 10/group) were randomized into either the ENDS exposure group or the control group. Mice in the ENDS group were exposed to e-cigarette vapor for 30 min daily at a frequency of 5 times per week for a total duration of 8 weeks as shown in **Figure 1A**. Mice were placed in a smoking chamber attached to an inExpose Smoking Robot (SCIREQ, Montreal, QC, Canada) with an attached e-cigarette accessory (ECX JoyeTech E-Vic Mini, SCIREQ, Canada) for the administration of vaporized S brand e-cigarette liquid containing nicotine at 50 mg/ml with caramel flavoring. After 8 weeks of e-cigarette vapor exposure, animals were euthanized within 24 h after the last e-cigarette vapor exposure using CO_2. Then, bronchoalveolar lavage (BAL) fluid, and lung tissues were collected for analysis as described below.

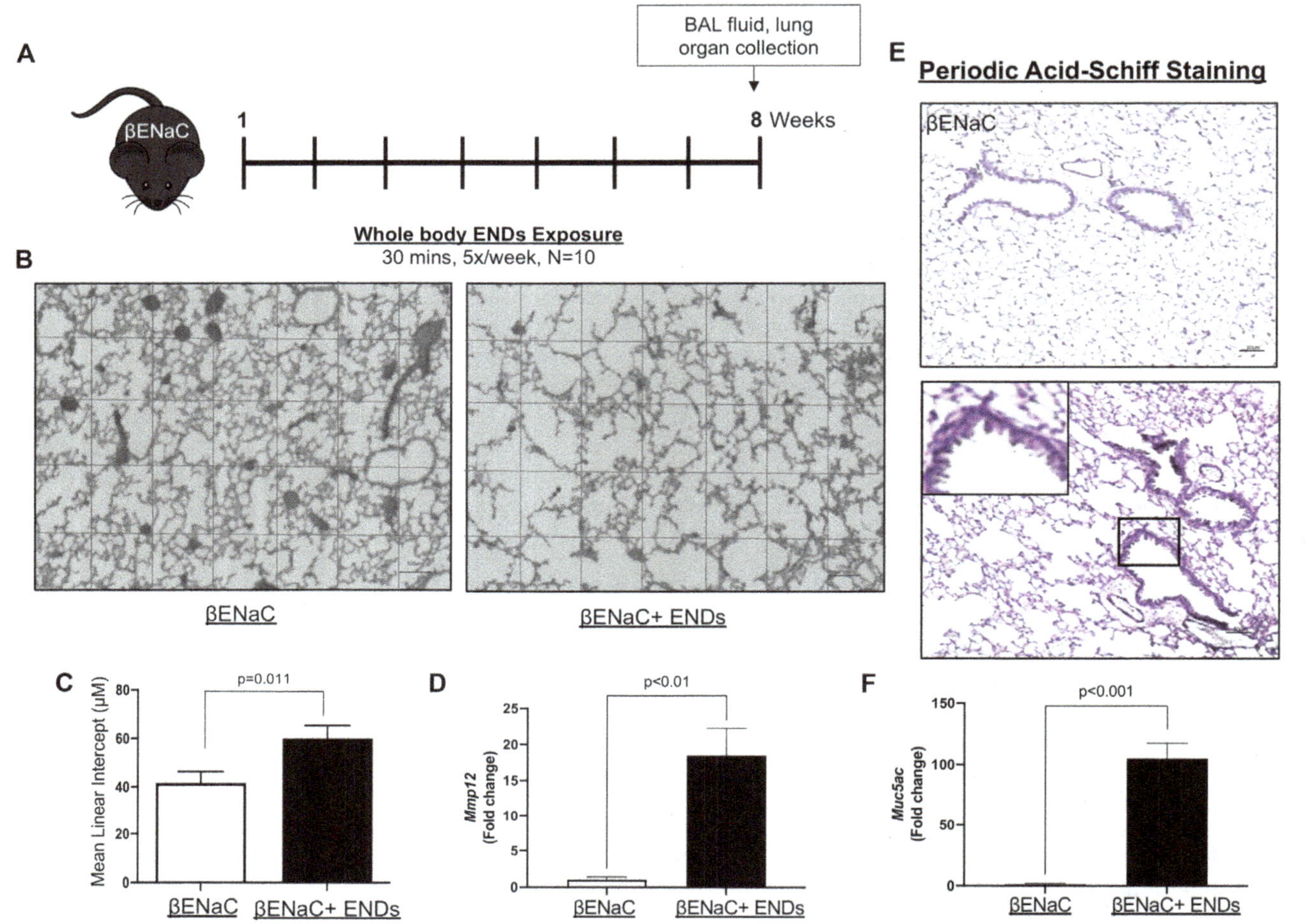

FIGURE 1 | E-cigarette exposure aggravates COPD in βENaC mice. **(A)** Experimental schematic of whole body ENDS exposure in βENaC mice. **(B)** ENDS exposure caused emphysematous phenotypes changes in βENaC mice. Representative data of H&E staining images using lung sections of sham air (left) (n = 4) or ENDS exposed (right) (n = 4) mice. **(C)** Quantification of the free distance between gas exchange surfaces in lungs of βENaC mice with or without ENDS exposure. **(D,F)** Determination of mRNA levels of COPD-related proteins MMP12 **(D)** and Muc5ac **(F)** in lung tissues from βENaC mice with or without ENDS exposure by qPCR. **(E)** Representative images of Periodic Acid-Schiff staining in lung sections of βENaC mice with or without ENDS exposure. The inset indicates the enlarged image of the boxed area showing positive staining. All data presented at mean ± SEM.

Cell Counts and Cytokine Measurements in Bronchoalveolar Lavage Fluid

After the mice were euthanized, tracheostomy was performed, and lungs were immediately flushed with 1 ml ice-cold phosphate-buffered saline (PBS) twice for collection of BAL fluid. Total cells from the BAL were centrifuged and counted using Countess™ II Automated Cell Counter (Invitrogen, Carlsbad, CA) as previously described (Mall et al., 2004). Total immune cell count (5,000 cells/slide) was performed on Shandon cytospin slides (Thermo Shandon, Pittsburgh, PA) stained with Diff-Quik (Dade Bering, Newark, DE). The BAL supernatants were stored at −80°C until analysis.

Morphometric Assessment

In order to determine the effects of ENDS exposure on the development of emphysema, we did a morphometric assessment according to the previous protocol (Bartalesi et al., 2005; Mall et al., 2008). Briefly, the mouse lungs were inflated with 1% low melting-point agarose to 25 cm of H_2O pressure. After 48 h of fixation, lungs were paraffin-embedded, sectioned, and stained with hematoxylin and eosin (H&E). The paraffin slides were baked at 60°C for 2 h, then deparaffinized with xylene and rehydrated with graded ethanol solutions. Next, the slides were incubated with Mayer's Hematoxylin for 10 min and washed under tap water for 10 min. Slides were then immersed in Eosin for 30 s and washed under tap water, after which, the slides were dehydrated and mounted with a mounting medium. Mean linear intercepts were determined and calculated (Dunnill, 1962).

Immunohistochemistry

The mouse lungs were inflated with 1% low melting-point agarose to 25 cm of fixative pressure and then fixed with 4%

neutral buffered formalin for 48 h. Later, these tissue samples were embedded in paraffin, and sectioned into 4 μm sections using a rotary microtome. For immunohistochemical analysis, tissue sections were deparaffinized with xylene and rehydrated with graded concentrations of ethanol, followed by antigen retrieval in 10 mM citric acid solution (pH = 6) for 20 min using a pressure cooker. Endogenous peroxidase activity was blocked by 3% hydrogen peroxide. After blocking with 5% BSA for 30 min, the slides were incubated with the primary antibodies against the following proteins at 4°C overnight: α-smooth muscle actin (α-SMA) 1:500 (Ab5694; Abcam); Arginase I 1:1,000 (sc-20150; Santa Cruz). After washing, the sections were incubated with the appropriate HRP polymers and developed with 3–3′ diaminobenzidine solution (DAB substrate kit; Vector Laboratories). After counterstaining with hematoxylin, the slides were dehydrated and mounted with a mounting medium.

Periodic-Acid Schiff Staining

Periodic-acid Schiff (PAS; Sigma Aldrich, Saint Louis, MO) staining was used to evaluate mucus accumulation and immune cell infiltration. The Periodic-acid Schiff staining was performed following the manufacturer's instructions. All images were taken at 20x magnification using Keyence Fluorescent Microscope (Keyence, Itasca, IL).

Sirius Red Staining

Sirius Red staining was performed with Novaultra Sirius Red Stain Kit (IW-3012, IHC world) following the instructions of the manufacturer. In brief, the paraffin-embedded slides were deparaffinized in xylene and hydrated in gradient concentrations of ethanol. The slides were stained with Weigert's hematoxylin for 8 min, followed by picro-sirius red for 1 h. After two washes in acidified water, slides were dehydrated, mounted in a resinous medium, and covered by cover slides.

Cell Culture

Raw264.7 cells were purchased from ATCC and cultured in DMEM media supplied with 10% fetal bovine serum. Raw264.7 cells were maintained in a cell culture incubator at 37°C and 5% CO_2. To test whether ENDS can induce macrophage polarization, Raw264.7 were incubated with DMSO or ENDS with nicotine (50 mg/ml) or IL-4+IL-13 (IL-4 20 ng/ml; IL-13 20 ng/ml) for 48 h and harvested for analysis of protein expression by western blot.

Flow Cytometry

Freshly harvested lung tissues were minced and dissociated using collagenase D (Sigma 11088858001, 0.5 mg/ml) and DNase I for 20 min at 37°C on a shaker. Cell suspensions were subsequently passed through a 40 μm cell strainer to get a single cell suspension. Non-specific Fc-mediated interactions were blocked by incubating cells with CD16/CD32 antibodies (Thermofisher, 14–0161–82). Cells were labeled with fluorophore-conjugated antibodies, including CD45-FITC (BioLegend 103,108), F4/80-PE/Cy5 (BioLegend, 123111), CD11b-APC (Thermofisher, 17–0112–82), Ly6G-BV421(BioLegend, 127627), CD206-e450 (Thermofisher, 48–2061–82). At the last step, Cells were resuspended in FACS staining buffer and acquired using LSRFortessa flow cytometer (BD Biosciences). Data were analyzed by FlowJo software (Tree Star).

RNA Isolation and RT-qPCR Analysis

The expressions of inflammatory cytokines, proteins, and growth factors were assessed with qPCR using lung tissues. The total RNA was isolated using the RNeasy Plus mini kit (Qiagen) according to the manufacturer's instructions. For RT-qPCR, 0.5 μg of total RNA was reverse-transcribed to cDNA using Maxima First Strand cDNA Synthesis Kit (Thermo Fisher K1641). Real-time qPCR was then performed using 2 μL of cDNA using Luna Universal qPCR Master Mix (NEB M3003) with SYBR® Green as the fluorescent dye and the 7,500 Fast Real-Time PCR System (Life Technologies). The primer pairs are used at a final concentration of 250 nM. Primer sequences are listed in the box below (**Table 1**). Cyclophilin was used as the reference gene. The relative transcript abundance of target genes compared with the reference gene was expressed in the cycle threshold (ΔCt) as ΔCt = Ct(target)—Ct(reference). The relative difference in transcript levels of the treated group compared with the control group was expressed as ΔΔCt = ΔCt(treated)—ΔCt(control). The relative fold changes in the transcript level were represented as $2^{-\Delta\Delta Ct}$.

Data Analysis

In the case of only two groups, two-tail *t*-tests were performed to assess the differences. All analyses were carried out using Prism7.0 software (GraphPad Software Inc., San Diego, CA). Values are represented as mean ± SEM. Levels of significance designated as $p < 0.05$ unless otherwise indicated.

RESULTS

E-Cigarette Exposure Aggravates Chronic Obstructive Pulmonary Disease in βENaC Mice

In our study, the *β*ENaC mice were given whole-body ENDS exposure as indicated (**Figure 1A**). At the end of the treatment, the mice were sacrificed, and organs were collected for further analysis. We observed that lung morphology was changed, and the lung normal structure integrity was damaged after ENDS exposure (**Figure 1B**). Further assessment of airspace size by mean linear intercept indicated that the free distance between gas exchange surfaces was significantly increased in ENDS-exposed mice by more than 40%, indicating that there were emphysematous changes to lungs (**Figures 1B,C**). Moreover, we observed a significant accumulation of mucus in bronchi after ENDS exposure (**Figure 1E**). Additionally, the expression levels of Muc5ac and Mmp12, which are highly involved in COPD (Caramori et al., 2009; Hunninghake et al., 2009; Churg et al., 2012; Li and Ye, 2020), were also increased after ENDS exposure (**Figures 1D,F**). Overall, the lung emphysema and mucus

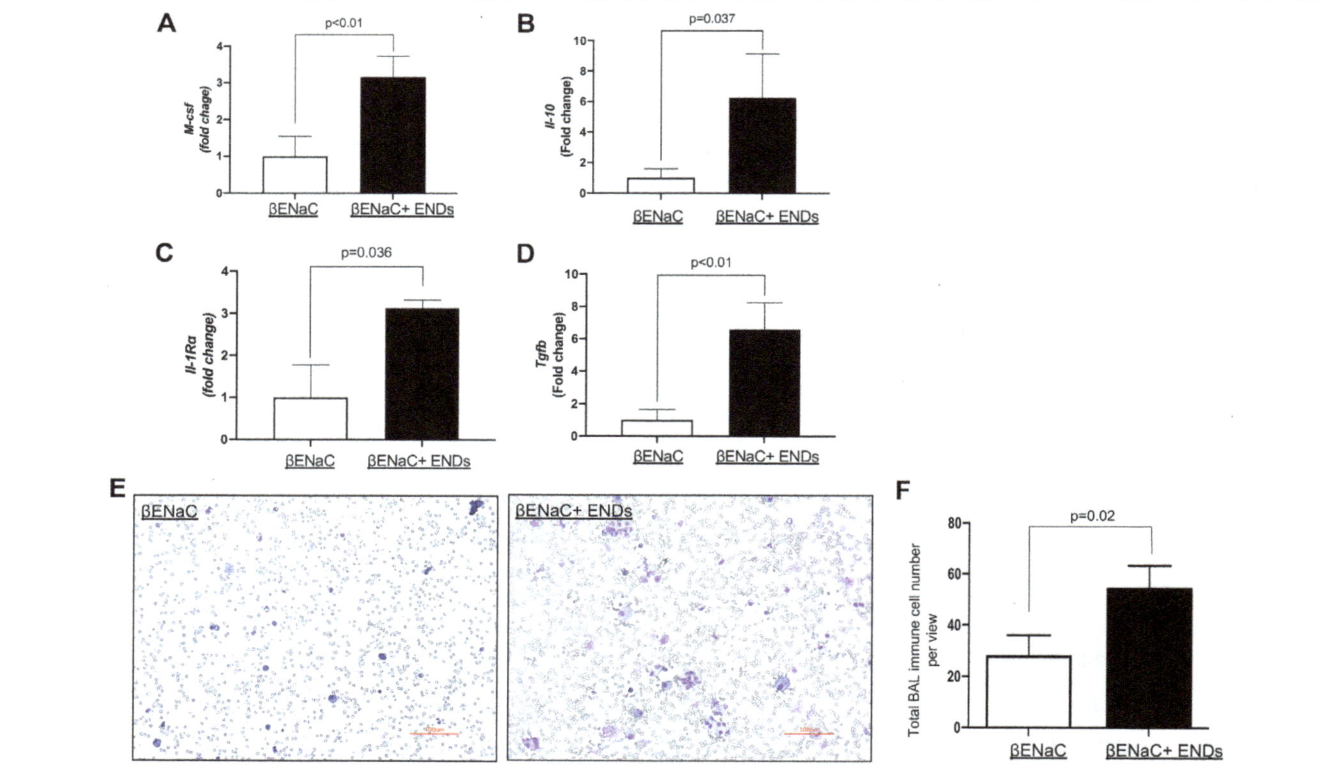

FIGURE 2 | E-cigarette exposure elevates inflammatory response. **(A–D)** Determination of mRNA levels of inflammatory cytokines in lung tissues from βENaC mice with or without ENDS exposure by qPCR. **(E)** Representative images of Diff-Quik staining of BAL from βENaC mice with or without ENDS exposure (n = 4 per group). **(F)** Quantification of Diff-Quik staining as in (E) (n = 4 per group). All data presented at mean ± SEM.

overproduction after ENDS exposure suggested ENDS aggravate COPD phenotype in βENaC mice background.

E-Cigarette Exposure Elevates the Inflammatory Response

COPD is characterized by lung inflammation, leading to progressive and irreversible airflow obstruction (King, 2015). Next, we determined the cytokine production in mice with or without exposure to ENDS. We measured the production of major cytokines by real-time qPCRs using lungs from mice of different groups. The results showed that the ENDS exposure significantly increased the production of multiple cytokines, including M-CSF, IL-1rα, IL-10, and TGF-β1(**Figures 2A–D**). In addition, the number of immune cells in BAL fluid collected from mice with ENDS exposure was remarkedly higher than that from mice without ENDS exposure (**Figures 2E,F**). Together, the ENDS elevate multiple cytokine production, indicating a skewed inflammation response.

E-Cigarette Increases Macrophage Numbers in Lungs

Since ENDS exposure significantly augmented levels of cytokines, which are predominantly secreted by immune cells, for instance, macrophages, so our next question was asked as to whether ENDS exposure modulated populations of immune cells. We then assessed the numbers of macrophages and neutrophils with FACS and found that ENDS exposure increased the numbers of macrophages (**Figures 3A,B**), but did not change that of neutrophils (**Figures 3C,D**).

E-Cigarette Increases the Population of M2 Phenotype of Macrophages

Macrophages have two subtypes, M1 and M2. M1 and M2 macrophages have different functions and distinct cytokine profiles. The qPCR results showed ENDS promoted the productions of multiple cytokines including M-CSF, IL-1rα, IL-10, and TGF-β1. Notably, IL-1rα, IL-10, and TGF-β1 are typical cytokines of the M2 phenotype of macrophages, especially IL-10, which is predominantly secreted by M2 macrophages (Martinez and Gordon, 2014; Da Silva et al., 2015; Rőszer, 2015). Therefore, we wondered whether ENDS exposure affected the M2 phenotype population. We used FACS to separate the non-M2 and M2 macrophage populations. The single cells were dissociated from lung tissues treated with and without ENDS and labeled by CD45, F4/80, and CD206. M2 macrophages were identified as $F4/80^{+}CD45^{+}CD206^{+}$ population while non-M2 macrophages as $F4/80^{+}$ $CD45^{+}CD206^{-}$ population

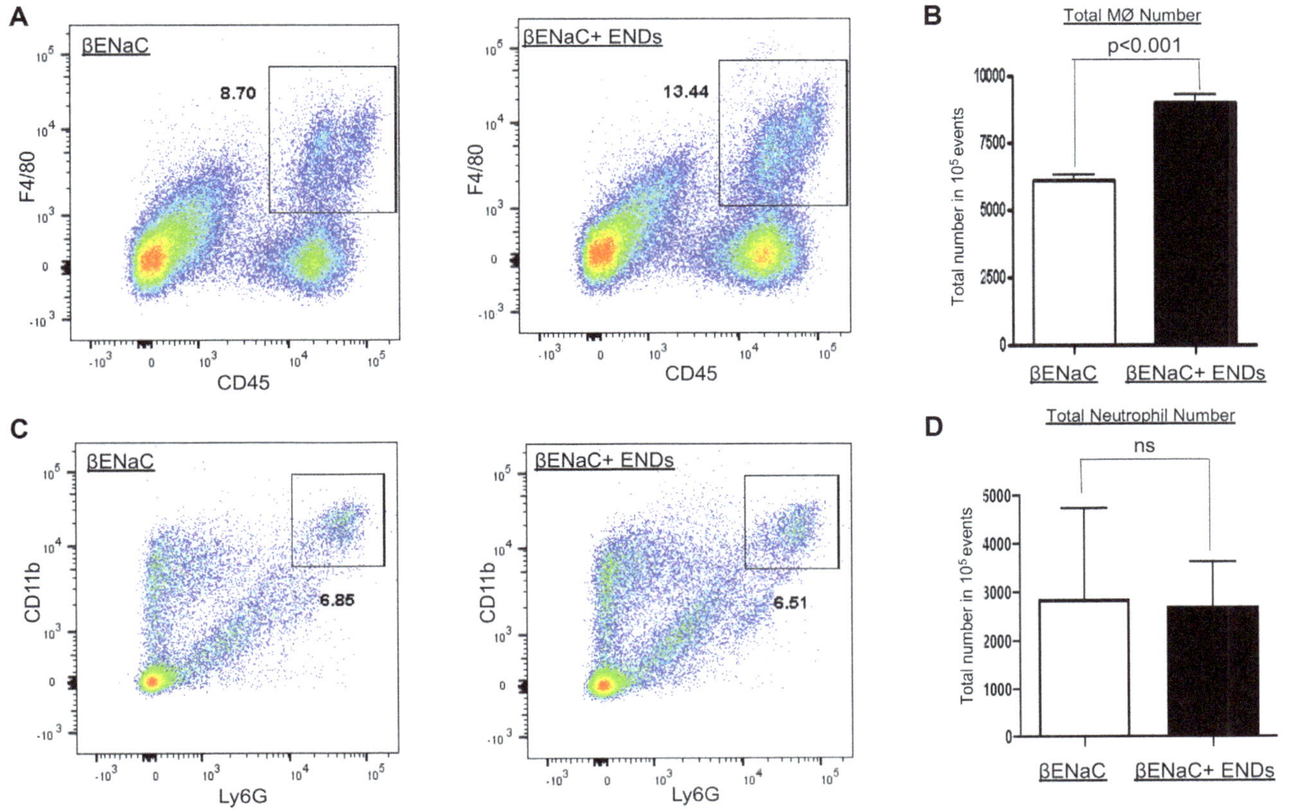

FIGURE 3 | E-cigarette increases macrophage numbers in lungs. **(A,C)** FACS analysis of cell population of $CD45^+F4/80^+$ macrophages and $CD11b^+Ly6G^+$ neutrophils in lung tissues of βENaC mice with or without ENDS exposure (*n* = 3 per group). **(B,D)** Quantification of FCAS analysis of macrophage and neutrophil population as in **(A)** and **(C)**, respectively. All data presented at mean ± SEM.

(**Figure 4A**). The results showed that both non-M2 and M2 populations were significantly increased by ~25 and ~50% respectively after ENDS exposure (**Figures 4B,C**). Notably, the increase in the M2 population was larger compared to the increase in the non-M2 population. We further quantified the percentage of M2 in total macrophages and found that the percentage of M2 in total macrophages was remarkably elevated after ENDS treatment (**Figure 4D**). In addition, we further assessed M2 macrophages by performing immunohistochemical staining of Arginase 1, a commonly used marker for M2 macrophages, in lungs from mice with and without ENDS exposure. The results showed that the staining of Arginase 1^+ M2 macrophages was significantly enriched in ENDS-treated mice (**Figures 4E,F**). Therefore, our results suggested ENDS exposure resulted in a phenotype alteration of macrophages towards M2 in mouse lungs.

Since we observed that ENDS increased the M2 macrophage population, then we asked whether ENDS directly induced M2 macrophages polarization. We tested our hypothesis using murine macrophage cell line Raw264.7. We treated Raw264.7 with DMSO, ENDS, or IL-4+IL-13 and then harvested cells for immunoblots of M2 marker Arginase 1. IL-4+IL-13, which are well-known to induce M2 macrophage polarization, are used as a positive control. Immunoblot results demonstrated that ENDS treatment did not increase Arginase 1 expression compared to DMSO treatment, while IL-4+IL-13 upregulated expression of Arginase 1 in Raw264.7 (**Figure 4G**). Our results suggest that ENDS do not induce M2 macrophage polarization directly in the cultured murine macrophage cell line.

E-Cigarette Exposure Enhances Fibrotic Phenotypes in the Lungs

Substantial studies have shown that M2 macrophages promote lung fibrosis (Song et al., 2000; Bargagli et al., 2011; Hou et al., 2018); and ENDS elevate extracellular matrix accumulation and profibrotic progress (Chapman et al., 2019; Shi et al., 2019; Wang et al., 2019; Wang et al., 2020), we next questioned whether fibrotic phenotypes were enhanced in the lungs after exposure to ENDS. We assessed collagen content using Sirius Red staining and found that ENDS exposure dramatically increased collagen levels in mice (**Figures 5A,B**). The collagen is predominantly produced by myofibroblasts, a group of key effector cells in fibrosis progression which is considered as a hallmark of fibrosis (Hinz, 2007; Hinz et al., 2007; Kendall and Feghali-Bostwick, 2014). We then stained myofibroblasts in lung

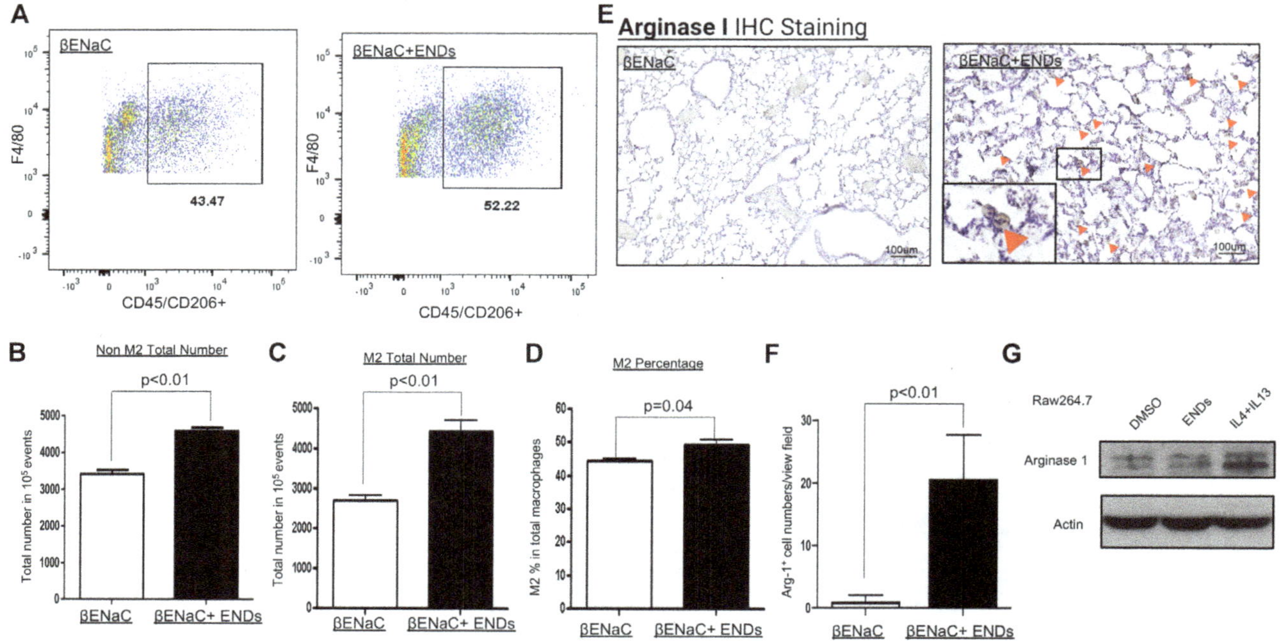

FIGURE 4 | E-cigarette increases the population of M2 phenotype of macrophages. **(A)** FACS analysis of the cell population of F4/80$^+$CD206$^+$ M2 macrophages in lung tissues of βENaC mice with or without ENDS exposure (n = 3 per group). The M2 macrophages were pre-gated on live CD45$^+$ cells. **(B)** Quantification of FACS analysis of CD45$^+$F4/80$^+$CD206$^-$ non-M2 macrophage cell number in lung tissues of βENaC mice with or without ENDS exposure. **(C)** Quantification of FACS analysis of CD45$^+$F4/80$^+$CD206$^+$ M2 macrophage cell number in lung tissues of βENaC mice with or without ENDS exposure. **(D)** Quantification of FACS analysis of CD206$^+$CD45$^+$F4/80$^+$ M2 phenotype percentage in CD45$^+$F4/80$^+$ total macrophages in lung tissues of βENaC mice with or without ENDS exposure. **(E)** Representative images of immunohistochemical (IHC) staining of Arginase I in lung tissues of βENaC mice with or without ENDS exposure. The inset indicates the enlarged image of the boxed area showing positive staining. **(F)** Quantification of IHC staining of Arginase I as in **(E)**. The positive staining areas were calculated as percentages of total area, using five randomly selected sections per mouse, a total of four mice in each group. **(G)** Representative blots showing the expression level of Arginase I after indicated treatments. Actin was used as an internal control. Raw264.7 were treated with DMSO or ENDS (50 mg/ml) or IL-4+IL-13 (IL-4 20 ng/ml; IL-13 20 ng/ml) for 48 h and harvested for analysis of protein expression by western blot. Columns and error bars represent means ± SEM.

tissues from mice with or without ENDS delivery, using a commonly used marker α-Smooth Muscle Actin (α-SMA). The result showed that ENDS treatment increased *the* α-SMA$^+$ myofibroblast population in the lungs (**Figures 5C,D**). In addition, the hydroxyproline contents were also remarkably increased in mice receiving ENDS treatment (**Figure 5E**). These results demonstrate that ENDS enhance lung fibrotic phenotypes in COPD mice.

DISCUSSION

Smoking is the leading cause of COPD, which accounts for as much as 90% of COPD risk. ENDS are considered as a safe replacement for cigarette smoking. However, increasing concerns have been raised in recent years as ENDS use shows a high correlation with COPD occurrence (Bowler et al., 2017; Perez et al., 2019), the underneath mechanisms of which have not been fully understood. Here we report that ENDS rewired cytokine production in lungs of COPD mice caused by ENDS exposure. Increasing evidence indicates that chronic inflammatory and immune responses play key roles in the development and progression of COPD (Rovina et al., 2013). Our study is the first one to elucidate that ENDS shaped an anti-inflammatory environment by increasing levels of several important anti-inflammatory cytokines and augmenting the population of the anti-inflammatory M2 phenotype of macrophages. We also found that ENDS increased fibrosis in COPD mice. It has been reported that the development of fibrosis in COPD results in a reduction in lung elasticity, which further worsens COPD (Rovina et al., 2013).

We demonstrated that ENDS exposure elevated inflammation response and enhanced lung fibrosis. Lung inflammation and fibrosis are both essentially implicated in the development and progression of COPD; and they also are closed correlated (Ward and Hunninghake, 1998; Rao et al., 2020). Observations that lung tissues from patients with lung fibrosis display significant inflammation are widely documented, suggesting that the inflammatory process could result in lung fibrosis (Ward and Hunninghake, 1998; Bringardner et al., 2008). Intensive investigations reveal that fibrosis seems to be the end outcome of unresolved chronic inflammatory reactions induced by a variety of stimuli and tissue injury (Wynn, 2008). Specifically, in COPD, the pathogenesis usually starts with an inflammatory process (Cornwell et al., 2010). Under certain circumstances, inflammation reactions are not resolved. Such a chronic,

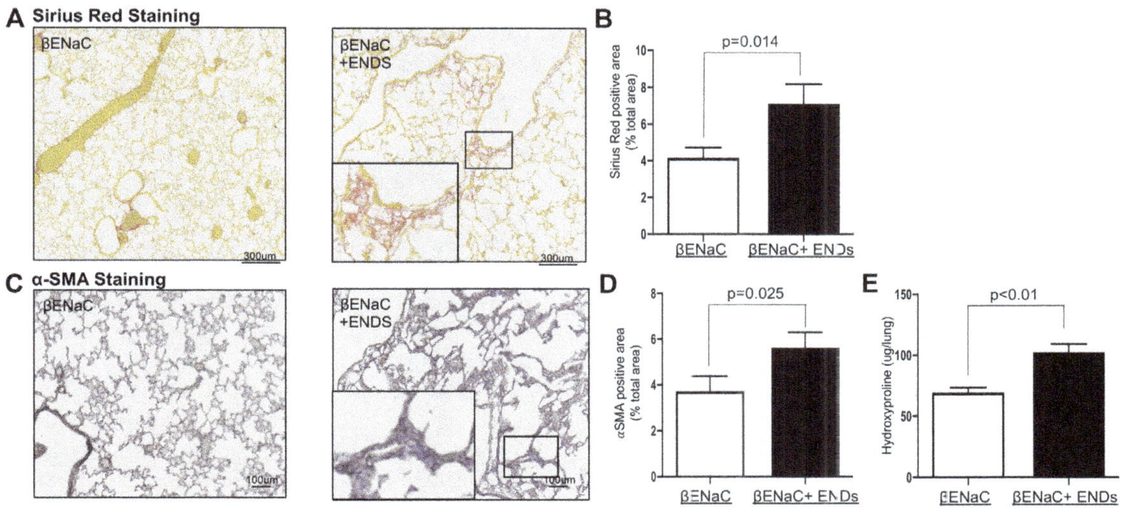

FIGURE 5 | E-cigarette exposure enhances fibrosis in the lungs. **(A)** Representative images of Pico-Sirius Red staining in lung sections from βENaC mice with or without ENDS exposure ($n = 4$ per group). The inset indicates the enlarged image of the boxed area showing positive staining. **(B)** Quantitative analysis of Pico-Sirius Red staining as in **(A)**. The positive staining areas were calculated as percentages of total area, using five randomly selected sections per mouse, a total of four mice in each group. **(C)** Representative images of α-SMA IHC staining in lung sections from βENaC mice with or without ENDS exposure ($n = 4$ per group). The inset indicates the enlarged image of the boxed area showing positive staining. **(D)** Quantitative analysis of α-SMA IHC staining as in **(C)**. The positive staining areas were calculated as percentages of total area, using five randomly selected sections per mouse, a total of four mice in each group. **(E)** Measurement of collagen contents by hydroxyproline assay using lung tissues of βENaC mice with or without ENDS exposure ($n = 4$ per group). Columns and error bars represent means ± SEM.

TABLE 1 | PCR primers used in this study.

Gene	Species	Forward sequence	Reverse sequence
Cyclophilin	Mouse	CTTCGAGCTGTTTGCAGACAA AGT	AGATGCCAGGACCTGTATGCT
SCNN1B	Mouse	CCTCCAAGAGTTCAACTACCG	TCTACCAGCTCAGCCACAGTG
M-CSF	Mouse	ATGAGCAGGAGTATTGCCAAGG	TCCATTCCCAATCATGTGGCTA
IL-1Rα	Mouse	GCTCATTGCTGGGTACTTACAA	CCAGACTTGGCACAAGACAGG
IL-10	Mouse	GCTCTTACTGACTGGCATGAG	CGCAGCTCTAGGAGCATGTG
MMP12	Mouse	CGCAGCTCTAGGAGCATGTG	TGGGCTAGTGTACCACCTTTG
Muc5ac	Mouse	GGACTTCAATATCCAGCTACGC	CAGCTCAACAACTAGGCCATC
TGFβ-1	Mouse	CTCCCGTGGCTTCTAGTGC	GCCTTAGTTTGGACAGGATCTG

persistent inflammatory response results in extensive fibrosis, and consequently, causes an exacerbation of COPD conditions (Barnes, 2014; Barnes, 2019). In the current study, we found that ENDS exposure elevated inflammation response by increasing multiple cytokine production and enhanced pro-fibrotic activity by augmenting M2 macrophage numbers, both of which worsen the COPD symptoms in mice.

We observed ENDS exposure remarkedly elevated the population of M2 macrophages. The balance of M1/M2 macrophages is well-recognized to control the fate of an organ in inflammation or fibrosis (Patel et al., 2017; Chen et al., 2020). M1 macrophages are known as a pro-inflammatory or anti-fibrotic phenotype as they trigger inflammatory responses by producing proinflammatory cytokines and contribute to tissue destruction (Byrne et al., 2016). Conversely, M2 macrophages are known as an anti-inflammatory or pro-fibrotic phenotype, which are implicated in the aberrant wound-healing process during fibrosis by producing pro-fibrotic cytokines (Byrne et al., 2016; Shapouri-Moghaddam et al., 2018). M2 macrophage numbers are reported to be elevated during fibrotic disease; and excessive M2 macrophages contribute to a pathological fibroproliferative response and consequently promote lung fibrosis found in the later phase of acute lung injury and acute respiratory distress syndrome (Janssen et al., 2011; Xiang et al., 2016). Our finding showing that ENDS elevated M2 macrophage numbers suggests ENDS could lead to a fibrotic amplification which may exacerbate COPD in patients.

We further intended to uncover the underlying mechanisms of how ENDS promoted the alteration of macrophage phenotype. We asked whether ENDS directly regulated the M2 phenotype switch. ENDS is commonly made up of four basic ingredients: water, nicotine, flavorings, and propylene glycol (PG) and/or vegetable glycerin base (VG). Nicotine is usually thought to be the major toxic component in ENDS. It has been shown that cigarette smoke extract (CSE) and pure nicotine can induce M2 phenotype change (Lu et al., 2017; Alqasrawi et al., 2020), so we hypothesized that ENDS may directly induce macrophage M2 polarization *via* nicotine.

However, murine macrophage Raw264.7 did not display an increase in Arginase 1 expression level after the treatment of nicotine-containing ENDS juice, which means the ENDS might not directly induce macrophage M2 polarization. This suggests the importance of vaping smoking in causing the M2 macrophage phenotype. Our results elucidated that anti-inflammatory cytokines were increased after ENDS delivery. Such change in cytokines profile is reported as a stimulus to induce macrophage polarization in murine models of emphysema (Kohler et al., 2019). So, the change in cytokine profile, instead of being a consequence of M2 macrophage polarization, might be the cause of M2 macrophage phenotype change.

Myofibroblasts are major effector cells during lung injury and repair. Our results showed that ENDS exposure increased the number of α-SMA$^+$ myofibroblasts. The crosstalk between myofibroblast and macrophages has been well-recognized in fibrotic diseases and cancer (Comito et al., 2014; Van Linthout et al., 2014; Fernando et al., 2016; Hou et al., 2018; Johnson et al., 2018; An et al., 2020). Macrophages, especially M2 macrophages release abundant TGF-β1 which is a major driver of the activation of myofibroblasts (Hou et al., 2018). On the other hand, myofibroblasts are active in the secretion of a number of cytokines and chemokines, which are reported to enhance the recruitment and activity of macrophages (Bagalad et al., 2017; Monteran and Erez, 2019). Therefore, another plausible mechanism is that ENDS altered macrophage phenotype through myofibroblast-secreted mediators indirectly, which needs further investigations.

Besides, a typical feature of widespread peribronchiolar fibrosis with collagen deposition in COPD patients suggests fibrosis is probably the earliest and an important mechanism for COPD progression, which however has been long neglected with very few studies (Mcdonough et al., 2011; Hogg et al., 2017; Koo et al., 2018; Barnes, 2019). In this study, we have also investigated fibrotic phenotypes in mice after ENDS exposure. We observed a significant increase in collagen accumulation and α-SMA positive myofibroblast population, indicating ENDS enhanced fibrotic phenotypes in COPD mice. It is plausible that the increase in M2 macrophages induced by ENDS results in the augment of fibrotic phenotypes.

In addition, a notable phenomenon in our study is that ENDS remarkably enriched the myofibroblast population, suggesting ENDS might induce the activation of myofibroblasts. The myofibroblast is the predominant cell type that is responsible for the deposition of extracellular matrix and is considered as a hallmark of fibrotic diseases (Hinz et al., 2007; Hinz, 2016; Pakshir et al., 2020). And we observed lung fibrosis was enhanced in mice who received ENDS exposure. It would be interesting to understand whether ENDS can stimulate the differentiation of fibroblasts to myofibroblasts. This might uncover another potential risk of ENDS as it might promote lung fibrosis development *via* inducing myofibroblasts differentiation.

In conclusion, our study elucidates that ENDS exposure elevates COPD features and causes inflammatory response alteration with an increase in M2 macrophage number. The changes in inflammatory response resulted from ENDS further lead to an enhancement in lung fibrosis. Our study provides us a deeper understanding of the mechanism how ENDS affects COPD. Lastly, though βENaC-overexpressing mice serve as a good species exposed to ENDS for induction of animal model of COPD, the effect of ENDS on wild type mice still requires further investigations.

AUTHOR CONTRIBUTIONS

HH, GP, MM, and XJ planned and designed experiments and wrote the manuscript. HH, GP, and MM carried out the animal studies performed molecular and cell biology experiments. HH and GP acquired histology analysis. GP performed flow cytometry and FACs analysis. HY, JY, M-HZ, Z-RL, and XJ provided intellectual oversight and reviewed the manuscript. HY provided pathological support and statistical analyses.

ACKNOWLEDGMENTS

We thank Jian-dong Li (Georgia State University) for his useful discussions.

REFERENCES

Alqasrawi, D., Abdelli, L. S., and Naser, S. A. (2020). Mystery Solved: Why Smoke Extract Worsens Disease in Smokers with Crohn's Disease and Not Ulcerative Colitis? Gut MAP!. *Microorganisms* 8, 666. doi:10.3390/microorganisms8050666

An, Y., Liu, F., Chen, Y., and Yang, Q. (2020). Crosstalk between Cancer-associated Fibroblasts and Immune Cells in Cancer. *J. Cel Mol Med* 24, 13–24. doi:10.1111/jcmm.14745

Bagalad, B., Mohan Kumar, K., and Puneeth, H. (2017). Myofibroblasts: Master of Disguise. *J. Oral Maxillofac. Pathol.* 21, 462–463. doi:10.4103/jomfp.jomfp_146_15

Bargagli, E., Prasse, A., Olivieri, C., Muller-Quernheim, J., and Rottoli, P. (2011). Macrophage-Derived Biomarkers of Idiopathic Pulmonary Fibrosis. *Pulm. Med.* 2011, 717130. doi:10.1155/2011/717130

Barnes, P. J. (2014). Cellular and Molecular Mechanisms of Chronic Obstructive Pulmonary Disease. *Clin. Chest Med.* 35, 71–86. doi:10.1016/j.ccm.2013.10.004

Barnes, P. J. (2016). Inflammatory Mechanisms in Patients with Chronic Obstructive Pulmonary Disease. *J. Allergy Clin. Immunol.* 138, 16–27. doi:10.1016/j.jaci.2016.05.011

Barnes, P. J. (2019). Small Airway Fibrosis in COPD. *Int. J. Biochem. Cel Biol.* 116, 105598. doi:10.1016/j.biocel.2019.105598

Bartalesi, B., Cavarra, E., Fineschi, S., Lucattelli, M., Lunghi, B., Martorana, P. A., et al. (2005). Different Lung Responses to Cigarette Smoke in Two Strains of Mice Sensitive to Oxidants. *Eur. Respir. J.* 25, 15–22. doi:10.1183/09031936.04.00067204

Belok, S. H., Parikh, R., Bernardo, J., and Kathuria, H. (2020). E-cigarette, or Vaping, Product Use-Associated Lung Injury: a Review. *Pneumonia* 12, 1–8. doi:10.1186/s41479-020-00075-2

Bhatt, J. M., Ramphul, M., and Bush, A. (2020). An Update on Controversies in E-Cigarettes. *Paediatric Respir. Rev.* 36, 75. doi:10.1016/j.prrv.2020.09.003

Bhatta, D. N., and Glantz, S. A. (2020). Association of E-Cigarette Use with Respiratory Disease Among Adults: a Longitudinal Analysis. *Am. J. Prev. Med.* 58, 182–190. doi:10.1016/j.amepre.2019.07.028

Bowler, R. P., Hansel, N. N., Hansel, N. N., Jacobson, S., Graham Barr, R., Make, B. J., et al. (2017). Electronic Cigarette Use in US Adults at Risk for or with COPD: Analysis from Two Observational Cohorts. *J. Gen. Intern. Med.* 32, 1315–1322. doi:10.1007/s11606-017-4150-7

Breland, A., Soule, E., Lopez, A., Ramôa, C., El-Hellani, A., and Eissenberg, T. (2017). Electronic Cigarettes: what Are They and what Do They Do?. *Ann. N.Y. Acad. Sci.* 1394, 5–30. doi:10.1111/nyas.12977

Bringardner, B. D., Baran, C. P., Eubank, T. D., and Marsh, C. B. (2008). The Role of Inflammation in the Pathogenesis of Idiopathic Pulmonary Fibrosis. *Antioxid. Redox Signaling* 10, 287–302. doi:10.1089/ars.2007.1897

Byrne, A. J., Maher, T. M., and Lloyd, C. M. (2016). Pulmonary Macrophages: A New Therapeutic Pathway in Fibrosing Lung Disease?. *Trends Mol. Med.* 22, 303–316. doi:10.1016/j.molmed.2016.02.004

Caramori, G., Casolari, P., Di Gregorio, C., Saetta, M., Baraldo, S., Boschetto, P., et al. (2009). MUC5AC Expression Is Increased in Bronchial Submucosal Glands of Stable COPD Patients. *Histopathology* 55, 321–331. doi:10.1111/j.1365-2559.2009.03377.x

Chapman, D. G., Casey, D. T., Ather, J. L., Aliyeva, M., Daphtary, N., Lahue, K. G., et al. (2019). The Effect of Flavored E-Cigarettes on Murine Allergic Airways Disease. *Scientific Rep.* 9, 13671. doi:10.1038/s41598-019-50223-y

Chávez-Galán, L., Olleros, M. L., Vesin, D., and Garcia, I. (2015). Much More Than M1 and M2 Macrophages, There Are Also CD169(+) and TCR(+) Macrophages. *Front. Immunol.* 6, 263. doi:10.3389/fimmu.2015.00263

Chen, X., Tang, J., Shuai, W., Meng, J., Feng, J., and Han, Z. (2020). Macrophage Polarization and its Role in the Pathogenesis of Acute Lung Injury/acute Respiratory Distress Syndrome. *Inflamm. Res.* 69, 883–895. doi:10.1007/s00011-020-01378-2

Cherian, S. V., Kumar, A., and Estrada-Y-Martin, R. M. (2020). E-cigarette or Vaping Product-Associated Lung Injury: a Review. *Am. J. Med.* 133, 657–663. doi:10.1016/j.amjmed.2020.02.004

Churg, A., Zhou, S., and Wright, J. L. (2012). Matrix Metalloproteinases in COPD. *Eur. Respir. J.* 39, 197–209. doi:10.1183/09031936.00121611

Comito, G., Giannoni, E., Segura, C. P., Barcellos-De-Souza, P., Raspollini, M. R., Baroni, G., et al. (2014). Cancer-associated Fibroblasts and M2-Polarized Macrophages Synergize during Prostate Carcinoma Progression. *Oncogene* 33, 2423–2431. doi:10.1038/onc.2013.191

Cornwell, W., Kim, V., Song, C., and Rogers, T. (2010). Pathogenesis of Inflammation and Repair in Advanced COPD. *Semin. Respir. Crit. Care Med.* 31, 257–266. doi:10.1055/s-0030-1254066

Da Silva, C. O., Gicquel, T., Daniel, Y., Bartholo, T., Vene, E., Loyer, P., et al. (2020). Alteration of Immunophenotype of Human Macrophages and Monocytes after Exposure to Cigarette Smoke. *Scientific Rep.* 10, 1–13. doi:10.1038/s41598-020-68753-1

Da Silva, M. D., Bobinski, F., Sato, K. L., Kolker, S. J., Sluka, K. A., and Santos, A. R. S. (2015). IL-10 Cytokine Released from M2 Macrophages Is Crucial for Analgesic and Anti-inflammatory Effects of Acupuncture in a Model of Inflammatory Muscle Pain. *Mol. Neurobiol.* 51, 19–31. doi:10.1007/s12035-014-8790-x

Das, A., Sinha, M., Datta, S., Abas, M., Chaffee, S., Sen, C. K., et al. (2015). Monocyte and Macrophage Plasticity in Tissue Repair and Regeneration. *Am. J. Pathol.* 185, 2596–2606. doi:10.1016/j.ajpath.2015.06.001

Dunnill, M. S. (1962). Quantitative Methods in the Study of Pulmonary Pathology. *Thorax* 17, 320–328. doi:10.1136/thx.17.4.320

Eapen, M. S., Hansbro, P. M., Mcalinden, K., Kim, R. Y., Ward, C., Hackett, T. L., et al. (2017a). Abnormal M1/M2 Macrophage Phenotype Profiles in the Small Airway wall and Lumen in Smokers and Chronic Obstructive Pulmonary Disease (COPD). *Sci. Rep.* 7, 13392. doi:10.1038/s41598-017-13888-x

Eapen, M. S., Myers, S., Walters, E. H., and Sohal, S. S. (2017b). Airway Inflammation in Chronic Obstructive Pulmonary Disease (COPD): a True Paradox. *Expert Rev. Respir. Med.* 11, 827–839. doi:10.1080/17476348.2017.1360769

Eisner, M. D., Anthonisen, N., Coultas, D., Kuenzli, N., Perez-Padilla, R., Postma, D., et al. (2010). An Official American Thoracic Society Public Policy Statement: Novel Risk Factors and the Global burden of Chronic Obstructive Pulmonary Disease. *Am. J. Respir. Crit. Care Med.* 182, 693–718. doi:10.1164/rccm.200811-1757st

Fernando, M. R., Giembycz, M. A., and Mckay, D. M. (2016). Bidirectional Crosstalk via IL-6, PGE2 and PGD2 between Murine Myofibroblasts and Alternatively Activated Macrophages Enhances Anti-inflammatory Phenotype in Both Cells. *Br. J. Pharmacol.* 173, 899–912. doi:10.1111/bph.13409

Funes, S. C., Rios, M., Escobar-Vera, J., and Kalergis, A. M. (2018). Implications of Macrophage Polarization in Autoimmunity. *Immunology* 154, 186–195. doi:10.1111/imm.12910

Garcia-Arcos, I., Geraghty, P., Baumlin, N., Campos, M., Dabo, A. J., Jundi, B., et al. (2016). Chronic Electronic Cigarette Exposure in Mice Induces Features of COPD in a Nicotine-dependent Manner. *Thorax* 71, 1119–1129. doi:10.1136/thoraxjnl-2015-208039

Gilpin, W. (2019). Cellular Automata as Convolutional Neural Networks. *Phys. Rev. E* 100, 032402. doi:10.1103/physreve.100.032402

Gordon, S., and Martinez, F. O. (2010). Alternative Activation of Macrophages: Mechanism and Functions. *Immunity* 32, 593–604. doi:10.1016/j.immuni.2010.05.007

Hiemstra, P. S. (2013). Altered Macrophage Function in Chronic Obstructive Pulmonary Disease. *Ann. ATS* 10, S180–S185. doi:10.1513/annalsats.201305-123aw

Hinz, B. (2007). Formation and Function of the Myofibroblast during Tissue Repair. *J. Invest. Dermatol.* 127, 526–537. doi:10.1038/sj.jid.5700613

Hinz, B. (2016). Myofibroblasts. *Exp. Eye Res.* 142, 56–70. doi:10.1016/j.exer.2015.07.009

Hinz, B., Phan, S. H., Thannickal, V. J., Galli, A., Bochaton-Piallat, M.-L., and Gabbiani, G. (2007). The Myofibroblast. *Am. J. Pathol.* 170, 1807–1816. doi:10.2353/ajpath.2007.070112

Hogg, J. C., Paré, P. D., and Hackett, T.-L. (2017). The Contribution of Small Airway Obstruction to the Pathogenesis of Chronic Obstructive Pulmonary Disease. *Physiol. Rev.* 97, 529. doi:10.1152/physrev.00025.2015

Hou, J., Shi, J., Chen, L., Lv, Z., Chen, X., Cao, H., et al. (2018). M2 Macrophages Promote Myofibroblast Differentiation of LR-MSCs and Are Associated with Pulmonary Fibrogenesis. *Cell Commun. Signaling* 16, 89. doi:10.1186/s12964-018-0300-8

Hunninghake, G. M., Cho, M. H., Tesfaigzi, Y., Soto-Quiros, M. E., Avila, L., Lasky-Su, J., et al. (2009). MMP12,Lung Function, and COPD in High-Risk Populations. *N. Engl. J. Med.* 361, 2599–2608. doi:10.1056/nejmoa0904006

Janssen, W. J., Barthel, L., Muldrow, A., Oberley-Deegan, R. E., Kearns, M. T., Jakubzick, C., et al. (2011). Fas Determines Differential Fates of Resident and Recruited Macrophages during Resolution of Acute Lung Injury. *Am. J. Respir. Crit. Care Med.* 184, 547–560. doi:10.1164/rccm.201011-1891oc

Johannesson, B., Hirtz, S., Schatterny, J., Schultz, C., and Mall, M. A. (2012). CFTR Regulates Early Pathogenesis of Chronic Obstructive Lung Disease in βENaC-overexpressing Mice. *PloS one* 7, e44059. doi:10.1371/journal.pone.0044059

Johnson, Z. I., Lopresti, S., Lantonio, B., Wells, A., Ismail, N., Brown, B. N., et al. (2018). Bi-directional Macrophage-Fibroblast Crosstalk Directs Wound Resolution Factors. *FASEB J.* 32, 412–414. doi:10.1096/fasebj.2018.32.1_supplement.414.2

Kapellos, T. S., Bassler, K., Aschenbrenner, A. C., Fujii, W., and Schultze, J. L. (2018). Dysregulated Functions of Lung Macrophage Populations in COPD. *J. Immunol. Res.* 2018, 2349045. doi:10.1155/2018/2349045

Kendall, R. T., and Feghali-Bostwick, C. A. (2014). Fibroblasts in Fibrosis: Novel Roles and Mediators. *Front. Pharmacol.* 5, 123. doi:10.3389/fphar.2014.00123

King, P. T. (2015). Inflammation in Chronic Obstructive Pulmonary Disease and its Role in Cardiovascular Disease and Lung Cancer. *Clin. translational Med.* 4, 68. doi:10.1186/s40169-015-0068-z

Kohler, J. B., Cervilha, D. A. B., Riani Moreira, A., Santana, F. R., Farias, T. M., Alonso Vale, M. I. C., et al. (2019). Microenvironmental Stimuli Induce Different Macrophage Polarizations in Experimental Models of Emphysema. *Biol. Open* 8, bio040808. doi:10.1242/bio.040808

Koo, H.-K., Vasilescu, D. M., Booth, S., Hsieh, A., Katsamenis, O. L., Fishbane, N., et al. (2018). Small Airways Disease in Mild and Moderate Chronic Obstructive Pulmonary Disease: a Cross-Sectional Study. *Lancet Respir. Med.* 6, 591–602. doi:10.1016/s2213-2600(18)30196-6

Li, J., and Ye, Z. (2020). The Potential Role and Regulatory Mechanisms of MUC5AC in Chronic Obstructive Pulmonary Disease. *Molecules* 25, 4437. doi:10.3390/molecules25194437

Lu, J., Xie, L., Liu, C., Zhang, Q., and Sun, S. (2017). PTEN/PI3k/AKT Regulates Macrophage Polarization in Emphysematous Mice. *Scand. J. Immunol.* 85, 395–405. doi:10.1111/sji.12545

Mall, M. A., Harkema, J. R., Trojanek, J. B., Treis, D., Livraghi, A., Schubert, S., et al. (2008). Development of Chronic Bronchitis and Emphysema in β-Epithelial

Na+Channel-Overexpressing Mice. *Am. J. Respir. Crit. Care Med.* 177, 730–742. doi:10.1164/rccm.200708-1233oc

Mall, M., Grubb, B. R., Harkema, J. R., O'neal, W. K., and Boucher, R. C. (2004). Increased Airway Epithelial Na+ Absorption Produces Cystic Fibrosis-like Lung Disease in Mice. *Nat. Med.* 10, 487–493. doi:10.1038/nm1028

Mantovani, A., Biswas, S. K., Galdiero, M. R., Sica, A., and Locati, M. (2013). Macrophage Plasticity and Polarization in Tissue Repair and Remodelling. *J. Pathol.* 229, 176–185. doi:10.1002/path.4133

Mantovani, A., Sica, A., Sozzani, S., Allavena, P., Vecchi, A., and Locati, M. (2004). The Chemokine System in Diverse Forms of Macrophage Activation and Polarization. *Trends Immunology* 25, 677–686. doi:10.1016/j.it.2004.09.015

Martinez, F. O., and Gordon, S. (2014). The M1 and M2 Paradigm of Macrophage Activation: Time for Reassessment. *F1000prime Rep.* 6, 13. doi:10.12703/p6-13

Mcalinden, K. D., Eapen, M. S., Lu, W., Sharma, P., and Sohal, S. S. (2020). The Rise of Electronic Nicotine Delivery Systems and the Emergence of Electronic-Cigarette-Driven Disease. *Am. J. Physiol. Lung Cel Mol Physiol* 319, L585–L595. doi:10.1152/ajplung.00160.2020

Mcdonough, J. E., Yuan, R., Suzuki, M., Seyednejad, N., Elliott, W. M., Sanchez, P. G., et al. (2011). Small-airway Obstruction and Emphysema in Chronic Obstructive Pulmonary Disease. *N. Engl. J. Med.* 365, 1567–1575. doi:10.1056/nejmoa1106955

Monteran, L., and Erez, N. (2019). The Dark Side of Fibroblasts: Cancer-Associated Fibroblasts as Mediators of Immunosuppression in the Tumor Microenvironment. *Front. Immunol.* 10, 1835. doi:10.3389/fimmu.2019.01835

Mosser, D. M., and Edwards, J. P. (2008). Exploring the Full Spectrum of Macrophage Activation. *Nat. Rev. Immunol.* 8, 958–969. doi:10.1038/nri2448

Pakshir, P., Noskovicova, N., Lodyga, M., Son, D. O., Schuster, R., Goodwin, A., et al. (2020). The Myofibroblast at a Glance. *J. Cel Sci.* 133, jcs227900. doi:10.1242/jcs.227900

Patel, U., Rajasingh, S., Samanta, S., Cao, T., Dawn, B., and Rajasingh, J. (2017). Macrophage Polarization in Response to Epigenetic Modifiers during Infection and Inflammation. *Drug Discov. Today* 22, 186–193. doi:10.1016/j.drudis.2016.08.006

Perez, M. F., Atuegwu, N. C., Mead, E. L., Oncken, C., and Mortensen, E. M. (2019). Adult E-Cigarettes Use Associated with a Self-Reported Diagnosis of COPD. *Int. J. Environ. Res. Public Health* 16, 3938. doi:10.3390/ijerph16203938

Polosa, R., Morjaria, J. B., Caponnetto, P., Prosperini, U., Russo, C., Pennisi, A., et al. (2016). Evidence for Harm Reduction in COPD Smokers Who Switch to Electronic Cigarettes. *Respir. Res.* 17, 166. doi:10.1186/s12931-016-0481-x

Polosa, R., Morjaria, J. B., Prosperini, U., Busà, B., Pennisi, A., Malerba, M., et al. (2020). COPD Smokers Who Switched to E-Cigarettes: Health Outcomes at 5-year Follow up. *Ther. Adv. Chronic Dis.* 11, 2040622320961617. doi:10.1177/2040622320961617

Quaderi, S., and Hurst, J. (2018). The Unmet Global burden of COPD. *Glob. Health Epidemiol. Genom* 3, e4. doi:10.1017/gheg.2018.1

Rao, W., Wang, S., Duleba, M., Niroula, S., Goller, K., Xie, J., et al. (2020). Regenerative Metaplastic Clones in COPD Lung Drive Inflammation and Fibrosis. *Cell* 181, 848–864.e818. doi:10.1016/j.cell.2020.03.047

Rovina, N., Koutsoukou, A., and Koulouris, N. G. (2013). Inflammation and Immune Response in COPD: where Do We Stand?. *Mediators Inflamm.* 2013, 413735. doi:10.1155/2013/413735

Rőszer, T. (2015). Understanding the Mysterious M2 Macrophage through Activation Markers and Effector Mechanisms. *Mediators Inflamm.* 2015, 816460. doi:10.1155/2015/816460

Seys, L. J., Verhamme, F. M., Dupont, L. L., Desauter, E., Duerr, J., Agircan, A. S., et al. (2015). Airway Surface Dehydration Aggravates Cigarette Smoke-Induced Hallmarks of COPD in Mice. *PLoS One* 10, e0129897. doi:10.1371/journal.pone.0129897

Shapouri-Moghaddam, A., Mohammadian, S., Vazini, H., Taghadosi, M., Esmaeili, S. A., Mardani, F., et al. (2018). Macrophage Plasticity, Polarization, and Function in Health and Disease. *J. Cel Physiol* 233, 6425–6440. doi:10.1002/jcp.26429

Shi, H., Fan, X., Horton, A., Haller, S. T., Kennedy, D. J., Schiefer, I. T., et al. (2019). The Effect of Electronic-Cigarette Vaping on Cardiac Function and Angiogenesis in Mice. *Scientific Rep.* 9, 4085. doi:10.1038/s41598-019-40847-5

Shields, P. G., Berman, M., Brasky, T. M., Freudenheim, J. L., Mathe, E., Mcelroy, J. P., et al. (2017). A Review of Pulmonary Toxicity of Electronic Cigarettes in the Context of Smoking: a Focus on Inflammation. *Cancer Epidemiol. Biomarkers Prev.* 26, 1175–1191. doi:10.1158/1055-9965.epi-17-0358

Shuto, T., Kamei, S., Nohara, H., Fujikawa, H., Tasaki, Y., Sugahara, T., et al. (2016). Pharmacological and Genetic Reappraisals of Protease and Oxidative Stress Pathways in a Mouse Model of Obstructive Lung Diseases. *Scientific Rep.* 6, 1–15. doi:10.1038/srep39305

Song, E., Ouyang, N., Hörbelt, M., Antus, B., Wang, M., and Exton, M. S. (2000). Influence of Alternatively and Classically Activated Macrophages on Fibrogenic Activities of Human Fibroblasts. *Cell Immunol.* 204, 19–28. doi:10.1006/cimm.2000.1687

Traboulsi, H., Cherian, M., Abou Rjeili, M., Preteroti, M., Bourbeau, J., Smith, B. M., et al. (2020). Inhalation Toxicology of Vaping Products and Implications for Pulmonary Health. *Int. J. Mol. Sci.* 21, 3495. doi:10.3390/ijms21103495

Van Linthout, S., Miteva, K., and Tschöpe, C. (2014). Crosstalk between Fibroblasts and Inflammatory Cells. *Cardiovasc. Res.* 102, 258–269. doi:10.1093/cvr/cvu062

Wang, Q., Ahmad Khan, N., Muthumalage, T., Lawyer, G. R., Mcdonough, S. R., Chuang, T. D., et al. (2019). Dysregulated Repair and Inflammatory Responses by E-cigarette-derived Inhaled Nicotine and Humectant Propylene Glycol in a Sex-dependent Manner in Mouse Lung. *FASEB BioAdvances* 1, 609–623. doi:10.1096/fba.2019-00048

Wang, Q., Lucas, J. H., Sundar, I., and Rahman, I. (2020). Electronic-Cigarette Induces Dysregulated Repair Response and Extracellular Matrix Remodeling in Mouse Lung via ±7 Nicotinic Acetylcholine Receptor. 21 (1), 154. doi:10.21203/rs.2.23829/v1

Ward, P. A., and Hunninghake, G. W. (1998). Lung Inflammation and Fibrosis. *Am. J. Respir. Crit. Care Med.* 157, S123–S129. doi:10.1164/ajrccm.157.4.nhlbi-10

Wynn, T. (2008). Cellular and Molecular Mechanisms of Fibrosis. *J. Pathol.* 214, 199–210. doi:10.1002/path.2277

Xiang, J., Cheng, S., Feng, T., Wu, Y., Xie, W., Zhang, M., et al. (2016). Neotuberostemonine Attenuates Bleomycin-Induced Pulmonary Fibrosis by Suppressing the Recruitment and Activation of Macrophages. *Int. Immunopharmacology* 36, 158–164. doi:10.1016/j.intimp.2016.04.016

Xie, Z., Ossip, D. J., Rahman, I., and Li, D. (2020). Use of Electronic Cigarettes and Self-Reported Chronic Obstructive Pulmonary Disease Diagnosis in Adults. *Nicotine Tob. Res.* 22, 1155–1161. doi:10.1093/ntr/ntz234

12

The Extracellular Matrix Enriched with Exosomes for the Treatment on Pulmonary Fibrosis in Mice

*Yanzhen Yu[1,2], Xingzhi Liu[1,2], Zhe Zhao[2], Zhongjuan Xu[1,2], Yong Qiao[2], Yuanshuai Zhou[3], Hong Qiao[4], Junjie Zhong[5], Jianwu Dai[6] and Guangli Suo[2]**

[1]School of Nano-Tech and Nano-Bionics, University of Science and Technology of China, Hefei, China, [2]CAS Key Laboratory of Nano-Bio Interface, Suzhou Institute of Nano-Tech and Nano-Bionics, Chinese Academy of Sciences, Suzhou, China, [3]Jiangsu Key Lab of Medical Optics, Suzhou Institute of Biomedical Engineering and Technology, Chinese Academy of Sciences, Suzhou, China, [4]Department of Molecular Biosciences, the University of Texas at Austin, Austin, TX, United States, [5]Department of Neurosurgery, Fudan University Huashan Hospital, National Key Laboratory of Medical Neurobiology, Institutes of Brain Science, Shanghai Medical College, Fudan University, Shanghai, China, [6]State Key Laboratory of Molecular, Developmental Biology, Institute of Genetics and Developmental Biology, Chinese Academy of Sciences, Beijing, China

***Correspondence:**
Guangli Suo
glsuo2013@sinano.ac.cn

Pulmonary fibrosis (PF) is a severe respiratory disease caused by lung microenvironment changes. TGF-β/Smad3 signaling pathway plays a critical role in the fibrotic process. MicroRNA-29 (miR-29) has proved to alleviate the occurrence of PF by downregulating TGF-β/Smad3 signaling pathway. The miRNA application encounters obstacles due to its low stability in body and no targeting to lesions. Exosomes can be used for therapeutic delivery of miRNA due to their favorable delivery properties. However, low efficiency of separation and production impedes the therapeutic application of exosomes. In this study, we developed a liquid natural extracellular matrix (ECM) enriched with miR-29-loaded exosomes for PF treatment. The collagen-binding domain (CBD)-fused Lamp2b (CBD-Lamp2b) and miR-29 were overexpressed in human foreskin fibroblast (HFF) host cells for the entrapment of miR-29-loaded exosomes in ECM of the cells. The repeated freeze-thaw method was performed to prepare the liquid ECM enriched with exosomes without destroying the exosomal membrane. In summary, this study developed a novel functional ECM biomaterial for therapy of PF, and also provided a promising gene therapy platform for different diseases by treatment with liquid ECM that is, enriched with exosomes loaded with different functional miRNAs.

Keywords: pulmonary fibrosis, extracellular matrix, miR-29, exosome, collagen-binding domain

INTRODUCTION

Pulmonary fibrosis (PF) is a model fibrotic disease mainly caused by microenvironmental lung changes (Parker et al., 2014). Fibroblasts and myofibroblasts play essential roles in the pathological process *via* secreting growth factors, such as transforming growth factor (TGF-β), and excessive collagens (Yang et al., 2013). The inhibition of TGF-β1/Smad3 signaling has been reported to alleviate PF (Wang et al., 2016). For example, the TGF-β1/Smad3 signaling pathway was inhibited by microRNAs for the treatment of lung PF (Yang et al., 2013; Wang et al., 2016). Previous studies suggest that the microRNA-29 (miR-29) is one of the known TGF-β1-associated microRNAs involved in PF because it can regulate the expression levels of extracellular matrix (ECM) proteins such as collagen1a1 (Col1a1) and collagen3a1 (Col3a1) (Xiao et al., 2012; Montgomery et al., 2014).

Although miR-29 has shown excellent advantages in treating PF, its clinical application faces some challenges, such as easy degradation by RNA enzyme, no targeting, and low stability *in vivo*. Recently, many powerful nano delivery systems have been developed for stable and efficient RNA delivery, such as viruses, liposomes, polymer nanoparticles, and exosomes (Paroo and Corey, 2004; Davis et al., 2009; Zhang et al., 2013; Li and Rana, 2014; Shu et al., 2014; Yang et al., 2014; Borna et al., 2015; Maghsoudnia et al., 2020). They have shown many advantages on low dose, high efficacy, stability and targeting.

Exosomes, nano-sized vesicles with diameters of 40–150 nm, are secreted by most eukaryotic cells and circulated in the extracellular environment (Wortzel et al., 2019; Duan et al., 2020; Miao et al., 2021). The exosomes play a functional role in cell-to-cell signaling interactions for the main contains the exosomes can deliver, including nucleic acids (RNA and DNA), proteins, lipids, and metabolites. When exosomes are uptaken by recipient cells, various biomolecules carried by exosomes are transferred to the recipient cells. This causes the response and even changes the functions of recipient cells (Wu et al., 2020). Exosomes have attracted extensive interest in the field of therapeutic applications due to their favorable properties for the delivery of RNAs (Lu and Huang, 2020). So far, exosomes-associated gene delivery has shown its therapeutic effects on brain liver diseases, cardiovascular diseases, and other diseases (Duan et al., 2020). But low efficiency of separation and production, difficulty in drug loading and targeting are common problems for therapeutic application of exosomes (Li P. et al., 2017; Lu and Huang, 2020; Zhang et al., 2020).

Extracellular matrix (ECM), a non-cellular three-dimensional macromolecular network secreted by cells and distributed surrounding the cells, plays a vital role in maintaining microenvironment for cells. Its main molecular complexes contain fibronectin, laminins, elastin, proteoglycans/glycosaminoglycans, collagens, and glycoproteins (Theocharis et al., 2016; Bhattacharjee et al., 2019; Zhang et al., 2019). ECM components form a complex network by binding each other as well as cell adhesion receptors. Cell surface receptors transduce signals into cells from ECM, which regulates diverse cellular functions such as survival, growth, migration, and differentiation. ECM has been applied as an ideal biomaterial to mimic cellular microenvironment for tissue engineering research and diseases treatment for its merits such as neutrality, good biocompatibility, degradability, and controllability. ECM was used to create a suitable bony microenvironment with cell-derived ECM and biodegradable β-tricalcium phosphate (β-TCP) (Kang et al., 2011). It was also used to form a dynamic microenvironment for stem cell niche (Gattazzo et al., 2014), to control cell culture (Barthes et al., 2015; Lin et al., 2020), and to maintain hematopoietic microenvironment (Klein, 1995). In our previous study, we developed a liquid natural ECM biomaterial enriched with insulin-degrading enzyme (IDE) and membrane metalloendopeptidase (MME) to reduce amyloid-beta (Aβ) peptide accumulation and Tau phosphorylation in Alzheimer's disease cell models (Zhang et al., 2019). The ECM and exosomes are both synthesized and secreted by cells. Thereby, it is possible to modify the exosome membrane proteins to link exosomes to ECM by means of genetic engineering for the purpose of exosomes enrichment.

In this study, we developed a functional ECM biomaterial for PF treatment. We overexpressed collagen-binding domain (CBD)-fused Lamp2b (CBD-Lamp2b) and miR-29 in human foreskin fibroblast (HFF) cells, and further produced liquid ECM in which the exosomes loaded with miR-29 were remarkably enriched relying on the binding between CBD on exosomal membrane and collagen I in ECM. Our study demonstrated that this miR-29-loaded exosomes-enriched ECM (mi29-Exo-ECM) inhibited TGF-β1/Smad3 signaling pathway *in vitro*, and effectively alleviated the accumulation of PF *in vivo*. This study developed a type of novel functional ECM biomaterial that may hopefully facilitate PF therapy. In addition, a promising platform for gene therapy was developed to potentially treat different diseases with the liquid ECM that is, enriched with exosomes loaded with different functional miRNA.

MATERIALS AND METHODS

Cell Culture

Human foreskin fibroblast (HFF) and human embryonic kidney cells (HEK 293T) were cultured in Dulbecco's modified Eagle medium (DMEM) (GIBCO, ThermoFisher, Waltham, MA, United States) supplemented with 10% pre-selected fetal bovine serum (FBS) (GIBCO, ThermoFisher, Waltham, MA, United States), 1% penicillin and streptomycin (GIBCO, ThermoFisher, Waltham, MA, United States) in a 37°C humidified incubator with 5% CO_2. Human umbilical cord mesenchymal stem cells (hUCMSCs) were cultured in Dulbecco's modified Eagle's medium/nutrient mixture F-12 HAM (1:1) (DMEM/F12, GIBCO, ThermoFisher, Waltham, MA, United States) containing 10% FBS and 1% penicillin/streptomycin in a 37°C humidified incubator with 5% CO_2.

NIH 3T3 cells were maintained in DMEM with 10% FBS and kept in a 37°C incubator with a 5% CO_2 air atmosphere, and TGF-β (Novoprotein, China) was added with 2 ng/ml. The total proteins of cells were harvested 24 h post-treatment.

Plasmid Construction, Lentivirus Production, and Transduction

The cDNA encoding the lysosome-associated membrane protein-2b (Lamp2b) was cloned from HFF cells by polymerase chain reaction (PCR). The fused gene CBD-Lamp2b was generated by PCR using cDNA of Lamp2b as template. The DNA fragment of CBD-Lamp2b was subcloned into the reading frame of pLVX-IRES-Puro lentiviral vector (Clontech Laboratories, Mountain View, CA), and the new formed construct was named as pLVX-CBD-Lamp2b. MiR-29 oligos purchased from Genewiz (Jiangsu, China) were cloned into pLKO.1 (Addgene, United States) to form new construct named as pLKO.1-miR-29. All primers with restriction sites were listed in **Supplementary Table S1**.

For lentivirus production, HEK 293T cells were cultured to 70% confluence in 60 mm dishes and were co-transfected with packaging plasmids (pMD2.G and psPAX2) and lentiviral vectors (pLVX-CBD-Lamp2b) using lipofectamine 2000 (Invitrogen, Carlsbad, CA, United States). After 6 h of transduction, the medium was replaced with fresh medium. After 48 h of culture, the virus-containing supernatant was collected and filtered through a 0.22 μm pore size filter. The virus stocks were used to infect HFF cells with the presence of 8 μg/ml polybrene to form HFF-pLVX, HFF-pLVX-Lamp2b, HFF-pLVX-CBD-Lamp2b cell lines. After transfection, those cells were selected by 1 μg/ml of puromycin for 7 days to get the stable transfected cell lines. In order to overexpress miR-29 in exosomes, HFF-pLVX-CBD-Lamp2b cells were cultured to 80% confluence in 100 mm dish and co-transfected with pLKO.1-miR-29 using lipofectamine 2000. After 6 h of culture, the medium was replaced with fresh medium.

Quantitative Real-Time Polymerase Chain Reaction

The qRT-PCR was performed according to previously reported method (Qiao et al., 2020) to confirm the overexpression of CBD-Lamp2b in HFF and the overexpression of miR-29 in exosomes from mi29-Exo-ECM. Briefly, total RNA was extracted from HFF-pLVX, HFF-pLVX-Lamp2b, HFF-pLVX-CBD-Lamp2b using TRIzol Reagent (Invitrogen, ThermoFisher, Waltham, MA, United States). The total RNA of exosomes was extracted with miRNeasy Mini Kit (Qiagen, Germany). The RNA was subsequently reverse transcribed to cDNA using High Capacity cDNA Reverse Transcription Kit (Thermo Fisher, Waltham, MA, United States), and miR-29 was reverse transcribed with specialized reverse primers (**Supplementary Table S1**). The qRT-PCR was performed with the Power SYBR Green PCR Master Mix (Applied Biosystems, TheomoFisher, Walltham, MA, United States) on 7,500 real time thermocycle instrument (Applied Biosystems, ThermoFisher, Walltham, MA, United States). The relative expression levels were expressed in arbitrary units (a.u.) while the Ct value of the gene of interest was normalized to that of β-actin or U6. The qRT-PCR primers for target genes (Lamp2b and miR-29) were designed using the Primer Express software (Version 2.0, Applied Biosystems, Walltham, MA, United States) and showed in **Supplementary Table S1**.

Liquid ECM Material Preparation by Repeated Freeze-Thaw Method

The repeated freeze-thaw method was used for liquid ECM preparation (Lu et al., 2011, 2012; Xing et al., 2015; Fernández-Pérez and Ahearne, 2019; Li et al., 2019). Briefly, the cells were expanded to confluence in culture dish and continuously cultured for 14 days in DMEM containing 10% FBS, 50 μM ascorbic acid, and 1% penicillin/streptomycin in a 37°C humidified incubator with 5% CO_2. After washing with phosphate-buffered saline (PBS) for three times, the cells were frozen in −80°C refrigerator for 2 h and then thawed in 37°C incubator for 5 min. This freeze-thaw process was repeated three times to rupture the cell membrane. Finally, the cell contents were removed by gently rinsing with PBS for three times. Subsequently, the decellularized ECM was dissolved in PBS and centrifuged at 10,000 g for 20 min at 4°C to sufficiently remove the cell membrane fragments; the supernatant was collected as the liquid ECM that was named as Exo-ECM. Western blot, transmission electron microscopy (TEM), scanning electron microscope (SEM) and nanoparticle tracking analysis (NTA) were performed to characterize the ECM biomaterials containing exosomes.

Western Blot Analysis

Cells or exosomes were harvested and lysed in RIPA lysis buffer. The lysates were centrifuged at 12,000 g for 20 min at 4°C, and proteins in the supernatants were quantitated using the Lowry Protein Assay quantitation Kit (Beyotime, Shanghai, China). Lysates were fractionated on 10% SDS-PAGE gels and transferred to polyvinylidene difluoride (PVDF) membranes. After blocked with 5% bovine serum albumin (BSA) for 1.5 h, PVDF membranes were incubated with primary antibodies overnight at 4°C and HRP-conjugated secondary antibody for 2 h at room temperature. Finally, the membranes were visualized by chemiluminescence following standard protocols and photographed by Fujifilm LAS 4000 luminescent image analyzer (Fujifilm Life Science, Japan). The densities of protein bands were measured using ImageJ software. The antibodies against following protein were purchased from Cell Signaling Technology (Beverly, MA, United States): Smad3 (C67H9) Rabbit mAb, β-actin, GAPDH, Phospho-Smad3 (Ser423/425) (C25A9) Rabbit mAb, Alix (3A9) Mouse mAb, COL1A1 (E8I9Z) Rabbit mAb, α-Smooth Muscle Actin (D4K9N) XP® Rabbit mAb, E-Cadherin (24E10) Rabbit mAb. The antibodies against following protein were purchased from Proteintech (United States): CD63 Polyclonal Antibody, HSP90 Monoclonal Antibody, LAMP2 Monoclonal Antibody, Collagen Type IV Polyclonal Antibody, Fibronectin Polyclonal Antibody, laminin, Aggrecan Polyclonal Antibody, Elastin Polyclonal Antibody, ATP1A1 Polyclonal Antibody, TGF Beta 1 Polyclonal Antibody. The antibody against TSG 101 was purchased from abcam (Cambridge, CB2 0AX, UK). The goat anti-rabbit or anti-mouse HRP conjugated secondary antibodies were purchased from Cell Signaling Technology (Beverly, MA, United States).

Transmission Electron Microscopy and Scanning Electron Microscope

The scanning electron microscopy was used to observe and assess the entrapment of exosomes in ECM surrounding cells. The cells were expanded to confluence in glass slide and continuously cultured for 14 days in DMEM containing 10% FBS, 50 μM ascorbic acid, and 1% penicillin/streptomycin in a 37°C humidified incubator with 5% CO_2. Then the cells were fixed in 2.5% glutaraldehyde in PBS (pH 7.4) overnight. After dehydration, critical point drying and spraying, the cells were analyzed with a scanning electron microscope (Hitachi SU8010, Japan). The morphological images of HFF cells were acquired, and the number of exosomes with diameter ranging from 40 to 150 nm surrounding cells was counted.

The transmission electron microscopy was used to observe the morphology of exosomes isolated from liquid ECM by ultracentrifugation. Exosomes were fixed in 2.5% glutaraldehyde in PBS (pH 7.4) overnight. Then the samples were rinsed in PBS and refixed in 1% osmium tetroxide at 4°C overnight. After dehydrated in increasing concentrations of acetone, samples were embedded in epoxy resin. Ultrathin sections were prepared and adsorbed to formvar-coated copper grids. Samples were stained with uranyl acetate and lead citrate and then photographed using Tecnai transmission electron microscope (FEI, United States).

Nanoparticle Tracking Analysis

Exosomes were diluted with PBS to reach the recommended measurement range (10^6 to 10^9 particles/mL) and were analyzed using NanoSight NS300 instruments (Malvern Instruments, Inc., UK). The light scattered by the exosomes with laser illumination was captured by a camera and a video file of exosomes moving under Brownian motion was created. The NTA software tracked and analyzed particles individually from 10 to 2000 nm and the Strokes-Einstein equation was used to calculate their particle sizes together with an estimate of the concentration (Dragovic et al., 2011).

Exosomal miRNA Analysis *via* Next-Generation Sequencing Technology

The next-generation sequencing technology was used to investigate the difference of RNAs content among the different types of exosomes from the media of HFF cells, HFF-Lamp2b cells and hUCMSCs, and from the ECM of HFF-CBD-Lamp2b cells. Small RNA sequencing was serviced by LC Sciences (Hangzhou, Zhejiang, China). The experimental process was performed under the standard steps provided by Illumina, including library preparation and sequencing experiments. Total RNA was extracted and purified using the mirVanaTM miRNA Isolation Kit without phenol (Ambion, United States). TruSeq Small RNA Sample Prep Kits (Illumina, San Diego, United States) were used to construct miRNA sequencing libraries. Total RNAs were ligated with the ligate 3′ and 5′ adapter using T4 RNA ligase (Epicentre, United States) at 28°C for 1 h. The adapter-ligated miRNAs were used as templates to perform PCR amplification and the cDNAs were purified with 6% TBE PAGE gels. The completed libraries' quality and correctness were evaluated with qRT-PCR, and the high-throughput sequencing of the cDNA was performed on the HiSeq 2,500 (Illumina, United States). Raw reads were subjected to an in-house program ACGT101-miR (LC Sciences, Houston, Texas, United States) to remove adapter dimers, junk, low complexity, common RNA families (rRNA, tRNA, snRNA, snoRNA) and repeats. Then the clean reads were used for the analysis of small RNA data. The spearman's correlation analysis, principal component analysis (PCA) and heat map analysis were performed to compare the miRNA differences in exosomes from each group.

The Development of PF Model and the Treatment With ECM

C57BL/6 mice (~25 g, male) were anesthetized by placing them in a chamber containing paper towels soaked with 40% isoflurane solution, and 2 mg/kg mouse of bleomycin (Selleck, United States) in 50 μL of 0.9% saline was administered intratracheally. To study the effect of materials on early fibrosis, we administered total 600 μg liquid ECM with about 25 pmol exosomes with or without miR-29 enrichment in one mouse at the 3rd day after bleomycin treatment and sacrificed the mice at the 14th day. The lungs were harvested for histological, immunohistochemical (IHC) and Western blot analysis.

Histologic, Masson, and Immunohistochemical Analyses

Histologic, Masson and IHC analyses were performed according to the previously reported methods (Qiao et al., 2020) with modifications. For histological analysis, lung sections were stained with haematoxylin and eosin (H&E) and Masson. The antibodies against α-SMA (CST, Beverly, MA, United States), TGF-β (Proteintech, United States) were used for IHC staining in lung tissue sections, the percentage of TGF-β and α-SMA positive area (%) from IHC were quantified by ImageJ software. The stained sections were observed and the images were acquired using a microscope (ZEISS AXIO microscope, Axio Scope A1, United States).

Quantify Degree of Fibrosis With Ashcroft Scoring System

The Ashcroft score was performed according to previously reported method (Ashcroft et al., 1988) to estimate severity of PF. Briefly, a paraffin section of lung stained by haematoxylin and eosin method, was systematically scanned in a microscope using a 10X objective. Each successive field was individually assessed for severity of interstitial fibrosis and allotted a score between 0 and 8 using a predetermined scale of severity. "0" represented normal lung; "1" and "2" represented minimal fibrous thickening of alveolar or bronchiolar walls; "3" and "4" represented moderate thickening of walls without obvious damage to lung architecture; "5" and "6" represented increased fibrosis with definite damage to lung structure and formation of fibrous bands or small fibrous masses; "7" represented severe distortion of structure and large fibrous areas; "8" represented total fibrous obliteration of the field. After examining the whole section the mean score of all the fields was taken as the fibrosis score for the section and was expressed correct to two decimal places.

Hydroxyproline Assay

A HYP assay kit (Nanjing Jiancheng Bioengineering Institute) was used to measure the concentration of HYP in lung tissue samples. The experimental procedure was performed according the instruction. Briefly, the lung tissue (30 mg) was homogenized in 1 ml hydrolysate (95°C water bath for 20 min). After

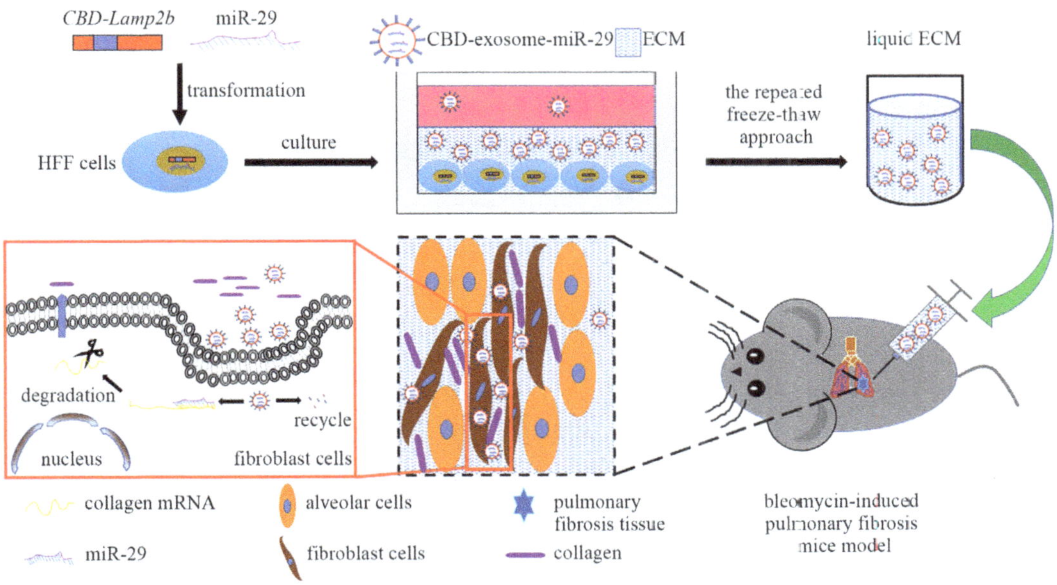

FIGURE 1 | The scheme of this study includes four main steps: 1) construction of HFF cell lines that stably expressing CBD-Lamp2b and miR-29; 2) enrichment of CBD-exosomes in ECM; 3) production of liquid ECM; 4) treatment of pulmonary fibrosis mice with mi29-Exo-ECM biomaterial.

neutralizing the hydrolysates with NaOH, the mixture was diluted to 10 ml with water. Subsequently, the absorbance values of the prepared samples were detected at 550 nm. The results were expressed as μg hydroxyproline/mg wet lung.

Statistical Analysis

All experiments were independently repeated 3 times and all measurements were done at least in triplicates. Statistical significance was determined by unpaired two-tailed student's *t*-test ($p < 0.05$) and one-way ANOVA. $p < 0.05$ was considered statistically significant. All statistical analyses were performed using GraphPad Prism 5 (GraphPad Software, Inc., La Jolla, CA, United States).

RESULTS

In this study, we attempted to develop a kind of functional biomaterial containing ECM microenvironment enriched with exosomes for repair of PF. The scheme of this study was shown in **Figure 1**. First, we overexpressed the fusion protein CBD-Lamp2b in HFF cells to entrap the secreted exosomes in ECM surrounding the cells by the binding of CBD on exosomal membrane with the collagen I in ECM. The expression cassette of the modified Lamp2b protein was shown in **Supplementary Figure S1**. Second, to obtain the liquid exosomes-enriched ECM without destroying the exosomal membrane, we performed repeated freeze-thaw method to remove cell contents and dissolve the decellularized ECM in PBS. Third, to endow the function of this biomaterial on PF therapy, we overexpressed miR-29 into the host HFF cells from which the miR-29-loaded exosomes (mi29-Exo) were generated. Finally, miR-29-loaded exosomes-enriched ECM (mi29-Exo-ECM) biomaterial was produced and applied for PF repair *in vivo*.

Enrichment of Exosomes Surrounding the Host Cells

To entrap exosomes in ECM of host cells, according to the methods from previous researches (Alvarez-Erviti et al., 2011; Zhang et al., 2019), we fused a targeting peptide CBD with the extra-exosomal N-terminus of Lamp2b and overexpressed this fusion protein in host cells (**Supplementary Figure S1**). Since the heptapeptide CBD derived from collagenase can specifically bind to collagen I in ECM, we expect that the fused CBD in exosome membrane protein Lamp2b can lead to the entrapment of exosomes in ECM. The overexpression of CBD-Lamp2b fusion protein in HFF was confirmed by the results of qRT-PCR and Western blot analysis (**Figures 2A–C**).

To investigate whether modified exosomes could be entrapped and enriched into the ECM surrounding HFF cells, we first assessed and measured the number of exosomes surrounding the host HFF cells exhibited in morphological images acquired by SEM (**Figure 2D**). We found that more exosomes (extracellular vesicles with 40–150 nm of diameter) were attached on the surface of HFF-CBD-Lamp2b cells than them on surfaces of the HFF-Lamp2b and HFF cells (**Figure 2E**). In addition, we further examined the expression levels of exosomes markers (Hsp90, TSG101, and CD63) in the whole proteins of cells by Western blot. We found that the expression levels of Hsp90, TSG101, and CD63 were higher in HFF-CBD-Lamp2b cells than them in HFF cells and HFF-Lamp2b cells when the protein levels of ECM markers (fibronectin, collagen I, laminin, and aggrecan) and internal control of β-actin are almost same (**Figure 2F** and **Supplementary Figure**

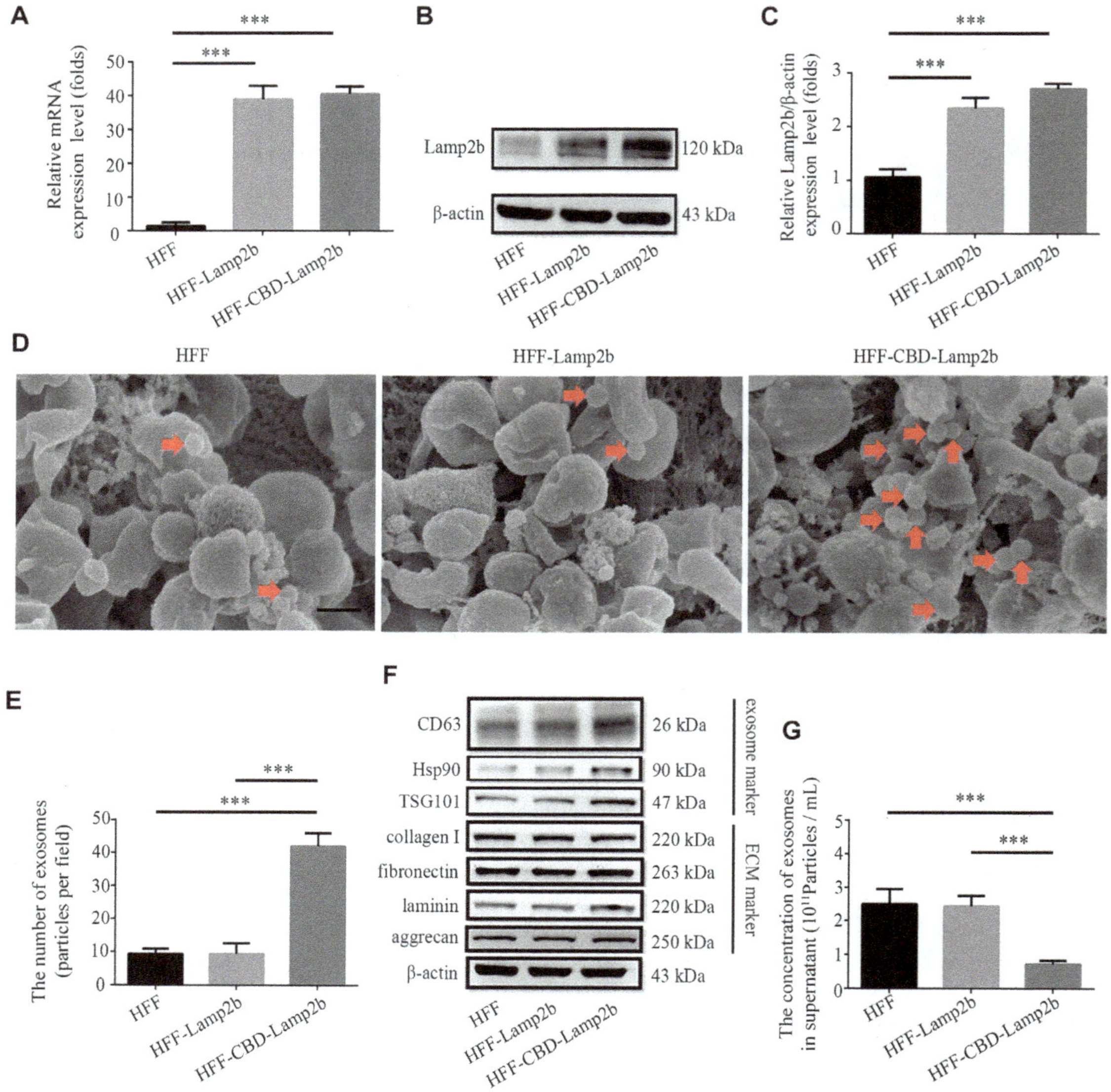

FIGURE 2 | Enrichment of exosomes surrounding the host cells. Overexpression of Lamp2b in HFF cells determined by **(A)** qRT-PCR and **(B)** Western blot. **(C)** Relative expression level of Lamp2b was quantified. The β-actin was used as an internal control. **(D)** Representative SEM images of indicated cell surface. The red arrows indicate the exosomes surrounding the host cells. Scale bar = 250 nm. **(E)** The number of exosomes in the view. **(F)** Western blot analysis of exosomal markers and ECM markers in indicated cells. **(G)** The NTA analysis of exosomal number in cell culture supernatants. Data are represented as mean ± SD (n = 3). ANOVA was performed; "***": $p < 0.001$.

S2). The exosomal particle number measurement by NTA showed that there were less number of exosomes in the supernatant of HFF-CBD-Lamp2b cells than them in the supernatants of HFF cells and HFF-Lamp2b cells (**Figure 2G**). These results suggest that the CBD-Lamp2b fusion protein preferentially entraps the exosomes in the ECM around host cells.

Preparation and Characterization of Exosomes Enriched in ECM

To verify that the ectopic expression of CBD-Lamp2b fusion protein can entrap the exosomes into the ECM of host cells and the exosomes can be enriched by liquid ECM preparation, we developed a repeated freeze-thaw approach to obtain the liquid ECM without destroying the membrane structure of exosomes (Lu et al., 2011, 2012; Fernández-Pérez and Ahearne, 2019; Li et al., 2019). The results from Western blot confirmed that the liquid ECM was successfully prepared by assessment of the ECM components such as collagen I, collagen IV, fibronectin, laminin, aggrecan and elastin from liquid ECM and whole cell protein (**Figure 3A**). Since the GAPDH is a conserved protein localized in cytoplasm, the lack of GAPDH expression in ECM indicated the success of decellularization (**Figure 3A**).

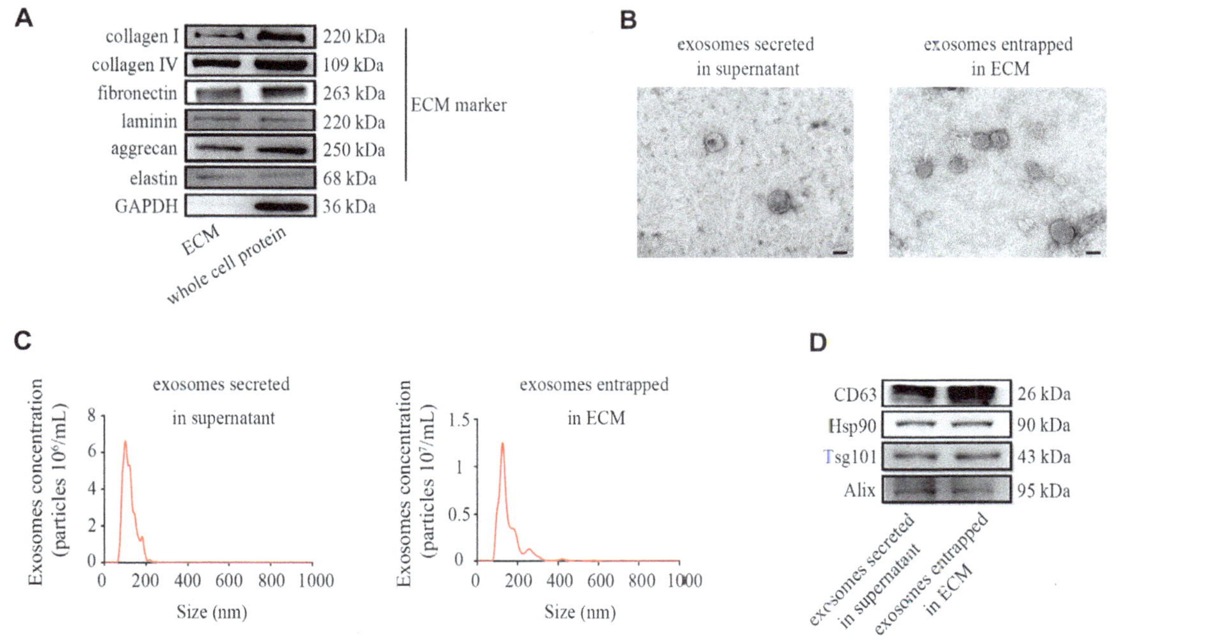

FIGURE 3 | Preparation and characterization of exosomes enriched in ECM. **(A)** The markers of liquid ECM were determined by Western blot. **(B)** TEM images for exosome morphology. **(C)** NTA analysis of particle size, and **(D)** Western blot analysis for exosomal markers of exosomes entrapped in ECM from HFF-CBD-Lamp2b cells and those secreted in supernatant from HFF cells. Scale bar = 100 nm.

To verify the quality of exosomes in the liquid ECM, we characterized the exosomes entrapped in ECM from HFF-CBD-Lamp2b cells compared to those secreted in supernatant from HFF cells by the analysis of Western blot, TEM and NTA. The results from TEM image and NTA analysis showed that the particle of exosomes enriched in ECM has the size around 130 nm diameters that was almost the same as the size of exosomes secreted in medium. Exosomes in both ECM and medium had the similar biofilm structures that were consistent with those previously reported (**Figures 3B,C**) (Alvarez-Erviti et al., 2011; Wu et al., 2020). The results from Western blot confirmed the enrichment of exosomes in ECM by the detection of exosomal markers such as CD63, Hsp90, Tsg101, and Alix (**Figure 3D**).

To further investigate the quality of exosomes enriched in ECM, we profiled the exosomal miRNAs using next-generation sequencing technology and compared the miRNAs in ECM exosomes from HFF-CBD-Lamp2b cells with those in medium exosomes from HFF cells, HFF-Lamp2b cells and hUCMSCs by spearman correlation analysis, principal component analysis (PCA) and heatmap analysis. The results from spearman correlation analysis showed the correlation coefficients between any two exosome samples from HFF cells medium, HFF-Lamp2b cells medium and from HFF-CBD-Lamp2b cells ECM had a high correlation ($R > 0.75$); however, the exosomes from HFF-CBD-Lamp2b cells ECM, from the media of HFF and HFF-Lamp2b had a low correlation ($R < 0.5$) with the exosomes from the medium of hUCMSCs (**Figure 4A**). The PCA showed that the distribution of exosomes from the media of HFF cells and HFF-Lamp2b cells, and the ECM of HFF-CBD-Lamp2b cells were different from the exosomes from hUCMSCs medium. The exosomes from hUCMSCs medium strayed far from the other three types of exosomes (**Figure 4B**). These results indicated that the miRNAs from these three types of exosomes were similar and high correlation. The results from heatmap analysis (**Figure 4C**) also demonstrated that the exosomes from the media of HFF and HFF-Lamp2b cells, and from the ECM of HFF-CBD-Lamp2b showed similar expression pattern compared to the exosomes from hUCMSCs medium. We found that the expression levels of 154 kinds of miRNAs from exosomes in the media of HFF and HFF-Lamp2b cells, and in the ECM of HFF-CBD-Lamp2b were significantly different compared with miRNAs levels from exosomes in hUCMSCs medium. Among the differentially expressed miRNAs, 104 miRNAs were up-regulated (fold change > 2) and 50 miRNAs were down-regulated (fold change < 0.5) in exosomes from hUCMSCs medium as compared to the other three exosomes (**Figure 4C**). The heatmap of miRNA expression showed high inter-group similarity for the exosomes from the media of HFF and HFF-Lamp2b cells, and the exosomes from ECM of HFF-CBD-Lamp2b. Overall, overexpression of CBD-Lamp2b will not change the quality of exosomes enriched in ECM compared to the exosomes in the media of HFF host cells.

Mi29-Exo-ECM Biomaterial Inhibited TGF-β-Induced Accumulation of Collagen I *in Vitro*

PF is associated with an excessive accumulation of collagens (He et al., 2013). It is well-known that the miR-29 is a major regulator of genes associated with PF (Xiao et al., 2012; Montgomery et al.,

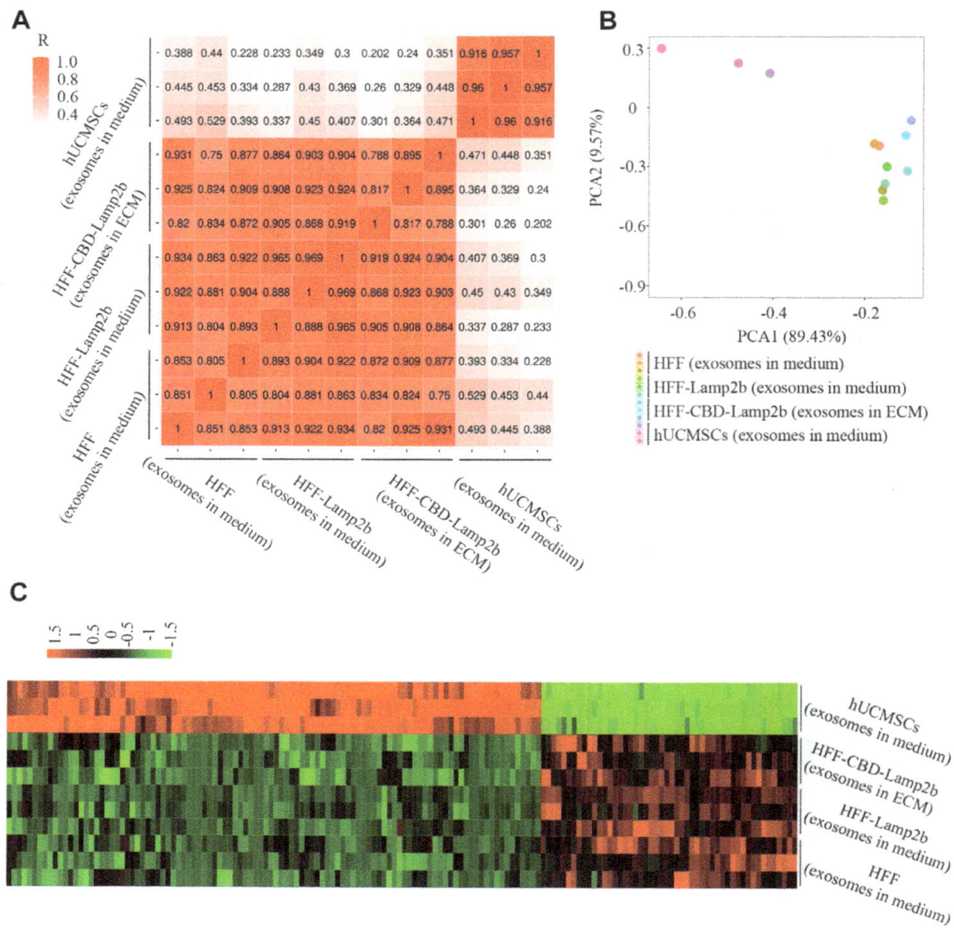

FIGURE 4 | The comparison of exosomal miRNAs from ECM or media derived from HFF-CBD-Lamp2b cells, HFF cells, HFF-Lamp2b cells and hUCMSCs. **(A)** Spearman's correlation analysis. **(B)** Principal component analysis was used to investigate the differences of exosomal miRNA from indicated samples. **(C)** The heatmap was used to show the expression of different miRNAs from indicated samples (red color means upregulation; green color means downregulation).

2014). Overexpression of miR-29 can negatively regulate TGF-β expression and Smad3 signaling activation that are correlated with the severity of the fibrosis (Cushing et al., 2011; He et al., 2013). Here, the miR-29 was overexpressed in HFF-CBD-Lamp2b cells to produce the liquid mi29-Exo-ECM. The result from qRT-PCR analysis (**Figure 5A**) showed that the expression levels of miR-29 in mi29-Exo-ECM were significantly higher than them in control Exo-ECM that was derived from HFF-CBD-Lamp2b cells without miR-29 ectopic expression. To evaluate whether mi29-Exo-ECM biomaterial can function on PF, we first investigate its function on reduction of collagen I, α-SMA (alpha-smooth muscle actin) expression and inactivation of Smad3 in TGF-β-induced NIH 3T3 cells. The TGF-β treatment clearly increased the expression of collagen I, α-SMA and phosphorylation of Smad3 (p-Smad3) in NIH 3T3 cells; only the mi29-Exo-ECM effectively reduced the levels of p-Smad3, collagens I and α-SMA in TGF-β-induced NIH 3T3 cells compared to the Exo-ECM (**Figures 5B–E** and **Supplementary Figures S3A,B**). Meanwhile, mi29-Exo-ECM could significantly down regulate the mRNA levels of Col1a1 and Col3a1 that were generally highly expressed in NIH 3T3 cells (**Supplementary Figures S3C,D**).

Local Administration of Liquid mi29-Exo-ECM Efficiently Reduce PF *in Vivo*

To confirm the therapeutic potential of mi29-Exo-ECM for PF *in vivo*, bleomycin-induced PF mice were intratracheally administered with total 600 μg liquid ECM with about 25 pmol exosomes with or without miR-29 enrichment, mi29-Exo-ECM or Exo-ECM. After 11 days of treatment, the mice were sacrificed and the lung tissues were harvested for H&E, Masson and IHC staining, and Western blot analysis. The upregulations of TGF-β and α-SMA are well known critical markers of tissue epithelial-mesenchymal transition (EMT) and PF (Cushing et al., 2011; Lemoinne et al., 2016). The results from H&E, Masson staining, and IHC analysis for TGF-β and α-SMA showed that the bleomycin treatment successfully caused the fibrosis and

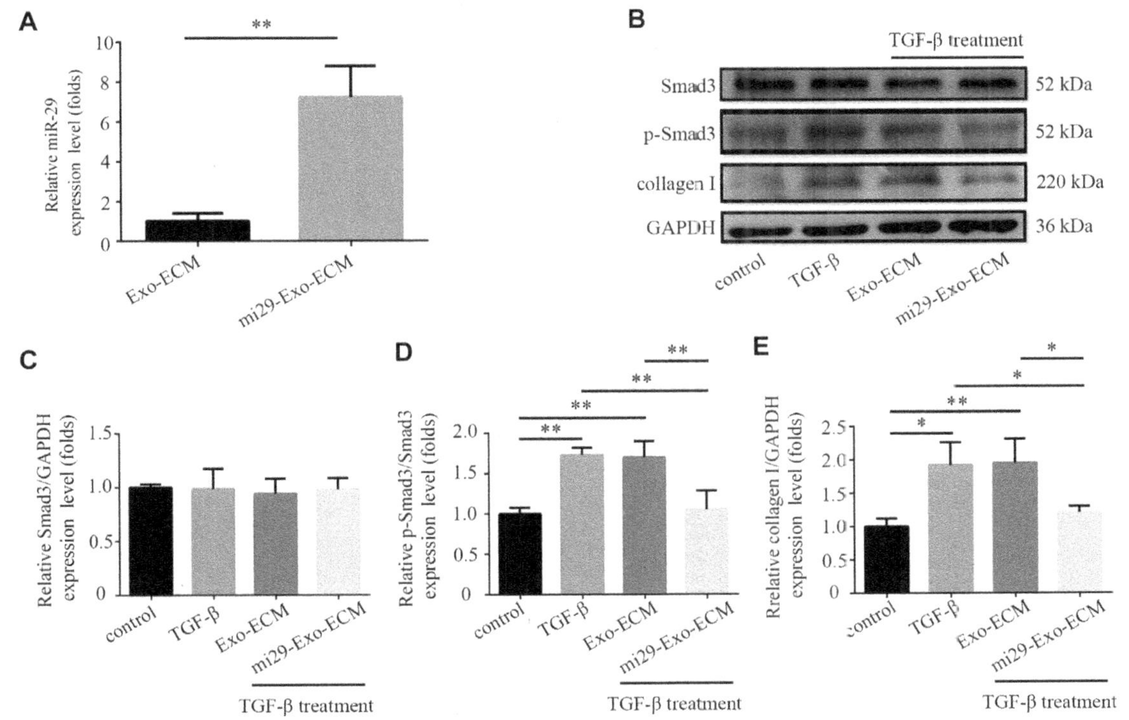

FIGURE 5 | Mi29-Exo-ECM inhibited TGF-β-induced accumulation of collagen I in NIH 3T3 cells. **(A)** Expression level of miR-29 in mi29-Exo-ECM was determined by qRT-PCR. "Exo-ECM": exosomes from ECM of HFF-CBD-Lamp2b cells; "mi29-Exo-ECM": exosomes from mi29-Exo-ECM. Data are represented as mean ± SD ($n = 3$). Student's t-test was performed; "**": $p < 0.01$. **(B)** The changes of collagen I protein levels and phosphorylation levels of Smad3 were analyzed by Western blot. Relative expression levels of Smad3 **(C)**, *p*-Smad3/Smad3 **(D)**, collagen I **(E)** were quantified. The GAFDH was used as an internal control. "Control": NIH 3T3 cells; "TGF-β": TGF-β-induced NIH 3T3 cells; "Exo-ECM": Exo-ECM treatment; "mi29-Exo-ECM": mi29-Exo-ECM treatment; Data are represented as mean ± SD ($n = 3$). ANOVA was performed; "*": $p < 0.05$; "**": $p < 0.01$.

upregulation of TGF-β and α-SMA in lung lesion areas in mice, and mi29-Exo-ECM treatment dramatically restored lung textures from fibrosis and decreased the expression levels of TGF-β and α-SMA compared to Exo-ECM treatment (**Figure 6A** and **Supplementary Figure S7**). The Western blot assay further demonstrated that the mi29-Exo-ECM reduced the expression levels of collagen I, TGF-β and α-SMA in PF tissues of mice (**Figures 6B–E**). Treatment with mi29-Exo-ECM lowered the Ashcroft scores significantly and down-regulated the levels of HYP in lungs in bleomycin-induced PF mice (**Supplementary Figures S5, S6**). These results were consistent with those observed in the pathological sections, which suggested that the mi29-Exo-ECM treatment restored lung textures from fibrosis. Overall, the results from **Figure 6**; **Supplementary Figures S5, S6** indicated that mi29-Exo-ECM showed the good repair effect on PF *in vivo* due to the enriched exosomes loaded with miR-29.

DISCUSSION

In this study, we successfully developed a type of functional ECM biomaterial enriched with miR-29-loaded exosomes and investigated the therapeutic effect of the biomaterials on PF. This biomaterial has some features as follows: 1) the liquid ECM biomaterial can entrap and enrich exosomes and provide an appropriate environment for exosomes to maintain the stability and to function; 2) as a carrier, exosomes can deliver small RNAs and protect them from degradation; 3) the overexpressed miR-29 can be recruited in and delivered by exosomes to function on the lesion of PF.

PF is a high mortality lung disease and no current treatment has proved effective to cure the disease. Many studies demonstrated that PF is associated with the abnormal activity of alveolar epithelial cells (AECs). These cells produce myofibroblast foci *via* stimulating the epithelial to mesenchymal transition (EMT) (Korfei et al., 2008; King Jr et al., 2011). In myofibroblast foci, the fibroblast secretes excessive amounts of ECM, mainly collagens, leading to scarring and destruction of the lung architecture (Gross and Hunninghake, 2001; King Jr et al., 2011; Martinez et al., 2017; Richeldi et al., 2017; Lederer and Martinez, 2018). Since TGF-β/Smad3 signaling is a critical factor for ECM gene expression, regulation of this signaling has been considered a potential approach for treatment of PF (Cushing et al., 2011; Xiao et al., 2012; He et al., 2013; Montgomery et al., 2014). For example, TGF-β antisense oligonucleotides has been delivered and targeted to lung to treat PF (Kim et al., 2020). In PF, TGF-β suppressed the level of miR-29 leading to the overexpression of collagens-related

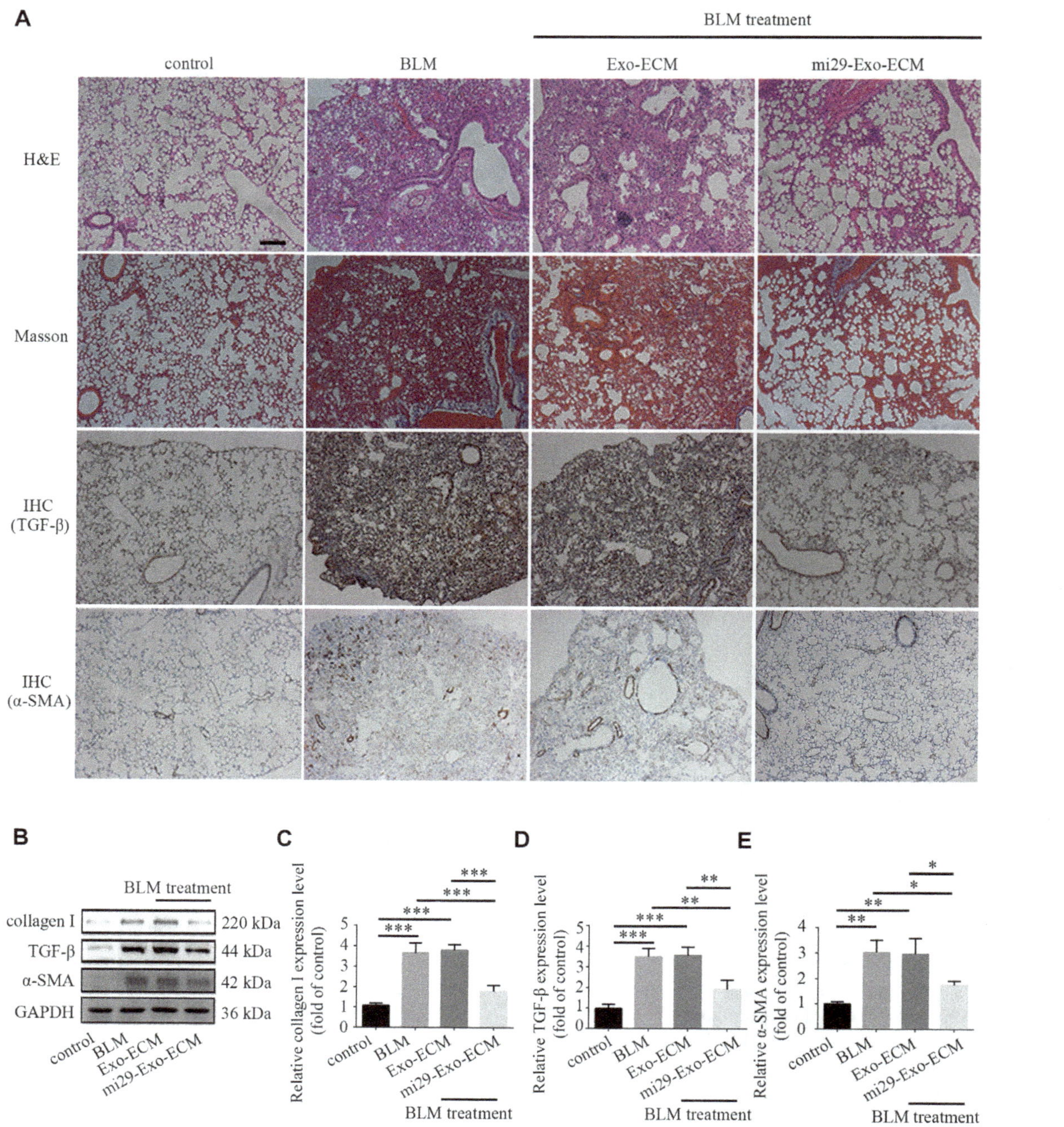

FIGURE 6 | Pulmonary fibrosis therapeutic potential of mi29-Exo-ECM biomaterial. **(A)** H&E staining, Masson staining and IHC of lung tissues from mice treated with BLM, Exo-ECM biomaterial, mi29-Exo-ECM biomaterial. Scale bar = 1,000 μm. **(B)** The changes of collagen I, TGF-β and α-SMA protein levels in pulmonary fibrosis mice after treated with mi29-Exo-ECM biomaterial. Relative expression levels of collagen I **(C)**, TGF-β **(D)**, α-SMA **(E)** were quantified. "Control": no treatment mice; "BLM": bleomycin-induced pulmonary fibrosis mice model; "Exo-ECM": Exo-ECM treatment; "mi29-Exo-ECM": mi29-Exo-ECM treatment; Data are represented as mean ± SD (n = 5). ANOVA was performed; "*": $p < 0.05$; "**": $p < 0.01$; "***": $p < 0.001$.

genes suggesting that miR-29 is an important mediator of TGF-β/Smad3 signaling. Moreover, it was reported that there was a complex feedback regulatory relationship between miR-29 and TGF-β/Smad3 signaling (Cushing et al., 2015). Sleeping beauty (SB)-mediated miR-29 gene transfection has proved effective to prevent and treat PF induced by bleomycin in mice (Xiao et al., 2012). Recent studies showed that miR-29 could regulate ECM production and deposition to alleviate PF treatment (Cushing et al., 2011; Cushing et al., 2015). According to the past studies, miR-29 has been proved to act as a "master fibro-miRNA" regulator to be involved in fibrosis (Deng et al., 2017). In PF, the down regulation of miR-29 level is negatively related to fibrosis and the expression level of profibrotic genes, such as Col1a1 and Col3a1 (Cushing et al., 2011; Xiao et al., 2012). MiR-29 plays a critical role in TGF-β-induced ECM production by activating the phosphatidyl inositol 3-kinase (*PI3K*)/protein kinase B (*AKT*) pathway and the Wnt/β-catenin pathway in human lung fibroblasts (Deng et al., 2017). Many previous studies showed that therapeutic delivery of miR-29 for PF decreased collagen expression and reversed PF (Cushing et al., 2011; Montgomery et al., 2014). MiR-29 is likely to become a new target in the diagnosis and evaluation of PF, as well as a new perspective and direction in which to search for new therapeutic targets of fibrosis.

It is well known that miRNAs have great potential for clinical therapy. However, direct administration of miRNAs in the body would face the problems of rapid diffusion and RNA enzyme degradation, which leads to shorter treatment duration. Therefore, package by liposomes, polymer nanoparticles, or virus can protect miRNAs from enzyme degradation and diffusion, and can prolong and enhance its function (Sercombe et al., 2015; Ha et al., 2016). Unlike typical nanoparticulate systems such as liposomes, polymeric nanoparticles or virus, exosomes are natural carriers for microRNA delivery and can deliver cargoes such as small RNAs directly into the cytoplasm potentially avoiding the endosomal pathway and lysosomal degradation, and therefore enhanced the transfection efficiency of small RNAs (Ha et al., 2016). For this great merit, exosomes have proved to offer a potential new paradigm in treatment of diseases.

Exosomes were secreted by most cells and distributed in different bodily fluids (e.g., blood, urine, and saliva) (Boriachek et al., 2018). However, how to isolate exosome remains an obstacle for it application. Existing methods for exosome isolation mainly rely on a large collection of medium and heavy ultracentrifugation. Although the ultracentrifugation-based methods were currently considered as the gold standard of exosome isolation, it had some disadvantages such as high equipment cost, time-consuming, large sample volume required, low recovery, and purity (Li P. et al., 2017). Other separation methods currently developed include sucrose-gradient centrifugation, coprecipitation, size-exclusion chromatography, and field flow fractionation. Their advantages have been reported, such as easy and user-friendly processing, high yield, wide variety of eluents and broad separation range. However, they also faced the problems of lengthy duration and fractionation equipment required (Xu et al., 2016; Coumans et al., 2017; Shao et al., 2018). To optimize exosome isolation, we attempted to develop a novel method to entrap and enrich the secreted exosomes to ECM of cell surface and to reduce their diffusion in the medium during long time cell culture. CBD is a heptapeptide (TKKTLRT) derived from collagenase and could specifically bind to collagen I, one of the main compounds in ECM (Jiang et al., 2019; Zhang et al., 2019). In our previous study, we overexpressed fusion proteins CBD-IDE and CBD-MME in HFF cells and developed a type of liquid ECM biomaterial enriched with CBD-IDE and CBD-MME relying on the binding of CBD and collagen I in ECM. This biomaterial successfully reduced the Aβ accumulation and Tau phosphorylation in AD cell models (Zhang et al., 2019). Lamp2b was a protein found abundantly in exosomal membranes (Alvarez-Erviti et al., 2011). By fusing CBD to the extra-exosomal N terminus of Lamp2b, the secreted exosomes were entrapped in ECM surrounding the host cells *via* the binding of CBD on external membrane of exosomes and collagen I in ECM. In this case, exosomes can be enriched in ECM and easily isolated by collecting the liquid ECM.

In this study, we enriched the miR-29 into exosomes and entrapped exosomes into ECM by overexpressing miR-29 and CBD-Lamp2b in HFF host cells, and produced the functional ECM biomaterial enriched with miR-29-loaded exosomes through the repeated freeze-thaw method without destroying the exosome membrane. Finally, this composite mi29-Exo-ECM was used for the repair of PF and showed a good treatment effect. This novel mi29-Exo-ECM biomaterial has the following merits: 1) miR-29 is a potential regulator for therapy of PF; 2) as a natural vehicle, exosome can prevent miRNA from enzymatic hydrolysis, facilitate the spread of RNA over long distance, and increase the duration of RNA function; 3) ECM plays a positive role in improving the disease microenvironment and contributes to the repair of tissue wound (Hou et al., 2016; Li J. et al., 2017; Zhang et al., 2019); 4) ECM provides appropriate environment for the collection and function of exosomes.

Although the liquid mi29-Exo-ECM had a good effect on the treatment of PF, there were still some problems that need to be further solved in the future, such as multiple dosing modalities and intervals to achieve optimal treatment outcomes, and the quantification of miR-29 in exosomes to facilitate drug administration consistency. In this study, to preserve the integrity of exosomes enriched in the ECM around HFF cells, the repeated freeze-thaw method was used to prepare the decellularized ECM. Our results confirmed the integrity and enrichment of exosomes in liquid ECM. However, the cell membrane components are hardly removed completely, which may affect the quality assessment of mi29-Exo-ECM. In this study, the miR-29 was enriched in exosomes by simply overexpressing miR-29 in the host cells. In the future, more efficient approaches should be developed for orientated enrichment by the specific binding between special peptide fused in inner membrane proteins of exosome and RNA fragment integrated in miR-29

CONCLUSION

In conclusion, our proof-of-concept study first demonstrated that exosomes could be enriched in ECM by overexpression of fusion gene CBD-Lamp2b in host cells. Based on this novel strategy, we developed a kind of functional biomaterial containing liquid natural ECM enriched with miR-29-loaded exosomes for PF treatment. The liquid ECM provides an appropriate microenvironment for exosomes function in the foci of damaged tissues, and the exosome is ideal natural carrier for miRNAs delivery for therapeutic purpose. This functional biomaterial provides a promising platform for gene therapy that could potentially be applied to treat different diseases by loading different functional miRNAs in exosomes that can be enriched in the liquid ECM.

AUTHOR CONTRIBUTIONS

YY and XL conceived and designed the experiments; YY, ZZ, and YQ performed the experiments and analyzed the data; YY and GS wrote the manuscript; ZX, YQ, YZ, HQ, and JZ provided technical guidance; JD and GS projected administration; GS provided the guidance for the research.

ACKNOWLEDGMENTS

LivingChip Inc. is acknowledged for the technical assistance.

REFERENCES

Alvarez-Erviti, L., Seow, Y., Yin, H., Betts, C., Lakhal, S., and Wood, M. J. (2011). Delivery of siRNA to the Mouse Brain by Systemic Injection of Targeted Exosomes. *Nat. Biotechnol.* 29, 341–345. doi:10.1038/nbt.1807

Ashcroft, T., Simpson, J. M., and Timbrell, V. (1988). Simple Method of Estimating Severity of Pulmonary Fibrosis on a Numerical Scale. *J. Clin. Pathol.* 41, 467–470. doi:10.1136/jcp.41.4.467

Barthes, J., Vrana, N. E., Özçelik, H., Gahoual, R., François, Y. N., Bacharouche, J., et al. (2015). Priming Cells for Their Final Destination: Microenvironment Controlled Cell Culture by a Modular ECM-Mimicking Feeder Film. *Biomater. Sci.* 3, 1302–1311. doi:10.1039/c5bm00172b

Bhattacharjee, O., Ayyangar, U., Kurbet, A. S., Ashok, D., and Raghavan, S. (2019). Unraveling the ECM-Immune Cell Crosstalk in Skin Diseases. *Front. Cel Dev. Biol.* 7, 68. doi:10.3389/fcell.2019.00068

Boriachek, K., Islam, M. N., Möller, A., Salomon, C., Nguyen, N. T., Hossain, M. S. A., et al. (2018). Biological Functions and Current Advances in Isolation and Detection Strategies for Exosome Nanovesicles. *Small* 14, 1702153. doi:10.1002/smll.201702153

Borna, H., Imani, S., Iman, M., and Azimzadeh Jamalkandi, S. (2015). Therapeutic Face of RNAi: *In Vivo* Challenges. *Expert Opin. Biol. Ther.* 15, 269–285. doi:10.1517/14712598.2015.983070

Coumans, F. A. W., Brisson, A. R., Buzas, E. I., Dignat-George, F., Drees, E. E. E., El-Andaloussi, S., et al. (2017). Methodological Guidelines to Study Extracellular Vesicles. *Circ. Res.* 120, 1632–1648. doi:10.1161/CIRCRESAHA.117.309417

Cushing, L., Kuang, P., and Lü, J. (2015). The Role of miR-29 in Pulmonary Fibrosis. *Biochem. Cel Biol.* 93, 109–118. doi:10.1139/bcb-2014-0095

Cushing, L., Kuang, P. P., Qian, J., Shao, F., Wu, J., Little, F., et al. (2011). miR-29 Is a Major Regulator of Genes Associated with Pulmonary Fibrosis. *Am. J. Respir. Cel Mol Biol* 45, 287–294. doi:10.1165/rcmb.2010-0323OC

Davis, S., Propp, S., Freier, S. M., Jones, L. E., Serra, M. J., Kinberger, G., et al. (2009). Potent Inhibition of microRNA *In Vivo* without Degradation. *Nucleic Acids Res.* 37, 70–77. doi:10.1093/nar/gkn904

Deng, Z., He, Y., Yang, X., Shi, H., Shi, A., Lu, L., et al. (2017). MicroRNA-29: a Crucial Player in Fibrotic Disease. *Mol. Diagn. Ther.* 21, 285–294. doi:10.1007/s40291-016-0253-9

Dragovic, R. A., Gardiner, C., Brooks, A. S., Tannetta, D. S., Ferguson, D. J., Hole, P., et al. (2011). Sizing and Phenotyping of Cellular Vesicles Using Nanoparticle Tracking Analysis. *Nanomedicine* 7, 780–788. doi:10.1016/j.nano.2011.04.003

Duan, L., Xu, L., Xu, X., Qin, Z., Zhou, X., Xiao, Y., et al. (2020). Exosome-mediated Delivery of Gene Vectors for Gene Therapy. *Nanoscale* 13, 1387–1397. doi:10.1039/d0nr07622h

Fernández-Pérez, J., and Ahearne, M. (2019). The Impact of Decellularization Methods on Extracellular Matrix Derived Hydrogels. *Sci. Rep.* 9, 1–12. doi:10.1038/s41598-019-49575-2

Gattazzo, F., Urciuolo, A., and Bonaldo, P. (2014). Extracellular Matrix: a Dynamic Microenvironment for Stem Cell Niche. *Biochim. Biophys. Acta* 1840, 2506–2519. doi:10.1016/j.bbagen.2014.01.010

Gross, T. J., and Hunninghake, G. W. (2001). Idiopathic Pulmonary Fibrosis. *N. Engl. J. Med.* 345, 517–525. doi:10.1056/NEJMra003200

Ha, D., Yang, N., and Nadithe, V. (2016). Exosomes as Therapeutic Drug Carriers and Delivery Vehicles across Biological Membranes: Current Perspectives and Future Challenges. *Acta Pharm. Sin. B* 6, 287–296. doi:10.1016/j.apsb.2016.02.001

He, Y., Huang, C., Lin, X., and Li, J. (2013). MicroRNA-29 Family, a Crucial Therapeutic Target for Fibrosis Diseases. *Biochimie* 95, 1355–1359. doi:10.1016/j.biochi.2013.03.010

Hou, L., Coller, J., Natu, V., Hastie, T. J., and Huang, N. F. (2016). Combinatorial Extracellular Matrix Microenvironments Promote Survival and Phenotype of Human Induced Pluripotent Stem Cell-Derived Endothelial Cells in Hypoxia. *Acta Biomater.* 44, 188–199. doi:10.1016/j.actbio.2016.08.003

Jiang, P., Tang, X., Wang, H., Dai, C., Su, J., Zhu, H., et al. (2019). Collagen-binding Basic Fibroblast Growth Factor Improves Functional Remodeling of Scarred Endometrium in Uterine Infertile Women: a Pilot Study. *Sci. China Life Sci.* 62, 1617–1629. doi:10.1007/s11427-018-9520-2

Kang, Y., Kim, S., Khademhosseini, A., and Yang, Y. (2011). Creation of Bony Microenvironment with CaP and Cell-Derived ECM to Enhance Human Bone-Marrow MSC Behavior and Delivery of BMP-2. *Biomaterials* 32, 6119–6130. doi:10.1016/j.biomaterials.2011.05.015

Kim, J., Jeon, S., Kang, S. J., Kim, K. R., Thai, H. B. D., Lee, S., et al. (2020). Lung-targeted Delivery of TGF-β Antisense Oligonucleotides to Treat Pulmonary Fibrosis. *J. Control. Release* 322, 108–121. doi:10.1016/j.jconrel.2020.03.016

King, T. E., Jr, Pardo, A., and Selman, M. (2011). Idiopathic Pulmonary Fibrosis. *Lancet* 378, 1949–1961. doi:10.1016/S0140-6736(11)60052-4

Klein, G. (1995). The Extracellular Matrix of the Hematopoietic Microenvironment. *Experientia* 51, 914–926. doi:10.1007/BF01921741

Korfei, M., Ruppert, C., Mahavadi, P., Henneke, I., Markart, P., Koch, M., et al. (2008). Epithelial Endoplasmic Reticulum Stress and Apoptosis in Sporadic Idiopathic Pulmonary Fibrosis. *Am. J. Respir. Crit. Care Med.* 178, 838–846. doi:10.1164/rccm.200802-313OC

Lederer, D. J., and Martinez, F. J. (2018). Idiopathic Pulmonary Fibrosis. *N. Engl. J. Med.* 378, 1811–1823. doi:10.1056/NEJMra1705751

Lemoinne, S., Thabut, D., and Housset, C. (2016). Portal Myofibroblasts Connect Angiogenesis and Fibrosis in Liver. *Cell Tissue Res* 365, 583–589. doi:10.1007/s00441-016-2443-5

Li, J., Zhang, K., and Huang, N. (2017a). Engineering Cardiovascular Implant Surfaces to Create a Vascular Endothelial Growth Microenvironment. *Biotechnol. J.* 12, 1600401. doi:10.1002/biot.201600401

Li, P., Kaslan, M., Lee, S. H., Yao, J., and Gao, Z. (2017b). Progress in Exosome Isolation Techniques. *Theranostics* 7, 789–804. doi:10.7150/thno.18133

Li, M., Zhang, T., Jiang, J., Mao, Y., Zhang, A., and Zhao, J. (2019). ECM Coating Modification Generated by Optimized Decellularization Process Improves Functional Behavior of BMSCs. *Mater. Sci. Eng. C Mater. Biol. Appl.* 105, 110039. doi:10.1016/j.msec.2019.110039

Li, Z., and Rana, T. M. (2014). Therapeutic Targeting of microRNAs: Current Status and Future Challenges. *Nat. Rev. Drug Discov.* 13, 622–638. doi:10.1038/nrd4359

Lin, X., Patil, S., Gao, Y. G., and Qian, A. (2020). The Bone Extracellular Matrix in Bone Formation and Regeneration. *Front. Pharmacol.* 11, 757. doi:10.3389/fphar.2020.00757

Lu, H., Hoshiba, T., Kawazoe, N., and Chen, G. (2011). Autologous Extracellular Matrix Scaffolds for Tissue Engineering. *Biomaterials* 32, 2489–2499. doi:10.1016/j.biomaterials.2010.12.016

Lu, H., Hoshiba, T., Kawazoe, N., and Chen, G. (2012). Comparison of Decellularization Techniques for Preparation of Extracellular Matrix Scaffolds Derived from Three-Dimensional Cell Culture. *J. Biomed. Mater. Res. A.* 100, 2507–2516. doi:10.1002/jbm.a.34150

Lu, M., and Huang, Y. (2020). Bioinspired Exosome-like Therapeutics and Delivery Nanoplatforms. *Biomaterials* 242, 119925. doi:10.1016/j.biomaterials.2020.119925

Maghsoudnia, N., Eftekhari, R. B., Sohi, A. N., Zamzami, A., and Dorkoosh, F. A. (2020). Application of Nano-Based Systems for Drug Delivery and Targeting: a Review. *J. Nanopart. Res.* 22, 1–41. doi:10.1007/s11051-020-04959-8

Martinez, F. J., Collard, H. R., Pardo, A., Raghu, G., Richeldi, L., Selman, M., et al. (2017). Idiopathic Pulmonary Fibrosis. *Nat. Rev. Dis. Primers* 3, 17074–17119. doi:10.1038/nrdp.2017.74

Miao, C., Zhou, W., Wang, X., and Fang, J. (2021). The Research Progress of Exosomes in Osteoarthritis, with Particular Emphasis on the Mediating Roles of miRNAs and lncRNAs. *Front. Pharmacol.* 12, 685623. doi:10.3389/fphar.2021.685623

Montgomery, R. L., Yu, G., Latimer, P. A., Stack, C., Robinson, K., Dalby, C. M., et al. (2014). MicroRNA Mimicry Blocks Pulmonary Fibrosis. *EMBO Mol. Med.* 6, 1347–1356. doi:10.15252/emmm.201303604

Parker, M. W., Rossi, D., Peterson, M., Smith, K., Sikström, K., White, E. S., et al. (2014). Fibrotic Extracellular Matrix Activates a Profibrotic Positive Feedback Loop. *J. Clin. Invest.* 124, 1622–1635. doi:10.1172/JCI71386

Paroo, Z., and Corey, D. R. (2004). Challenges for RNAi *In Vivo*. *Trends Biotechnol.* 22, 390–394. doi:10.1016/j.tibtech.2004.06.004

Qiao, Y., Xu, Z., Yu, Y., Hou, S., Geng, J., Xiao, T., et al. (2020). Single Cell Derived Spheres of Umbilical Cord Mesenchymal Stem Cells Enhance Cell Stemness Properties, Survival Ability and Therapeutic Potential on Liver Failure. *Biomaterials* 227, 119573. doi:10.1016/j.biomaterials.2019.119573

Richeldi, L., Collard, H. R., and Jones, M. G. (2017). Idiopathic Pulmonary Fibrosis. *Lancet* 389, 1941–1952. doi:10.1016/S0140-6736(17)30866-8

Sercombe, L., Veerati, T., Moheimani, F., Wu, S. Y., Sood, A. K., and Hua, S. (2015). Advances and Challenges of Liposome Assisted Drug Delivery. *Front. Pharmacol.* 6, 286. doi:10.3389/fphar.2015.00286

Shao, H., Im, H., Castro, C. M., Breakefield, X., Weissleder, R., and Lee, H. (2018). New Technologies for Analysis of Extracellular Vesicles. *Chem. Rev.* 118, 1917–1950. doi:10.1021/acs.chemrev.7b00534

Shu, Y., Pi, F., Sharma, A., Rajabi, M., Haque, F., Shu, D., et al. (2014). Stable RNA Nanoparticles as Potential New Generation Drugs for Cancer Therapy. *Adv. Drug Deliv. Rev.* 66, 74–89. doi:10.1016/j.addr.2013.11.006

Theocharis, A. D., Skandalis, S. S., Gialeli, C., and Karamanos, N. K. (2016). Extracellular Matrix Structure. *Adv. Drug Deliv. Rev.* 97, 4–27. doi:10.1016/j.addr.2015.11.001

Wang, Y. C., Liu, J. S., Tang, H. K., Nie, J., Zhu, J. X., Wen, L. L., et al. (2016). miR-221 T-argets HMGA2 to I-nhibit B-leomycin-induced P-ulmonary F-ibrosis by R-egulating TGF-β1/Smad3-I-nduced EMT. *Int. J. Mol. Med.* 38, 1208–1216. doi:10.3892/ijmm.2016.2705

Wortzel, I., Dror, S., Kenific, C. M., and Lyden, D. (2019). Exosome-mediated Metastasis: Communication from a Distance. *Dev. Cel* 49, 347–360. doi:10.1016/j.devcel.2019.04.011

Wu, P., Zhang, B., Ocansey, D. K. W., Xu, W., and Qian, H. (2021). Extracellular Vesicles: A Bright star of Nanomedicine. *Biomaterials* 269, 120467. doi:10.1016/j.biomaterials.2020.120467

Xiao, J., Meng, X. M., Huang, X. R., Chung, A. C., Feng, Y. L., Hui, D. S., et al. (2012). miR-29 Inhibits Bleomycin-Induced Pulmonary Fibrosis in Mice. *Mol. Ther.* 20, 1251–1260. doi:10.1038/mt.2012.36

Xing, Q., Yates, K., Tahtinen, M., Shearier, E., Qian, Z., and Zhao, F. (2015). Decellularization of Fibroblast Cell Sheets for Natural Extracellular Matrix Scaffold Preparation. *Tissue Eng. Part. C Methods* 21, 77–87. doi:10.1089/ten.tec.2013.0666

Xu, R., Greening, D. W., Zhu, H. J., Takahashi, N., and Simpson, R. J. (2016). Extracellular Vesicle Isolation and Characterization: toward Clinical Application. *J. Clin. Invest.* 126, 1152–1162. doi:10.1172/JCI81129

Yang, H. W., Huang, C. Y., Lin, C. W., Liu, H. L., Huang, C. W., Liao, S. S., et al. (2014). Gadolinium-functionalized Nanographene Oxide for Combined Drug and microRNA Delivery and Magnetic Resonance Imaging. *Biomaterials* 35, 6534–6542. doi:10.1016/j.biomaterials.2014.04.057

Yang, T., Liang, Y., Lin, Q., Liu, J., Luo, F., Li, X., et al. (2013). miR-29 Mediates TGFβ1-Induced Extracellular Matrix Synthesis through Activation of PI3K-AKT Pathway in Human Lung Fibroblasts. *J. Cel. Biochem.* 114, 1336–1342. doi:10.1002/jcb.24474

Zhang, S., Xiao, T., Yu, Y., Qiao, Y., Xu, Z., Geng, J., et al. (2019). The Extracellular Matrix Enriched with Membrane Metalloendopeptidase and Insulin-Degrading Enzyme Suppresses the Deposition of Amyloid-Beta Peptide in Alzheimer's Disease Cell Models. *J. Tissue Eng. Regen. Med.* 13, 1759–1769. doi:10.1002/term.2906

Zhang, Y., Bi, J., Huang, J., Tang, Y., Du, S., and Li, P. (2020). Exosome: A Review of its Classification, Isolation Techniques, Storage, Diagnostic and Targeted Therapy Applications. *Int. J. Nanomedicine* 15, 6917–6934. doi:10.2147/IJN.S264498

Zhang, Y., Wang, Z., and Gemeinhart, R. A. (2013). Progress in microRNA Delivery. *J. Control. Release* 172, 962–974. doi:10.1016/j.jconrel.2013.09.015

13

Dihydromyricetin Alleviates Pulmonary Fibrosis by Regulating Abnormal Fibroblasts through the STAT3/p-STAT3/GLUT1 Signaling Pathway

Zhen Li[1], Jing Geng[1], Bingbing Xie[1], Jiarui He[1], Jing Wang[2], Liang Peng[3], Yinan Hu[1], Huaping Dai[1]* and Chen Wang[1]**

[1]Department of Pulmonary and Critical Care Medicine, Center of Respiratory Medicine, China-Japan Friendship Hospital; National Center for Respiratory Medicine; National Clinical Research Center for Respiratory Diseases; Institute of Respiratory Medicine, Chinese Academy of Medical Sciences, Peking Union Medical College, Beijing, China, [2]State Key Laboratory of Medical Molecular Biology, Department of Physiology, Institute of Basic Medical Sciences Chinese Academy of Medical Sciences, School of Basic Medicine Peking Union Medical College, Beijing, China, [3]Institute of Clinical Medical Sciences, China-Japan Friendship Hospital, Beijing, China

Correspondence:
Yinan Hu
403698131@qq.com
Huaping Dai
daihuaping@ccmu.edu.cn
Chen Wang
cyh-birm@263.net

Background: Idiopathic pulmonary fibrosis (IPF) is a chronic and progressive disorder with a poor prognosis. Although dihydromyricetin (DHM), extracted from vine tea and other Ampelopsis species, has been proven to have anti-inflammatory and antioxidant functions, the effects of DHM on IPF remain unclear.

Methods: The effects of DHM on the differentiation, migration, proliferation, and respiratory functions of primary mouse lung fibroblasts (PMLFs) and primary human lung fibroblasts (PHLFs) were detected by western blotting, the Transwell assay, EdU staining, and the Mito Stress test. Then, the impacts of DHM on bleomycin (BLM)-induced pulmonary fibrosis were evaluated by pathological staining, western blotting, and coimmunofluorescence staining. The signaling pathway influenced by DHM was also investigated.

Results: DHM could regulate the differentiation of fibroblasts to myofibroblasts and suppress the abnormal migration, proliferation, and respiratory functions of myofibroblasts induced by TGF-β1 or myofibroblasts from IPF patients. DHM could also alleviate pulmonary fibrosis induced by BLM. All these effects were achieved by regulating the STAT3/p-STAT3/GLUT1 signaling pathway.

Conclusion: DHM could regulate the abnormal functions of myofibroblasts induced by TGF-β1 and myofibroblasts from IPF patients and alleviate pulmonary fibrosis induced by BLM; thus, DHM might be a candidate medicinal treatment for IPF.

Keywords: idiopathic pulmonary fibrosis, dihydromyricetin, fibroblast, myofibroblast, GLUT1, glucose metabolism

INTRODUCTION

Idiopathic pulmonary fibrosis (IPF), characterized by chronic and progressive fibrosis of the interstitial lung tissue, is an irreversible and fatal lung disease with a poor prognosis (Richeldi et al., 2017). Historical clinical evidence suggests that the median survival of untreated IPF patients is approximately 2–3 years after diagnosis, and the mortality rate of IPF patients remains high, although some antifibrotic treatments (pirfenidone and nintedanib) have been adopted (Lederer and Martinez, 2018). Therefore, new drugs for the treatment of IPF patients are urgently needed.

The histopathological characteristics of IPF are the formation of fibroblast foci and deposition of disordered collagen and an extracellular matrix (ECM) (Wolters et al., 2014). Although the precise initiation factors that lead to these disorders remain unknown, it is widely recognized that the pathological process of IPF is related to fibroblasts and myofibroblasts (Chanda et al., 2019). Previous studies have suggested that various cytokines, such as the transform growth factor (TGF-β), and signaling pathways, such as the STAT/pSTAT3 pathway, can promote fibroblast differentiation into myofibroblasts and ultimately result in fibrosis of the lung tissue (Zehender et al., 2018). For this reason, restraining the differentiation of fibroblasts into myofibroblasts may block the initiation of fibrosis, while reversing this differentiation process might lead to a breakthrough treatment for IPF (Wei et al., 2019).

Dihydromyricetin (DHM, the structure of which is shown in **Figure 1**), a natural flavonoid extracted from vine tea and other Ampelopsis species, has anti-inflammatory and antioxidant effects and has been proven to inhibit liver fibrosis and diabetic nephropathy (Liu et al., 2019; Zhou et al., 2021). However, its effects on pulmonary fibrosis have not been determined. As inflammation and oxidative stress participate in the process of lung fibrosis (Heukels et al., 2019; Otoupalova et al., 2020), we hypothesized that DHM would be a good potential drug for the prevention and treatment of pulmonary fibrosis.

To test the feasibility of our hypothesis, we detected the effects of DHM on the differentiation, proliferation, and migration of primary fibroblasts from the lungs of IPF patients and control subjects or those from mice, and to explore whether the STAT3/p-STAT3/GLUT1 signaling pathway is involved in these effects, we also used bleomycin (BLM) to induce pulmonary fibrosis in male mice and confirmed the effects of DHM in the mouse model. Our findings suggest that DHM could alleviate pulmonary fibrosis in the mouse model and restrain the differentiation, proliferation, and migration of fibroblasts or myofibroblasts *via* the STAT3/pSTAT3/GLUT1 signaling pathways. Together, our studies suggest that DHM may be a novel treatment for IPF patients.

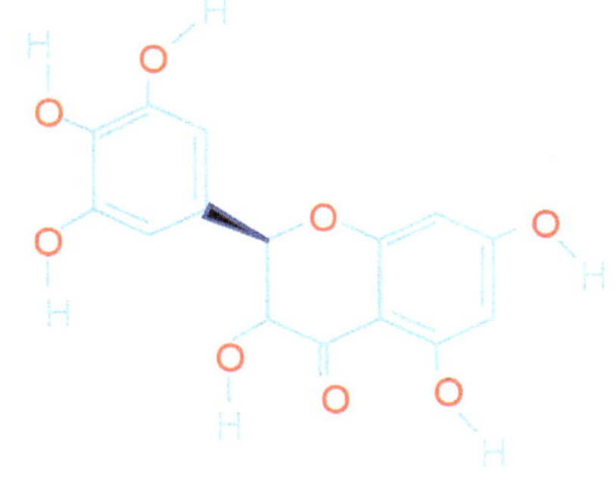

FIGURE 1 | Chemical structure of dihydromyricetin.

MATERIALS AND METHODS

Human Samples

Lung tissues were collected from IPF patients (n = 9) and donors (n = 6) during lung transplantation surgery. The diagnosis of IPF was made according to consensus diagnostic criteria from the American Thoracic Society (ATS)/European Respiratory Society (ERS) (Raghu et al., 2019). All patients provided informed written consent. The study was approved by the Human Assurance Committee of the China–Japan Friendship Hospital.

Animals

WT C57BL/6 male mice aged 8–10 weeks were purchased from GemPharmatech Co., Ltd. (Nanjing, China). All animals were bred in a specific pathogen-free environment at the China–Japan Friendship Hospital and randomly assigned to four groups: 1) the saline group, 2) the DHM group, 3) the BLM (Hanhui Pharmaceuticals Co., Ltd.) group, and 4) the BLM + DHM group. Pulmonary fibrosis was induced by BLM treatment. The mice in the BLM group and the BLM + DHM group were anesthetized with 1% pentobarbital sodium (50 mg/kg) and intratracheally administered 1.5 U/kg BLM in 50 μL of sterile saline. For mice in the saline group and the DHM group, BLM was replaced with the same volume of saline. DHM was administered by gavage to mice in the DHM group and the BLM + DHM group on day 14 after BLM administration and every day until day 27. Finally, the mice were euthanized on day 28 to analyze pulmonary fibrosis. All experimental procedures complied with the International Association of Veterinary Editors guidelines of 2010 and the Guide for the Care and Use of Laboratory Animals, 8th edition, 2011. All protocols were approved by the Institutional Animal Care and Use Committee of the China–Japan Friendship Hospital (zryhyy11-20-09-4).

Cell Culture

Primary mouse lung fibroblasts (PMLFs) were isolated from the lung tissue from wild-type (WT) C57BL/6 male mice at 2 weeks of age. Primary human lung fibroblasts (PHLFs) were isolated from the fibrotic lung tissue of IPF patients (IPF-HLF) or the normal lung tissue of donors (N-HLF) (Wang Q. et al., 2021). All cells were verified by coimmunofluorescence analysis with anti-fsp-1 (Proteintech, 66489-1-Ig, 1:200) and anti-alpha-smooth muscle actin (α-SMA) (Abcam, ab124964, 1:200). The purity of the cells used in our study was more than 90%. All the cells were cultured in Dulbecco's modified Eagle's

TABLE 1 | Information of the primary antibody used for cells and model mice.

Primary antibody	For cells	For model mice
Anti-β-ACTIN	Proteintech, 66009-1-Ig, 1:5000 42kd	
Anti-fibronectin	Proteintech,15613-1-AP, 1:1000 270kd	Abcam, ab2413, 1:1000 280kd
Anti-Col1a1	Proteintech, 66761-1-Ig, 1:1000 130kd	CST, 81375 1:1000 220kd
Anti-α-SMA	Proteintech, 14395-1-AP, 1:1000 42kd	
Anti-GLUT1	Proteintech, 66290-1-Ig, 1:1000 54kd	
Anti-STAT3	CST, 9139, 1:1000 86kd	Proteintech, 60199-1-Ig, 1:1000 88kd
Anti-p-STAT3	CST, 9145, 1:1000 86kd	

medium (DMEM) containing 20% fetal bovine serum (FBS) and penicillin/streptomycin at 37°C and 5% CO_2 and used between passages 3 and 5. PMLFs were stimulated with DHM (100 μM/ 200 μM/300 μM) (Ruifensi, Chengdu, China) or an equal amount of DMSO (Sigma, C6164) 1 h before treatment with mouse recombinant TGF-β1 (15 ng/ml) (MCE, HEK293) for 36 h, and IPF-HLFs and N-HLFs were treated with only DHM (100 μM/200 μM/300 μM) or an equal amount of DMSO for 36 h.

Cell Viability Assay

The viability of PMLFs and PHLFs was detected by the Cell Counting Kit-8 (CCK-8) assay (Beyotime, Shanghai, China) (Wang et al., 2020). Initially, 5 × 10^3 cells/well were seeded in 96-well plates and then treated with different concentrations of DHM (100 μM, 200 μM, 300 μM, 400 μM, or 500 μM) or 1‰ DMSO for 36 h. After the treatment was finished, 5 mg/ml CCK-8 reagent was added and incubated for 2 h, and cell viability was quantified by calorimetry.

Western Blotting and Antibodies

Lung tissues or fibroblasts were homogenized in RIPA lysis buffer (Beyotime, Shanghai, China), to which two kinds of protease inhibitor cocktails (MCE, HY-K0022) had also been added. The proteins were separated on polyacrylamide gels and finally detected with a chemiluminescence substrate system (Bio-Rad Laboratories, CA, United States and Tanon, Shanghai, China) (Miao et al., 2020). The antibodies used for western blotting were as follows (**Table 1**).

Cell Migration Assay

Cell migration was detected by using Transwell inserts with membranes with an 8.0 μM pore size (Corning, MA, United States) according to previously reported methods. A total of 3 × 10^4 cells were suspended in 2% FBS containing DMEM and seeded into the upper chambers. DMEM containing 20% FBS was added to the lower chambers as a chemoattractant for cells in the upper chambers. After incubation for 24 h, cells that had migrated through the membrane were stained with 1% crystal violet (Solarbio, Beijing, China).

Cell Proliferation Assay

PMLFs and PHLFs were cultured in 96-well plates at a density of 5 × 10^3 cells/well. Cell proliferation was detected by using the EdU proliferation assay (RiboBio, Guangzhou, China). After being seeded in plates and incubated with DHM or DHM combined with TGF-β1 for 18 h, the cells were labeled with EdU for 2 h at 37°C and 5% CO_2, subjected to Apollo staining and Hoechst 33342 staining, and observed by fluorescence microscopy (Leica, DMi8, Germany).

Seahorse XF Cell Mito Stress Test

The oxygen consumption rate (OCR) was detected with a Mito Stress test kit using a Seahorse XFe24 analyzer (Agilent Technologies). PHLFs were first seeded in XF24 cell culture plates at a density of 2×10^4 cells/well and treated with DHM for 36 h. After the treatment was finished, the Cell Mito Stress assay medium was prepared according to the assay instructions and added to the XF24 plate. Finally, the OCR was detected with a Seahorse instrument.

Histological Analysis

After inflation with 300 μL of 4% paraformaldehyde, the left lung of each mouse was removed and immersed in 4% paraformaldehyde for at least 24 h at room temperature. Then, the left lung was embedded in paraffin and sliced into 3 μM sections. The lung tissues were separately subjected to hematoxylin and eosin (H&E) staining, Sirius red staining, Masson staining, and immunohistochemistry. Assessment with the Ashcroft scoring system and immunohistochemistry were carried out as described previously (Wang Q. et al., 2021), and the severity of lung fibrosis was evaluated by the Ashcroft score (Ashcroft et al., 1988).

Immunofluorescence Analysis

Each slide containing the lung tissue was incubated with anti-collagen I (Proteintech, 66761-1-Ig, 1:200) and anti-α-SMA (Proteintech, 14395-1-AP, 1:200) antibodies overnight at 4°C. After incubation, the slide was washed three times with PBS and then incubated with HRP- or 488-conjugated anti-mouse antibody and Alexa Fluor 594-conjugated anti-rabbit antibody (ZSGB-BIO, ZF-0512/0516, 1:400) for 1 h at room temperature. The slide was finally embedded with 4,6-diamino-2-phenylindole (DAPI) and analyzed under a fluorescence microscope (Wang Y. et al., 2021).

Statistical Analysis

All experimental data were analyzed by using GraphPad Prism (San Diego, CA, United States). Other data are expressed as the mean ± standard error of the mean (SEM) or standard deviation

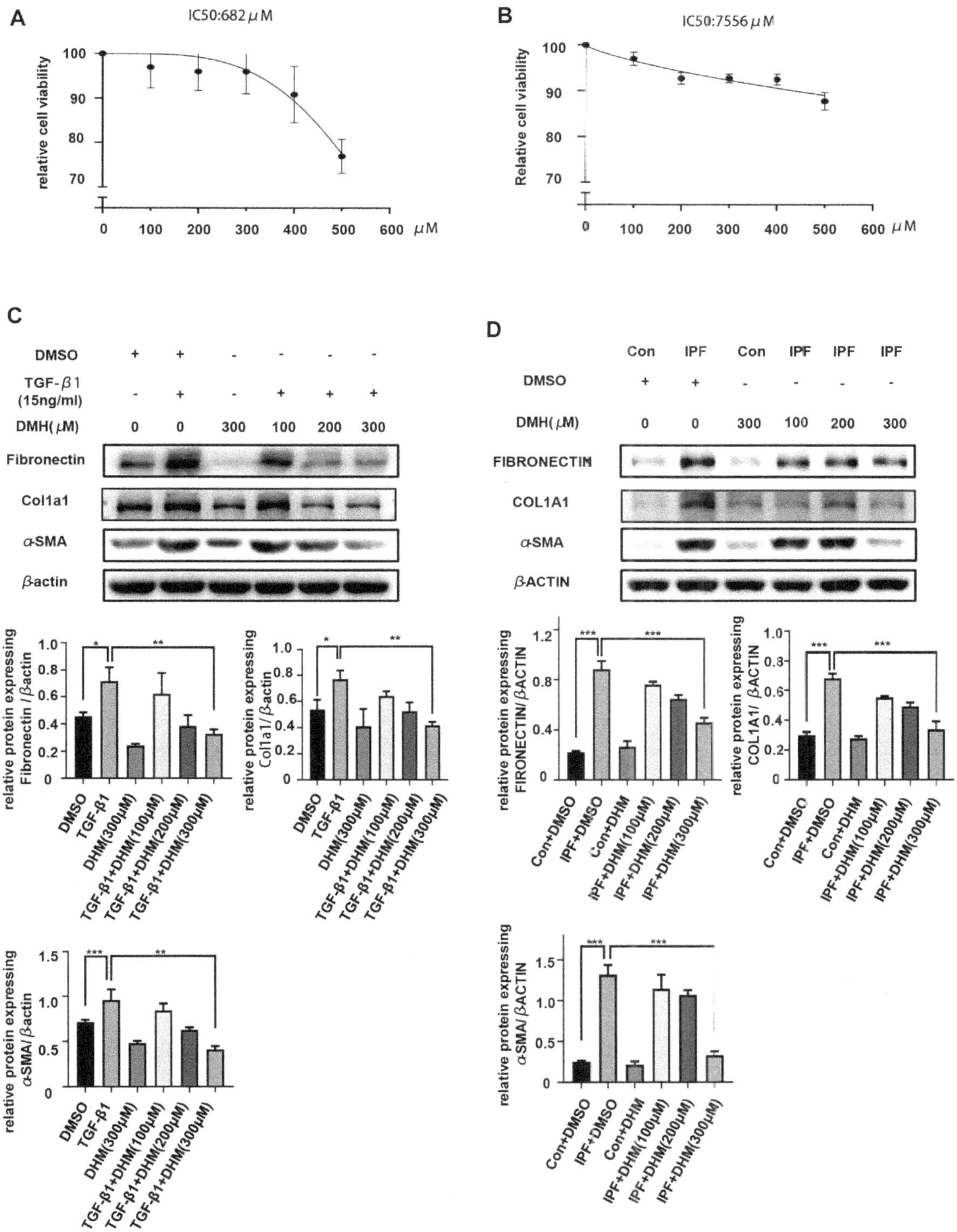

FIGURE 2 | Effects of DHM on the differentiation of fibroblasts. **(A)** Toxicity detection of DHM on PHLFs by the CCK-8 assay ($n = 6$). **(B)** Toxicity detection of DHM on PMLFs by the CCK-8 assay ($n = 4$). **(C)** Western blotting analysis of fibronectin, Col1a1, and α-SMA in PMLFs treated with DHM ($n = 5$). **(D)** Western blotting analysis of fibronectin, COL1A1, and α-SMA expression in PHLFs treated with DHM ($n = 5$). The data are represented as the mean ± SD of three independent experiments. Ordinary one-way ANOVA analysis was applied. *, $p < 0.05$; **, $p < 0.01$; ***, $p < 0.001$.

(SD), and an independent Student's t-test was administered to analyze the statistical significance of differences between two groups. The one-way analysis of variance (ANOVA), followed by Dunnett's t post-hoc test or Tukey's test, was also performed on raw data. If data were not normally distributed, the Kruskall–Wallis test was performed, followed by Dunn's multiple comparison test. $p < 0.05$ was used to indicate statistical significance. All data were tested for normalization before analysis.

RESULTS

In vitro Assessment of the Toxicity of Dihydromyricetin

To evaluate the toxicity of DHM *in vitro*, we treated PMLFs and PHLFs with increasing concentrations (100–500 μM) of DHM for 36 h. Notably, the CCK-8 assay revealed that the IC50 of DHM was 628 μM in PMLFs (**Figure 2A**) and 7556 μM in PHLFs (**Figure 2B**). These results also suggested that the population of cells was nearly unchanged when the concentration of DHM was below 400 μM. These results indicated that DHM may be safe for clinical applications.

Dihydromyricetin Regulates the Differentiation of Fibroblasts to Myofibroblasts

The differentiation of fibroblasts to myofibroblasts is pivotal in the onset of pulmonary fibrosis, and myofibroblasts play important roles in the progression of pulmonary fibrosis (Peyser et al., 2019). Therefore, we evaluated the effects of DHM on the TGF-β1-stimulated differentiation of PMLFs and IPF-HLFs. The results of western blotting demonstrated that TGF-β1 stimulation significantly increased expression of the differentiation markers fibronectin, Col1a1, and α-SMA in PMLFs (**Figure 2C**). More interestingly, when compared to those in the N-HLFs, the levels of FIBRONECTIN, COL1A1, and α-SMA were much higher in the IPF-HLFs (**Figure 2D**). Moreover, DHM markedly suppressed the levels of these proteins in PMLFs stimulated with TGF-β1 and in IPF-HLFs. Furthermore, the degree to which differentiation was alleviated was greater in the group treated with DHM at a high concentration (300 μM) (**Figures 2C,D**). All these results revealed that DHM could not only attenuate the differentiation of fibroblasts to myofibroblasts induced by TGF-β1 but also lead to the dedifferentiation of IPF-HLFs, indicating that DHM may be effective for preventing pulmonary fibrosis and restoring the fibrotic lung tissue in clinical applications.

Dihydromyricetin Facilitates Fibroblast Migration and Proliferation

In addition to the functional effect of DHM on differentiation, its functional effects on migration and proliferation were assessed by the Transwell assay and EdU staining, respectively. The results of the Transwell assay revealed that the migration ability was much higher in myofibroblasts than in fibroblasts, but DHM at 300 μM remarkably suppressed the migration of PMLFs (**Figure 3A**) and PHLFs (**Figure 3B**) across the Transwell membrane. As shown by the EdU staining test, fewer EdU-positive cells were noted in the DHM treatment groups than in the untreated groups of PMLFs stimulated with TGF-β1 (**Figure 3C**). A similar result was also observed in the IPF-HLFs (**Figure 3D**). The proliferation function of the IPF-HLFs was much higher than that of the N-HLFs, and DHM remarkably suppressed the proliferation function of the IPF-HLFs.

Dihydromyricetin Decreased the Increased Oxygen Consumption Rate in IPF-HLFs

Patients with IPF exhibit symptoms of dyspnea and need supplemental oxygen treatment, so the oxygen consumption of myofibroblasts in fibroblastic foci and those in healthy areas may differ. Thus, the OCR was detected by the Seahorse XF Cell Mito Stress test. As we hypothesized, the OCR (especially the basal respiration and maximal respiration stage) of the IPF-HLFs was much higher than that of the N-HLFs, and DHM significantly suppressed the basal and maximal respiration (**Figure 3E**) in both N-HLFs and IPF-HLFs. However, the suppression rate appeared to be higher in N-HLFs than IPF-HLFs.

Dihydromyricetin Treatment Alleviated Pulmonary Fibrosis in a BLM Mouse Model

DHM has been proven to suppress the TGF-β1-induced differentiation of fibroblasts to myofibroblasts and regulate the differentiation of IPF-HLFs *in vitro*. To assess the effects of DHM *in vivo*, we established BLM-induced pulmonary fibrosis in mice, treated the mice with DHM, and assessed the degree of pulmonary fibrosis (**Figure 4A**). Intratracheal injection of BLM induced the destruction of the normal lung architecture and the formation of lung fibrosis, but lesions in the lung tissue induced by BLM were alleviated in the DHM-treated group, as evidenced by H&E and Masson and Sirius Red staining (**Figure 4B**). Furthermore, the Ashcroft score of the DHM-treated group was lower than that of the untreated group (**Figure 4C**). Additionally, similar results were also observed by assessment of the survival curves, and the DHM-treated group had a higher survival rate than the BLM group (**Figure 4D**).

To further assess the effects of DHM on pulmonary fibrosis, we detected the levels of fibrotic markers (α-SMA, Col1a1, and fibronectin) by western blot analysis. Treatment with DHM markedly decreased the expression of fibrotic markers at the protein level in the BLM-induced mice (**Figure 5A**). Consistently, the same changes were also observed by immunohistochemistry (**Supplementary Figure S1**) and coimmunofluorescence (**Figure 5B**). The mice treated with BLM and DHM exhibited much lower levels of α-SMA, Col1a1, and fibronectin than those treated with BLM alone.

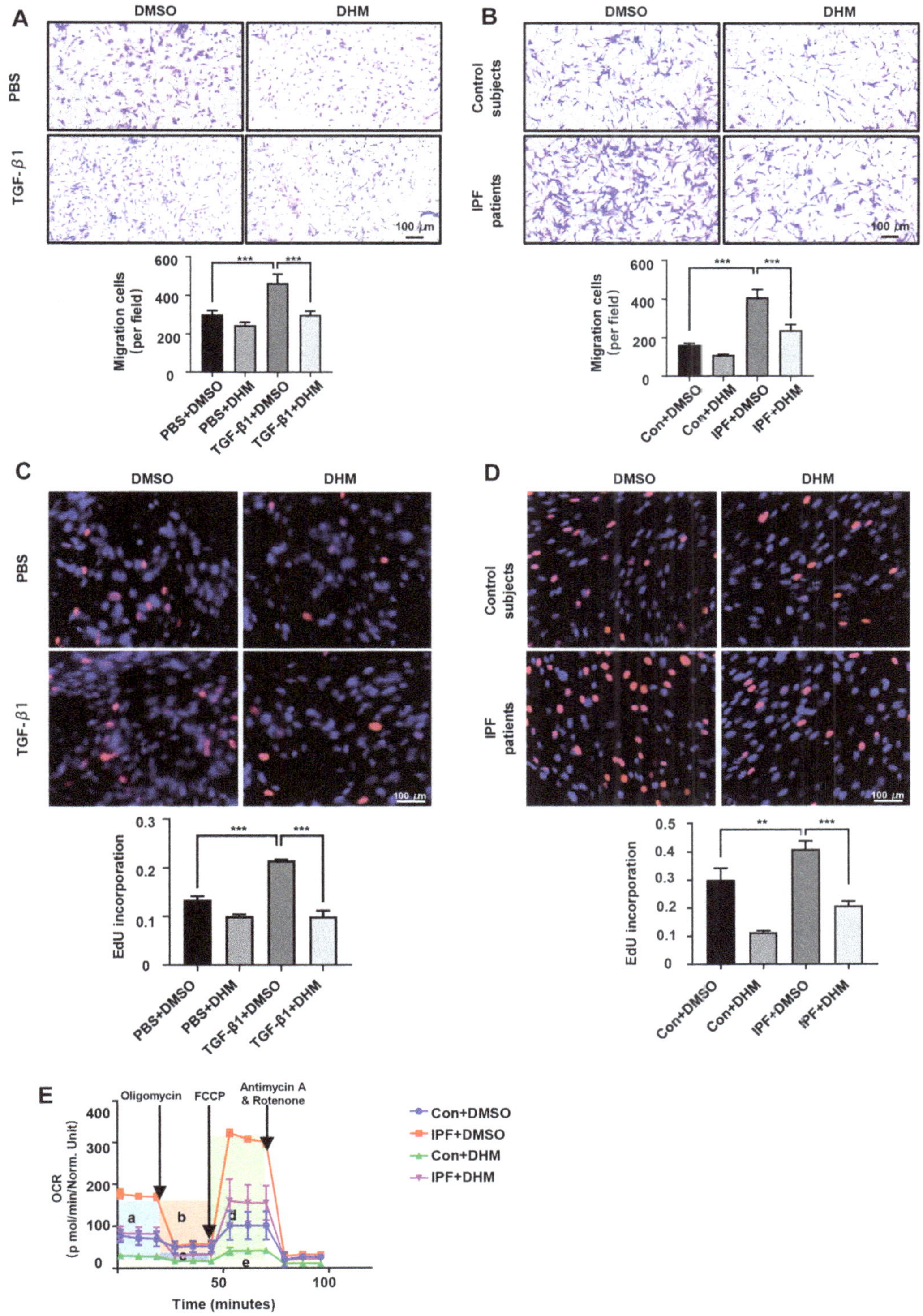

FIGURE 3 | Effects of DHM on the proliferation, migration, and respiratory functions of fibroblasts. **(A)** Results for the Transwell assay in PMLFs treated with DHM. Images were captured at 100 × magnification (n = 5). **(B)** Results for the Transwell assay in PHLFs treated with DHM. Images were captured at 100 × magnification (n = 5). **(C)** Results for EdU staining in PMLFs treated with DHM. Images were captured at 200 × magnification (n = 5). **(D)** Results for EdU staining in PHLFs treated with DHM. Images were captured at 200 × magnification (n = 5). **(E)** Cell Mito Stress test results of PLHMs with DHM (a: basal respiration, b: ATP production, c: proton leak, d: maximal respiration, e: nonmitochondrial respiration) (n = 3). The data are represented as the mean ± SD of three independent experiments. Ordinary one-way ANOVA analysis was applied. *, $p < 0.05$; **, $p < 0.01$; ***, $p < 0.001$.

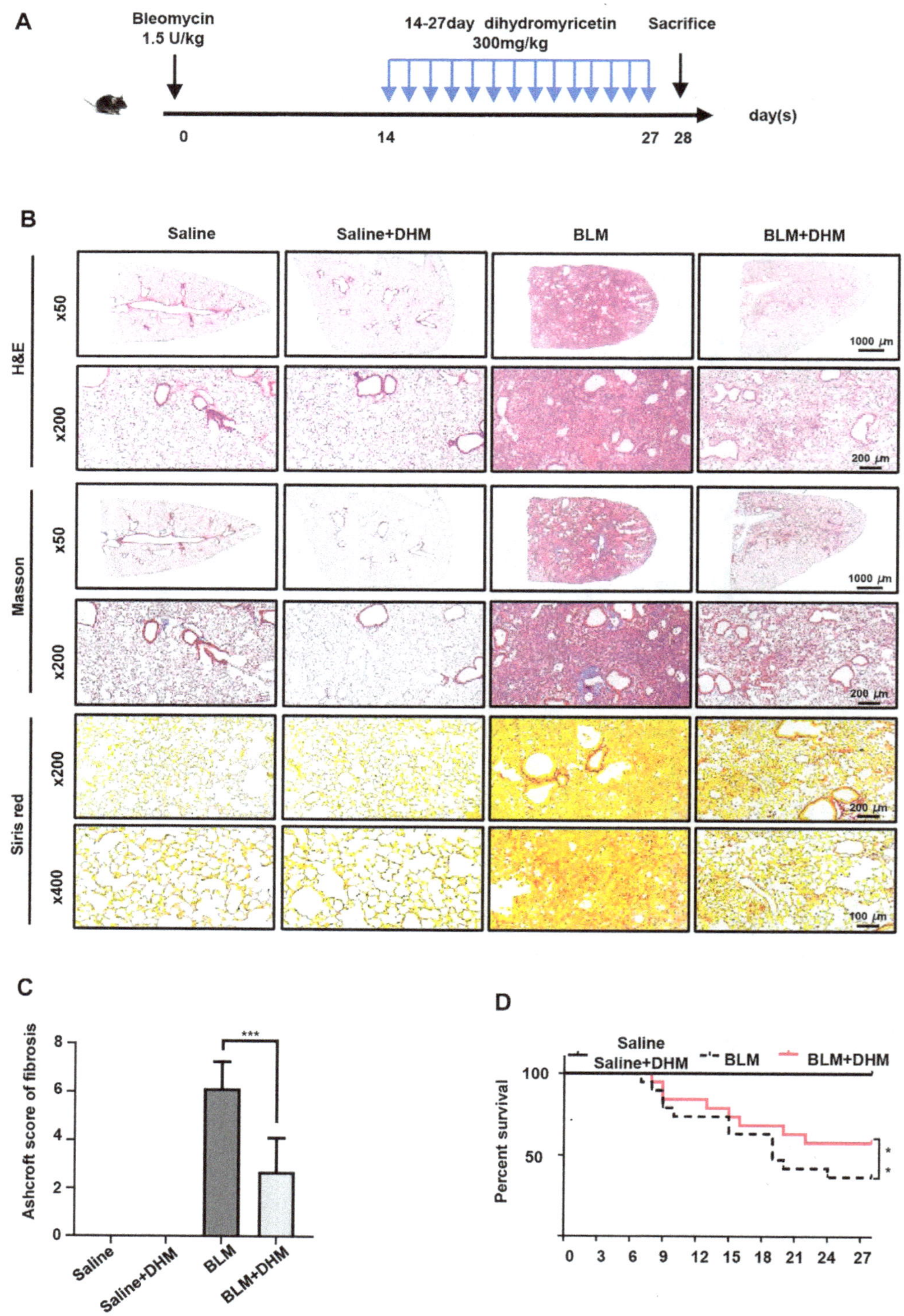

FIGURE 4 | Effects of DHM on the severity of lung fibrosis in mice after BLM induction. Saline $n = 6$, DHM $n = 6$, BLM $n = 6$, BLM + DHM $n = 6$. **(A)** Time course of BLM and DHM administration. **(B)** Histological analysis of the severity of lung fibrosis in mice after BLM induction. Images were captured at 50 ×, 200 ×, and 400 × magnification. **(C)** Ashcroft score in different groups of mice ($n = 6$). **(D)** Survival ratio in different groups of mice. The data are represented as the mean ± SD. Two-sided Student's t-test was applied. *, $p < 0.05$; **, $p < 0.01$; ***, $p < 0.001$.

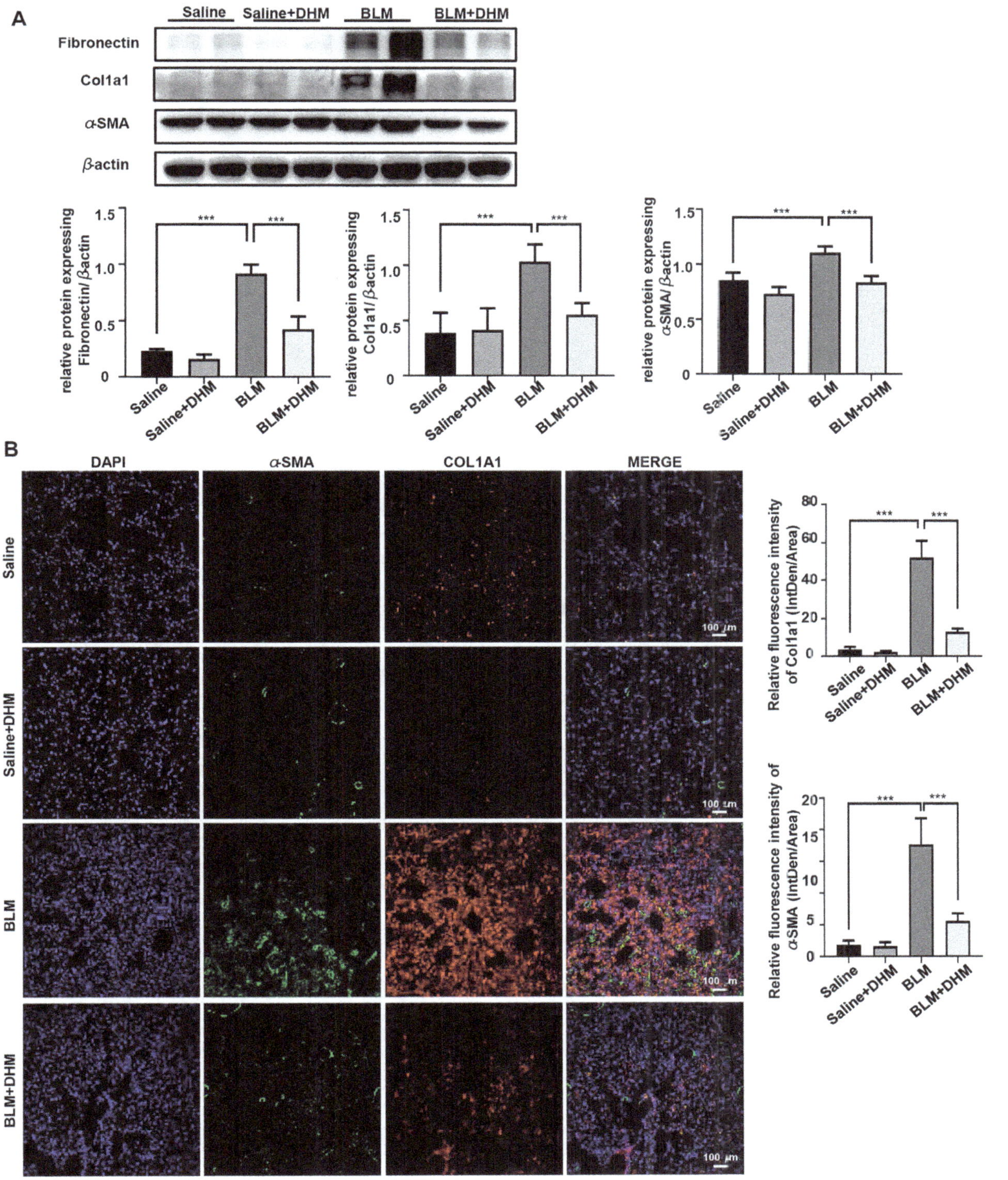

FIGURE 5 | Effects of DHM on fibrosis markers in mice after BLM induction. Saline $n = 6$, DHM $n = 6$, BLM $n = 6$, BLM + DHM $n = 6$. **(A)** Western blotting analysis of fibronectin, Col1a1, and α-SMA expression in the lung homogenate from different groups. **(B)** Coimmunostaining of Col1a1 and α-SMA in the lung sections from different groups. Images were captured at 200 × magnification. The data are represented as the mean ± SD. Ordinary one-way ANOVA analysis was applied. *, $p < 0.05$; **, $p < 0.01$; ***, $p < 0.001$.

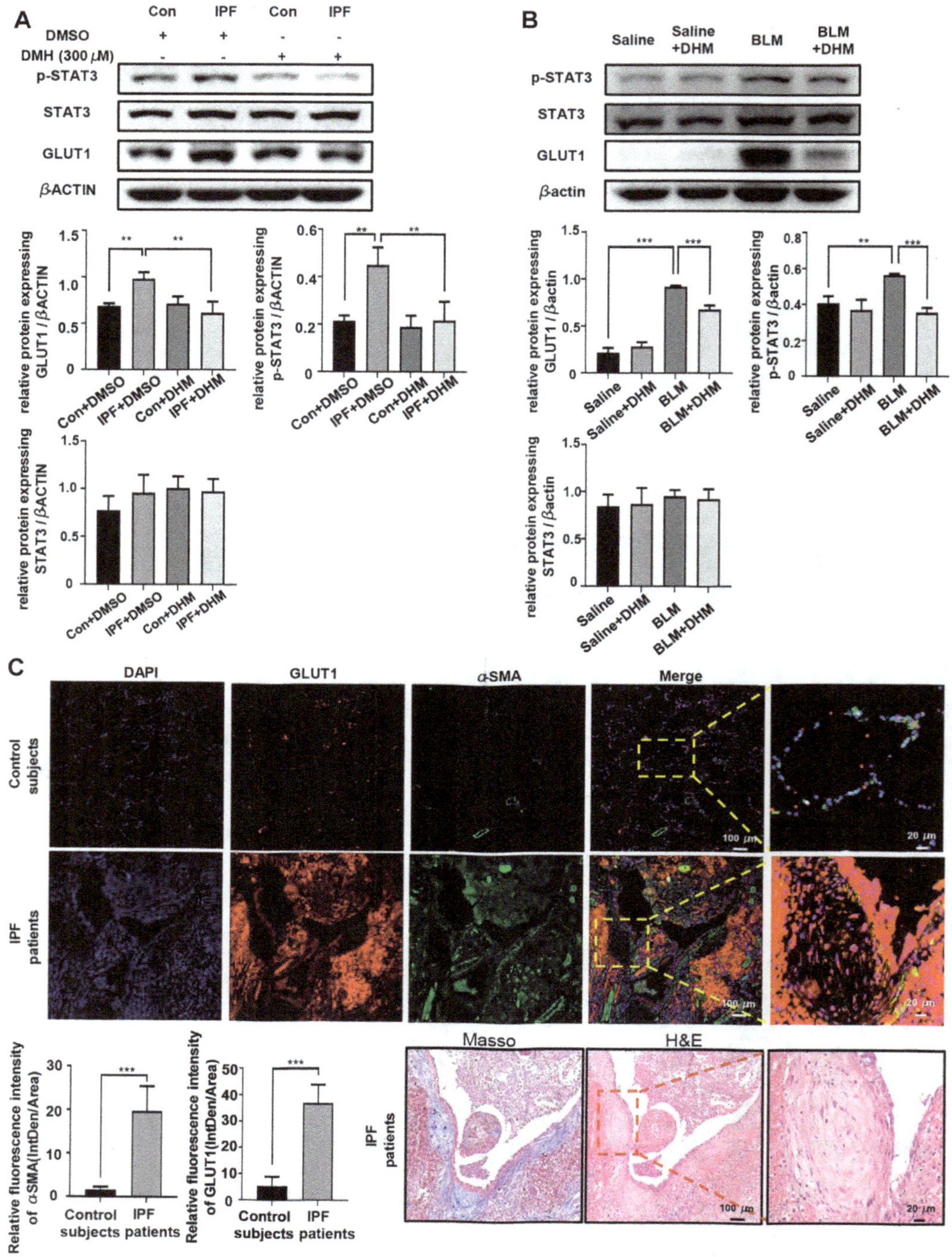

FIGURE 6 | DHM affects the expression of pSTAT3/GLUT1. **(A)** Western blotting analysis of the levels of STAT3/p-STAT3/GLUT1 in PHLFs treated with DHM (n = 5). **(B)** Western blotting analysis of the levels of STAT3/p-STAT3/GLUT1 in the DHM-treated mouse model (n = 5). **(C)** Representative images for coimmunostaining of GLUT1 and α-SMA in the lung sections from control subjects and IPF patients. Images were captured at 100 × and 400 × magnification (control subjects = 5, IPF = 8). Representative images for Masson and H&E stain of an IPF patient. The data are represented as the mean ± SD. Ordinary one-way ANOVA analysis was applied. *, $p < 0.05$; **, $p < 0.01$; ***, $p < 0.001$.

Although DHM was proven to be nontoxic *in vitro*, its toxic effects were also measured in mice. Excitingly, no obvious toxic effects of DHM on mice were observed, and no perceptible differences were found between the DHM group and the untreated group upon pathological staining of multiple organs, such as the heart, liver, spleen, and kidney (**Supplementary**

Figure S2A), and the determination of biochemical liver and kidney indices, such as aspartate aminotransferase (AST), aminotransferase (ALT), urea (UR), and serum creatinine (CR) levels (**Supplementary Figure S2B**). All these findings indicate that DHM was well tolerated and safe for treating pulmonary fibrosis in a BLM-induced mouse model.

Dihydromyricetin Regulates the STAT3/P-STAT3/GLUT1 Signaling Pathway

Because DHM could significantly suppress the increased OCR in myofibroblasts, DHM might regulate the glucose metabolism. Glucose transporter 1 (GLUT1), the most widely distributed glucose transporter in mammalian cells (Rylaarsdam et al., 2019), is critical for glycolysis and has been reported to be regulated by the STAT3/p-STAT3 signaling pathway (Shang et al., 2020). Previous studies have also demonstrated that the STAT3/p-STAT3 signaling pathway participates in the progression of fibrosis and that DHM can regulate the STAT3/p-STAT3 pathway (Li et al., 2017; Celada et al., 2018). Therefore, we hypothesized that the antifibrotic function of DHM might be achieved by regulation of the STAT3/pSTAT3/GLUT1 signaling pathway. To verify this hypothesis, western blotting was used to analyze the levels of STAT3, pSTAT3, and GLUT1. As expected, compared to those in N-HLFs, the levels of pSTAT3 and GLUT1 in IPF-HLFs were much higher, and DHM suppressed the expression of pSTAT3 and GLUT1 *in vitro* (**Figure 6A**). Similar results were also found *in vivo*. We observed that BLM administration remarkably induced the expression of pSTAT3 and GLUT1 in mouse lung tissues, while DHM treatment could effectively block this pathway and suppress the expression of both proteins (**Figure 6B**). To further confirm our findings, we tested the expression of GLUT1 in the lung tissues of IPF patients and control subjects by coimmunofluorescence (**Figure 6C**). The level of GLUT1 was significantly increased in IPF patients, especially GLUT1 levels in the fibrotic foci of lung tissues.

Colivelin, a brain-penetrant neuroprotective peptide and potent activator of p-STAT3 that was reported to significantly increase p-STAT3 protein levels in BV-2 cells (Fang and Zhang, 2021), was used to test the effects of DHM on the STAT3/p-STAT3/GLUT1 axis. Western blot analysis revealed that colivelin not only reversed the DHM-induced suppression of p-STAT3 and GLUT1 expression in IPF-HLFs but also promoted the expression of fibrotic markers (**Figure 7A**). As colivelin increased the expression of GLUT1, the OCR (**Figure 7B**) was also increased after treatment with colivelin. Further studies on the functions of IPF-HLFs found that the DHM-induced suppression of migration (**Figure 7C**) and proliferation (**Figure 7D**) was also abrogated after treatment with colivelin.

DISCUSSION

Our research showed that DHM could regulate the differentiation, migration, and proliferation functions of TGF-β1-stimulated fibroblasts and IPF-HLFs. DHM also alleviated BLM-induced pulmonary fibrosis in a mouse model (**Figure 8A**). Furthermore, regulation of the STAT3/p-STAT3/GLUT1 signaling pathway by DHM was found to be involved in this process (**Figure 8B**).

Before testing the effects of DHM on TGF-β1-induced fibroblasts and IPF-HLFs, we measured the toxicity of DHM in PMLFs and PHLFs. The CCK-8 assay was adopted to test the toxicity of DHM. Previous studies have suggested that the effective concentrations of DHM range from 1 to 200 μM *in vitro* and from 10 to 500 mg/kg/day *in vivo* (Zhang et al., 2018). Thus, in our research, five concentrations (100 μM, 200 μM, 300 μM, 400 μM, and 500 μM) were used. No obvious cell toxicity was observed at these concentrations. Interestingly, the toxicity of DHM was much lower in PHLFs than in PMLFs, suggesting that the activity in myofibroblasts might be greater than that in fibroblasts.

In recent studies on pulmonary fibrosis, TGF-β1 has been used to induce fibroblasts to differentiate into myofibroblasts. We also used 15 ng/ml TGF-β1 to stimulate PMLFs, and the concentration of DHM was set much lower than the IC50 value. Fibrotic markers (fibronectin, Col1a1, and α-SMA) were increased after TGF-β1 treatment, and these changes were suppressed by DHM in PMLFs. Although fibroblasts could be induced to differentiate into myofibroblasts by TGF-β1 *in vitro*, they did not completely imitate the functions of pulmonary myofibroblasts *in vivo* (Epstein et al., 2020). Then, we isolated IPF-HLFs and N-HLFs. Interestingly, the levels of fibrosis-associated proteins were much higher in IPF-HLFs than in N-HLFs, even without stimulation with TGF-β1. Treatment with DHM not only suppressed the expression of these proteins in PMLFs but also seemed to demonstrate stronger inhibitory effects in IPF-HLFs. These findings provide firm evidence that DHM did in fact regulate the differentiation of IPF-HLFs. In addition to differentiation, the abnormally elevated migration and proliferation of myofibroblasts are also considered important in the progression of pulmonary fibrosis (Wollin et al., 2015). In our research, we found that the proliferation and migration functions of IPF-HLFs were also much stronger than those of N-HLFs. DHM was also found to affect these functions. The increased migration and proliferation of TGF-β1-induced fibroblasts or IPF-HLFs were clearly attenuated with DHM treatment. Our findings obtained with PMLFs and PHLFs indicated that DHM could not only suppress the activation effects of TGF-β1 on fibroblasts but also regulate the functions of IPF-HLFs. All these results suggest DHM might be a multifunctional medicine for the prevention and treatment of pulmonary fibrosis.

Shortness of breath and increasing cough are the most common clinical symptoms of IPF in patients (Pleasants and Tighe, 2019). Both damage to the normal lung tissue and oxygen exchange dysfunction contribute to hypoxia and respiratory failure in these patients (Richeldi et al., 2017). Even though under hypoxic conditions, myofibroblasts in the lung tissue still maintain a highly proliferative state (Senavirathna et al., 2018), we wondered whether the abnormal metabolism is related to increased proliferation. As the main nutrient used in eukaryotic cell proliferation is glucose and the metabolism of

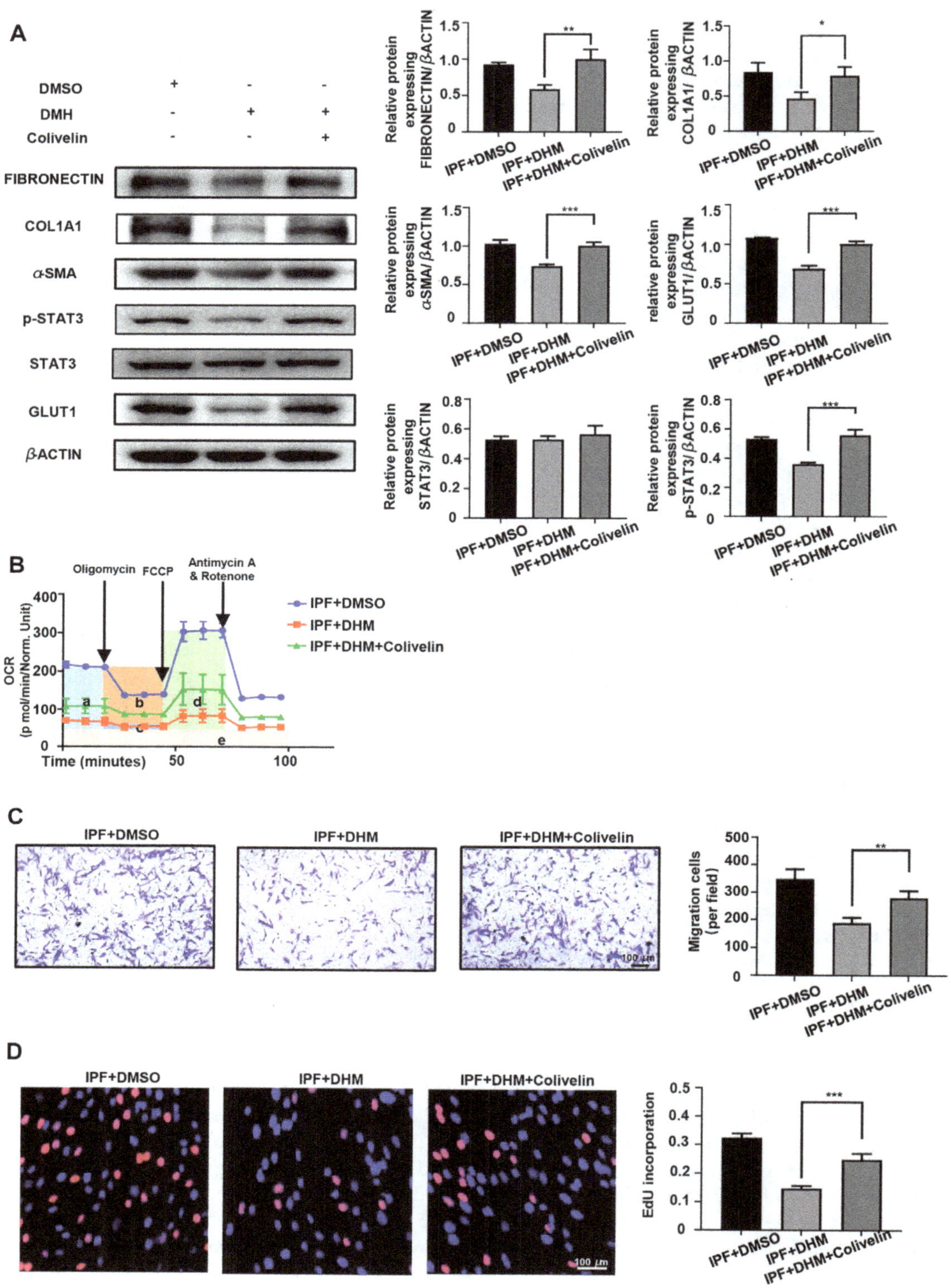

FIGURE 7 | Colivelin reversed the effect of DHM on PHLFs. **(A)** Western blotting analysis of the levels of fibronectin, COL1A1, α-SMA, and STAT3/p-STAT3/GLUT1 in colivelin-treated PHLFs (n = 5). **(B)** Cell Mito Stress test results of colivelin-treated PLHMs (a: basal respiration, b: ATP production, c: proton leak, d: maximal respiration, e: nonmitochondrial respiration) (n = 3). **(C)** Results for the Transwell assay in colivelin-treated PLHMs (n = 5). **(D)** Results for EdU staining in colivelin-treated PLHMs (n = 5). The data are represented as the mean ± SD of three independent experiments. Two-sided Student's t-test was applied. *, $p < 0.05$; **, $p < 0.01$; ***, $p < 0.001$.

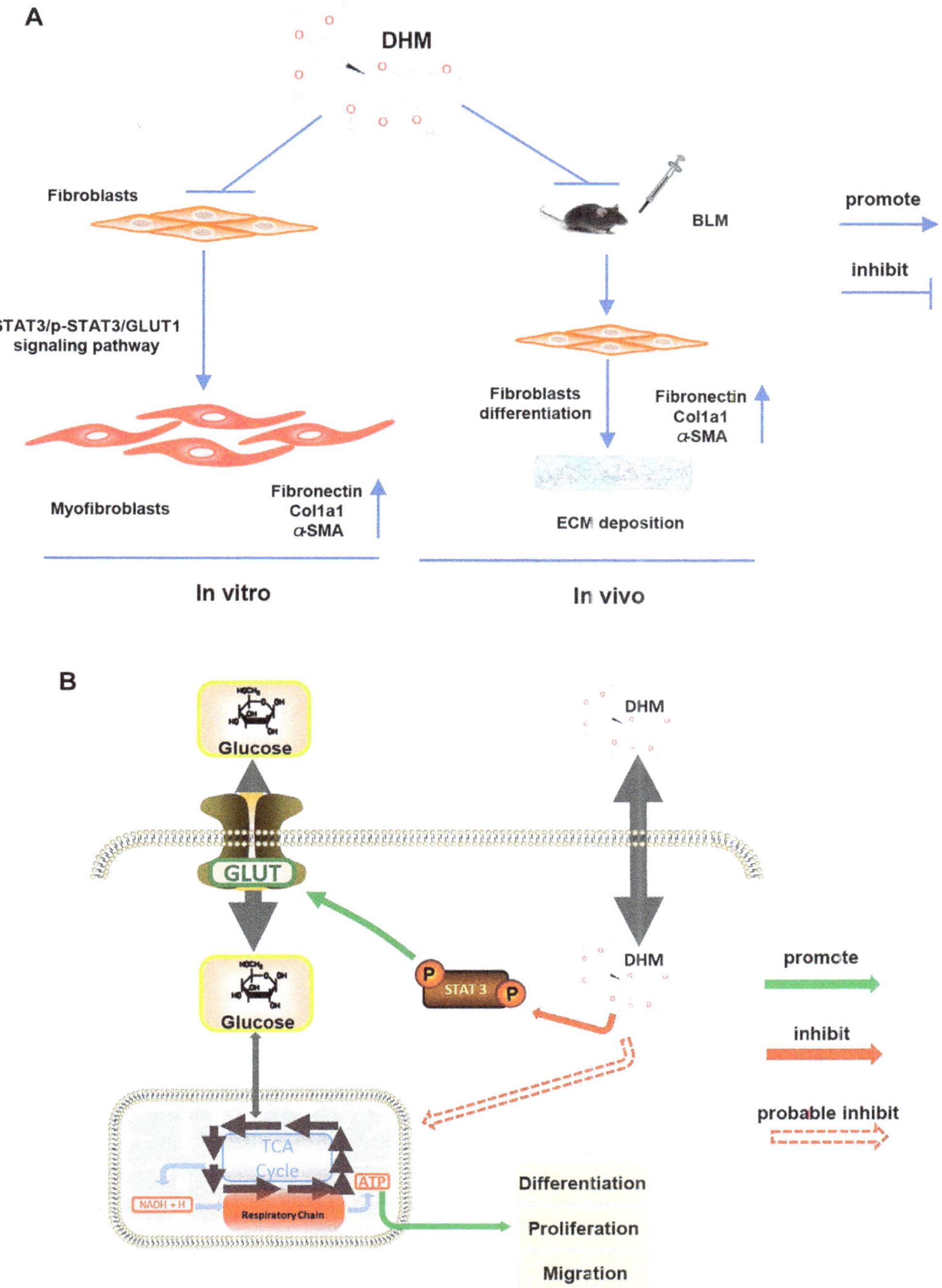

FIGURE 8 | Mechanism of DHM on pulmonary fibrosis. **(A)** Schematic presentation of the mechanism in pulmonary fibrosis affected by DHM: TGF-β1 could induce fibroblasts to differentiate into myofibroblasts and overexpress fibronectin, Col1a1, and α-SMA *in vitro*, while DHM could suppress this differentiation progress by inhibiting the STAT3/p-STAT3/Glut1 signaling pathway; DHM could also alleviate pulmonary fibrosis induced by BLM *via* suppressing the differentiation of fibroblasts in the mouse model. **(B)** Intracellular signaling pathway of DHM: phosphorylation of STAT3 could promote the expression of GLUT1 and enhance the production of ATP, which eventually lead to the differentiation, proliferation, and migration of fibroblasts; DHM could regulate these functions by inhibiting the phosphorylation of STAT3. DHM might also regulate the respiratory chain directly and lead to the suppression of differentiation, proliferation, and migration of fibroblasts.

glucose mainly occurs in the mitochondria, we used the Seahorse XF Cell Mito Stress test to detect the OCR in fibroblasts and myofibroblasts and the effects of DHM on the OCRs. As illustrated by the OCR results, basal respiration, ATP production, and maximal respiration were all increased in the IPF-HLFs compared with the N-HLFs. More importantly, DHM significantly attenuated these functions in both N-HLFs and IPF-HLFs. As previously mentioned, the N-HLFs were more suppressed than IPF-HLFs by DHM in the suppression rate, and this phenomenon might be caused by the antagonism between the antioxidative effects of DHM and the high expression of GLUT1 on IPF-HLFs. DHM might suppress the mitochondrial respiration directly on N-HLFs and IPF-HLFs (**Figure 8B**). However, on IPF-HLFs, the high expression of GLUT1 contributed to the increase of OCRs and weakened the suppression effects of DHM. This finding also suggested that GLUT1 might participate into the progression of pulmonary fibrosis by regulating mitochondrial respiratory.

After verifying the effects of DHM on TGF-β1-induced PMLFs and IPF-HLFs, we also detected the effects of DHM on BLM-induced pulmonary fibrosis in a mouse model. According to previous studies, DHM can suppress liver fibrosis and renal interstitial fibrosis by inhibiting inflammation and injury induced by TGF-β1. To determine the therapeutic effects of DHM on pulmonary fibrosis, DHM treatment was applied after the formation of pulmonary fibrosis in our experiment. As the expression of fibrogenic genes started increasing on the 7th day and peaked on the 14th day after intratracheal injection of BLM, DHM treatment was started at the fibrosis stage from the 14th day to the 27th day following BLM induction. The mice were sacrificed on the 28th day. To our delight, the mice in the BLM + DHM group demonstrated greater remission of pulmonary fibrosis than those in the BLM group. Notably, no differences in survival rates were observed between the BLM group and the treatment group over the first 14 days (the inflammation stage), but in the fibrosis stage, the treatment group exhibited higher survival rates than the BLM group. These results suggest that DHM treatment after the formation of fibrosis effectively alleviated pulmonary fibrosis and was well tolerated in the BLM-induced mouse model.

As found previously, an abnormal metabolism was present in IPF-HLFs, and the abnormal metabolism can drive myofibroblasts to proliferate and secrete ECM in excess, ultimately aggravating pulmonary fibrosis. This process is similar to the process by which growth and migration are driven by the aberrant metabolism in tumors (Park et al., 2020). Studies have found that the STAT3/p-STAT3/GLUT1 pathway is involved in the metabolism and proliferation of cancer cells (Xu et al., 2016; Nagarajan et al., 2017). In our study, DHM downregulated the levels of p-STAT3 and GLUT1 in myofibroblasts. Further investigation revealed that DHM also suppressed the increase in p-STAT3 and GLTU1 levels induced by BLM in the model mice. Many studies have demonstrated that TGF-β1 can promote fibrosis *via* the STAT3/p-STAT3 pathway (Chakraborty et al., 2017; Dees et al., 2020); however, few of these studies have explored the effects of abnormal STAT3/p-STAT3 expression on IPF-HLFs. Our research showed that even without TGF-β1 stimulation, the increase in p-STAT3 still aggravated the dysfunction of IPF-HLFs, and regulating the level of p-STAT3 modulated the functions of IPF-HLFs. Some research has indicated that upregulated expression of GLUT1 in fibroblasts and macrophages can exacerbate pulmonary fibrosis (El-Chemaly et al., 2013; Andrianifahanana et al., 2016), and the pathways in which GLUT1 is involved are mostly focused on inflammation. Hence, this might be the first study to show that GLUT1 is regulated by p-STAT3 in IPF-HLFs and that this regulation participates in the abnormal glucose metabolism. Coimmunofluorescence analysis of lung tissues from IPF patients illustrated that the expression of GLUT1 in myofibroblasts located in fibroblastic foci was remarkably increased; more interestingly, the blood supply around the fibroblastic foci was also remarkably increased. These abnormal lung tissue features also explain why even though IPF patients always suffer from hypoxia, the activity of myofibroblasts in their lung tissue remains at a high level and promotes the progression of fibrosis. To further confirm the regulatory effects of DHM on the STAT3/p-STAT3/GLUT1 pathway, colivelin was used to increase the expression of p-STAT3. As expected, colivelin specifically upregulated the expression of p-STAT3, and the expression of GLUT1 was subsequently increased. To our delight, the DHM-induced suppression of myofibroblast differentiation, proliferation, and migration was nearly reversed by colivelin in DHM and colivelin-treated cells. However, the suppressed respiration functions of IPF-HLFs by DHM were partially reversed by colivelin, and this might be related to the antioxidative effects of DHM and the direct effects of DHM on mitochondrial respiration. These findings suggest that the antifibrotic effects of DHM might mainly depend on the STAT3/p-STAT3/GLUT1 signaling pathway.

Although pirfenidone and nintedanib have been approved for the treatment of IPF, the outcomes of IPF patients are still not optimistic, and new treatments are urgently needed (Caminati et al., 2019). As traditional Chinese medicine has attracted increasing attention, studies have illustrated that some herbal extracts have antifibrotic effects by suppressing the inflammation and oxidative stress induced by cytokines such as IL-6 and TGF-β1 (Wang et al., 2020; Wang Z. et al., 2021), but few of these medicines have been proven effective in clinical IPF patients. In our study, we isolated IPF-HLFs from the lung tissues of IPF patients, and DHM effectively regulated the differentiation, migration, and proliferation of IPF-HLFs. This finding provides substantial evidence that DHM is a candidate medicinal treatment for IPF. More interestingly, our findings suggest that GLUT1 participates in the differentiation of fibroblasts in the development of pulmonary fibrosis. Similar changes were also found in cancer cells (Ancey et al., 2018) as GLUT1 was found to promote the proliferation and migration of cancer cells (Oh et al., 2017; Gonzalez-Menendez et al., 2018; Li et al., 2020) and the regulation of GLUT1 and the glucose metabolism could suppress the proliferation and migration of cancer cells (Liu et al., 2012; Zambrano et al., 2019; Heydarzadeh et al., 2020). All these findings have led to new targeted therapy for cancer treatment. Our findings suggest that DHM could alleviate pulmonary fibrosis by suppressing GLUT1 in mice and might also lead to a breakthrough in the treatment of IPF by regulating the glucose metabolism in fibroblasts.

Our study also has some limitations. Although no perceptible toxicities were detected *in vivo* or *in vitro* in our study, the blood concentration and pharmacokinetics of DHM remain unclear and should be investigated in the future. Second, DHM is a lipid-soluble drug, which limits the bioavailability of DHM. Thus, more research to improve the bioavailability of DHM is needed.

CONCLUSION

Our research suggests that DHM could alleviate pulmonary fibrosis *in vitro* and *in vivo via* the STAT3/p-STAT3/GLUT1 signaling pathway. The antifibrotic effects of DHM are achieved by regulating the abnormal glucose metabolism in myofibroblasts. This finding provides us with new insight indicating that metabolic therapy might be a breakthrough for IPF treatment. We would be delighted if our work could act as a sufficient theoretical basis for this new research direction.

AUTHOR CONTRIBUTIONS

ZL designed the study, made the experiments, collected and analyzed the data, and finished the manuscript. JG, BX, and JH participated in the collection of clinical data and samples of IPF patients and controls and the analysis of data. JW and LP participated in the design of the study and the analysis of data. YH participated the design of the study, the analysis of data, and the revision of the manuscript. CW and HD conceived the study, analyzed and interpreted the data, revised the article, and finally approved for the version to be published. All authors contributed to the article and approved the final version of the manuscript.

SUPPLEMENTARY MATERIAL

Supplementary Figure S1 | Immunohistochemistry of fibronectin, Col1a1, and α-SMA in the lung sections from different groups (n = 6).

Supplementary Figure S2 | Toxic effects of DHM on mice. **(A)** Histological analysis of the inflammation levels of multiorgans in different groups (n = 6). Images were captured at 100 × magnification. **(B)** Levels of biomarkers of the liver and kidney in different groups (n = 6). The data are represented as the mean ± SD. Two-sided Student's t-test was applied.

REFERENCES

Ancey, P. B., Contat, C., and Meylan, E. (2018). Glucose Transporters in Cancer - from Tumor Cells to the Tumor Microenvironment. *FEBS J.* 285 (16), 2926–2943. doi:10.1111/febs.14577

Andrianifahanana, M., Hernandez, D. M., Yin, X., Kang, J. H., Jung, M. Y., Wang, Y., et al. (2016). Profibrotic Up-Regulation of Glucose Transporter 1 by TGF-β Involves Activation of MEK and Mammalian Target of Rapamycin Complex 2 Pathways. *FASEB J.* 30 (11), 3733–3744. doi:10.1096/fj.201600428R

Ashcroft, T., Simpson, J. M., and Timbrell, V. (1988). Simple Method of Estimating Severity of Pulmonary Fibrosis on a Numerical Scale. *J. Clin. Pathol.* 41 (4), 467–470. doi:10.1136/jcp.41.4.467

Caminati, A., Lonati, C., Cassandro, R., Elia, D., Pelosi, G., Torre, O., et al. (2019). Comorbidities in Idiopathic Pulmonary Fibrosis: An Underestimated Issue. *Eur. Respir. Rev.* 28 (153), 190044. doi:10.1183/16000617.0044-2019

Celada, L. J., Kropski, J. A., Herazo-Maya, J. D., Luo, W., Creecy, A., Abad, A. T., et al. (2018). PD-1 Up-Regulation on CD4+ T Cells Promotes Pulmonary Fibrosis through STAT3-Mediated IL-17A and TGF-β1 Production. *Sci. Transl. Med.* 10 (460), eaar8356. doi:10.1126/scitranslmed.aar8356

Chakraborty, D., Šumová, B., Mallano, T., Chen, C. W., Distler, A., Bergmann, C., et al. (2017). Activation of STAT3 Integrates Common Profibrotic Pathways to Promote Fibroblast Activation and Tissue Fibrosis. *Nat. Commun.* 8 (1), 1130. doi:10.1038/s41467-017-01236-6

Chanda, D., Otoupalova, E., Smith, S. R., Volckaert, T., De Langhe, S. P., and Thannickal, V. J. (2019). Developmental Pathways in the Pathogenesis of Lung Fibrosis. *Mol. Aspects Med.* 65, 56–69. doi:10.1016/j.mam.2018.08.004

Dees, C., Pötter, S., Zhang, Y., Bergmann, C., Zhou, X., Luber, M., et al. (2020). TGF-β-Induced Epigenetic Deregulation of SOCS3 Facilitates STAT3 Signaling to Promote Fibrosis. *J. Clin. Invest.* 130 (5), 2347–2363. doi:10.1172/JCI122462

El-Chemaly, S., Malide, D., Yao, J., Nathan, S. D., Rosas, I. O., Gahl, W. A., et al. (2013). Glucose Transporter-1 Distribution in Fibrotic Lung Disease: Association with [^{18}F]-2-fluoro-2-Deoxyglucose-PET Scan Uptake, Inflammation, and Neovascularization. *Chest* 143 (6), 1685–1691. doi:10.1378/chest.12-1359

Epstein, S. G., Brook, E., Bardenstein-Wald, B., and Shitrit, D. (2020). TGF-β Pathway Activation by Idiopathic Pulmonary Fibrosis (IPF) Fibroblast Derived Soluble Factors Is Mediated by IL-6 Trans-Signaling. *Respir. Res.* 21 (1), 56. doi:10.1186/s12931-020-1319-0

Fang, Y. Y., and Zhang, J. H. (2021). MFG-E8 Alleviates Oxygen-Glucose Deprivation-Induced Neuronal Cell Apoptosis by STAT3 Regulating the Selective Polarization of Microglia. *Int. J. Neurosci.* 131 (1), 15–24. doi:10.1080/00207454.2020.1732971

Gonzalez-Menendez, P., Hevia, D., Alonso-Arias, R., Alvarez-Artime, A., Rodriguez-Garcia, A., Kinet, S., et al. (2018). GLUT1 Protects Prostate Cancer Cells from Glucose Deprivation-Induced Oxidative Stress. *Redox Biol.* 17, 112–127. doi:10.1016/j.redox.2018.03.017

Heukels, P., Moor, C. C., von der Thüsen, J. H., Wijsenbeek, M. S., and Kool, M. (2019). Inflammation and Immunity in IPF Pathogenesis and Treatment. *Respir. Med.* 147, 79–91. doi:10.1016/j.rmed.2018.12.015

Heydarzadeh, S., Moshtaghie, A. A., Daneshpoor, M., and Hedayati, M. (2020). Regulators of Glucose Uptake in Thyroid Cancer Cell Lines. *Cell Commun. Signal.* 18 (1), 83. doi:10.1186/s12964-020-00586-x

Lederer, D. J., and Martinez, F. J. (2018). Idiopathic Pulmonary Fibrosis. *N. Engl. J. Med.* 378 (19), 1811–1823. doi:10.1056/NEJMra1705751

Li, C., Chen, Q., Zhou, Y., Niu, Y., Wang, X., Li, X., et al. (2020). S100A2 Promotes Glycolysis and Proliferation *via* GLUT1 Regulation in Colorectal Cancer. *FASEB J.* 34 (10), 13333–13344. doi:10.1096/fj.202000555R

Li, Q., Wang, J., Zhu, X., Zeng, Z., Wu, X., Xu, Y., et al. (2017). Dihydromyricetin Prevents Monocrotaline-Induced Pulmonary Arterial Hypertension in Rats. *Biomed. Pharmacother.* 96, 825–833. doi:10.1016/j.biopha.2017.10.007

Liu, Y., Bi, X., Xiong, J., Han, W., Xiao, T., Xu, X., et al. (2019). MicroRNA-34a Promotes Renal Fibrosis by Downregulation of Klotho in Tubular Epithelial Cells. *Mol. Ther.* 27 (5), 1051–1065. doi:10.1016/j.ymthe.2019.02.009

Liu, Y., Cao, Y., Zhang, W., Bergmeier, S., Qian, Y., Akbar, H., et al. (2012). A Small-Molecule Inhibitor of Glucose Transporter 1 Downregulates Glycolysis, Induces Cell-Cycle Arrest, and Inhibits Cancer Cell Growth *In Vitro* and *In Vivo*. *Mol. Cancer Ther.* 11 (8), 1672–1682. doi:10.1158/1535-7163.MCT-12-0131

Miao, K., Pan, T., Mou, Y., Zhang, L., Xiong, W., Xu, Y., et al. (2020). Scutellarein Inhibits BLM-Mediated Pulmonary Fibrosis by Affecting Fibroblast Differentiation, Proliferation, and Apoptosis. *Ther. Adv. Chronic Dis.* 11, 2040622320940185. doi:10.1177/2040622320940185

Nagarajan, A., Dogra, S. K., Sun, L., Gandotra, N., Ho, T., Cai, G., et al. (2017). Paraoxonase 2 Facilitates Pancreatic Cancer Growth and Metastasis by Stimulating GLUT1-Mediated Glucose Transport. *Mol. Cel* 67 (4), 685–701. doi:10.1016/j.molcel.2017.07.014

Oh, S., Kim, H., Nam, K., and Shin, I. (2017). Glut1 Promotes Cell Proliferation, Migration and Invasion by Regulating Epidermal Growth Factor Receptor and Integrin Signaling in Triple-Negative Breast Cancer Cells. *BMB Rep.* 50 (3), 132–137. doi:10.5483/bmbrep.2017.50.3.189

Otoupalova, E., Smith, S., Cheng, G., and Thannickal, V. J. (2020). Oxidative Stress in Pulmonary Fibrosis. *Compr. Physiol.* 10 (2), 509–547. doi:10.1002/cphy.c190017

Park, J. H., Pyun, W. Y., and Park, H. W. (2020). Cancer Metabolism: Phenotype, Signaling and Therapeutic Targets. *Cells* 9 (10), 2308. doi:10.3390/cells9102308

Peyser, R., Macdonnell, S., Gao, Y., Cheng, L., Kim, Y., Kaplan, T., et al. (2019). Defining the Activated Fibroblast Population in Lung Fibrosis Using Single-Cell Sequencing. *Am. J. Respir. Cel Mol Biol* 61 (1), 74–85. doi:10.1165/rcmb.2018-0313OC

Pleasants, R., and Tighe, R. M. (2019). Management of Idiopathic Pulmonary Fibrosis. *Ann. Pharmacother.* 53 (12), 1238–1248. doi:10.1177/1060028019862497

Raghu, G., Remy-Jardin, M., Myers, J., Richeldi, L., and Wilson, K. C. (2019). The 2018 Diagnosis of Idiopathic Pulmonary Fibrosis Guidelines: Surgical Lung Biopsy for Radiological Pattern of Probable Usual Interstitial Pneumonia Is Not Mandatory. *Am. J. Respir. Crit. Care Med.* 200 (9), 1089–1092. doi:10.1164/rccm.201907-1324ED

Richeldi, L., Collard, H. R., and Jones, M. G. (2017). Idiopathic Pulmonary Fibrosis. *Lancet* 389 (10082), 1941–1952. doi:10.1016/S0140-6736(17)30866-8

Rylaarsdam, L. E., Johnecheck, G. N., Looyenga, B. D., and Louters, L. L. (2019). GLUT1 Is Associated with Sphingolipid-Organized, Cholesterol-Independent Domains in L929 Mouse Fibroblast Cells. *Biochimie* 162, 88–96. doi:10.1016/j.biochi.2019.04.010

Senavirathna, L. K., Huang, C., Yang, X., Munteanu, M. C., Sathiaseelan, R., Xu, D., et al. (2018). Hypoxia Induces Pulmonary Fibroblast Proliferation through NFAT Signaling. *Sci. Rep.* 8 (1), 2709. doi:10.1038/s41598-018-21073-x

Shang, R., Wang, M., Dai, B., Du, J., Wang, J., Liu, Z., et al. (2020). Long Noncoding RNA SLC2A1-AS1 Regulates Aerobic Glycolysis and Progression in Hepatocellular Carcinoma *via* Inhibiting the STAT3/FOXM1/GLUT1 Pathway. *Mol. Oncol.* 14 (6), 1381–1396. doi:10.1002/1878-0261.12666

Wang, Q., Liu, J., Hu, Y., Pan, T., Xu, Y., Yu, J., et al. (2021). Local Administration of Liposomal-Based Srpx2 Gene Therapy Reverses Pulmonary Fibrosis by Blockading Fibroblast-To-Myofibroblast Transition. *Theranostics* 11 (14), 7110–7125. doi:10.7150/thno.61085

Wang, Q., Yu, J., Hu, Y., Chen, X., Zhang, L., Pan, T., et al. (2020). Indirubin Alleviates Bleomycin-Induced Pulmonary Fibrosis in Mice by Suppressing Fibroblast to Myofibroblast Differentiation. *Biomed. Pharmacother.* 131, 110715. doi:10.1016/j.biopha.2020.110715

Wang, Y., Zhang, L., Wu, G.-R., Zhou, Q., Yue, H., Rao, L.-Z., et al. (2021). MBD2 Serves as a Viable Target against Pulmonary Fibrosis by Inhibiting Macrophage M2 Program. *Sci. Adv.* 7 (1), eabb6075. doi:10.1126/sciadv.abb6075

Wang, Z., Li, X., Chen, H., Han, L., Ji, X., Wang, Q., et al. (2021). Resveratrol Alleviates Bleomycin-Induced Pulmonary Fibrosis *via* Suppressing HIF-1α and NF-κB Expression. *Aging (Albany NY)* 13 (3), 4605–4616. doi:10.18632/aging.202420

Wei, P., Xie, Y., Abel, P. W., Huang, Y., Ma, Q., Li, L., et al. (2019). Transforming Growth Factor (TGF)-β1-Induced miR-133a Inhibits Myofibroblast Differentiation and Pulmonary Fibrosis. *Cell Death Dis* 10 (9), 670. doi:10.1038/s41419-019-1873-x

Wollin, L., Wex, E., Pautsch, A., Schnapp, G., Hostettler, K. E., Stowasser, S., et al. (2015). Mode of Action of Nintedanib in the Treatment of Idiopathic Pulmonary Fibrosis. *Eur. Respir. J.* 45 (5), 1434–1445. doi:10.1183/09031936.00174914

Wolters, P. J., Collard, H. R., and Jones, K. D. (2014). Pathogenesis of Idiopathic Pulmonary Fibrosis. *Annu. Rev. Pathol.* 9, 157–179. doi:10.1146/annurev-pathol-012513-104706

Xu, D. D., Zhou, P. J., Wang, Y., Zhang, L., Fu, W. Y., Ruan, B. B., et al. (2016). Reciprocal Activation between STAT3 and miR-181b Regulates the Proliferation of Esophageal Cancer Stem-Like Cells *via* the CYLD Pathway. *Mol. Cancer* 15 (1), 40. doi:10.1186/s12943-016-0521-7

Zambrano, A., Molt, M., Uribe, E., and Salas, M. (2019). Glut 1 in Cancer Cells and the Inhibitory Action of Resveratrol as A Potential Therapeutic Strategy. *Int. J. Mol. Sci.* 20 (13), 3374. doi:10.3390/ijms20133374

Zehender, A., Huang, J., Györfi, A. H., Matei, A. E., Trinh-Minh, T., Xu, X., et al. (2018). The Tyrosine Phosphatase SHP2 Controls TGFβ-Induced STAT3 Signaling to Regulate Fibroblast Activation and Fibrosis. *Nat. Commun.* 9 (1), 3259. doi:10.1038/s41467-018-05768-3

Zhang, J., Chen, Y., Luo, H., Sun, L., Xu, M., Yu, J., et al. (2018). Recent Update on the Pharmacological Effects and Mechanisms of Dihydromyricetin. *Front. Pharmacol.* 9, 1204. doi:10.3389/fphar.2018.01204

Zhou, X., Yu, L., Zhou, M., Hou, P., Yi, L., and Mi, M. (2021). Dihydromyricetin Ameliorates Liver Fibrosis *via* Inhibition of Hepatic Stellate Cells by Inducing Autophagy and Natural Killer Cell-Mediated Killing Effect. *Nutr. Metab. (Lond)* 18 (1), 64. doi:10.1186/s12986-021-00589-6

14

Obesity and the Development of Lung Fibrosis

Xia Guo[†]*, Christudas Sunil*[†] *and Guoqing Qian* *

Department of Cellular and Molecular Biology, The University of Texas Health Science Center at Tyler, The University of Texas at Tyler, Tyler, TX, United States

Correspondence:
Guoqing Qian
guoqing.qian@uthct.edu

[†]*These authors have contributed equally to this work*

Obesity is an epidemic worldwide and the obese people suffer from a range of respiratory complications including fibrotic changes in the lung. The influence of obesity on the lung is multi-factorial, which is related to both mechanical injury and various inflammatory mediators produced by excessive adipose tissues, and infiltrated immune cells. Adiposity causes increased production of inflammatory mediators, for example, cytokines, chemokines, and adipokines, both locally and in the systemic circulation, thereby rendering susceptibility to respiratory diseases, and altered responses. Lung fibrosis is closely related to chronic inflammation in the lung. Current data suggest a link between lung fibrosis and diet-induced obesity, although the mechanism remains incomplete understood. This review summarizes findings on the association of lung fibrosis with obesity, highlights the role of several critical inflammatory mediators (e.g., TNF-α, TGF-β, and MCP-1) in obesity related lung fibrosis and the implication of obesity in the outcomes of idiopathic pulmonary fibrosis patients.

Keywords: obesity, lung, fibrosis, inflammation, high-fat diet

INTRODUCTION

In the past three decades, the prevalence of obesity has been increasing worldwide. Those obese people suffer from a range of respiratory complications, including asthma, airway hyperresponsiveness, chronic obstructive pulmonary disease, and lung fibrosis (Dixon and Peters, 2018; Hales et al., 2018). The influence of obesity on the lung is multi-factorial that involves both mechanical injury and the roles of various inflammatory mediators produced by excessive adipose tissues and infiltrated immune cells. Adiposity causes increased production of inflammatory mediators, for example, cytokines, chemokines, and adipokines, both locally and in the systemic circulation, and thereby rendering susceptibility to respiratory diseases and altered responses. The effects of obesity on lung function (Salome et al., 2010; Dixon and Peters, 2018), asthma (Peters et al., 2018), and chronic obstructive pulmonary disease (COPD) (Hanson et al., 2014) have been reviewed previously and will not discussed here. In this review, we provide updates on the link between obesity and lung fibrosis with a focus on the critical role of several inflammatory mediators implicated in the development of lung fibrosis associated with obesity.

ASSOCIATION OF OBESITY WITH LUNG FIBROSIS

Obesity contributes to the fibrosis of different organs including the lung (Pessin and Kwon, 2012), the liver (Chiang et al., 2011), the heart (Cavalera et al., 2014), the kidney (Deji et al., 2009; Laurentius et al., 2019;

Abbreviations: DIO, diet-induced obesity; HFD, high-fat diet; HFHF, high-fat high-fructose diet; IPF, idiopathic pulmonary fibrosis; MCP-1, monocyte chemoattractant protein-1; TGF-β, transforming growth factor-β; TNF-α, tumor necrosis factor-α.

Liu et al., 2019), and the adipose tissue (Buechler et al., 2015; Marcelin et al., 2019). Pulmonary fibrosis is the progressive scarring of the lung, leading to lung structure remodeling, and respiratory functional impairment. High intake of saturated fatty acids and meat increases the risk of idiopathic pulmonary fibrosis (IPF) (Miyake et al., 2006), a most common form of interstitial lung disease. Observational studies suggest a significant link between obesity and IPF (Miyake et al., 2006; Lee et al., 2014; Pessin and Kwon, 2012). One study shows that IPF patients are approximately twice more frequent to have obesity compared to normal control subjects (Lee et al., 2014). In addition, several risk factors for IPF such as gastro-esophageal reflux, obstructive sleep apnea, and diabetes mellitus are also closely associated with obesity (Anand and Katz, 2010; Zaman and Lee, 2018). Chronic inflammation is considered important in the pathogenesis of lung fibrosis through regulating production of cytokines/chemokines (e.g., tumor necrosis factor-alpha (TNF-α), Interleukins (ILs), and monocyte chemoattractant protein-1 (MCP-1), etc.) and growth factors (e.g., transforming growth factor beta (TGF-β), connective tissue growth factor, and platelet-derived growth factor, etc.) from macrophages and modulating matrix (e.g., via MMP-2), vasculature, growth-factor receptor, and oxidative stress status (Bringardner et al., 2008; Sgalla et al., 2018). Increasing *in vivo* evidence has linked diet-induced obesity (DIO) with lung fibrosis, as determined by collagen deposition or hydroxyproline content (Naura et al., 2009; Ge et al., 2013; Yu et al., 2013, Song et al., 2015; Baack et al., 2016; Chu et al., 2019; Park et al., 2019; Vedova et al., 2019; Han et al., 2021; Hegab et al., 2021) (**Table 1**). Different inflammatory mediators as well as immune cells are involved in high-fat diet (HFD)-induced lung fibrosis. Recently, vitamin D deficiency has also been suggested as a link between obesity and pulmonary fibrosis. HFD decreased serum 25-hydroxyl vitamin D level and induced lung fibrosis as well as TGF-β1 and phosphorylated Smad2/3 in the lungs of mice. Vitamin D supplementation attenuated these changes caused by HFD in C57BL/6 mice. *In vitro* treatment of bronchial epithelial cells BEAS-2B with vitamin D also suppressed TGF-β1 protein expression (Han et al., 2021). The induction of lung fibrosis by diet also seems to be time dependent. For example, feeding mice with a HFD rich in palmitic acid for 2 weeks did not induce obvious pulmonary inflammation or fibrosis although it promoted bleomycin induced pulmonary fibrosis (Chu et al., 2019). Our recent work shows that a high-fat and high-fructose (HFHF) diet promotes inflammatory infiltration in the lungs of C56BL/6 mice after 10- and 20-weeks' treatment. Conversely, collagen deposition in the lung tissues as determined by Masson's staining and Western blotting analysis was found to be prominent only after 20 weeks but not 10 weeks (Qian et al., 2021).

The impact of maternal exposure to HFD on the development of lung in offspring is of emerging interest. Maternal exposure to high-fat diet has been shown to impair lung development in the rat offspring, however, no significant changes in fibrosis was observed in offspring at 3 weeks after birth (Baack et al., 2016). In contrast, another study by Song et al. reported opposite results (Song et al., 2015). Maternal Sprague-Dawley rats were given either high-fat diet or standard diet after weaning and throughout pregnancy and lactation. The offspring were maintained on regular diet and evaluated for the lung histology after 3 months. Offspring with maternal HFD feeding showed increased body weight at birth and at 3 months, enhanced inflammatory infiltration and collagen deposition as well as TGF-β1 expression in the lungs. The discrepancy might relate to the different timing of examination after birth. The effect of maternal obesity on lung fibrosis of offspring remains less understood and further research is needed.

ROLE OF INFLAMMATORY MEDIATORS IN DIET INDUCED LUNG FIBROSIS

Tumor Necrosis Factor-α

Mounting evidence show the elevated TNF-α in the adipose tissue and the lung in high-fat diet induced obesity. TNF-α plays a critical role in mediating insulin resistance associated with high-fat diet and targeting TNF-α increases insulin sensitivity (Hotamisligil et al., 1993; Tzanavari et al., 2010). The signaling of TNF-α through its receptors seems to be essential in pulmonary fibrosis development. Knockout of TNF-α receptor provides protection of mice against pulmonary fibrosis caused by bleomycin, asbestos, and silica (Liu et al., 1998; Ortiz et al., 1998; Ortiz et al., 1999). In addition, blocking TNF-α with quenching antibody attenuates pulmonary fibrosis induced by bleomycin and silica in mice (Piguet et al., 1989; Piguet et al., 1990). Soluble TNF-α was thought important for transition from inflammation to fibrosis in the lung that involves recruitment of lymphocytes (Oikonomou et al., 2006). In accord, a soluble receptor for TNF-α was shown to alleviate bleomycin-induced pulmonary fibrosis (Piguet and Vesin, 1994). Therefore, endogenous TNF-α and its receptors seem to be required for the development of lung fibrosis.

A previous study showed that overexpression of TNF-α induces mild pulmonary fibrosis in rats (Sime et al., 1998). Similarly, direct intratracheal administration of TNF-α into wild-type mice also results in the expression of ICAM-1, VCAM-1, IL-1β, MCP-1, as well as TGF-β1, and collagen type I (Naura et al., 2009), a pattern of changes in the lung resembling that found in ApoE−/− mice fed a high-fat diet, suggesting a potential role of TNF-α in lung injury, and fibrosis associated with obesity. On the other hand, conflicting evidence suggest an anti-fibrotic role of TNF-α in different contexts. For instance, the transgenic TNF-α mice that overexpress murine TNF-α under the control of the human surfactant protein C promoter (Miyazaki et al., 1995) are more tolerant to bleomycin or active TGF-β1 induced pulmonary fibrosis (Fujita et al., 2003). Administration of recombinant human TNF-α also attenuates bleomycin-induced pulmonary fibrosis in mice (Fujita et al., 2003). In addition, intratracheal delivery of TNF-α facilitates the resolution of established pulmonary fibrosis induced by bleomycin (Redente et al., 2014). The author proposed that locally increased TNF-α might cause apoptosis of profibrotic macrophages, important in pathogenesis of pulmonary fibrosis through secretion of TGF-β1, IGF-1, PDGF, and arginase I. These microphages could also contribute to the pool of myofibroblasts via trans-differentiation (Gibbons et al., 2011). The controversial role of TNF-α in lung fibrosis has been discussed previously (Distler et al., 2008). Some clues might help understand this discrepancy, e.g., the stage-specific changes in inflammation profile (early-stage inflammation versus late-stage resolution and fibrosis), the requirement of inflammation and importantly, TNF-α,

TABLE 1 | Summary of studies linking obesity and pulmonary fibrosis.

Author (year)	Study model	Main findings associated with HFD
Ge et al. (2013)	SD/HFD feeding of C57BL/6 mice for 12 weeks (60% kcal from fat), followed by challenge with cockroach allergen.	Elevated lung TGF-β, PAI-1 expression, lung collagen expression, and decreased lung function. Infiltrated immune cells, epithelial, and endothelial cells were found as a major source of TGF-β expression.
Park et al. (2019)	SD/HFD feeding of C57BL/6 mice for 12 weeks (60% kcal from fat).	Increased insulin resistance, AHR, peribranchial and perivascular fibrosis, and macrophages in the BAL; insulin stimulates TGF-β1 expression in bronchial epithelial cells *in vivo* and *in vitro*; Anti-TGF-β1 antibody attenuated HFD-induced lung fibrosis.
Hegab et al. (2021)	SD/HFD feeding (60% kcal from fat) for 4 weeks, followed by bleomycin challenge and examine after 3, 6, and 9 weeks.	No significant differences in inflammation and fibrosis severity between SD and HFD-fed flies after 3 weeks; HFD-induced a delay in alveolar repair and fibrosis resolution at 6 weeks following bleomycin treatment.
Naura et al. (2009)	SD/HFD feeding for 12 weeks (42% kcal from fat) in ApoE−/− mice; direct intratracheal TNF-α (100 ng/mouse) administration in ApoE−/− mice for 6 and 24 h.	Elevated TNF-α, IFN-γ, and MIP-1α and increased tissue distribution of TGF-β, recruitment of monocytes and macrophages, subepithelial, and perivascular collagen deposition and thickening in lungs of ApoE−/− mice. TNF-α induced proinflammatory cytokines similar as that of HFD and induced MCP-1, TGF-β1, IL-1β, and collagen type 1 expression.
Yu et al. (2013)	HFD (Lieber-DeCarli liquid diet) feeding of male Sprague-Dawley (SD) rats for 8 weeks	Increased TGF-β expression in lung tissues and deposition of collagen fibers at alveolar septa in HFD group.
Han et al. (2021)	SD/HFD feeding of C57BL/6 mice for 12 weeks (60% kcal from fat)	Increased BAL cell numbers; elevated lung TGF-β; increased collagen deposition, hydroxyproline content, and fibrosis; and decreased serum 25-hydroxyl vitamin D in mice received HFD.
Vedova et al. (2019)	SD/HFD (22% chicken fat) and with or without 10% fructose for 16 weeks.	HFD plus fructose additively enhanced pulmonary inflammation, oxidative stress, and pro-fibrotic changes.
Chu et al. (2019)	SD/HFD feeding of C57BL/6 mice (42% kcal from fat) for 2 weeks followed by bleomycin challenge (1.2 mg/kg) via oral aspiration. Lung tissues examined at 3, 7, and 21 days after bleomycin.	HFD for 5 weeks did not induce hydroxyproline in the lung, however, it significantly enhanced bleomycin-increased hydroxyproline content, mRNA levels of collagen 1 and fibronectin at 21 days. HFD induced apoptosis and a prolonged ER stress after bleomycin.
Baack et al. (2016)	Female SD rats fed HFD (40% kcal from fat) 4 weeks before mating, offspring examined at 3 weeks of age.	No difference in lung fibrosis in offspring at 3 weeks of age; increased perinatal mortality and decreased pulmonary vessels in maternal HFD-exposed offspring.
Song et al. (2015)	Female SD rats were fed a SD/HFD for 8 weeks, then bred with normal male rats, maintained on SD/HFD during pregnancy and lactation.	Maternal HFD exposed offspring showed significantly increased pulmonary inflammatory infiltration, collagen deposition, and increased TGF-β and α-smooth muscle actin expression in the lung.

Note: AHR, airway hyperreactivity; BAL, bronchoalveolar lavage; SD, standard diet; HFD, high-fat diet.

in the development of fibrosis, and the direct induction of TGF-β1 by TNF-α. The decision of complete resolution of inflammation or progression towards fibrosis remains unclear and further research is needed. The role of TNF-α in pulmonary fibrosis in the context of diet-induced obesity remains an open question and further research using genetic modified mice or approaches to manipulate the expression of TNF-α in the lung is deserved.

Transforming Growth Factor-β

Induction of Transforming Growth Factor-β by High-Fat Diet

In obesity, increased levels of TGF-β1 in the adipose tissue and/or in the lung have been observed in obese humans, mice, rats, and drosophila (Samad et al., 1997; Yadav et al., 2011, Jung et al., 2013; Sousa-Pinto et al., 2016; Lee, 2018; Park et al., 2019) (**Table 1**). High-fat diet has been shown to induce TGF-β1 expression in the bronchial epithelium (Park et al., 2019). This finding was thought to be related with insulin resistance, which is closely associated with high-fat diet in mammalian models. The authors demonstrated the induction of TGF-β1 by insulin in BEAS-2b cells and *in vivo* through intranasal administration of insulin to mice fed standard diet (Park et al., 2019). These findings implicate insulin in high-fat diet induced TGF-β1 expression in the lung. Activated macrophages in adipose tissue also contribute to the elevated TGF-β1 in obesity (Chow et al., 2005; Spencer et al., 2010). An alternative programmed macrophage, M2 macrophage, were found increased in fibrotic areas in adipose tissues from insulin-resistant subjects. Those macrophages express higher TGF-β1 and can be further promoted by co-culture with adipocytes (Spencer et al., 2010).

In addition, a role of TNF-α in direct induction of TGF-β1 has been suggested based on the findings that TNF-α induces mRNA levels of TGF-β1 in adipose tissues from lean mice *ex vivo* and in cultured adipocytes *in vitro* (Samad et al., 1997). In primary mouse lung fibroblasts and the Swiss 3T3 fibroblast cell line, TNF-α treatment also induces TGF-β1 expression at the transcriptional level through the activation of ERK (Sullivan et al., 2005), and AP-1 pathways (Sullivan et al., 2009).

Inhibition of ERK with pharmaceutical inhibitors (PD98059 and U0126) blocked TNF-α-induced stabilization of TGF-β1 mRNA; overexpression of active MEK1, an upstream activator of ERK, instead enhances TGF-β1 mRNA stability (Sullivan et al., 2005). Furthermore, TNF-α was also found to increase nuclear levels of c-Jun and its binding to the DNA promoter region of TGF-β1. Accordingly, inhibition of AP-1 signaling attenuates upregulation of TGF-β1 induced by TNF-α in the Swiss 3T3 fibroblasts (Sullivan et al., 2009).

It remains relevant that if the oxidized low-density lipoprotein (ox-LDL), frequently found to increase in obesity, also induces the expression of TGF-β1. A cross-sectional study suggests that ox-LDL is significantly correlated with TGF-β1 in the sera of type 2 diabetic patients (Nakhjavani et al., 2009). Previous studies have demonstrated a causal role of ox-LDL in inducing TGF-β1 in human glomerular epithelial and mesangial cells (Ding et al., 1997; Song et al., 2005; Song et al., 2008) and porcine endothelial cells with potential implication in renal pathogenesis induced by TGF-β1 (Chatauret et al., 2014). With regards to the lung, ox-LDL has been shown to induce TGF-β1 expression in human alveolar epithelial cells that requires the activation of the Ras/ERK/PLTP pathway (Guo et al., 2012). In macrophages, ox-LDL was reported to mildly induce TGF-β1 production, which can be exaggerated by co-exposure with silica (Hou et al., 2019). Taken together, multiple mechanisms are likely to be involved in the induction of TGF-β1 by ox-LDL in the lung and cell-type specific effects are anticipated. However, it needs to be noted that many other studies fail to show the induction of TGF-β1 in the lung or peripheral circulation. The reasons could be due to differences in diet fat content, duration of HFD exposure, as well as the method of detection.

Role of Transforming Growth Factor-β in the Development of Obesity

Increasing evidence support TGF-β as an important mediator for high-fat diet induced obesity and insulin resistance. Blockade of the TGF-β signaling through Smad3 knockout protects mice from high-fat diet induced obesity and insulin resistance (Tan et al., 2011; Tsurutani et al., 2011; Yadav et al., 2011). Conversely, overexpression of *glass bottom boat* (*gbb*), a drosophila homologue of mammalian TGF-β1, induces obesity and insulin resistance similarly as that induced by high-fat diet whereas inhibiting *gbb* leads to the opposite effects (Hong et al., 2016). These several lines of evidence point to a crucial role of TGF-β in regulating adipose tissue differentiation (adipogenesis) and energy metabolism. Indeed, altered expression of genes responsible for adipogenesis, fat accumulation, and fatty acid oxidation were observed in Smad3 deficient mice. A more detailed discussion of the crucial role of TGF-β/Smad signaling in obesity can be referred to a previous review (Tan et al., 2012).

3.2.3 Role of Transforming Growth Factor-β in Obesity Related Pulmonary Fibrosis

The critical role of TGF-β in high-fat diet associated lung fibrosis has been assessed with the use of genetic modified animal models and pharmaceutical approaches targeting TGF-β/Smad3 signaling. Inhibition of TGF-β signaling through knockout of Smad3, the key mediator of TGF-β canonical pathway, successfully abolishes pulmonary fibrosis induced by high-fat diet (Tan et al., 2011; Yadav et al., 2011). In accord, the administration of TGF-β1 neutralizing antibody demonstrates similar protecting effects against HFD-induced peribronchial and perivascular fibrosis (Park et al., 2019). In addition, airway hyperreactivity and fibrosis associated with HFD are suggested to be attributed to enhanced airway TGF-β1 expression. One study showed that asthmatic patients exhibited elevated TGF-β1 in airways which correlated with the severity of asthmatics as well as infiltration of eosinophils and that the subepithelial airways fibrosis also correlated with the severity of asthmatics (Minshall et al., 1997), suggesting an important role of eosinophil-derived TGF-β in airway fibrosis, and AHR. Similar correlation between TGF-β and subepithelial fibrosis in asthmatic patients was reported and further, both eosinophils and fibroblasts were found to account for the increased TGF-β1 synthesis (Vignola et al., 1997). Other cell types including epithelial cells, macrophages, and neutrophils may also contribute to airway remodeling in asthmatics (Al-Alawi et al., 2014). In contrast, Jung et al. reported that mice with mild obesity induced by high-fat diet did not develop AHR or eosinophilic infiltration in the lung (Jung et al., 2013), suggesting that the severity of obesity may play a role in the development of AHR or fibrosis.

Monocyte Chemoattractant Protein-1

MCP-1 is a potent chemokine that induces the infiltration of macrophages into the site of inflammation. In obesity, adipose tissue produces increased levels of MCP-1 that is released into the peripheral blood. Elevated MCP-1 levels have been reported in both obese adults (Catalan et al., 2007) and obese children (Breslin et al., 2012). Further, obese children with lung fibrosis were reported to have significantly higher MCP-1 levels in the bronchoalveolar lavage (BAL) (Hartl et al., 2005). In an experimental fibrosis model, MCP-1 level was significantly increased between 3 and 10 days after bleomycin treatment. Targeting MCP-1 using overexpression of a mutant form of MCP-1, accordingly, attenuates pulmonary fibrosis induced by bleomycin in C57BL/6 mice (Inoshima et al., 2004). Despite these findings, evidence supporting the role of MCP-1 in lung fibrosis especially in the context of obesity remains scarce. More research is needed before any conclusion can be made.

Interleukins

Interleukins are a type of cytokines crucial for modulating inflammatory response and immune functions that are derived from various cell types including macrophages, lymphocytes, mast cells, fibroblasts, and epithelial cells, etc. (Akdis et al., 2016). Aberrant levels of cytokines from IPF patients has been reported and the role of interleukins in the pathogenesis of pulmonary fibrosis has been reviewed recently (She et al., 2021), among the upregulated interleukins in serum or bronchoalveolar lavage fluid (BALF) include IL-1β, IL-2, IL-8, IL-10, IL-12, IL-17A, and IL-33. While a common role in regulation inflammation exists, they act differently in terms of collagen synthesis or fibrosis. For example, the favorable group for pulmonary fibrosis includes IL-1β, IL-4, IL-6, IL11, IL-13, IL-17A, IL-15, and IL-33; in contrast, the other group with anti-

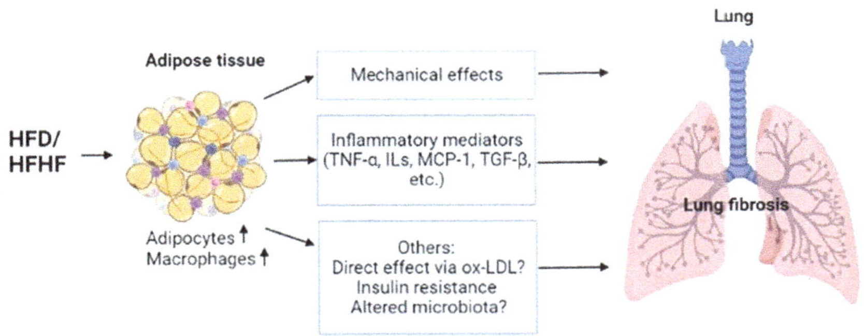

FIGURE 1 | A Proposed model of obesity caused lung fibrosis.

fibrotic function has IL-7, IL-10, IL-12, and IL-27 (Borthwick, 2016; Steen et al., 2020; She et al., 2021). In obesity, both adipocytes and infiltrated inflammatory cells release interleukins in the adipose tissue and the blood stream (Bastard et al., 2006; Um et al., 2011; Tateya et al., 2013). Therefore, there is a potential role of interleukins in the IPF development associated with obesity.

INTERACTION OF HIGH-FAT DIET WITH BLEOMYCIN-INDUCED PULMONARY FIBROSIS

Of note, high-fat diet contributes to increased severity of experimental pulmonary fibrosis induced by bleomycin. A recent study shows that administration of palmitic acid (PA), one kind of saturated fatty acid, significantly increased pulmonary fibrosis in mice challenged with bleomycin compared to bleomycin challenged mice fed a standard diet (Chu et al., 2019). The interaction is likely due to increased apoptosis and endoplasmic reticulum (ER) stress in the lung epithelial cells. Downregulation of CD36, a fatty acid transporter, attenuated the effects of PA on apoptosis, and ER stress induction in the lung epithelial cells. These data suggest a link between epithelial lipotoxicity on the development of pulmonary fibrosis. Hegab et al. also reported that HFD delayed the resolution of lung fibrosis and alveolar repair following bleomycin administration in mice (Hegab et al., 2021). The epithelial repair, e.g., infiltration of alveolar type-2 cells and bronchioalveolar stem cell into the fibrotic foci, was dampened by HFD. The enhanced fatty acid oxidation due to high-fat diet is proposed and inhibition of FAO abolished HFD-induced a delay in alveolar repair and fibrosis resolution *in vivo*. It is noteworthy that the same group also reported that HFD increases the activation and number of alveolar type 2 cells in the lungs (Hegab et al., 2018). Such increase is suggested to be an indirect effect that is possibly linked with chronic inflammation. However, it remains elusive about the mechanisms underlying the impaired infiltration of alveolar type-2 cells and bronchioalveolar stem cells into fibrotic areas. The exploring of other cell types including the lung fibroblasts, and macrophages, etc., in the contribution of HFD to bleomycin-induced pulmonary fibrosis might be worthwhile for future studies.

IMPLICATION OF OBESITY IN THE OUTCOMES OF IDIOPATHIC PULMONARY FIBROSIS PATIENTS

Accumulating evidence suggest that obesity is an independent predictor for the outcomes of IPF patients. A higher body mass index (BMI) in IPF patients has also been recently shown to improve the mortality, although the overall morbidity is more prevalent in obese IPF patients (Mujahid et al., 2020). Similar paradoxical findings of obesity in IPF patients have also been reported in another IPF cohort conducted in the Appalachian area. An increase in BMI was found to predict better prognosis in IPF patients (Sangani et al., 2021). Acute exacerbation of IPF (AE-IPF) represents the leading cause of mortality in IPF patients. Recently, researchers in Japan evaluated the relationship between BMI and in-hospital mortality in patients with AE-IPF using a large retrospective cohort consisting of 14,783 patients. In those AE-IPF patients, the underweight subgroup showed higher mortality rate than the obese subgroup (Awano et al., 2021) Consistently, those IPF patients who experienced body weight loss (≥5%) within the first year of diagnosis show a worst prognosis compared to those without body weight loss (Nakatsuka et al., 2018). In general, these studies demonstrate a protective effect of obesity on the disease burden of IPF. In contrast, obesity seems to be adversely associated with the mortality of IPF patients who undergo bilateral lung transplant. The obese IPF patients have been reported to have increased waitlist and 90-days post-transplant mortality, i.e., those IPF patients with a BMI >30 kg/m^2 are at 1.71 more risk of mortality within 3 months after bilateral lung transplant compared to those with BMIs from 18.5 to 30 kg/m^2 (Gries et al., 2015). Similarly, another study showed that IPF patients who are obese (BMI >30 kg/m^2) were 1.71 times more likely to die within 1 year compared to nonobese IPF patients (Lederer et al., 2009). These observations resemble the paradoxical effects of obesity on acute lung inflammation and injury and the outcomes (Zhi et al., 2016). The systematic low-grade inflammation might prime the lung and attenuate the immune responses resulting from insults from bacterial, viral, or chemical origin.

CONCLUDING REMARKS AND PERSPECTIVES

Obesity is an increasing epidemic worldwide and it has considerable effects on the inflammatory infiltration and remodeling of the lung. A proposed model of the relationship between obesity and lung fibrosis is shown in **Figure 1**. High-fat diet induced inflammatory mediators (TNF-α, MCP-1, and TGF-β) from adipose tissues involving adipocytes and macrophages are important for the development of lung fibrosis. Mechanic effects of accumulating fat impairs lung function and induces fibrotic changes in the diaphragm (Buras et al., 2019), which may play a role in the fibrosis of the lung through inflammatory changes. Other factors related with obesity are likely being involved to promote lung fibrosis, such as a potential direct effect through oxidized LDL (Qian et al., 2021), indirect conditions such as insulin resistance (Park et al., 2019) and altered microbiota in the lung (Chioma et al., 2021). Inflamed lung also propagates the secretion of those mediators from diverse cell types locally, further leading to a transition towards profibrotic changes. Identification of inflammatory mediators that are important for both obesity and lung fibrosis might hold promise for the treatment or prevention of obesity-related lung fibrosis. Better understanding of the relationship between obesity and lung fibrosis may require further research using both a cell-specific approach and a systemic method to elucidate the roles of important inflammatory mediators/regulators implicated in both obesity and lung fibrosis, which may eventually lead to the identification of novel intervention or therapeutic strategies for lung fibrosis associated with obesity.

AUTHOR CONTRIBUTIONS

XG, GQ, and CS prepared the original draft; CS drew the figure; XG and GQ conceptualized the article and provided critical review.

REFERENCES

Akdis, M., Aab, A., Altunbulakli, C., Azkur, K., Costa, R. A., Crameri, R., et al. (2016). Interleukins (From IL-1 to IL-38), Interferons, Transforming Growth Factor β, and TNF-α: Receptors, Functions, and Roles in Diseases. *J. Allergy Clin. Immunol.* 138, 984–1010. doi:10.1016/j.jaci.2016.06.033

Al-Alawi, M., Hassan, T., and Chotirmall, S. H. (2014). Transforming Growth Factor β and Severe Asthma: a Perfect Storm. *Respir. Med.* 108, 1409–1423. doi:10.1016/j.rmed.2014.08.008

Anand, G., and Katz, P. O. (2010). Gastroesophageal Reflux Disease and Obesity. *Gastroenterol. Clin. North. Am.* 39, 39–46. doi:10.1016/j.gtc.2009.12.002

Awano, N., Jo, T., Yasunaga, H., Inomata, M., Kuse, N., Tone, M., et al. (2021). Body Mass index and In-Hospital Mortality in Patients with Acute Exacerbation of Idiopathic Pulmonary Fibrosis. *ERJ Open Res.* 7, 00037-2021. doi:10.1183/23120541.00037-2021

Baack, M. L., Forred, B. J., Larsen, T. D., Jensen, D. N., Wachal, A. L., Khan, M. A., et al. (2016). Consequences of a Maternal High-Fat Diet and Late Gestation Diabetes on the Developing Rat Lung. *PLoS One* 11, e0160818. doi:10.1371/journal.pone.0160818

Bastard, J. P., Maachi, M., Lagathu, C., Kim, M. J., Caron, M., Vidal, H., et al. (2006). Recent Advances in the Relationship between Obesity, Inflammation, and Insulin Resistance. *Eur. Cytokine Netw.* 17, 4–12.

Borthwick, L. A. (2016). The IL-1 Cytokine Family and its Role in Inflammation and Fibrosis in the Lung. *Semin. Immunopathol.* 38, 517–534. doi:10.1007/s00281-016-0559-z

Breslin, W. L., Johnston, C. A., Strohacker, K., Carpenter, K. C., Davidson, T. R., Moreno, J. P., et al. (2012). Obese Mexican American Children Have Elevated MCP-1, TNF-α, Monocyte Concentration, and Dyslipidemia. *Pediatrics* 129, e1180–6. doi:10.1542/peds.2011-2477

Bringardner, B. D., Baran, C. P., Eubank, T. D., and Marsh, C. B. (2008). The Role of Inflammation in the Pathogenesis of Idiopathic Pulmonary Fibrosis. *Antioxid. Redox Signal.* 10, 287–301. doi:10.1089/ars.2007.1897

Buechler, C., Krautbauer, S., and Eisinger, K. (2015). Adipose Tissue Fibrosis. *World J. Diabetes* 6, 548–553. doi:10.4239/wjd.v6.i4.548

Buras, E. D., Converso-Baran, K., Davis, C. S., Akama, T., Hikage, F., Michele, D. E., et al. (2019). Fibro-Adipogenic Remodeling of the Diaphragm in Obesity-Associated Respiratory Dysfunction. *Diabetes* 68, 45–56. doi:10.2337/db18-0209

Catalán, V., Gómez-Ambrosi, J., Ramirez, B., Rotellar, F., Pastor, C., Silva, C., et al. (2007). Proinflammatory Cytokines in Obesity: Impact of Type 2 Diabetes Mellitus and Gastric Bypass. *Obes. Surg.* 17, 1464–1474. doi:10.1007/s11695-008-9424-z

Cavalera, M., Wang, J., and Frangogiannis, N. G. (2014). Obesity, Metabolic Dysfunction, and Cardiac Fibrosis: Pathophysiological Pathways, Molecular Mechanisms, and Therapeutic Opportunities. *Transl Res.* 164, 323–335. doi:10.1016/j.trsl.2014.05.001

Chatauret, N., Favreau, F., Giraud, S., Thierry, A., Rossard, L., Le Pape, S., et al. (2014). Diet-induced Increase in Plasma Oxidized LDL Promotes Early Fibrosis in a Renal Porcine Auto-Transplantation Model. *J. Transl Med.* 12, 76. doi:10.1186/1479-5876-12-76

Chiang, D. J., Pritchard, M. T., and Nagy, L. E. (2011). Obesity, Diabetes Mellitus, and Liver Fibrosis. *Am. J. Physiol. Gastrointest. Liver Physiol.* 300, G697–G702. doi:10.1152/ajpgi.00426.2010

Chioma, O. S., Hesse, L. E., Chapman, A., and Drake, W. P. (2021). Role of the Microbiome in Interstitial Lung Diseases. *Front. Med. (Lausanne)* 8, 595522. doi:10.3389/fmed.2021.595522

Chow, F. Y., Nikolic-Paterson, D. J., Ozols, E., Atkins, R. C., and Tesch, G. H. (2005). Intercellular Adhesion Molecule-1 Deficiency Is Protective against Nephropathy in Type 2 Diabetic Db/db Mice. *J. Am. Soc. Nephrol.* 16, 1711–1722. doi:10.1681/ASN.2004070612

Chu, S. G., Villalba, J. A., Liang, X., Xiong, K., Tsoyi, K., Ith, B., et al. (2019). Palmitic Acid-Rich High-Fat Diet Exacerbates Experimental Pulmonary Fibrosis by Modulating Endoplasmic Reticulum Stress. *Am. J. Respir. Cel. Mol. Biol.* 61, 737–746. doi:10.1165/rcmb.2018-0324OC

Deji, N., Kume, S., Araki, S., Soumura, M., Sugimoto, T., Isshiki, K., et al. (2009). Structural and Functional Changes in the Kidneys of High-Fat Diet-Induced Obese Mice. *Am. J. Physiol. Ren. Physiol.* 296, F118–F126. doi:10.1152/ajprenal.00110.2008

Ding, G., van Goor, H., Ricardo, S. D., Orlowski, J. M., and Diamond, J. R. (1997). Oxidized LDL Stimulates the Expression of TGF-Beta and Fibronectin in Human Glomerular Epithelial Cells. *Kidney Int.* 51, 147–154. doi:10.1038/ki.1997.18

Distler, J. H., Schett, G., Gay, S., and Distler, O. (2008). The Controversial Role of Tumor Necrosis Factor Alpha in Fibrotic Diseases. *Arthritis Rheum.* 58, 2228–2235. doi:10.1002/art.23645

Dixon, A. E., and Peters, U. (2018). The Effect of Obesity on Lung Function. *Expert Rev. Respir. Med.* 12, 755–767. doi:10.1080/17476348.2018.1506331

Fujita, M., Shannon, J. M., Morikawa, O., Gauldie, J., Hara, N., and Mason, R. J. (2003). Overexpression of Tumor Necrosis Factor-Alpha Diminishes Pulmonary Fibrosis Induced by Bleomycin or Transforming Growth

Factor-Beta. *Am. J. Respir. Cel. Mol. Biol.* 29, 669–676. doi:10.1165/rcmb.2002-0046OC

Ge, X. N., Greenberg, Y., Hosseinkhani, M. R., Long, E. K., Bahaie, N. S., Rao, A., et al. (2013). High-fat Diet Promotes Lung Fibrosis and Attenuates Airway Eosinophilia after Exposure to Cockroach Allergen in Mice. *Exp. Lung Res.* 39, 365–378. doi:10.3109/01902148.2013.829537

Gibbons, M. A., MacKinnon, A. C., Ramachandran, P., Dhaliwal, K., Duffin, R., Phythian-Adams, A. T., et al. (2011). Ly6Chi Monocytes Direct Alternatively Activated Profibrotic Macrophage Regulation of Lung Fibrosis. *Am. J. Respir. Crit. Care Med.* 184, 569–581. doi:10.1164/rccm.201010-1719OC

Gries, C. J., Bhadriraju, S., Edelman, J. D., Goss, C. H., Raghu, G., and Mulligan, M. S. (2015). Obese Patients with Idiopathic Pulmonary Fibrosis Have a Higher 90-day Mortality Risk with Bilateral Lung Transplantation. *J. Heart Lung Transpl.* 34, 241–246. doi:10.1016/j.healun.2014.09.031

Guo, L. L., Chen, Y. J., Wang, T., An, J., Wang, C. N., Shen, Y. C., et al. (2012). Ox-LDL-induced TGF-β1 Production in Human Alveolar Epithelial Cells: Involvement of the Ras/ERK/PLTP Pathway. *J. Cel. Physiol.* 227, 3185–3191. doi:10.1002/jcp.24005

Hales, C. M., Fryar, C. D., Carroll, M. D., Freedman, D. S., and Ogden, C. L. (2018). Trends in Obesity and Severe Obesity Prevalence in US Youth and Adults by Sex and Age, 2007-2008 to 2015-2016. *JAMA.* 319, 1723–1725. doi:10.1001/jama.2018.3060

Han, H., Chung, S. I., Park, H. J., Oh, E. Y., Kim, S. R., Park, K. H., et al. (2021). Obesity-induced Vitamin D Deficiency Contributes to Lung Fibrosis and Airway Hyperresponsiveness. *Am. J. Respir. Cel. Mol. Biol.* 64, 357–367. doi:10.1165/rcmb.2020-0086OC

Hanson, C., Rutten, E. P., Wouters, E. F., and Rennard, S. (2014). Influence of Diet and Obesity on COPD Development and Outcomes. *Int. J. Chron. Obstruct Pulmon Dis.* 9, 723–733. doi:10.2147/COPD.S50111

Hartl, D., Griese, M., Nicolai, T., Zissel, G., Prell, C., Reinhardt, D., et al. (2005). A Role for MCP-1/CCR2 in Interstitial Lung Disease in Children. *Respir. Res.* 6, 93. doi:10.1186/1465-9921-6-93

Hegab, A. E., Ozaki, M., Meligy, F. Y., Kagawa, S., Ishii, M., and Betsuyaku, T. (2018). High Fat Diet Activates Adult Mouse Lung Stem Cells and Accelerates Several Aging-Induced Effects. *Stem Cel Res* 33, 25–35. doi:10.1016/j.scr.2018.10.006

Hegab, A. E., Ozaki, M., Kagawa, S., and Fukunaga, K. (2021). Effect of High Fat Diet on the Severity and Repair of Lung Fibrosis in Mice. *Stem Cell Dev* 30, 908–921. doi:10.1089/scd.2021.0050

Hong, S. H., Kang, M., Lee, K. S., and Yu, K. (2016). High Fat Diet-Induced TGF-β/Gbb Signaling Provokes Insulin Resistance through the Tribbles Expression. *Sci. Rep.* 6, 30265. doi:10.1038/srep30265

Hotamisligil, G. S., Shargill, N. S., and Spiegelman, B. M. (1993). Adipose Expression of Tumor Necrosis Factor-Alpha: Direct Role in Obesity-Linked Insulin Resistance. *Science* 259, 87–91. doi:10.1126/science.7678183

Hou, X., Summer, R., Chen, Z., Tian, Y., Ma, J., Cui, J., et al. (2019). Lipid Uptake by Alveolar Macrophages Drives Fibrotic Responses to Silica Dust. *Sci. Rep.* 9, 399. doi:10.1038/s41598-018-36875-2

Inoshima, I., Kuwano, K., Hamada, N., Hagimoto, N., Yoshimi, M., Maeyama, T., et al. (2004). Anti-monocyte Chemoattractant Protein-1 Gene Therapy Attenuates Pulmonary Fibrosis in Mice. *Am. J. Physiol. Lung Cel. Mol. Physiol.* 286, L1038–L1044. doi:10.1152/ajplung.00167.2003

Jung, S. H., Kwon, J. M., Shim, J. W., Kim, D. S., Jung, H. L., Park, M. S., et al. (2013). Effects of Diet-Induced Mild Obesity on Airway Hyperreactivity and Lung Inflammation in Mice. *Yonsei Med. J.* 54, 1430–1437. doi:10.3349/ymj.2013.54.6.1430

Laurentius, T., Raffetseder, U., Fellner, C., Kob, R., Nourbakhsh, M., Floege, J., et al. (2019). High-fat Diet-Induced Obesity Causes an Inflammatory Microenvironment in the Kidneys of Aging Long-Evans Rats. *J. Inflamm. (Lond)* 16, 14. doi:10.1186/s12950-019-0219-x

Lederer, D. J., Wilt, J. S., D'Ovidio, F., Bacchetta, M. D., Shah, L., Ravichandran, S., et al. (2009). Obesity and Underweight Are Associated with an Increased Risk of Death after Lung Transplantation. *Am. J. Respir. Crit. Care Med.* 180, 887–895. doi:10.1164/rccm.200903-0425OC

Lee, A. S., Mira-Avendano, I., Ryu, J. H., and Daniels, C. E. (2014). The burden of Idiopathic Pulmonary Fibrosis: an Unmet Public Health Need. *Respir. Med.* 108, 955–967. doi:10.1016/j.rmed.2014.03.015

Lee, M. J. (2018). Transforming Growth Factor Beta Superfamily Regulation of Adipose Tissue Biology in Obesity. *Biochim. Biophys. Acta Mol. Basis Dis.* 1864, 1160–1171. doi:10.1016/j.bbadis.2018.01.025

Liu, J. Y., Brass, D. M., Hoyle, G. W., and Brody, A. R. (1998). TNF-alpha Receptor Knockout Mice Are Protected from the Fibroproliferative Effects of Inhaled Asbestos Fibers. *Am. J. Pathol.* 153, 1839–1847. doi:10.1016/s0002-9440(10)65698-2

Liu, K., Zhou, S., Liu, J., Wang, Y., Zhu, F., and Liu, M. (2019). Silibinin Attenuates High-Fat Diet-Induced Renal Fibrosis of Diabetic Nephropathy. *Drug Des. Devel. Ther.* 13, 3117–3126. doi:10.2147/DDDT.S209981

Marcelin, G., Silveira, A. L. M., Martins, L. B., Ferreira, A. V., and Clément, K. (2019). Deciphering the Cellular Interplays Underlying Obesity-Induced Adipose Tissue Fibrosis. *J. Clin. Invest.* 129, 4032–4040. doi:10.1172/JCI129192

Minshall, E. M., Leung, D. Y., Martin, R. J., Song, Y. L., Cameron, L., Ernst, P., et al. (1997). Eosinophil-Associated TGF-Beta1 mRNA Expression and Airways Fibrosis in Bronchial Asthma. *Am. J. Respir. Cel. Mol. Biol.* 17, 326–333. doi:10.1165/ajrcmb.17.3.2733

Miyake, Y., Sasaki, S., Yokoyama, T., Chida, K., Azuma, A., Suda, T., et al. (2006). Dietary Fat and Meat Intake and Idiopathic Pulmonary Fibrosis: a Case-Control Study in Japan. *Int. J. Tuberc. Lung Dis.* 10, 333–339.

Miyazaki, Y., Araki, K., Vesin, C., Garcia, I., Kapanci, Y., Whitsett, J. A., et al. (1995). Expression of a Tumor Necrosis Factor-Alpha Transgene in Murine Lung Causes Lymphocytic and Fibrosing Alveolitis. A Mouse Model of Progressive Pulmonary Fibrosis. *J. Clin. Invest.* 96, 250–259. doi:10.1172/JCI118029

Mujahid, H., Sangani, R. G., Catherman, K., Patel, Z., and Zulfikar, R. (2020). Obesity and Idiopathic Pulmonary Fibrosis (IPF): Defining Relationship, an Experience from a Rural Appalachian Tertiary Center. *Am. J. Respir. Crit. Care Med.* A3358. doi:10.1164/ajrccm-conference.2020.201.1_meetingabstracts.a3358

Nakatsuka, Y., Handa, T., Kokosi, M., Tanizawa, K., Puglisi, S., Jacob, J., et al. (2018). The Clinical Significance of Body Weight Loss in Idiopathic Pulmonary Fibrosis Patients. *Respiration* 96, 338–347. doi:10.1159/000490355

Nakhjavani, M., Esteghamati, A., Asgarani, F., Khalilzadeh, O., Nikzamir, A., and Safari, R. (2009). Association of Oxidized Low-Density Lipoprotein and Transforming Growth Factor-Beta in Type 2 Diabetic Patients: a Cross-Sectional Study. *Transl. Res.* 153, 86–90. doi:10.1016/j.trsl.2008.11.009

Naura, A. S., Hans, C. P., Zerfaoui, M., Errami, Y., Ju, J., Kim, H., et al. (2009). High-fat Diet Induces Lung Remodeling in ApoE-Deficient Mice: an Association with an Increase in Circulatory and Lung Inflammatory Factors. *Lab. Invest.* 89, 1243–1251. doi:10.1038/labinvest.2009.98

Oikonomou, N., Harokopos, V., Zalevsky, J., Valavanis, C., Kotanidou, A., Szymkowski, D. E., et al. (2006). Soluble TNF Mediates the Transition from Pulmonary Inflammation to Fibrosis. *PLoS One* 1, e108. doi:10.1371/journal.pone.0000108

Ortiz, L. A., Lasky, J., Hamilton, R. F., Jr., Holian, A., Hoyle, G. W., Banks, W., et al. (1998). Expression of TNF and the Necessity of TNF Receptors in Bleomycin-Induced Lung Injury in Mice. *Exp Lung Res.* 24, 721–743. doi:10.3109/01902149809099592

Ortiz, L. A., Lasky, J., Lungarella, G., Cavarra, E., Martorana, P., Banks, W. A., et al. (1999). Upregulation of the P75 but Not the P55 TNF-Alpha Receptor mRNA after Silica and Bleomycin Exposure and protection from Lung Injury in Double Receptor Knockout Mice. *Am. J. Respir. Cel. Mol. Biol.* 20, 825–833. doi:10.1165/ajrcmb.20.4.3193

Park, Y. H., Oh, E. Y., Han, H., Yang, M., Park, H. J., Park, K. H., et al. (2019). Insulin Resistance Mediates High-Fat Diet-Induced Pulmonary Fibrosis and Airway Hyperresponsiveness through the TGF-β1 Pathway. *Exp. Mol. Med.* 51, 1–12. doi 10.1038/s12276-019-0258-7

Pessin, J. E., and Kwon, H. (2012). How Does High-Fat Diet Induce Adipose Tissue Fibrosis? *J. Investig. Med.* 60, 1147–1150. doi:10.2310/JIM.0b013e318271fdb9

Peters, U., Dixon, A. E., and Forno, E. (2018). Obesity and Asthma. *J. Allergy Clin. Immunol.* 141, 1169–1179. doi:10.1016/j.jaci.2018.02.004

Piguet, P. F., and Vesin, C. (1994). Treatment by Human Recombinant Soluble TNF Receptor of Pulmonary Fibrosis Induced by Bleomycin or Silica in Mice. *Eur. Respir. J.* 7, 515–518. doi:10.1183/09031936.94.07030515

Piguet, P. F., Collart, M. A., Grau, G. E., Kapanci, Y., and Vassalli, P. (1989). Tumor Necrosis Factor/cachectin Plays a Key Role in Bleomycin-Induced Pneumopathy and Fibrosis. *J. Exp. Med.* 170, 655–663. doi:10.1084/jem.170.3.655

Piguet, P. F., Collart, M. A., Grau, G. E., Sappino, A. P., and Vassalli, P. (1990).

Requirement of Tumour Necrosis Factor for Development of Silica-Induced Pulmonary Fibrosis. *Nature* 344, 245–247. doi:10.1038/344245a0

Qian, G., Adeyanju, O., Sunil, C., Huang, S. K., Chen, S. Y., Tucker, T. A., et al. (2021). Dedicator of Cytokinesis 2 (DOCK2) Deficiency Attenuates Lung Injury Associated with Chronic High-Fat and High-Fructose Diet-Induced Obesity. *Am. J. Pathol.* S0002-9440 (21), 00474–0. doi:10.1016/j.ajpath.2021.10.011

Redente, E. F., Keith, R. C., Janssen, W., Henson, P. M., Ortiz, L. A., Downey, G. P., et al. (2014). Tumor Necrosis Factor-α Accelerates the Resolution of Established Pulmonary Fibrosis in Mice by Targeting Profibrotic Lung Macrophages. *Am. J. Respir. Cel. Mol. Biol.* 50, 825–837. doi:10.1165/rcmb.2013-0386OC

Salome, C. M., King, G. G., and Berend, N. (2010). Physiology of Obesity and Effects on Lung Function. *J. Appl. Physiol. (1985)* 108, 206–211. doi:10.1152/japplphysiol.00694.2009

Samad, F., Yamamoto, K., Pandey, M., and Loskutoff, D. J. (1997). Elevated Expression of Transforming Growth Factor-Beta in Adipose Tissue from Obese Mice. *Mol. Med.* 3, 37–48. doi:10.1007/bf03401666

Sangani, R. G., Ghio, A. J., Mujahid, H., Patel, Z., Catherman, K., Wen, S., et al. (2021). Outcomes of Idiopathic Pulmonary Fibrosis Improve with Obesity: A Rural Appalachian Experience. *South. Med. J.* 114, 424–431. doi:10.14423/SMJ.0000000000001275

Sgalla, G., Iovene, B., Calvello, M., Ori, M., Varone, F., and Richeldi, L. (2018). Idiopathic Pulmonary Fibrosis: Pathogenesis and Management. *Respir. Res.* 19, 32. doi:10.1186/s12931-018-0730-2

She, Y. X., Yu, Q. Y., and Tang, X. X. (2021). Role of Interleukins in the Pathogenesis of Pulmonary Fibrosis. *Cell Death Discov* 7, 52. doi:10.1038/s41420-021-00437-9

Sime, P. J., Marr, R. A., Gauldie, D., Xing, Z., Hewlett, B. R., Graham, F. L., et al. (1998). Transfer of Tumor Necrosis Factor-Alpha to Rat Lung Induces Severe Pulmonary Inflammation and Patchy Interstitial Fibrogenesis with Induction of Transforming Growth Factor-Beta1 and Myofibroblasts. *Am. J. Pathol.* 153, 825–832. doi:10.1016/s0002-9440(10)65624-6

Song, C. Y., Kim, B. C., Hong, H. K., and Lee, H. S. (2005). Oxidized LDL Activates PAI-1 Transcription through Autocrine Activation of TGF-Beta Signaling in Mesangial Cells. *Kidney Int.* 67, 1743–1752. doi:10.1111/j.1523-1755.2005.00271.x

Song, C. Y., Kim, B. C., and Lee, H. S. (2008). Lovastatin Inhibits Oxidized Low-Density Lipoprotein-Induced Plasminogen Activator Inhibitor and Transforming Growth Factor-Beta1 Expression via a Decrease in Ras/extracellular Signal-Regulated Kinase Activity in Mesangial Cells. *Transl Res.* 151, 27–35. doi:10.1016/j.trsl.2007.09.008

Song, Y., Yu, Y., Wang, D., Chai, S., Liu, D., Xiao, X., et al. (2015). Maternal High-Fat Diet Feeding during Pregnancy and Lactation Augments Lung Inflammation and Remodeling in the Offspring. *Respir. Physiol. Neurobiol.* 207, 1–6. doi:10.1016/j.resp.2014.12.003

Sousa-Pinto, B., Gonçalves, L., Rodrigues, A. R., Tomada, I., Almeida, H., Neves, D., et al. (2016). Characterization of TGF-β Expression and Signaling Profile in the Adipose Tissue of Rats Fed with High-Fat and Energy-Restricted Diets. *J. Nutr. Biochem.* 38, 107–115. doi:10.1016/j.jnutbio.2016.07.017

Spencer, M., Yao-Borengasser, A., Unal, R., Rasouli, N., Gurley, C. M., Zhu, B., et al. (2010). Adipose Tissue Macrophages in Insulin-Resistant Subjects Are Associated with Collagen VI and Fibrosis and Demonstrate Alternative Activation. *Am. J. Physiol. Endocrinol. Metab.* 299, E1016–E1027. doi:10.1152/ajpendo.00329.2010

Steen, E. H., Wang, X., Balaji, S., Butte, M. J., Bollyky, P. L., and Keswani, S. G. (2020). The Role of the Anti-Inflammatory Cytokine Interleukin-10 in Tissue Fibrosis. *Adv. Wound Care (New Rochelle)* 9, 184–198. doi:10.1089/wound.2019.1032

Sullivan, D. E., Ferris, M., Pociask, D., and Brody, A. R. (2005). Tumor Necrosis Factor-Alpha Induces Transforming Growth Factor-Beta1 Expression in Lung Fibroblasts through the Extracellular Signal-Regulated Kinase Pathway. *Am. J. Respir. Cel. Mol. Biol.* 32, 342–349. doi:10.1165/rcmb.2004-0288OC

Sullivan, D. E., Ferris, M., Nguyen, H., Abboud, E., and Brody, A. R. (2009). TNF-Alpha Induces TGF-Beta1 Expression in Lung Fibroblasts at the Transcriptional Level via AP-1 Activation. *J. Cel. Mol. Med.* 13, 1866–1876. doi:10.1111/j.1582-4934.2009.00647.x

Tan, C. K., Leuenberger, N., Tan, M. J., Yan, Y. W., Chen, Y., Kambadur, R., et al. (2011). Smad3 Deficiency in Mice Protects against Insulin Resistance and Obesity Induced by a High-Fat Diet. *Diabetes* 60, 464–476. doi:10.2337/db10-0801

Tan, C. K., Chong, H. C., Tan, E. H., and Tan, N. S. (2012). Getting 'Smad' about Obesity and Diabetes. *Nutr. Diabetes* 2, e29. doi:10.1038/nutd.2012.1

Tateya, S., Kim, F., and Tamori, Y. (2013). Recent Advances in Obesity-Induced Inflammation and Insulin Resistance. *Front. Endocrinol. (Lausanne)* 4, 93. doi:10.3389/fendo.2013.00093

Tsurutani, Y., Fujimoto, M., Takemoto, M., Irisuna, H., Koshizaka, M., Onishi, S., et al. (2011). The Roles of Transforming Growth Factor-β and Smad3 Signaling in Adipocyte Differentiation and Obesity. *Biochem. Biophys. Res. Commun.* 407, 68–73. doi:10.1016/j.bbrc.2011.02.106

Tzanavari, T., Giannogonas, P., and Karalis, K. P. (2010). TNF-Alpha and Obesity. *Curr. Dir. Autoimmun.* 11, 145–156. doi:10.1159/000289203

Um, J. Y., Rim, H. K., Kim, S. J., Kim, H. L., and Hong, S. H. (2011). Functional Polymorphism of IL-1 Alpha and its Potential Role in Obesity in Humans and Mice. *PLoS One* 6, e29524. doi:10.1371/journal.pone.0029524

Vedova, M. C. D., Soler Garcia, F. M., Muñoz, M. D., Fornes, M. W., Gomez Mejiba, S. E., Gómez, N. N., et al. (2019). Diet-Induced Pulmonary Inflammation and Incipient Fibrosis in Mice: a Possible Role of Neutrophilic Inflammation. *Inflammation* 42, 1886–1900. doi:10.1007/s10753-019-01051-9

Vignola, A. M., Chanez, P., Chiappara, G., Merendino, A., Pace, E., Rizzo, A., et al. (1997). Transforming Growth Factor-Beta Expression in Mucosal Biopsies in Asthma and Chronic Bronchitis. *Am. J. Respir. Crit. Care Med.* 156, 591–599. doi:10.1164/ajrccm.156.2.9609066

Yadav, H., Quijano, C., Kamaraju, A. K., Gavrilova, O., Malek, R., Chen, W., et al. (2011). Protection from Obesity and Diabetes by Blockade of TGF-β/Smad3 Signaling. *Cel. Metab* 14, 67–79. doi:10.1016/j.cmet.2011.04.013

Yu, H. Z., Wu, Q., Du, Z. Z., Sun, X., Wang, C. Z., and Li, L. (2013). High-Fat Diet Induces Pulmonary Fibrosis in Rats and Inhibitory Effects of N-Acetylcysteine. *Zhonghua Yi Xue Za Zhi* 93, 3547–3550.

Zaman, T., and Lee, J. S. (2018). Risk Factors for the Development of Idiopathic Pulmonary Fibrosis: A Review. *Curr. Pulmonol Rep.* 7, 118–125. doi:10.1007/s13665-018-0210-7

Zhi, G., Xin, W., Ying, W., Guohong, X., and Shuying, L. (2016). "Obesity Paradox" in Acute Respiratory Distress Syndrome: Asystematic Review and Meta-Analysis. *PLoS One* 11, e0163677. doi:10.1371/journal.pone.0163677

15

Laryngopharyngeal pH Monitoring in Patients with Idiopathic Pulmonary Fibrosis

*Yiliang Su†, Li Shen†, Fen Zhang†, Xing Jiang, Xiaofeng Jin, Yuan Zhang, Yang Hu, Ying Zhou, Qiuhong Li and Huiping Li**

Department of Respiratory and Critical Care Medicine, Shanghai Pulmonary Hospital, School of Medicine, Tongji University, Shanghai, China

Correspondence:
Huiping Li
liw2013@126.com

†These authors have contributed equally to this work

Background: Patients with idiopathic pulmonary fibrosis (IPF) often have irritating persistent dry cough. Possible correlations between dry cough and laryngopharyngeal reflux (LPR) remain unclear.

Methods: 44 patients with IPF and 30 healthy individuals underwent 24 h laryngopharyngeal pH monitoring. Ryan index score was calculated. Patients' demographic and clinical data were collected.

Results: 44 patients with IPF and 30 healthy individuals were included. The proportions of men and smokers were significantly higher in IPF group than control group (All $p < 0.01$). The average laryngopharyngeal pH value for 24 h was similar in the IPF (7.11 ± 0.08) group and control group (7.09 ± 0.06). According to the percentage duration of pH < 6.5, pH6.5–7.5, and pH > 7.5 in the overall measure duration, the patients were classified into three pH groups. In entire pH monitoring duration, the proportion of pH > 7.5 group in IPF patients was higher than control group; at upright position, the proportion of pH > 7.5 group in IPF patients was higher than control group; at supine position, the proportion of pH < 6.5 group in IPF patients was higher than control group (All $p < 0.01$). Seven patients had Ryan index score>9.41 at upright position. All patients had Ryan index score<6.79 at supine position. Four patients showed significantly higher and one patient had significantly lower average pH at coughing than the overall average pH (All $p < 0.05$).

Conclusions: Patients with IPF may have LPR. Basic and acidic LPR may likely occur at upright and supine position, respectively. Ryan index may not accurately reflect LPR in patients with IPF.

Keywords: interstitial lung diseases, idiopathic pulmonary fibrosis, laryngopharyngeal reflux, ryan index, cough

INTRODUCTION

Interstitial lung diseases (ILDs) refer to a group of lung diseases characterized in alveolar inflammation and interstitial fibrotic lesions (Travis et al., 2013). The etiology of ILDs is complex and diverse. Idiopathic pulmonary fibrosis (IPF) and connective tissue disease-related interstitial lung disease (CTD-ILD) are the most common types of ILD (Hu et al., 2016). The main respiratory symptoms of IPF include irritating cough and breathing difficulty.

Gastroesophageal reflux disease (GERD) is caused by the reflux of gastric acid and other stomach contents into the esophagus, and one of its typical clinical symptoms is cough (Cohen et al., 2002;

Hom and Vaezi, 2013; Lai et al., 2013). GERD has been recognized as a common cause for chronic cough (Lai et al., 2013). International diagnosis and treatment guidelines for IPF suggest an association between GERD and IPF onset and thus recommend anti-acid treatments for patients with IPF (Raghu et al., 2006; Lee et al., 2011; Raghu et al., 2011; Raghu et al., 2015). However, a previous report has shown that anti-acid treatments do not reduce the all-cause mortality and the rate of hospitalization of patients with IPF (Lee et al., 2013). Moreover, Raghu and colleagues have found that approximately half of patients with IPF did not present gastroesophageal reflux (GER) symptoms, such as heartburn and sour regurgitation (Raghu et al., 2011). Extraesophageal reflux (EER) or laryngopharyngeal reflux (LPR) is the reflux of stomach contents into the throat and larynx, and patients with LPR usually do not present the classic symptoms of GERD (Hom and Vaezi, 2013). An accurate diagnosis of LPR remains challenging in clinical practice.

LPR is the reflux of stomach contents into the area above the upper esophageal sphincter, such as the nasal cavity, mouth, throat, trachea, and lung (Koufman, 2002). Patients with LPR disease (LPRD) often presents cough, laryngopharyngeal discomfort, and breathing difficulty (Cohen et al., 2002; Koufman, 2002; Ayazi et al., 2009). Similar to GERD, LPRD can also cause chronic cough. Gaseous refluxate in the airway reduces the pH of the upper airway to <6.5, which activates the pepsin that is from the refluxate and deposited on the airway mucosal epithelial cells and consequently induces nonspecific inflammation in the airway mucosa (Cohen et al., 2002; Koufman, 2002). Previous studies have demonstrated that 32–84% of patients with bronchial asthma had GERD and 50% of the patients with GERD did not present any obvious reflux symptoms such as heartburn and sour regurgitation (Harding et al., 2000; Mastronarde et al., 2009). GERD can exacerbate asthma. Antacids and gastric pro-motility drugs can alleviate asthma symptoms in patients with GERD (Sharma et al., 2007; DiMango et al., 2009; Liang et al., 2013). The association between LPR and IPF remains unclear, and monitoring upper airway pH in patients with IPF is essential to understand such association and may shed light on therapeutic strategies for LPR in patients with IPF.

MATERIALS AND METHODS

Study Design

This single-center prospective study was conducted in Shanghai Pulmonary Hospital of Tongji University in Shanghai China. A total of 44 patients with IPF treated in Shanghai Pulmonary Hospital from November 2016 to September 2017 were included in this study. The study protocol has been approved by the Ethics Committee of Shanghai Pulmonary Hospital (Approval No: K16-296). The study was registered on the Chinese Clinical Trial Registry (http://www.chictr.org.cn/abouten.aspx, ChiCTR-ODC-16009478). Written informed consent was obtained from all the study participants prior to inclusion in the study.

Study Participants

Patients with a confirmed diagnosis of IPF were enrolled. Patients with the following clinical characteristics were excluded: 1) had a malignancy or a history of malignancy; 2) were using glucocorticoid and/or immunosuppressants (including azathioprine, cyclophosphamide, mycophenolate mofetil, and cyclosporin A); 3) had serious systemic diseases and organ dysfunction; 4) refuse to do laryngophary reflux 24 h monitor; 5) had incomplete clinical data. A total of 30 age-matched healthy individuals, who had routine physical examination in Shanghai Pulmonary Hospital, were included as controls.

Disease Diagnostic Criteria

IPF was diagnosed according to the 2013 American Thoracic Society/European Respiratory Society statement (Travis et al., 2013).

Twenty Four-Hour Laryngopharyngeal pH Monitoring

The Restech® pH sensor (Respiratory Technology Corp., San Diego, CA) was first calibrated using two standard buffer solutions at pH 7 and pH 4, respectively. The nasal passage was topically anesthetized using Q-tips soaked with 2% lidocaine. The sensor was inserted into the nasal cavity and moved toward the throat until the flashing LED of the sensor was visible in the back of the throat, and then the sensor was positioned so that the flashing light was 5–10 mm below the uvula. The 5 mm-long LED light serves as a guide for the placement of the pH sensor. The catheter was first secured as close to the nares as possible on the face using a Tegaderm™ and then passed over the ear and secured on the neck using another Tegaderm™. The transmitter at the end of the catheter was either taped to the skin or attached to the study participant's clothing using a clip-on case. The data recorder was attached to the study participant's belt. The study participants were prohibited from taking a shower or bath during the recording period and were required to keep a diary to record meal periods and the time staying at supine and upright positions. The meal periods were excluded from data analyses. The data collected by the Restech® recorder and the information from the dairy were analyzed (Ayazi et al., 2009; Sun et al., 2009).

Ryan Index Calculation

Based on the data collected from the Dx-pH 24 h laryngopharyngeal pH monitoring, a LPR episode was defined as a pharyngeal pH < 5.5 at upright position and/or <5.0 at supine position. The number of LPR episodes, the longest duration of a LPR episode, and the proportion of total duration of LPR episodes in the total recording duration (episodes % time) were calculated, and the differences in these parameters between study participants and healthy population were determined according to a previous description (Cohen et al., 2002). The data analysis software of the Restech® recorder calculates patients' Ryan index based on the number of LPR episodes, duration of the longest LPR episode, and LPR episodes % time (Cohen et al., 2002).

TABLE 1 | Chest HRCT scoring criteria.

Score	Lesions and lung segments
Severity score	Parenchymal abnormalities
1	Ground glass opacities
2	Irregularities in the pleural margins
3	Septal/Subpleural lines
4	Honeycombing
5	Subpleural cysts
Extent score	Number of lung segments
1	1–3
2	4–9
3	>9

HRCT score = severity score + extent score (0–30). HRCT: high resolution computed tomography.

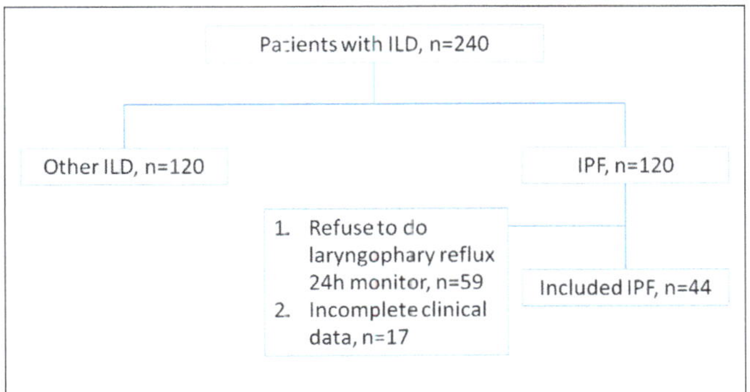

FIGURE 1 | Patient flow chart.

TABLE 2 | Cough symptom scoring criteria.

Score	Daytime cough symptom score	Night-time cough symptom score
0	no cough during the day	no cough during the night
1	cough for infrequent short periods	short cough when falling asleep/infrequent nocturnal cough
2	frequent coughing, which did interfere with usual daytime activities	mildly interfere with nocturnal sleep due to coughs
3	frequent coughing, which did severely interfere with usual daytime activities	severely interfere with nocturnal sleep due to coughs

Total cough symptom score = Daytime cough symptom score + Night-time cough symptom score.

Blood Tests and Arterial Blood Gas Test

Blood tests were performed to evaluate liver and kidney function, C-reactive protein (CRP) levels, and erythrocyte sedimentation rate (ESR). Partial pressure of oxygen (PaO_2), partial pressure of carbon dioxide ($PaCO_2$), and oxygen saturation (SaO_2) were also measured.

Chest High-Resolution Computed Tomography Score

The scoring criteria for chest HRCT followed a previous description and are described in **Table 1** (Su et al., 2017). One radiologist and two pulmonologists scored chest HRCT results separately, and the average score was used for data analyses.

Pulmonary Function Test

Force vital capacity (FVC), FVC expressed as a percentage of predicted (FVC % pred), and carbon monoxide diffusing capacity of the lung expressed as a percentage of predicted (D_LCO % pred) were determined to assess study participants' pulmonary function.

Cough Symptom Score

Cough symptom score (CSS) was determined according to a previous description and the criteria are displayed in **Table 2** (Chung, 2006). Two pulmonologists independently evaluated daytime CSS, nighttime CSS, and total CSS. The average scores from the two pulmonologists were used for data analysis.

TABLE 3 | Patient general clinical data.

	IPF (n = 44)	Control (n = 30)
Men/women (ratio)	40/4 (10:1)[a]	14/16
Age (mean ± SD), year	62 ± 8	61 ± 9
Smoker, n (%)	33 (75.0)[a]	5 (16.7)
Disease duration (mean ± SD),week	28 ± 21	NA
CRP (mg/L)	7.5 ± 11.3	NA
ESR (mm/h)	32 ± 23	NA
PaO_2 (mmHg)	80.5 ± 15.2	NA
$PaCO_2$ (mmHg)	39.0 ± 3.8	NA
SaO_2 (%)	95.1 ± 5.1	NA
FVC (L)	2.15 ± 0.90	NA
FVC, % pred	76.5 ± 28.2	NA
DLCO, % pred	58.2 ± 26.6	NA
Chest HRCT score	17.5 ± 7.6	NA
Daytime cough symptom score	1.26 ± 0.45	NA
Nighttime cough symptom score	0.65 ± 0.57	NA
Total cough symptom score	1.91 ± 0.90	NA

Control: healthy individuals. IPF = idiopathic pulmonary fibrosis, CRP = c-reactive protein, ESR = erythrocyte sedimentation rate, PaO_2 = partial pressure of oxygen, $PaCO_2$ = partial pressure of carbon dioxide, SaO_2 = oxygen saturation, FVC = force vital capacity, FVC % pred = force vital capacity expressed as a percentage of predicted, D_LCO % pred = carbon monoxide diffusing capacity of the lung expressed as a percentage of predicted, NA = not applicable, SD = standard deviation.

[a]Represent significant difference of the IPF group versus the control group, $p < 0.01$.

Statistical Analysis

The statistical analysis software SPSS 16.0 was used. Measurement variables are presented as mean ± standard deviation (SD). Inter-group comparison was examined by independent t-test. One sample t-test was used to compare the

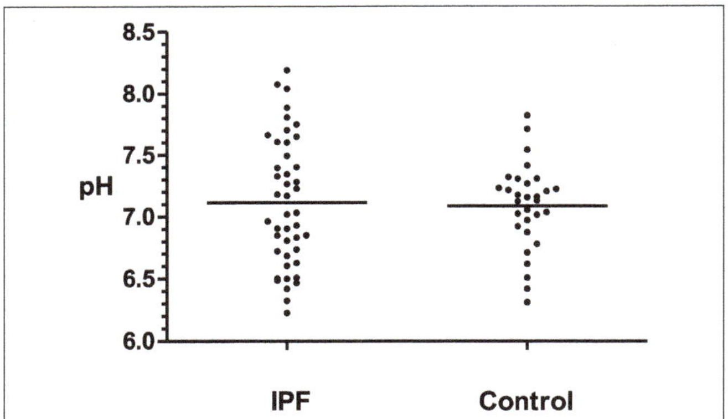

FIGURE 2 | Overall mean laryngopharyngeal pH values of IPF and control groups Control: healthy individuals. IPF = idiopathic pulmonary fibrosis. The overall average laryngopharyngeal pH of two groups were similar (IPF: 7.11 vs Control 7.09, $p > 0.05$, Kruskal-Wallis test).

average pH at coughing versus the overall average pH. $p < 0.05$ was considered statistically significant. The constituent ratios of different pH range (pH < 6.5, pH 6.5–7.5, and pH > 7.5) were analysed by chi-square test.

RESULTS

General Clinical Data

The patient flowchart is displayed in **Figure 1**. A total of 44 patients with IPF were included in the study. The control group included 30 age-matched healthy individuals. The IPF group had significantly higher proportions of men (90.9 vs 46.7%) and smokers (75.0 vs 16.7%) than the control group (All $p < 0.01$, **Table 3**). The average age was similar in two groups (IPF group: 62 ± 8 years, Control group: 61 ± 9 years) (**Table 3**).

TABLE 4 | Proportions of patients in different pH groups.

	pH < 6.5, *n* (%)	pH 6.5–7.5, *n* (%)	pH > 7.5, *n* (%)
Entire pH monitoring duration			
Control, *n* = 30	1 (3.3)	28 (93.4)	1 (3.3)
IPF, *n* = 44	5 (11.4)	27 (61.3)	12 (27.3)[a]
At upright position			
Control, *n* = 30	1 (3.3)	28 (93.4)	1 (3.3)
IPF, *n* = 44	3 (6.8)	28 (63.6)	13 (29.6)[a]
At supine position			
Control, *n* = 30	1 (3.3)	27 (90.0)	2 (6.7)
IPF, *n* = 44	12 (27.3)[a]	24 (54.5)	8 (18.2)

Control: healthy individuals. IPF = idiopathic pulmonary fibrosis.
[a]Represent significant difference of the IPF group versus the control group, p < 0.01.

Twenty-Four-hour Laryngopharyngeal pH Monitoring Results of the Three Groups

The average laryngopharyngeal pH value for 24 h was similar in the IPF (7.11 ± 0.08) group and control group (7.09 ± 0.06) (**Figure 2**). The typical results of 24 h laryngopharyngeal pH monitoring of one patient with IPF are presented in **Figure 3**. We calculated the percentage duration of pH < 6.5, pH 6.5–7.5, and pH > 7.5 in the overall measurement time of every patient and allocated the 44 IPF patients and 30 healthy individuals into pH < 6.5, pH 6.5–7.5, and pH > 7.5 groups according to the highest percentage duration. When the entire pH measurement duration was used as the denominator to calculate the percentage duration, 11.4, 61.3, and 27.3% of the 44 IPF patients were in pH < 6.5, pH 6.5–7.5, and pH > 7.5 group, respectively. 3.3, 93.4, and 3.3% of the 30 healthy individuals were in each respective group. The proportion of pH > 7.5 group in IPF patients was higher than control group ($p < 0.01$); when the duration of upright position was used for the calculation, 6.8, 63.6, and 29.6% of the 44 IPF patients were in each respective group. 3.3, 93.4, and 3.3% of the

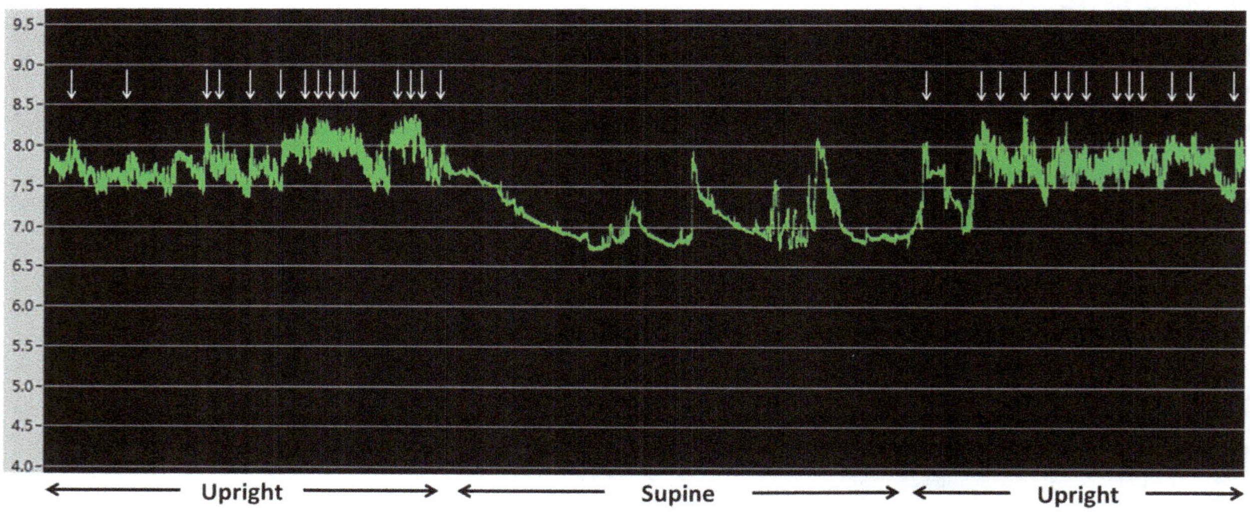

FIGURE 3 | Results of 24 h pharyngeal pH monitoring of a patient with IPF The upright and supine periods can be identified easily by the pattern of the pH recording. pH was more than 7.5 for the majority of the monitoring time. ↓ represent cough events. Cough occurred when pH was >7.5.

TABLE 5 | Seven patients showing abnormal Ryan index score.

Patient no	Disease	Ryan index score	
		At the upright position	At the supine position[a]
1	IPF	65.33	2.17
2	IPF	11.5	2.17
3	IPF	59.82	2.17
4	IPF	11.91	2.17
5	IPF	32.15	2.17
6	IPF	17.5	2.17
7	IPF	23.91	2.17

IPF = idiopathic pulmonary fibrosis.
[a]*When Ryan index score at the supine position was <6.79, the results from the calculation by the software were presented as 2.17.*

TABLE 6 | Five patients showing significant changes in pH values at coughing.

Patient no	Disease	Overall average pH	Average pH at coughing	*p* value
1	IPF	7.6083 ± 0.2953	7.6992 ± 0.1093	0.015
2	IPF	7.1698 ± 0.4367	7.4450 ± 0.3122	0.021
3	IPF	6.7369 ± 0.3188	7.0700 ± 0.1950	0.009
4	IPF	7.3443 ± 0.2719	7.5490 ± 0.1906	0.008
5	IPF	6.8064 ± 0.4245	5.8867 ± 0.3667	0.049

IPF = idiopathic pulmonary fibrosis

30 healthy individuals were in each respective group. The proportion of pH > 7.5 group in IPF patients was higher than control group ($p < 0.01$); when the duration of supine position was used, the proportions of 44 IPF patients in pH < 6.5, pH 6.5–7.5, and pH > 7.5 group were 27.3, 54.5, and 18.2%. The proportions of 30 healthy individuals in each respective group were 3.3, 90.0, and 6.7%. The proportion of pH < 6.5 group in IPF patients was higher than control group (**Table 4**). Overall, 7 patients showed abnormal Ryan index score at upright position (Ryan index score >9.41). None of the 44 patients showed abnormal Ryan index score at supine position (**Table 5**). Abnormal Ryan index score was defined as > 6.79.

Correlation Between pH Value and Cough

No heart burn event occurred in the 44 IPF patients and 30 healthy individuals during the 24 h laryngopharyngeal pH monitoring. Comparison of the average pH value during coughing versus the overall average pH value showed that 4 IPF patients had significantly higher average pH at coughing than the overall average pH and one patient had significantly lower average pH at coughing (All $p < 0.05$, **Table 6**).

DISCUSSION

IPF is a progressive lung disease with an unknown etiology. The pathology of IPF is characterized by slowly progressive diffuse alveolar inflammation and/or alveolar structural disorders, which eventually damage alveolar structure and result in pulmonary fibrosis and honeycomb lung. IPF has a poor prognosis and the survival time of patients with IPF is approximately 3–5 years (Loomis-King et al., 2013). IPF ultimately lead to scars in lung tissues.

Previous studies have suggested that IPF may be highly associated with GERD [(Raghu et al., 2011), (Lee et al., 2011)]. Chronic inhalation of gaseous refluxate is a risk factor for airway and pulmonary inflammation and could induce or exacerbate IPF. Antacids, such as proton pump inhibitors and histamine H2-receptor antagonists, have been found to reduce the risk of GER-associated pulmonary damages (Raghu et al., 2006; Lee et al., 2011). Clinicians have routinely prescribed anti-acid drugs for patients with IPF (Raghu et al., 2011; Raghu et al., 2015). GER is caused by abnormal lower esophageal sphincter relaxation, which allows stomach contents to flow back to the esophagus. The majority of the stomach contents in GER are liquid and stay inside the esophagus. Patients with GER and LPR may experience gaseous reflux into the upper airway. LPR is caused by abnormal upper esophageal sphincter relaxation and is mainly gaseous reflux into the throat, nose, and ear. The gaseous refluxate can then enter the lower airway and alveoli during breathing. Thus, compared with GER, LPR appears more likely to adversely affect the lower airway and lung parenchyma and exacerbate IPF.

The etiology of GERD is associated with the dysfunction of gastric cardia and lower part of the esophagus. The clinical presentations of GERD are mainly digestive tract symptoms and occasional airway symptoms. The pathophysiology of GERD is characterized by acidic or basic gastric liquid and gaseous reflux into the esophagus and into the airway in severe cases. The etiology of LPR is associated with gastric empty dysfunction. LPR causes pathological changes in the airway. The clinical presentations of LPR are mainly airway symptoms but not digestive tract symptoms. The pathophysiology of LPR is characterized by acidic or basic gaseous reflux into the airway. Only 20% of patients with LPRD and GERD show low esophageal pH (the duration of pH < 4.0 is more than 4% of the total measurement time). Therefore, only monitoring esophageal pH could miss the diagnosis of LPRD in 80% of patients with LPRD (Ford, 2005; Yuksel and Vaezi, 2013). The 24 h laryngopharyngeal pH monitoring (DX-pH) has been used to diagnose LPRD (Sun et al., 2009; Wiener et al., 2009; Vailati et al., 2013). The diagnostic criteria for LPR based on DX-pH are the Ryan index at upright position >9.41 and/or at supine position >6.79.

In the current study, we monitored the laryngopharyngeal pH of 44 patients with IPF and 30 healthy individuals for 24 h and explored the association between IPF and LPR. The analysis of the overall 24 h laryngopharyngeal pH showed that 61.3, 27.3, and 11.4% of the 44 IPF patients had neutral, basic, and acidic laryngopharyngeal pH, respectively. 93.4, 3.3, and 3.3% of the 30 healthy individuals had neutral, basic, and acidic laryngopharyngeal pH. The proportion of pH > 7.5 group in IPF patients was higher than control group. The normal pH in the lower airway is 7.0–7.5. Thus, both basic reflux (pH > 7.5) and acidic reflux (pH < 6.5) appear to occur in patients with IPF. According to the diagnostic criteria for LPR (Ryan index at upright position >9.41), only 7 IPF patients met the criteria.

The normal pH in the lung is 7.0–7.5. pH > 7.5 may reduce enzyme activity in the lung tissues or even denature enzymes.

Thus, basic reflux could affect lung function adversely, particularly for patients with IPF, who often have poor pulmonary elasticity because of lung fibrosis. Patients with IPF may have to inhale deeply to expand the alveoli because of the poor pulmonary elasticity. The deep inhalation may cause excessive negative pressure in the chest, which in turn may cause the basic contents including bile and pancreatic juice flow from the duodenal to the throat. The speed of this basic reflux may be too fast to allow the basic contents to be neutralized by gastric acid and to be cleared from the throat. The contents of basic refluxate and the adverse effects of basic refluxate on the laryngopharyngeal mucosa, the lower airway, and the lung need to be further investigated. Acidic reflux could activate the pepsin that has been deposited on the lower airway mucosa and alveoli and consequently result in nonspecific inflammation and trigger IPF.

The analysis of the pH at supine position showed that 54.5, 27.3, and 18.2% of the 44 IPF patients had neutral, acidic, and basic laryngopharyngeal pH, respectively. 90.0, 6.7, and 3.3% of the 30 healthy individuals had neutral, acidic, and basic laryngopharyngeal pH. The proportion of pH < 6.5 group in ILD patients was higher than control group. The supine position may actually facilitate gastric acid reflux into the throat. We found that using Ryan index only diagnosed 7 cases of LPR. For the entire pH monitoring duration and the duration at upright position, about 30% of the patients showed basic laryngopharyngeal pH, whereas for the duration at supine position, approximately 30% of the patients had acidic laryngopharyngeal pH. These findings indicate that the cut-off value of Ryan index for positive LPR (pH < 5.5 at upright position and/or pH < 5.0 at supine position) may not reflect LPR effectively in patients with IPF. In addition, we found that only five of the 44 patients showed significant difference between the average pH at coughing and the overall average pH. This suggests that cough appears more likely to be associated with IPF but not with LPR in patients with IPF. But it is not definitely clear whether the correlation between chronic cough and laryngopharyngeal pH changes is the causal effect or just correlation. We will further explore it in our future study. This study is an exploratory research. The sample size was relatively small. Idiopathic pulmonary fibrosis is a rare disease. Researches about laryngopharyngeal pH monitoring in patients with IPF were rarer. However, we still got some valuable findings in a limited number of study participants. Although the interpretation of the data is limited by small number of study participants, the current study was first to explore the possible association between LPR and IPF. In addition, we will investigate the composition of gaseous refluxate and study possible mechanism underlying the adverse effects of LPR on IPF initiation and development in our future study.

CONCLUSION

We found that 50–60% of the patients had neutral laryngopharyngeal pH and did not need anti-acid treatments. Basic LPR may likely occur at upright position, whereas acidic LPR may probably occur at supine position. Patients with acidic LPR may use antacids (Park et al., 2005; Sato, 2006; Naik and Vaezi, 2013) and gastric pro-motility drugs (Glicksman et al., 2014). Patients with basic LPR may only need gastric pro-motility drugs. Ryan index score calculated based on acidic LPR may not reflect LPR accurately in patients with IPF.

AUTHOR CONTRIBUTIONS

HL, YS, LS, and FZ participated in the conception, hypothesis and design of the study. YS, LS, FZ, XJ and XJ performed the experiments. YZ, YH, YZ and QL carried out the statistical analyses. All authors contributed to interpretation of the data. YS, LS, FZ and HL wrote the manuscript and all authors made critical revisions. All authors read and approved the final manuscript.

REFERENCES

Ayazi, S., Lipham, J. C., Hagen, J. A., Tang, A. L., Zehetner, J., Leers, J. M., et al. (2009). A new technique for measurement of pharyngeal pH: normal values and discriminating pH threshold. *J. Gastrointest. Surg.* 13 (8), 1422–1429. doi:10.1007/s11605-009-0915-6

Chung, K. F. (2006). Measurement of cough. *Respir. Physiol. Neurobiol.* 152 (3), 329–339. doi:10.1016/j.resp.2006.02.001

Cohen, J. T., Bach, K. K., Postma, G. N., and Koufman, J. A. (2002). Clinical manifestations of laryngopharyngeal reflux. *Ear Nose Throat J.* 81 (9 Suppl. 2), 19–23.

DiMango, E., Holbrook, J. T., Simpson, E., Reibman, J., Richter, J., Narula, S., et al. (2009). Effects of asymptomatic proximal and distal gastroesophageal reflux on asthma severity. *Am. J. Respir. Crit. Care Med.* 180 (9), 809–816. doi:10.1164/rccm.200904-0625oc

Ford, C. N. (2005). Evaluation and management of laryngopharyngeal reflux. *JAMA* 294 (12), 1534–1540. doi:10.1001/jama.294.12.1534

Glicksman, J. T., Mick, P. T., Fung, K., and Carroll, T. L. (2014). Prokinetic agents and laryngopharyngeal reflux disease: Prokinetic agents and laryngopharyngeal reflux disease: a systematic review. *The Laryngoscope* 124 (10), 2375–2379. doi:10.1002/lary.24738

Harding, S. M., Guzzo, M. R., and Richter, J. E. (2000). The prevalence of gastroesophageal reflux in asthma patients without reflux symptoms. *Am. J. Respir. Crit. Care Med.* 162 (1), 34–39. doi:10.1164/ajrccm.162.1.9907072

Hom, C., and Vaezi, M. F. (2013). Extra-esophageal manifestations of gastroesophageal reflux disease: diagnosis and treatment. *Drugs* 73 (12), 1281–1295. doi:10.1007/s40265-013-0101-8

Hu, Y., Wang, L.-S., Wei, Y.-R., Du, S.-S., Du, Y.-K., He, X., et al. (2016). Clinical Characteristics of Connective Tissue Disease-Associated Interstitial Lung Disease in 1,044 Chinese Patients. *Chest* 149 (1), 201–208. doi:10.1378/chest.15-1145

Koufman, J. A. (2002). Laryngopharyngeal reflux 2002: a new paradigm of airway disease. *Ear Nose Throat J.* 81 (9 Suppl. 2), 2–6.

Lai, K., Chen, R., Lin, J., Huang, K., Shen, H., Kong, L., et al. (2013). A prospective, multicenter survey on causes of chronic cough in China. *Chest* 143 (3), 613–620. doi:10.1378/chest.12-0441

Lee, J. S., Collard, H. R., Anstrom, K. J., Martinez, F. J., Noth, I., Roberts, R. S., et al. (2013). Anti-acid treatment and disease progression in idiopathic pulmonary fibrosis: an analysis of data from three randomised controlled trials. *Lancet Respir. Med.* 1 (5), 369–376. doi:10.1016/s2213-2600(13)70105-x

Lee, J. S., Ryu, J. H., Elicker, B. M., Lydell, C. P., Jones, K. D., Wolters, P. J., et al. (2011). Gastroesophageal reflux therapy is associated with longer survival in patients with idiopathic pulmonary fibrosis. *Am. J. Respir. Crit. Care Med.* 184, 1390–1394. doi:10.1164/rccm.201101-0138oc

Liang, B., Yi, Q., and Feng, Y. (2013). Association of gastroesophageal reflux disease with asthma control. *Dis. Esophagus* 26 (8), 794–798. doi:10.1111/j.1442-2050.2012.01399.x

Loomis-King, H., Flaherty, K. R., and Moore, B. B. (2013). Pathogenesis, current treatments and future directions for idiopathic pulmonary fibrosis. *Curr. Opin. Pharmacol.* 13, 377–385. doi:10.1016/j.coph.2013.03.015

Mastronarde, J. G., Mastronarde, J. G., Anthonisen, N. R., Castro, M., Holbrook, J. T., Leone, F. T., et al. (2009). Efficacy of esomeprazole for treatment of poorly controlled asthma. *N. Engl. J. Med.* 360 (15), 1487–1499. doi:10.1056/NEJMoa0806290

Naik, R. D., and Vaezi, M. F. (2013). Extra-esophageal manifestations of GERD: who responds to GERD therapy?. *Curr. Gastroenterol. Rep.* 15 (4), 318. doi:10.1007/s11894-013-0318-4

Park, W., Hicks, D. M., Khandwala, F., Richter, J. E., Abelson, T. I., Milstein, C., et al. (2005). Laryngopharyngeal reflux: prospective cohort study evaluating optimal dose of proton-pump inhibitor therapy and pretherapy predictors of response. *The Laryngoscope* 115 (7), 1230–1238. doi:10.1097/01.mlg.0000163746.81766.45

Raghu, G., Collard, H. R., Egan, J. J., Martinez, F. J., Behr, J., Brown, K. K., et al. (2011). An official ATS/ERS/JRS/ALAT statement: idiopathic pulmonary fibrosis: evidence-based guidelines for diagnosis and management. *Am. J. Respir. Crit. Care Med.* 183 (6), 788–824. doi:10.1164/rccm.2009-040gl

Raghu, G., Freudenberger, T. D., Yang, S., Curtis, J. R., Spada, C., Hayes, J., et al. (2006). High prevalence of abnormal acid gastro-oesophageal reflux in idiopathic pulmonary fibrosis. *Eur. Respir. J.* 27, 136–142. doi:10.1183/09031936.06.00037005

Raghu, G., Rochwerg, B., Zhang, Y., Garcia, C. A. C., Azuma, A., Behr, J., et al. (2015). An Official ATS/ERS/JRS/ALAT Clinical Practice Guideline: Treatment of Idiopathic Pulmonary Fibrosis. An Update of the 2011 Clinical Practice Guideline. *Am. J. Respir. Crit. Care Med.* 192 (2), e3–e19. doi:10.1164/rccm.201506-1063st

Sato, K. (2006). Laryngopharyngeal reflux disease with nocturnal gastric acid breakthrough while on proton pump inhibitor therapy. *Eur. Arch. Otorhinolaryngol.* 263 (12), 1121–1126. doi:10.1007/s00405-006-0117-8

Sharma, B., Sharma, M., and Daga, M. K. (2007). Effect of omeprazole and domperidone on adult asthmatics with gastroesophageal reflux. *Wjg* 13 (11), 1706–1710. doi:10.3748/wjg.v13.i11.1706

Su, Y., Gu, H., Weng, D., and Zhou, Y. (2017). Association of serum levels of laminin, type IV collagen, procollagen III N-terminal peptide, and hyaluronic acid with the progression of interstitial lung disease. *Medicine* 96 (18), e6617. doi:10.1097/md.0000000000006617

Sun, G., Muddana, S., Slaughter, J. C., Casey, S., Hill, E., Farrokhi, F., et al. (2009). A new pH catheter for laryngopharyngeal reflux: Normal values. *The Laryngoscope* 119 (8), 1639–1643. doi:10 1002/lary.20282

Travis, W. D., Costabel, U., Hansell, D. M., King, T. E., Jr, Lynch, D. A., Nicholson, A. G., et al. (2013). An official American Thoracic Society/European Respiratory Society statement: Update of the international multidisciplinary classification of the idiopathic interstitial pneumonias. *Am. J. Respir. Crit. Care Med.* 188, 733–748. doi:10.1164/rccm.201308-1483st

Vailati, C., Mazzoleni, G., Bondi, S., Bussi, M., Testoni, P. A., and Passaretti, S. (2013). Oropharyngeal pH Monitoring for Laryngopharyngeal Reflux: Is It a Reliable Test Before Therapy? *J. Voice* 27 (1), 84–89. doi:10.1016/j.jvoice.2012.08.006

Wiener, G. J., Tsukashima, R., Kelly, C., Wolf, E., Schmeltzer, M., Bankert, C., et al. (2009). Oropharyngeal pH Monitoring for the Detection of Liquid and Aerosolized Supraesophageal Gastric Reflux. *J. Voice* 23 (4), 498 504. doi:10.1016/j.jvoice.2007.12.005

Yuksel, E. S., and Vaezi, M. F. (2013). Therapeutic Strategies for Laryngeal Manifestations of Gastroesophageal Reflux Disease. *J. Clin. Gastroenterol.* 47 (3), 195–204. doi:10.1097/mcg.0b013e31827458f9

16

Long-Term Follow-Up of Patients with Idiopathic Pulmonary Fibrosis Treated with Pirfenidone or Nintedanib

Paolo Cameli, Rosa Metella Refini, Laura Bergantini, Miriana d'Alessandro, Valerio Alonzi, Carlo Magnoni, Paola Rottoli, Piersante Sestini and Elena Bargagli*

Respiratory Diseases Unit, Department of Medicine, Surgery and Neurosciences, University of Siena, Siena, Italy

Correspondence:
Paolo Cameli
paolocameli88@gmail.com

Background: Pirfenidone and nintedanib are the sole pharmacological therapies currently approved for idiopathic pulmonary fibrosis (IPF). Limited comparison data is available in literature, despite they are both prescribed for mild-to-moderate disease. Here, we describe our almost 10 years real-life experience with antifibrotic treatment to investigate potential differences in terms of efficacy.

Population and Methods: We retrospectively recruited patients diagnosed with IPF and treated with pirfenidone or nintedanib at Siena Referral Center. Clinical, functional, safety and radiological data was collected at baseline and during the follow-up, according to our Center protocol.

Results: We retrospectively recruited 263 IPF patients (139 treated with pirfenidone and 124 with nintedanib) in the study. After 885.3 ± 559.5 days of observation, the median survival was 1224 days. No significant differences were found between pirfenidone and nintedanib in terms of survival and time to decline of forced vital capacity >10% (p = 0.8786 and p = 0.1677, respectively). A smaller lung diffusion for carbon monoxide (DL_{CO}) decrease was found after 1 year of therapy with nintedanib in respect to pirfenidone (p = 0.0167). Overall, 21 patients permanently discontinued antifibrotic treatment due to side effects (14 with pirfenidone, 7 with nintedanib); no fatal adverse events were recorded.

Discussion: Our results showed a similar effectiveness between pirfenidone and nintedanib in terms of mortality and functional disease progression. Both drugs confirmed their good tolerability profile and no new safety alerts were observed. Nintedanib was associated with a smaller reduction of DL_{CO} after 1 year of follow-up compared with pirfenidone, maybe due to its antiangiogenic properties.

Keywords: idiopathic pulmonary fibrosis, real-life, pirfenidone, nintedanib, disease progression, mortality

INTRODUCTION

Idiopathic pulmonary fibrosis (IPF) is a chronic fibrosing lung disease, characterized by dry cough and progressive exertional dyspnea, invariably leading to respiratory failure and death within 3–5 years of diagnosis (Raghu et al., 2018). Pathogenesis is characterized by aberrant overexpression of profibrotic pathways, triggered by oxidative-nitrosative stress and alveolar epithelial injury refractory to anti-inflammatory and immunosuppressant treatments (Wolters et al., 2014; Sgalla et al., 2018; Cameli et al., 2019, 2020). Today, an "antifibrotic" approach is widely accepted and the only drugs approved for the treatment of IPF are pirfenidone and nintedanib. Randomized clinical trials of both drugs have demonstrated similar efficacy in slowing functional deterioration (expressed as decline in FVC percentages) and the risk of hospitalization for respiratory

Abbreviations: DL_{co}, diffusing capacity of the lung for CO; FEV1, forced expiratory volume in 1 second; I FVC, forced vital capacity; HRCT, high resolution computed tomography; PF, idiopathic pulmonary fibrosis.

TABLE 1 | Demographic, functional and radiological features of the study population.

	Study population	Pirfenidone	Nintedanib	*p*-value*
N°	263	139	124	
Male (%)	203 (77.1)	107 (76.9)	96 (77.4)	0.8360 Chi square: 0.04285, df 1
Age (years)	70.9 ± 8.6	68.1 ± 7.7	74.1 ± 8.5	<0.0001
Smoking history (pack/year)	24.1 ± 17.9	24 ± 19.5	24.7 ± 12.3	0.8953
Current smoker (%)	9 (3.4)	5 (3.6)	4 (3.2)	0.1265 Chi-square: 4.134, df 2
Former smoker (%)	168 (63.8)	81 (58.2)	87 (70.1)	0.1265 Chi-square: 4.134, df 2
Never smoker (%)	86 (32.6)	53 (38.1)	33 (26.6)	0.1265 Chi-square: 4.134, df 2
Familial history positive for ILD (%)	53 (20.1)	29 (20.8)	24 (19.3)	0.8778
Time from diagnosis to treatment (months)	7.8 ± 14.9	8.6 ± 12.4	5.1 ± 6.6	0.1512
Previous treatments				
Steroids (%)	59 (22.4)	35 (25.1)	24 (19.3)	0.3008
N-acetyl cysteine (%)	20 (7.6)	15 (10.7)	5 (4)	0.0601
Azathioprine (%)	3 (1.1)	3 (2.1)		n.a.
Comorbidities				
Emphysema (%)	35 (13.3)	20 (14.3)	15 (12.1)	0.7165
Lung cancer (%)	7 (2.6)	3 (2.1)	4 (3.2)	0.9055
Pulmonary arterial hypertension (%)	18 (6.8)	10 (7.1)	8 (6.4)	1.000
Gastroesophageal reflux disease (%)	119 (44.8)	67 (48.2)	52 (41.9)	0.3232
Arterial Hypertension (%)	167 (63.4)	87 (62.5)	80 (64.5)	0.7095
Ischemic heart disease (%)	79 (30)	41 (29.4)	38 (30.6)	0.8941
Diabetes mellitus (%)	32 (12.1)	20 (14.3)	12 (9.6)	0.1899
PFTs				
FVC% predicted value	78.2 ± 20.1	82.6 ± 19.7	73.1 ± 19.9	0.0004
(l)	(2.5 ± 0.7)	(2.7 ± 0.8)	(2.3 ± 0.7)	0.0002
FEV1% predicted value	81 ± 19	85.5 ± 18.6 (2.2 ± 0.6)	76.2 ± 18.9 (1.8 ± 0.5)	0.0004
(l)	(2 ± 0.6)			0.0001
FEV1/FVC	80.9 ± 7.6	81 ± 7.5	80.8 ± 7.7	0.8834
TLC% predicted value	76.4 ± 17.1	80.5 ± 17.2 (4.7 ± 1.3)	72.1 ± 17.4 (4.4 ± 1.2)	0.0015
(l)	(4.6 ± 1.2)			0.0504
DL_{CO}% predicted value	44.9 ± 16	50.2 ± 15.2	38.6 ± 14.7	<0.0001
KCO% predicted value	72.8 ± 19.9	77 ± 17.7	67.6 ± 21.4	0.0013
HRCT scan pattern				
Typical UIP (%)	199 (75.6)	110 (79.1)	89 (71.7)	0.3917
Probable UIP (%)	64 (24.3)	29 (20.8)	35 (28.2)	0.3917
Emphysema (%)	70 (26.6)	36 (25.8)	34 (27.4)	0.7820

**Comparison between pirfenidone and nintedanib subgroups. ILD, interstitial lung disease; PFTs, pulmonary function tests; FVC, forced vital capacity; FEV1, forced expiratory volume in the first second; TLC, total lung capacity; DL_{CO}, lung diffusion capacity for carbon monoxide; KCO carbon monoxide transfer coefficient; HRCT, high resolution computed tomography; UIP, usual interstitial pneumonia.*

problems (Noble et al., 2011; King et al., 2014; Richeldi et al., 2014). Real-life studies have confirmed the effectiveness of pirfenidone and nintedanib in slowing the progression of IPF, suggesting an improvement in survival rate (Fisher et al., 2017; Margaritopoulos et al., 2018; Lancaster et al., 2019) but without any substantial effect on quality of life.

Few evidences regarding the comparison of the efficacy of pirfenidone and nintedanib are currently available in the literature. A metanalysis published in 2016 failed to find any significant differences in safety or concerning progression between the two drugs, whereas nintedanib appeared to be more effective in reducing acute exacerbations and mortality risk (Rogliani et al., 2016). Two other retrospective observational studies confirmed the substantial similarity of the two antifibrotic drugs in terms of effectiveness and tolerability, albeit with a relatively short follow-up (Bargagli et al., 2019; Cerri et al., 2019).

Here we describe our almost 10 year experience with antifibrotic treatment at our Regional Referral Center for Rare Lung Diseases and lung transplant, assessing the effectiveness and safety of pirfenidone and nintedanib in a real-life cohort of IPF patients monitored over a long observation period.

MATERIALS AND METHODS

Study Population and Design

All IPF patients treated with pirfenidone and nintedanib at the Regional Referral Center for Rare Lung Diseases, Siena, from 2011 to June 2019 were retrospectively enrolled in the study. Diagnosis of IPF was according to international guidelines (Raghu et al., 2011, 2018). High-resolution computed tomography (HRCT) of the chest was performed in all patients for diagnostic purposes. The diagnosis of IPF was confirmed by multidisciplinary discussion. Demographic and clinical data, including comorbidities, family history, lung function parameters and radiological features were collected from medical records and entered in an electronic database for statistical analysis. We included serial assessment of all clinical and functional data collected regularly every 12 months. If available, we also included lung function test (LFT) parameters 1 year before starting antifibrotic therapy. Survival data and all causes of death were obtained by systematic revision of the medical records of our Center. Adverse effects related to treatment were also collected.

Patients were considered lost to follow-up in the case of death, lung transplant or interruption of treatment. Functional deterioration was defined as a decrease in FVC of 10% or more.

The study was conducted according the principles of the Declaration of Helsinki. All patients gave their written informed consent to participation in the study. The study was approved by our local ethical committee C.E. A. V. S. E. (code number 180712).

LFTs

Lung function tests were performed according to ATS/ERS standards (Miller et al., 2005; Graham et al., 2017) using a Jaeger body plethysmograph with corrections for temperature and barometric pressure. Forced expiratory volume in the first second (FEV1) and lung diffusing capacity for carbon monoxide (DLco) were recorded.

Statistical Analysis

Data was expressed as mean ± standard deviation, unless otherwise specified. Parametric tests (*T*-test and one-way ANOVA) were used to compare groups. Statistical analysis and graphs were performed and plotted using GraphPad Prism version 5.0 software for Windows (GraphPad Software, La Jolla, CA). Unadjusted survival and disease progression outcome estimates were obtained using Kaplan-Meier curves. Time-to-event endpoints were compared using a two-sided log-rank test. A $p \leq 0.05$ was considered significant.

RESULTS

Clinical and Functional Features of Study Population

A total of 263 patients (203 males, age 70.9 ± 8.6 years) affected with IPF were included in the study. Demographic characteristics, clinical-functional data and radiological features of the population are reported in **Table 1**. As expected, the majority of our patients were males and current/former smokers. On average, functional assessment at baseline showed mild restrictive impairment of lung volumes, associated with a moderate reduction in DLco percentages. DLco at baseline was available for 203 patients (105 treated with pirfenidone), who were able to perform the procedure and were not on oxygen therapy.

Fifty-six patients (21.2%, 43 treated with nintedanib) showed advanced stage disease at diagnosis and were treated on compassionate grounds (pirfenidone FVC < 50% and/or DLco < 35%; nintedanib FVC < 50% and DLco < 35% of predicted values). Twenty-two (8.3%) of them had been on long-term oxygen therapy (LTOT) due to chronic respiratory failure before starting antifibrotic treatment.

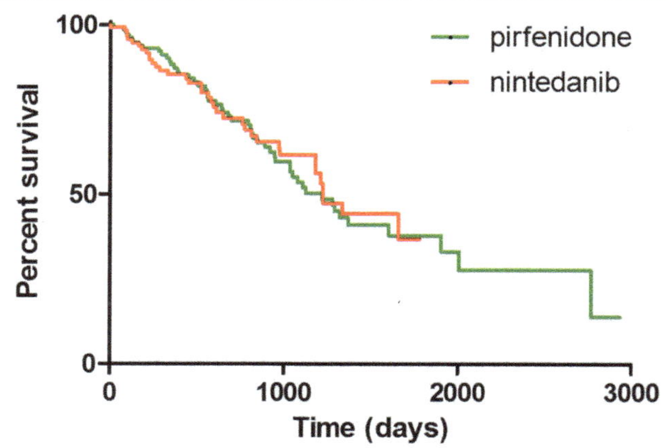

FIGURE 1 | Kaplan Meier curves for survival analysis between IPF patients treated with pirfenidone and nintedanib.

TABLE 2 | FVC and DLCO progression rate of IPF patients in pretreatment period, at baseline (initiation of antifibrotic therapy) and during the follow-up.

Parameters	Pre- treatment	Baseline (time 0)	12 months	24 months	36 months	48 months	60 months
Days from time 0	370.5 ± 100.4		363.7 ± 62.8	717.4 ± 98.5	1083.4 ± 89.6	1447.9 ± 107.5	1790.6 ± 58.2
Pirfenidone ($n°$)	44	139	134	87	40	21	7
Nintedanib ($n°$)	22	124	101	54	27	13	5
FVC%	82.7 ± 21.4	78.2 ± 20.1	78.1 ± 22.3	77.6 ± 22.5	76.4 ± 22	77.8 ± 22.3	72.8 ± 12.7
ΔFVC%*	+ 6.4 ± 9.1		−2.4 ± 8.1	−5.9 ± 11.2	−8.4 ± 12.1	−11.7 ± 12.8	−16.6 ± 9.9
FVC (ml)	2667.3 ± 838	2540.8 ± 79	2463.3 ± 824	2395.3 ± 871.8	2173.6 ± 780.5	2089.5 ± 714.1	2416 ± 542.9
ΔFVC (ml)*	+ 202.5 ± 27.1	4.4	−90.6 ± 244	−209.8 ± 329.3	−269.2 ± 266.6	−296.8 ± 292.4	−534 ± 296.7
DL_{CO}%	45.7 ± 18.3	44.9 ± 16	44.2 ± 17.4	44.3 ± 17.2	42.6 ± 16.6	36.2 ± 10.5	35.3 ± 8.5
ΔDL_{CO}%*	+ 5.4 ± 7.7		−3.8 ± 9.3	−8.2 ± 10.8	−11.6 ± 11.8	−18.2 ± 8.1	−17.2 ± 7.6

Difference against baseline values. FVC, forced vital capacity; FEV1, forced expiratory volume in the first second; DL_{CO}, lung diffusion capacity for carbon monoxide.

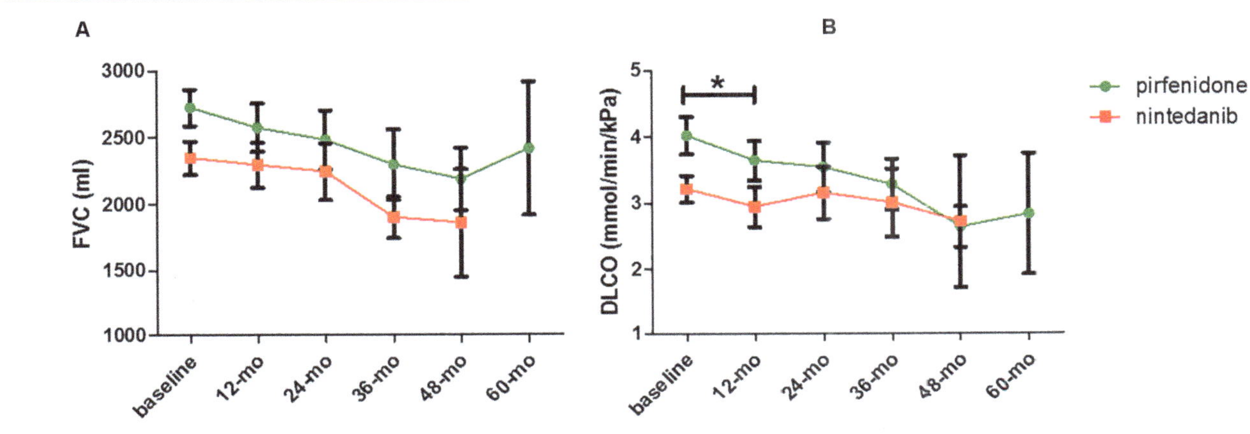

FIGURE 2 | Comparison of FVC **(A)** and DL_{CO} **(B)** decrease rate between pirfenidone and nintedanib subgroup (*p = 0.0201).

The study population was stratified by antifibrotic treatment: 139 patients (107 males) treated with pirfenidone, 124 (96 males) treated with nintedanib. Patients treated with nintedanib were significantly older ($p < 0.0001$) than the pirfenidone group at the start of antifibrotic therapy and showed worse FVC and DLco percentages ($p = 0.0004$ and $p < 0.0001$, respectively).

Outcome Analysis

At 1st January 2020 (885.3 ± 559.5 days of observation), median of survival was 1224 days. During follow-up, 59 patients died (22.4%, 29 pirfenidone, 30 nintedanib), 7 patients underwent lung transplant (2.6%, 6 pirfenidone, 1 nintedanib) and 21 (7.9%) discontinued treatment due to incoercible drug-related adverse effects (14 pirfenidone, 7 nintedanib). No significant differences in mortality rate were found between treatment groups (log rank test 0.02333, $p = 0.8786$) (**Figure 1**).

Concerning functional deterioration, mean time to FVC decline > 10% (TTD10) was 495.3 ± 263 days in the overall population. Pre-treatment LFTs and DLco were available in 66 and 52 patients, 44 on pirfenidone, 22 on nintedanib, respectively. In general, FVC and DLco reduction rates slowed significantly after 1 year of antifibrotic therapy ($p = 0.0062$ and $p = 0.0075$, respectively). Accordingly, the percentage of patients reaching

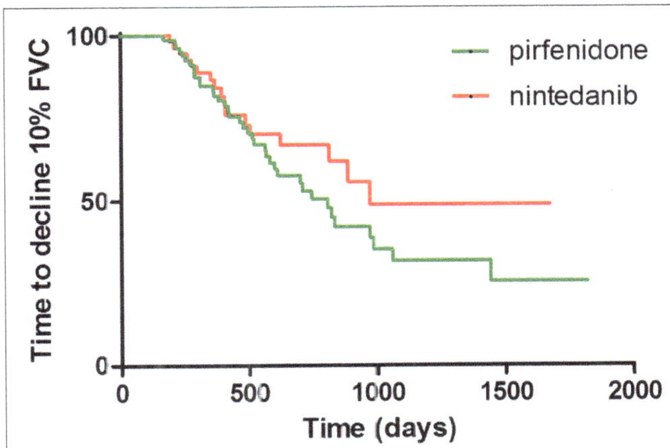

FIGURE 3 | Difference of time to decline of FVC > 10% between pirfenidone and nintedanib subgroups, expressed with Kaplan-Meier curves.

TTD10 was significantly higher in the pre-treatment period than after 1 year of therapy ($p = 0.0012$). FVC and DLco reduction rates during follow-up are reported in **Table 2**. In the following years of therapy, FVC progression rate tended to accelerate, even though not reaching statistical significance ($p = 0.0567$).

TABLE 3 | Adverse events (AE) reported in our cohort.

Side effects	Pirfenidone	Nintedanib
***N*° of patients with AE (%)**	44 (31)	52 (41.9)
Interruption of treatment (%)	14 (10)	7 (5.6)
Hypertransaminasemia (%)	7 (5)	12 (9.6)
Time from start treatment (months)	4.2 ± 7.4	3.5 ± 6.3
NCI-CTC grade 1	6	5
NCI-CTC grade 2	1	5
NCI-CTC grade 3	0	1
NCI-CTC grade 4	0	1
NCI-CTC grade 5	0	0
Anorexia (%)	10 (7.2)	3 (2.4)
Time from start treatment (months)	6.4 ± 5.2	4.9 ± 4.1
NCI-CTC grade 1	7	3
NCI-CTC grade 2	3	0
NCI-CTC grade 3	0	0
NCI-CTC grade 4	0	0
NCI-CTC grade 5	0	0
Weight loss (%)	25 (17.9)	17 (13.7)
Time from start treatment (months)	4.1 ± 6.6	4.8 ± 5.1
NCI-CTC grade 1	18	15
NCI-CTC grade 2	7	2
NCI-CTC grade 3	0	0
NCI-CTC grade 4	0	0
NCI-CTC grade 5	0	0
Nausea (%)	10 (7.2)	5 (4)
Time from start treatment (months)	2.9 ± 4.4	2.5 ± 2
NCI-CTC grade 1	8	2
NCI-CTC grade 2	2	3
NCI-CTC grade 3	0	0
NCI-CTC grade 4	0	0
NCI-CTC grade 5	0	0
Pyrosis (%)	13 (9.3)	9 (7.2)
Time from start treatment (months)	2.8 ± 3.9	2.5 ± 2.8
NCI-CTC grade 1	10	5
NCI-CTC grade 2	3	4
NCI-CTC grade 3	0	0
NCI-CTC grade 4	0	0
NCI-CTC grade 5	0	0
Diarrhea (%)	3 (2.1)	44 (31.6)
Time from start treatment (months)	5.2 ± 4.8	2.2 ± 3.1
NCI-CTC grade 1	1	20
NCI-CTC grade 2	2	18
NCI-CTC grade 3	0	6
NCI-CTC grade 4	0	0
NCI-CTC grade 5	0	0
Constipation (%)	7 (5)	2 (1.6)
Time from start treatment (months)	4.6 ± 6.7	5.1 ± 3.2
NCI-CTC grade 1	5	2
NCI-CTC grade 2	2	0
NCI-CTC grade 3	0	0
NCI-CTC grade 4	0	0
NCI-CTC grade 5	0	0
Photosensitivity (%)	16 (11.5)	0
Time from start treatment (months)	3.2 ± 5.1	
NCI-CTC grade 1	0	
NCI-CTC grade 2	4	
NCI-CTC grade 3	12	
NCI-CTC grade 4	0	
NCI-CTC grade 5	0	
Skin rash (%)	19 (13.6)	2 (1.6)
Time from start treatment (months)	2.6 ± 4.5	3.6 ± 4.2
NCI-CTC grade 1	9	0
NCI-CTC grade 2	10	2
NCI-CTC grade 3	1	0
NCI-CTC grade 4	0	0
NCI-CTC grade 5	0	0
Itch (%)	2 (1.4)	2 (1.6)
Time from start treatment (months)	6.7 ± 4.3	8.1 ± 5.4
NCI-CTC grade 1	0	1
NCI-CTC grade 2	1	1
NCI-CTC grade 3	1	0
NCI-CTC grade 4	0	0
NCI-CTC grade 5	0	0
Dizziness (%)	1 (0.7)	0
Time from start treatment (months)	1.5	
NCI-CTC grade 1	0	
NCI-CTC grade 2	1	
NCI-CTC grade 3	0	
NCI-CTC grade 4	0	
NCI-CTC grade 5	0	

NCI-CTC, National Cancer Institute Common Terminology Criteria.

Concerning comparisons between the pirfenidone and nintedanib groups, no statistically significant difference in terms of FVC deterioration rate ($p = 0.9396$ and $p = 0.6907$ for absolute and percentage values, respectively) (**Figure 2**) and TTD10 was observed during follow-up (log rank test 1.903, $p = 0.1677$) (**Figure 3**). After 1 year of antifibrotic treatment, we observed a more pronounced decrease in DLco in patients treated with pirfenidone than in those treated with nintedanib ($p = 0.0167$ and $p = 0.0201$ for absolute and percentage values), but this significant difference no longer emerged in subsequent years of follow-up (**Figure 2**).

Concerning tolerability, pirfenidone and nintedanib were both generally well tolerated: most adverse effects were mild to moderate and were readily managed with temporary discontinuation of therapy or with supporting treatments (**Table 3**). No drug-related fatal events were reported.

DISCUSSION

This observational real-life study of patients with IPF treated with nintedanib and pirfenidone offers a comparative evaluation of drug effectiveness after a long follow-up. Clinical, functional and survival data was collected for 60 months at our Regional Referral Center for Rare Lung Diseases, ensuring the homogeneity of data collection and the clinical management of patients. Although monocentric, this is the first real-life study to evaluate the safety and efficacy of the two antifibrotic treatments for a significantly longer follow-up than those reported in the international clinical trials and observational cohorts (Noble et al., 2011; King et al., 2014; Richeldi et al., 2014; Margaritopoulos et al., 2018). Only four previous studies have investigated the efficacy of pirfenidone over an observation period longer than 2 years in a real-life setting (Bando et al., 2016; Tzouvelekis et al., 2017; Zurkova et al., 2019; Vietri et al., 2020). The only evidence available for nintedanib comes from open-label extension studies of clinical trials; to our knowledge, no real-life data is available beyond 3 years of treatment (Richeldi et al., 2018; Crestani et al., 2019; Antoniou et al., 2020; Song et al., 2020).

As expected, our population showed a clear predominance of males and most patients were former smokers. The prevalence of males and smoking in our population, as well as the mean age of patients (over 65 years), are in line with epidemiological studies (Fernández-Fabrellas et al., 2019; Tran et al., 2020). Due to Italian prescription criteria for antifibrotic drugs, the patients treated with nintedanib were older than those treated with pirfenidone and had worse FVC and DLco percentage at baseline. This discrepancy is also related to the inclusion of patients treated with nintedanib on compassionate grounds, which allowed us to recruit and treat patients in an advanced stage of disease. Moreover, 8% of our patients were on oxygen therapy before starting antifibrotic treatment, in substantial conformity with other real-file IPF studies (Sköld et al., 2016; Bargagli et al., 2019). It is surely interesting that, despite the age discrepancy, no significant differences were found between pirfenidone and nintedanib subgroups in terms of progression-free survival and mortality. These findings further support the substantial efficacy of antifibrotic drugs and specifically of nintedanib, also in elderly age, as already reported in literature (Takeda et al., 2020).

Our results confirm the effectiveness of pirfenidone and nintedanib in slowing disease progression in terms of FVC reduction rate and in maintaining the effect in subsequent years of treatment. This result was emphasized by comparison of functional deterioration in the years before and after antifibrotic therapy, which showed a substantial halving of the FVC and DL_{CO} reduction rates. Similar results were recently reported by Vietri et al. (2020) for pirfenidone in a cohort of IPF patients. In our study, both antifibrotic molecules stabilized functional deterioration over many years of follow-up, suggesting their long-term effectiveness. Moreover, the deterioration of FVC and DL_{CO} was stabilized in the older population with advanced disease, further confirming previous studies that demonstrated that pirfenidone and nintedanib are also effective in advances stages of IPF (Wuyts et al., 2016; Nathan et al., 2019). Interestingly, the decrease in DLco was more pronounced after 1 year of pirfenidone than after 1 year of nintedanib treatment, although the significance tended to disappear after the first year of follow-up. Despite the limitations of our retrospective study, our results may suggest that nintedanib has a specific effect on slowing the decline in lung diffusion capacity with respect to pirfenidone, probably due to its well-known antiangiogenic properties (Hilberg et al., 2008; Reck, 2015). However, our nintedanib group showed older age and worse FVC and DLco values, aspects that likely influence our analysis, together with the relatively small sample size. Nevertheless, our results are certainly interesting and merit full assessment in a prospective study with larger cohorts.

Concerning mortality, our data showed a median survival of 1224 days, similar to that of previous reports (Margaritopoulos et al., 2018; Antoniou et al., 2020; Vietri et al., 2020). Despite the absence of a control group, comparison of our data with survival data of historical cohorts of patients reported in the literature confirmed the efficacy of nintedanib and pirfenidone in prolonging life expectancy in patients with IPF (Costabel et al., 2017; Fisher et al., 2017; Margaritopoulos et al., 2018; Lancaster et al., 2019). No significant differences were found in terms of survival between the pirfenidone and nintedanib groups. Although our data may be influenced by demographic discrepancies between the two groups, our results suggest that the two drugs have substantially the same performance in preventing functional deterioration and reducing mortality. These assumptions are in line with a recent paper by Cerri et al. (2019), although our study considered a larger cohort of patients (including those with advanced disease) and a much longer follow-up, further underlining the reliability of both antifibrotic drugs in the treatment of IPF.

Regarding drug tolerability, our results are in line with previous reports (Lancaster et al., 2017; Rodríguez-Portal, 2018). Despite the high prevalence of side effects (especially weight loss with pirfenidone and diarrhea with nintedanib), most (>90%) were mild and easily managed with supporting therapies and temporary dose reductions or discontinuation. No fatal events were reported in our cohort, confirming the good safety profile of the two drugs even in fragile patients, over a 5 year observation period.

In conclusion, this real-life retrospective comparison of the long-term effectiveness of the two currently approved pharmacological treatments for IPF showed similar efficacy in reducing functional deterioration and improving life expectancy, associated with acceptable tolerability, even in subjects with greater functional impairment. Long-term multicenter prospective studies, including populations of patients excluded from randomized clinical trials, are needed to confirm our findings. Future research will necessarily focus on identifying biomarkers to predict response to a specific drug, to enable a personalized therapeutic approach for IPF patients.

AUTHOR CONTRIBUTIONS

PC, RR, and EB: conception and study design, interpretation of results, writing of the manuscript. LB, Md'A, VA, and CM: data acquisition and analysis, revision of the study, interpretation of results. PC, EB, PR, and PS: statistical analysis, revision of the study. All authors approved the final version of the study and agreed to be accountable for all aspects of the work in ensuring that questions related to the accuracy or integrity of any part of the work are appropriately investigated and resolved.

REFERENCES

Antoniou, K., Markopoulou, K., Tzouvelekis, A., Trachalaki, A., Vasarmidi, E., Organtzis, J., et al. (2020*). Efficacy and safety of nintedanib in a Greek multicentre idiopathic pulmonary fibrosis registry: a retrospective, observational, cohort study. *ERJ Open Res.* 6:00172-2019. doi: 10.1183/23120541.00172-2019

Bando, M., Yamauchi, H., Ogura, T., Taniguchi, H., Watanabe, K., Azuma, A., et al. (2016). Clinical experience of the long-term use of pirfenidone for idiopathic pulmonary fibrosis. *Intern. Med.* 55, 443–448. doi: 10.2169/internalmedicine.55.5272

Bargagli, E., Piccioli, C., Rosi, E., Torricelli, E., Turi, L., Piccioli, E., et al. (2019). Pirfenidone and Nintedanib in idiopathic pulmonary fibrosis: real-life experience in an Italian referral centre. *Pulmonology* 25, 149–153. doi: 10.1016/j.pulmoe.2018.06.003

Cameli, P., Bergantini, L., Salvini, M., Refini, R. M., Pieroni, M., Bargagli, E., et al. (2019). Alveolar concentration of nitric oxide as a prognostic biomarker in idiopathic pulmonary fibrosis. *Nitric Oxide* 89, 41–45. doi: 10.1016/j.niox.2019.05.001

Cameli, P., Carleo, A., Bergantini, L., Landi, C., Prasse, A., and Bargagli, E. (2020). Oxidant/antioxidant disequilibrium in idiopathic pulmonary fibrosis pathogenesis. *Inflammation* 43, 1–7. doi: 10.1007/s10753-019-01059-1

Cerri, S., Monari, M., Guerrieri, A., Donatelli, P., Bassi, I., Garuti, M., et al. (2019). Real-life comparison of pirfenidone and nintedanib in patients with idiopathic pulmonary fibrosis: a 24-month assessment. *Respir. Med.* 159:105803. doi: 10.1016/j.rmed.2019.105803

Costabel, U., Albera, C., Lancaster, L. H., Lin, C.-Y., Hormel, P., Hulter, H. N., et al. (2017). An open-label study of the long-term safety of pirfenidone in patients with idiopathic pulmonary fibrosis (RECAP). *Respiration* 94, 408–415. doi: 10.1159/000479976

Crestani, B., Huggins, J. T., Kaye, M., Costabel, U., Glaspole, I., Ogura, T., et al. (2019). Long-term safety and tolerability of nintedanib in patients with idiopathic pulmonary fibrosis: results from the open-label extension study. INPULSIS-ON. *Lancet Respir. Med.* 7, 60–68. doi: 10.1016/s2213-2600(18)30339-4

Fernández-Fabrellas, E., Molina-Molina, M., Soriano, J. B., Portal, J. A. R., Ancochea, J., Valenzuela, C., et al. (2019). Demographic and clinical profile of idiopathic pulmonary fibrosis patients in Spain: the SEPAR national registry. *Respir. Res.* 20:127.

Fisher, M., Nathan, S. D., Hill, C., Marshall, J., Dejonckheere, F., Thuresson, P.-O., et al. (2017). Predicting life expectancy for pirfenidone in idiopathic pulmonary fibrosis. *J. Manag. Care Spec. Pharm.* 23(3-b Suppl.), S17–S24.

Graham, B. L., Brusasco, V., Burgos, F., Cooper, B. G., Jensen, R., Kendrick, A., et al. (2017). ERS/ATS standards for single-breath carbon monoxide uptake in the lung. *Eur. Respir. J.* 9:1600016. doi: 10.1183/13993003.00016-2016

Hilberg, F., Roth, G. J., Krssak, M., Kautschitsch, S., Sommergruber, W., Tontsch-Grunt, U., et al. (2008). BIBF 1120: triple angiokinase inhibitor with sustained receptor blockade and good antitumor efficacy. *Cancer Res.* 15, 4774–4782. doi: 10.1158/0008-5472.can-07-6307

King, T. E., Bradford, W. Z., Castro-Bernardini, S., Fagan, E. A., Glaspole, I., Glassberg, M. K., et al. (2014). A phase 3 trial of pirfenidone in patients with idiopathic pulmonary fibrosis. *N. Engl. J. Med.* 370, 2083–2092.

Lancaster, L., Crestani, B., Hernandez, P., Inoue, Y., Wachtlin, D., Loaiza, L., et al. (2019). Safety and survival data in patients with idiopathic pulmonary fibrosis treated with nintedanib: pooled data from six clinical trials. *BMJ Open Respir. Res.* 6:e000397. doi: 10.1136/bmjresp-2018-000397

Lancaster, L. H., de Andrade, J. A., Zibrak, J. D., Padilla, M. L., Albera, C., Nathan, S. D., et al. (2017). Pirfenidone safety and adverse event management in idiopathic pulmonary fibrosis. *Eur. Respir. Rev.* 26:170057. doi: 10.1183/16000617.0057-2017

Margaritopoulos, G. A., Trachalaki, A., Wells, A. U., Vasarmidi, E., Bibaki, E., Papastratigakis, G., et al. (2018). Pirfenidone improves survival in IPF: results from a real-life study. *BMC Pulm. Med.* 18:177. doi: 10.1186/s12890-018-0736-z

Miller, M. R., Crapo, R., Hankinson, J., Brusasco, V., Burgos, F., Casaburi, R., et al. (2005). General considerations for lung function testing. *Eur. Respir. J.* 26, 153–161. doi: 10.1183/09031936.05.00034505

Nathan, S. D., Costabel, U., Albera, C., Behr, J., Wuyts, W. A., Kirchgaessler, K.-U., et al. (2019). Pirfenidone in patients with idiopathic pulmonary fibrosis and more advanced lung function impairment. *Respir. Med.* 153, 44–51. doi: 10.1016/j.rmed.2019.04.016

Noble, P. W., Albera, C., Bradford, W. Z., Costabel, U., Glassberg, M. K., Kardatzke, D., et al. (2011). Pirfenidone in patients with idiopathic pulmonary fibrosis (CAPACITY): two randomised trials. *Lancet* 377, 1760–1769. doi: 10.1016/s0140-6736(11)60405-4

Raghu, G., Collard, H. R., Egan, J. J., Martinez, F. J., Behr, J., Brown, K. K., et al. (2011). An official ATS/ERS/JRS/ALAT statement: idiopathic pulmonary fibrosis: evidence-based guidelines for diagnosis and management. *Am. J. Respir. Crit. Care Med.* 183, 788–824. doi: 10.1164/rccm.2009-040gl

Raghu, G., Remy-Jardin, M., Myers, J. L., Richeldi, L., Ryerson, C. J., Lederer, D. J., et al. (2018). Diagnosis of idiopathic pulmonary fibrosis. An official ATS/ERS/JRS/ALAT clinical practice guideline. *Am. J. Respir. Crit. Care Med.* 198, e44–e68.

Reck, M. (2015). Nintedanib: examining the development and mechanism of action of a novel triple angiokinase inhibitor. *Expert Rev. Anticancer. Ther.* 15, 579–594. doi: 10.1586/14737140.2015.1031218

Richeldi, L., du Bois, R. M., Raghu, G., Azuma, A., Brown, K. K., Costabel, U., et al. (2014). Efficacy and safety of nintedanib in idiopathic pulmonary fibrosis. *N. Engl. J. Med.* 370, 2071–2082.

Richeldi, L., Kreuter, M., Selman, M., Crestani, B., Kirsten, A.-M., Wuyts, W. A., et al. (2018). Long-term treatment of patients with idiopathic pulmonary fibrosis with nintedanib: results from the TOMORROW trial and its open-label extension. *Thorax* 73, 581–583. doi: 10.1136/thoraxjnl-2016-209701

Rodríguez-Portal, J. A. (2018). Efficacy and safety of nintedanib for the treatment of idiopathic pulmonary fibrosis: an update. *Drugs R D.* 18, 19–25. doi: 10.1007/s40268-017-0221-9

Rogliani, P., Calzetta, L., Cavalli, F., Matera, M. G., and Cazzola, M. (2016). Pirfenidone, nintedanib and N-acetylcysteine for the treatment of idiopathic pulmonary fibrosis: a systematic review and meta-analysis. *Pulm. Pharmacol. Ther.* 40, 95–103. doi: 10.1016/j.pupt.2016.07.009

Sgalla, G., Iovene, B., Calvello, M., Ori, M., Varone, F., and Richeldi, L. (2018). Idiopathic pulmonary fibrosis: pathogenesis and management. *Respir. Res.* 19:32.

Sköld, C. M., Janson, C., Elf, ÅK., Fiaschi, M., Wiklund, K., and Persson, H. L. (2016). A retrospective chart review of pirfenidone-treated patients in Sweden: the REPRIS study. *Eur. Clin. Respir. J.* 3:32035. doi: 10.3402/ecrj.v3.32035

Song, J. W., Ogura, T., Inoue, Y., Xu, Z., Quaresma, M., Stowasser, S., et al. (2020). Long-term treatment with nintedanib in Asian patients with idiopathic pulmonary fibrosis: results from INPULSIS® -ON. *Respirology* 25, 410–416. doi: 10.1111/resp.13647

Takeda, T., Kunimatsu, Y., Tani, N., Hashimoto, I., Kurono, Y., and Hirose, K. (2020). Improvement in subjective symptoms and tolerability in response to nintedanib treatment in elderly patients with idiopathic pulmonary fibrosis. *J. Clin. Med.* 9:755. doi: 10.3390/jcm9030755

Tran, T., Šterclová, M., Mogulkoc, N., Lewandowska, K., Müller, V., Hájková, M., et al. (2020). The European MultiPartner IPF registry (EMPIRE): validating long-term prognostic factors in idiopathic pulmonary fibrosis. *Respir. Res.* 21:11.

Tzouvelekis, A., Karampitsakos, T., Ntolios, P., Tzilas, V., Bouros, E., Markozannes, E., et al. (2017). Longitudinal 'Real-World' outcomes of pirfenidone in idiopathic pulmonary fibrosis in greece. *Front. Med.* 4:213. doi: 10.3389/fmed.2017.00213

Vietri, L., Cameli, P., Perruzza, M., Cekorja, B., Bergantini, L., d'Alessandro, M., et al. (2020). Pirfenidone in idiopathic pulmonary fibrosis: real-life experience in the referral centre of Siena. *Ther. Adv. Respir. Dis.* 14:1753466620906326.

Wolters, P. J., Collard, H. R., and Jones, K. D. (2014). Pathogenesis of idiopathic pulmonary fibrosis. *Annu. Rev. Pathol.* 9, 157–179.

Wuyts, W. A., Kolb, M., Stowasser, S., Stansen, W., Huggins, J. T., and Raghu, G. (2016). First data on efficacy and safety of nintedanib in patients with idiopathic pulmonary fibrosis and forced vital capacity of =50 % of predicted value. *Lung* 94, 739–743. doi: 10.1007/s00408-016-9912-1

Zurkova, M., Kriegova, E., Kolek, V., Lostakova, V., Sterclova, M., Bartos, V., et al. (2019). Effect of pirfenidone on lung function decline and survival: 5-yr experience from a real-life IPF cohort from the Czech EMPIRE registry. *Respir. Res.* 20:16.

17

TRAF6 Suppresses the Development of Pulmonary Fibrosis by Attenuating the Activation of Fibroblasts

*Jiali Min[1], Qiao Li[1], Suosi Liu[1], Qianrong Wang[1], Min Yin[1], Yan Zhang[1], Jun Yan[2], Bing Cui[3] and Shanshan Liu[1]**

[1]National Clinical Research Center for Metabolic Diseases, Key Laboratory of Diabetes Immunology, Ministry of Education, Department of Metabolism and Endocrinology, The Second Xiangya Hospital of Central South University, Changsha, China, [2]Beijing Institute of Brain Disorders, Capital Medical University, Beijing, China, [3]State Key Laboratory of Bioactive Substance and Function of Natural Medicines, Institute of Materia Medica, Chinese Academy of Medical Sciences and Peking Union Medical College, Beijing, China

***Correspondence:**
Shanshan Liu
lss0625@csu.edu.cn

Pulmonary fibrosis (PF) has a high mortality rate, and its pathogenesis is unknown. TNF receptor-associated factor 6 (TRAF6), a signal transducer for inflammatory signaling, plays crucial roles in the pathogenesis of immune diseases. However, its function in PF remains unknown. Herein, we demonstrated that lungs from mice with bleomycin (BLM)-induced PF were characterized by decreased expression of TRAF6 in lung fibroblasts. Enhancing TRAF6 expression protected mice from BLM-induced PF coupled with a significant reduction in fibroblast differentiation. Furthermore, we demonstrated that overexpression of TRAF6 reversed the activation of myofibroblasts from PF mice by reducing the expression of Wnt3a and subsequently suppressing Wnt/β-catenin signaling. Additionally, the abundance of Tribbles pseudokinase 3 (TRIB3), a stress sensor, was negatively correlated with the abundance of TRAF6 in lung fibroblasts. TRIB3 overexpression decreased TRAF6 abundance by reducing TRAF6 stability in lung fibroblasts during PF. Mechanistic studies revealed that TRIB3 bound to TRAF6 and accelerated basal TRAF6 ubiquitination and degradation. Collectively, our data indicate that reduced TRAF6 expression in fibroblasts is essential for the progression of PF, and therefore, genetically increasing TRAF6 expression or disrupting the TRIB3-TRAF6 interaction could be potential therapeutic strategies for fibroproliferative lung diseases in clinical settings.

Keywords: pulmonary fibrosis, TRAF6, lung fibroblast, TRIB3, ubiquitination, protein degradation, Wnt3a

INTRODUCTION

Pulmonary fibrosis (PF) is a type of chronic, progressive, and irreversible fibrotic lung disease characterized by an excess of extracellular matrix (ECM), destruction of normal lung architecture, and ultimately, respiratory failure (Sgalla et al., 2019; George et al., 2020). To date, only two therapies, pirfenidone and nintedanib, have been approved for use in PF. However, neither treatment is known to be curative. Lung transplantation remains the final and life-saving therapeutic option for PF. The lack of a successful treatment of PF is due to a lack of understanding of the underlying cellular and molecular mechanisms. Therefore, an in-depth investigation of the molecular pathogenesis of PF is urgently needed.

Although the cause of PF remains unclear, existing evidence suggests that lung fibroblasts play a crucial role in the pathogenesis of PF (Hinz and Lagares, 2020; Liu G. et al., 2021). Upon stimulation of fibrotic factors, such as chemokine (C-C motif) ligand 1 (CCL1), transforming growth factor-β1 (TGF-β1), and platelet-derived growth factor (PDGF), fibroblasts differentiate into myofibroblasts, which secrete excessive amounts of ECM proteins, including type I collagen, and fibronectin (Lo Re et al., 2011; Frangogiannis, 2020; Liu S. S. et al., 2021). Increased accumulation of ECM obliterates functional alveolar units, thereby decreasing gas exchange and reducing lung function. It is critically important to identify the key mediators contributing to the activation of myofibroblasts during PF development.

TRAF6 (TNF receptor-associated factor 6), a member of the TRAF protein family, plays a pivotal role in immune signal transduction pathways triggered by members of the TNF receptor superfamily and the IL-1 receptor superfamily (Cao et al., 1996; Walsh et al., 2015). By acting as a ubiquitin ligase (E3) catalyzing the formation of Lys63-linked polyubiquitin on itself and its substrates, TRAF6 participates in many biological processes, such as the operation of the innate immune system, lymph node organogenesis, and osteoclast formation (Naito et al., 1999; Wu and Arron, 2003; Yang et al. 2009). TRAF6 contains a RING-finger domain in the N-terminus, which is responsible for its E3 ligase activity, followed by several zinc-finger domains and a conserved C-terminal TRAF domain that enables interaction with receptors and adaptor proteins. Recent studies have revealed the role of

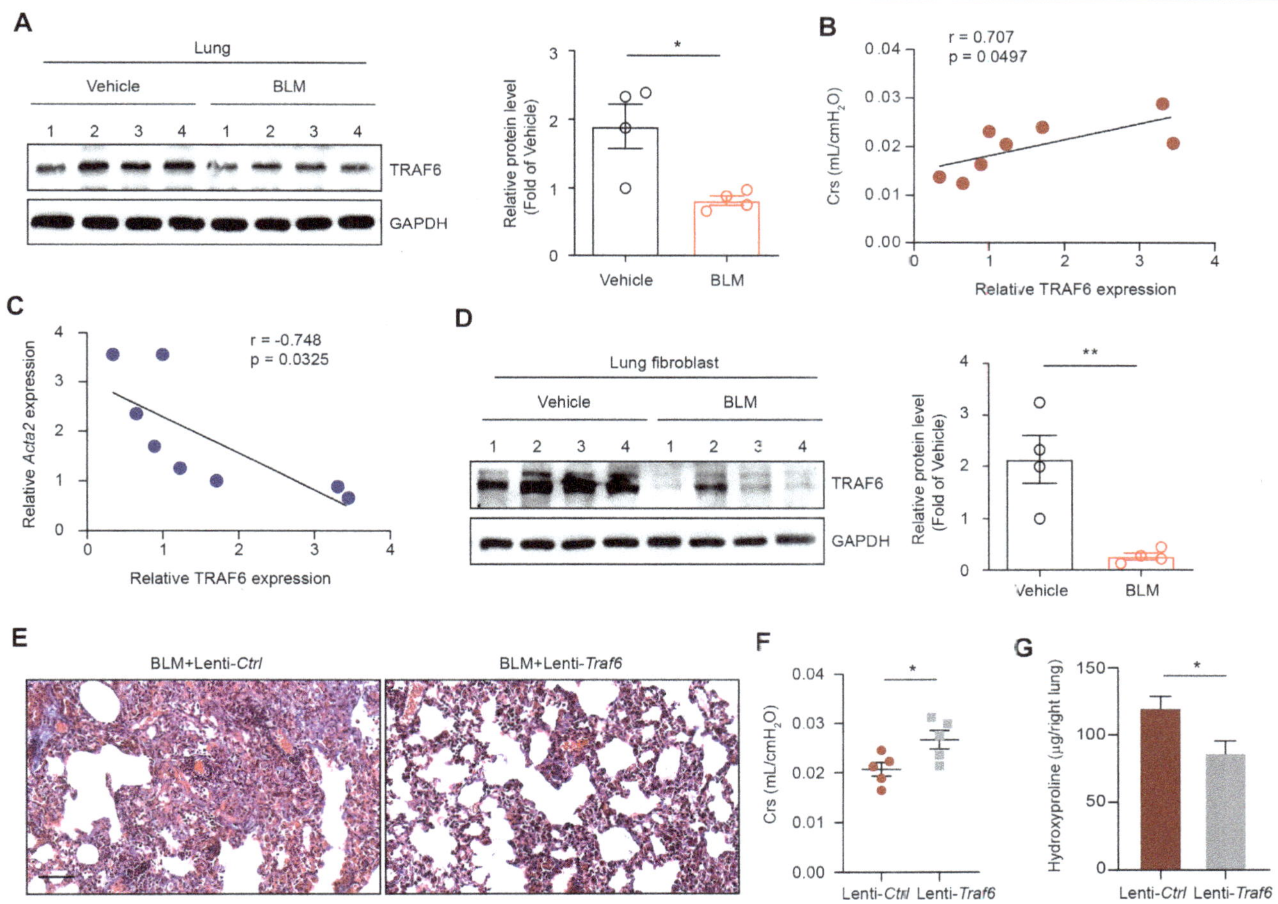

FIGURE 1 | TRAF6 expression in lung fibroblasts is negatively correlated with PF progression. **(A)** Western blot analysis of TRAF6 expression in the lungs of mice following BLM induction. **(B)** Correlation analysis between TRAF6 expression in the lungs of PF mice and respiratory system compliance (Crs) in mice. Each point represents the value of one mouse. Spearman's rank correlation test was employed to determine statistical significance. **(C)** Correlation analysis between TRAF6 expression and *Acta2* expression in the lungs of PF mice. Each point represents the value of one mouse. Spearman's rank correlation test was employed to determine statistical significance. **(D)** Western blot analysis of TRAF6 expression in lung fibroblasts isolated from the lungs of mice following BLM induction. **(E)** Masson staining was performed to evaluate fibrotic changes in the indicated mice (Group 1: BLM + Lenti-Ctrl, Group 2: BLM + Lenti-Traf6; n = 5 per group). Scale bars, 100 μm. Crs **(F)** and hydroxyproline content in the right lung **(G)** were assessed to evaluate pulmonary fibrosis and lung function (Group 1: BLM + Lenti-Ctrl, Group 2: BLM + Lenti-Traf6; $n = 5$ per group). Data are representative of 3 independent experiments. Data represent means ± SEM Statistical significance: $^*p < 0.05$ or $^{**}p < 0.01$.

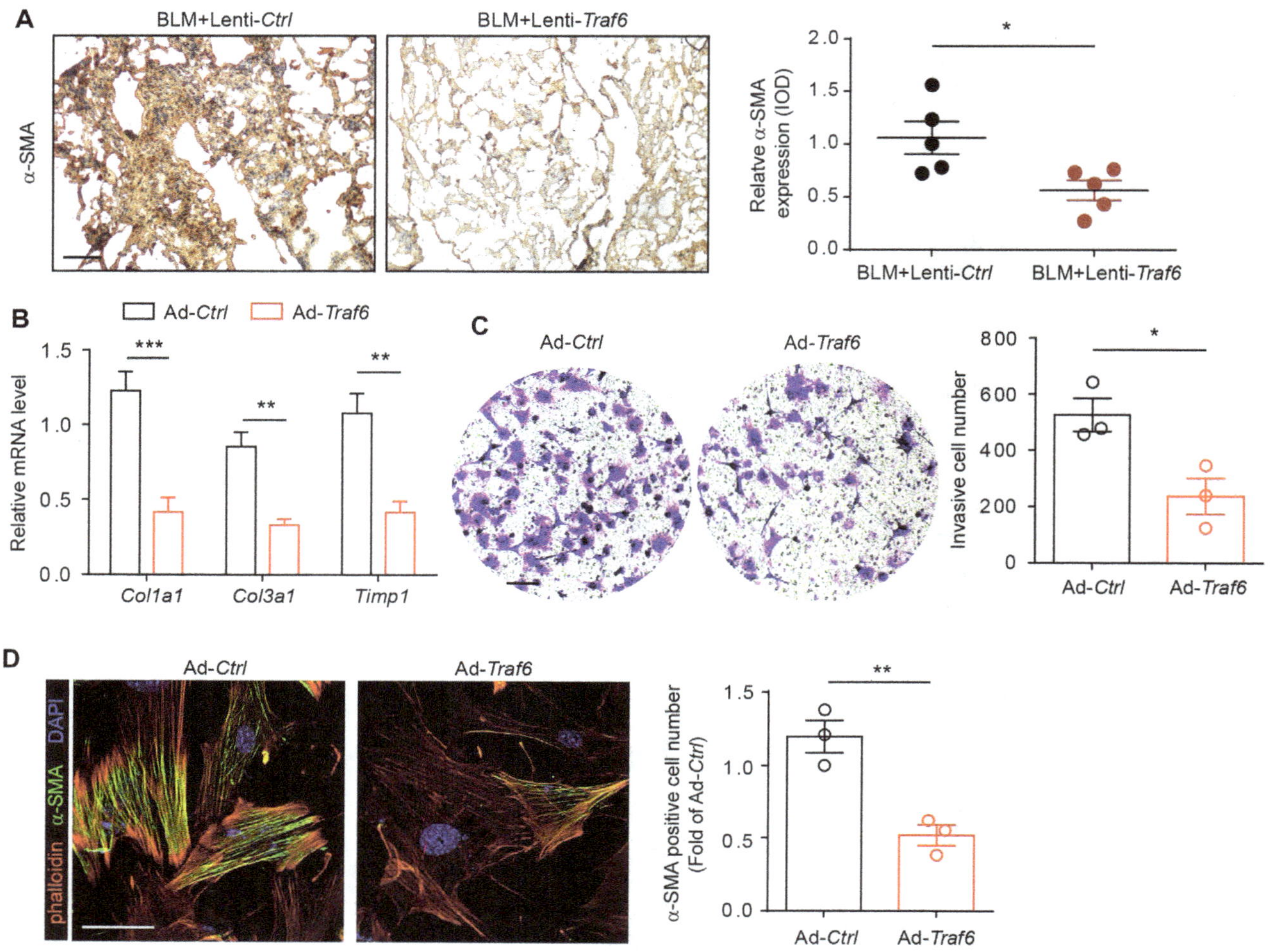

FIGURE 2 | Overexpression of TRAF6 suppresses fibroblast activation. **(A)** IHC staining showing the expression of α-SMA in lung tissues. Representative data and quantified results are shown (Group 1: BLM + Lenti-*Ctrl*, Group 2: BLM + Lenti-*Traf6*; $n = 5$ per group). Scale bar, 100 μm. **(B)** mRNA expression of fibrosis genes in mouse PF lung fibroblasts with or without TRAF6 overexpression. **(C)** Representative images and quantification of the invasion experiment results for mouse PF lung fibroblasts with or without TRAF6 overexpression. Scale bars, 100 μm. **(D)** Representative images and quantification of α-SMA immunostaining in mouse PF fibroblasts with or without TRAF6 overexpression. Scale bars, 50 μm. Data are representative of 3 independent experiments. Data represent means ± SEM Statistical significance: $^{*}p < 0.05$, $^{**}p < 0.01$ or $^{***}p < 0.001$.

TRAF6 in fibrosis (Wang et al., 2020; Zhang et al., 2021). TRAF6 overexpression in hepatocytes promotes ubiquitination-dependent activation of ASK1, contributing to the pathogenesis of hepatic fibrosis during the progression of nonalcoholic steatohepatitis (NASH) (Wang et al., 2020). However, it remains unclear whether TRAF6 plays any important roles in the pathogenesis of PF.

In the present study, we observed reduced protein levels of TRAF6 in the lungs of PF mice, supporting a role for TRAF6 in PF development. Using the classical bleomycin (BLM)-induced PF mouse model, we found that overexpression of TRAF6 reduced BLM-induced PF changes. Using gain- and loss-of-function approaches *in vitro*, we demonstrated that the downregulation of TRAF6 expression is induced by the upregulation of expression of TRIB3 in lung fibroblasts during chronic lung injury. Furthermore, the loss of TRAF6 aggravated the progression of PF by acting as a novel negative regulator of Wnt3a, thereby activating lung fibroblasts into myofibroblasts. Collectively, our findings revealed a critical role for TRAF6 in suppressing the activation of lung fibroblasts and preventing the development of PF.

MATERIALS AND METHODS

Antibodies and Reagents

Antibodies against TRAF6 and TRIB3 were purchased from Abcam (Cambridge, MA, United States); antibodies against Axin 2, c-Myc, and cyclin D1 were obtained from Cell Signaling Technology (Danvers, MA, United States); an antibody against α-SMA was purchased from BOSTER (Wuhan, China); and antibodies against DDK, Myc and HA were obtained from MBL BIOTECH (Beijing, China). CoraLite® 594-phalloidin was obtained from Proteintech

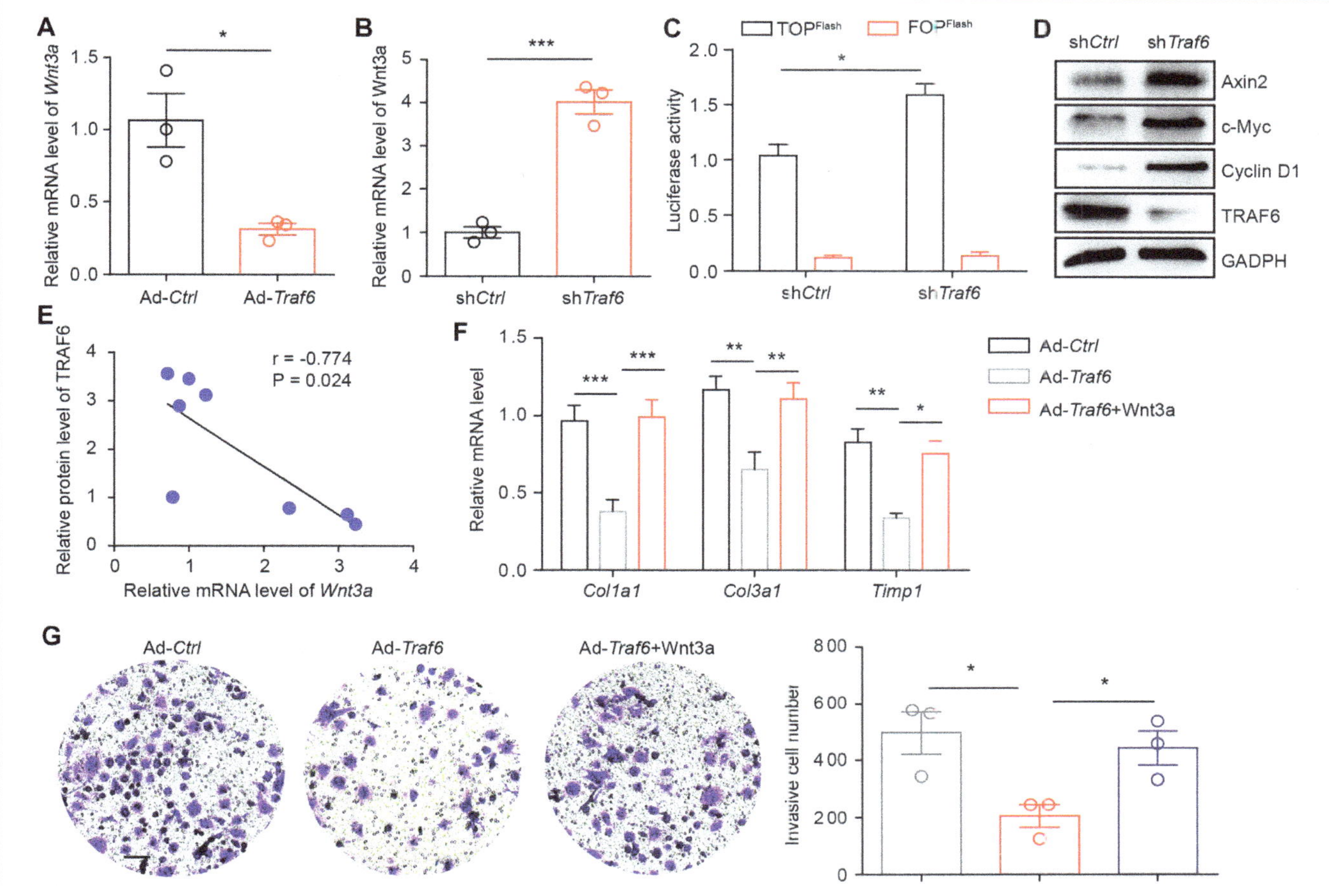

FIGURE 3 | TRAF6 suppresses fibroblast activation by reducing Wnt3a expression. **(A)** mRNA levels of *Wnt3a* as measured by qRT–PCR in TRAF6-overexpressing lung fibroblasts. **(B)** mRNA levels of *Wnt3a* as measured by qRT–PCR in TRAF6-depleted lung fibroblasts. **(C)** Wnt-reporter luciferase activity in PF lung fibroblasts with or without TRAF6 depletion. **(D)** Western blot analysis of β-catenin target gene expression in PF lung fibroblasts with or without TRAF6 depletion. **(E)** Correlation analysis of TRAF6 protein expression and *Wnt3a* mRNA levels in mouse PF lung fibroblasts. **(F)** qRT–PCR analysis of the expression of fibrosis genes in TRAF6-overexpressing mouse lung fibroblasts with or without Wnt3a stimulation. **(G)** Transwell assay for the evaluation of the invasion of TRAF6-overexpressing lung fibroblasts with or without Wnt3a stimulation. Scale bars, 100 μm. Data are representative of 3 independent experiments. Data represent means ± SEM Statistical significance: $^{*}p < 0.05$, $^{**}p < 0.01$ or $^{***}p < 0.001$.

(Wuhan, China). CHX was purchased from Sigma (St Louis, MO, United States). Bleomycin (BLM), MG132, and 3-Methyladenine (3-MA) were obtained from MCE (Shanghai, China).

Bleomycin (BLM) Induction of Pulmonary Fibrosis

C57BL/6J male mice (8 weeks old) were purchased from SJA Laboratory Animal Co., Ltd. (Hunan, China). The mouse PF model was induced as previously reported (Liu et al., 2019). In brief, mice were anesthetized with 400 mg/kg avertin (Sigma–Aldrich) via intraperitoneal injection and then treated with 1 mg/kg BLM in 50 μl PBS via intratracheal injection. This was conducted 6 times, with 14 days between each challenge. Mice were sacrificed by excessive anesthesia at Day 40 after the last BLM challenge, and then lungs were obtained for immunoblotting and RT–PCR analysis.

Lentiviral Treatment in Vivo

For lentivirus administration, lentiviruses (5×10^7 I.U.) overexpressing *Traf6* in 50 μl of PBS were administered to mice via intratracheal instillation for a total of two treatments at 2-weeks intervals beginning on Day 10 after the last BLM administration.

Isolation of Lung Fibroblasts

Lung fibroblasts were obtained from mice as reported previously (Liu S. S. et al., 2021). The chests of mice sacrificed by excessive anesthesia were cut open, and the lungs were removed, rinsed with sterile PBS and cut into 1 mm^3 pieces in culture medium. After centrifugation at 1,500 rpm for 10 min, the tissue suspension was suspended in DMEM containing 15% FBS and spread evenly in a 10-cm dish. After 5–7 days of culture, the adherent fibroblasts were harvested for passage or for assays.

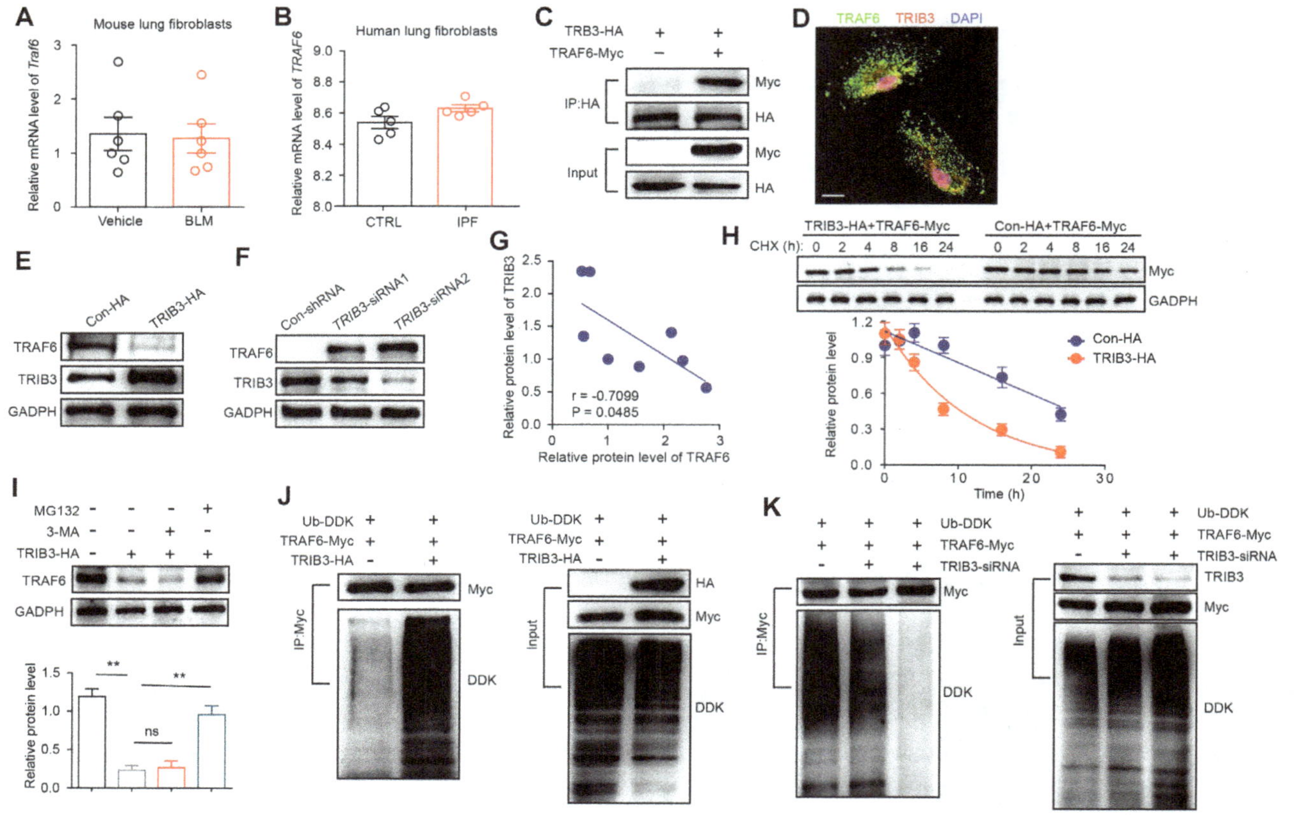

FIGURE 4 | TRIB3 decreases the expression of TRAF6 by promoting its degradation. **(A)** mRNA levels of *Traf6* as measured by qRT–PCR in lung fibroblasts from vehicle- and BLM-challenged mice. **(B)** *TRAF6* mRNA expression in lung fibroblasts of IPF patients compared with normal controls based on the reanalysis of a published dataset (GSE129164). **(C)** The interaction between TRAF6 and TRIB3 was evaluated by co-IP assays. HEK293T cell extracts were subjected to IP with an HA antibody and blotted with a Myc antibody. **(D)** Colocalization of TRAF6 and TRIB3 was evaluated in primary lung fibroblasts. Scale bars, 10 μm. **(E)** Sample immunoblot analyses of the expression of TRAF6 after TRIB3 overexpression in MRC5 cells. **(F)** Sample immunoblot analyses of the expression of TRAF6 after TRIB3 silencing in MRC5 cells. **(G)** Correlation analysis of TRAF6 protein expression and TRIB3 protein expression in mouse PF lung fibroblasts. **(H)** TRAF6 degradation in HEK293T cells with or without TRIB3 overexpression was determined by western blotting. **(I)** Analysis of the TRAF6 degradation pathway. Lung fibroblasts were incubated with CHX (20 μM), CHX plus 3-Methyladenine (3-MA, 5 mM), or MG132 (10 μM) for the indicated times. TRAF6 expression was detected by immunoblotting. **(J)** Immunoblots of ubiquitinated TRAF6 after TRIB3 overexpression. **(K)** Immunoblots of ubiquitinated TRAF6 after TRIB3 deletion. Data are representative of 3 independent experiments. Data represent means ± SEM Statistical significance: $^{**}p < 0.01$.

Cell Lines

MRC5 fibroblasts were cultured in minimal essential medium supplemented with 10% FCS, penicillin, streptomycin, and non-essential amino acid (NEAA) at 37°C in a humidified 5% CO_2 incubator.

Cell Transfection

Plasmids were transfected into cells with Lipofectamine 3,000 (Invitrogen) according to the manufacturer's instructions. siRNAs were transfected using Lipofectamine RNAiMAX (Invitrogen) according to the manufacturer's instructions.

Invasion Assays

Fibroblasts were cultured in serum-free DMEM for 24 h prior to cell invasion assays. Transwell invasion assays were performed using Transwell chambers with filter membranes of 8 μm pore size (Corning). The lower surface of the chambers was precoated with 10 μg ml^{-1} fibronectin, and the upper chambers were coated with BD Matrigel™ Basement Membrane Matrix (40 μl per well). Then, the chambers were inserted into 24-well culture plates. Single-cell suspensions were seeded into the upper chamber (1×10^4 cells per well in 0.4% FBS in DMEM), and the bottom chamber contained DMEM with 10% FBS. After 12 h, the medium was removed, and noninvasive cells were removed using cotton swabs. The invaded cells were fixed with 4% paraformaldehyde in PBS and stained with crystal violet staining solution. Invasive cells from 3 nonoverlapping fields of each membrane were imaged and counted using brightfield microscopy under 40x magnification.

RNA Extraction and Real-Time Polymerase Chain Reaction

Total RNA was isolated from cells and tissues using the Eastep® Super Total RNA Extraction Kit (Promega) according to the manufacturer's instructions. RNA was quantified using a

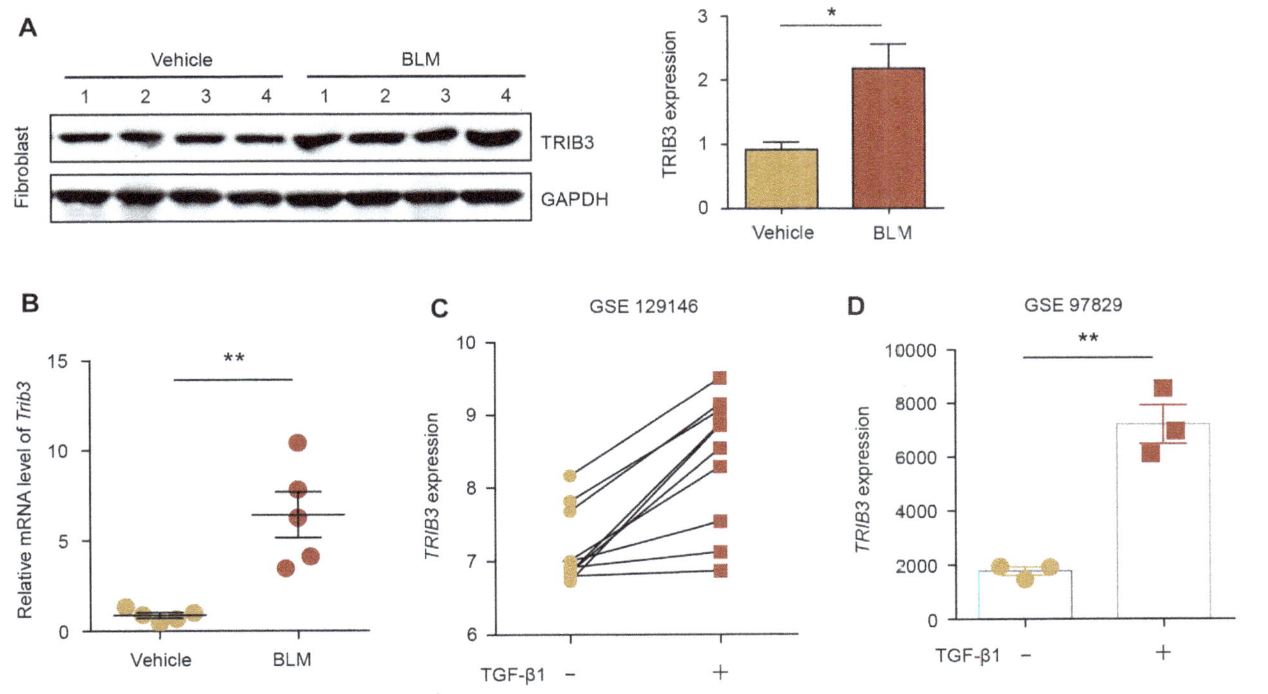

FIGURE 5 | TRIB3 expression is increased in PF lung fibroblasts. **(A)** Western blot analysis of TRIB3 expression in lung fibroblasts isolated from the lungs of mice following BLM induction. **(B)** mRNA levels of *Trib3* as measured by qRT–PCR in lung fibroblasts from vehicle- and BLM-challenged mice. **(C)** *TRIB3* mRNA expression in lung fibroblasts of IPF patients and normal controls treated with or without TGF-β1 based on the reanalysis of a published dataset (GSE129164). **(D)** *TRIB3* mRNA expression in lung fibroblasts treated with or without TGF- β1 based on the reanalysis of a published dataset (GSE97829). Data are representative of 3 independent experiments. Data represent means ± SEM Statistical significance: $^{*}p < 0.05$ or $^{**}p < 0.01$.

NanoDrop spectrophotometer. Reverse transcription was carried out with 1 mg of purified RNA using M-MLV reverse transcriptase (Transgen Biotech). Quantitative real-time PCR (qRT–PCR) was performed using the KAPA SYBR FAST RT–PCR Master Mix (2×) Kit (Kappa Biosystem, United States) and conducted by a LineGene 9,620 apparatus (Bioer). All primer details are listed in **Supplementary Table S1**.

Immunoblot

Tissues and cultured cells were lysed in RIPA buffer (Beyotime) containing protein inhibitors (Selleck). The protein concentration was determined by a BCA protein assay (Applygen Technologies Inc.). Proteins were mixed with 5× SDS sample loading buffer and incubated at 95°C for 10 min. Then, proteins were separated by SDS–PAGE gel, transferred to PVDF membranes (Millipore), and incubated with appropriate primary antibodies coupled with a horseradish peroxidase-conjugated secondary antibody. Images were visualized using ECL western blotting detection reagents (Tanon).

Coimmunoprecipitation (Co-IP)

Cells were washed twice in cold PBS and lysed in IP buffer (150 mmol/L NaCl, 25 mmol/L Tris-HCl (pH 7.4), 2.5 mmol/L $MgCl_2$, 0.5% NP-40, 0.5 mmol/L EDTA, and 5% glycerol) with protease inhibitors. Cell extracts were incubated with the indicated primary antibodies overnight at 4°C and then with Protein A/G Plus-Agarose (Santa Cruz, United States) at 4°C for 2 h. The beads were washed five times with wash buffer (IP buffer without NP-40), eluted in 2× SDS sample loading buffer, and then subjected to electrophoresis.

Immunostaining

For α-SMA immunostaining, cells cultured on coverslips were fixed with 4% (v/v) formaldehyde at room temperature for 10 min, permeabilized with 0.5% Triton X-100 at room temperature for 20 min, and blocked with 3% BSA at room temperature for 30 min. The slides were incubated with antibodies against α-SMA at 4°C overnight, followed by staining with Alexa Fluor 488-conjugated anti-mouse antibodies and CoraLite® 594-phalloidin for 2 h at room temperature. Finally, the slides were mounted with medium containing DAPI.

Luciferase Reporter Assay

For the luciferase reporter assay, MRC5 cells were cotransfected with TOP Flash or FOP Flash luciferase reporter. At 48 h post-transfection, the cells were collected and lysed with lysis buffer. The internal control used was pTK-Renilla. Firefly luciferase and Renilla luciferase activities were quantified using the dual-luciferase reporter assay system according to the manufacturer's instructions (Promega, Madison, WI).

Statistical Analysis

Statistical significance was calculated using GraphPad Prism 6 software. Data are representative and/or the mean ± SEM of 3 assays. An unpaired two-sided Student's t test was used to compare two groups, and one-way ANOVA was used to compare multiple groups unless otherwise indicated. Correlations between groups were determined by Pearson's correlation test. All experiments were conducted with at least 3 biological replicates. In all cases, $p < 0.05$ was considered statistically significant.

RESULTS

TRAF6 Expression Was Downregulated in Lung Fibroblasts From PF Mice and TRAF6 Overexpression Protected Mice Against BLM-Induced PF

To address the role of TRAF6 in PF, we first examined TRAF6 expression in the lungs of mice following BLM-induced PF. Western blot analysis showed decreased TRAF6 protein levels in the lungs of PF mice compared to those of controls (**Figure 1A**). Moreover,

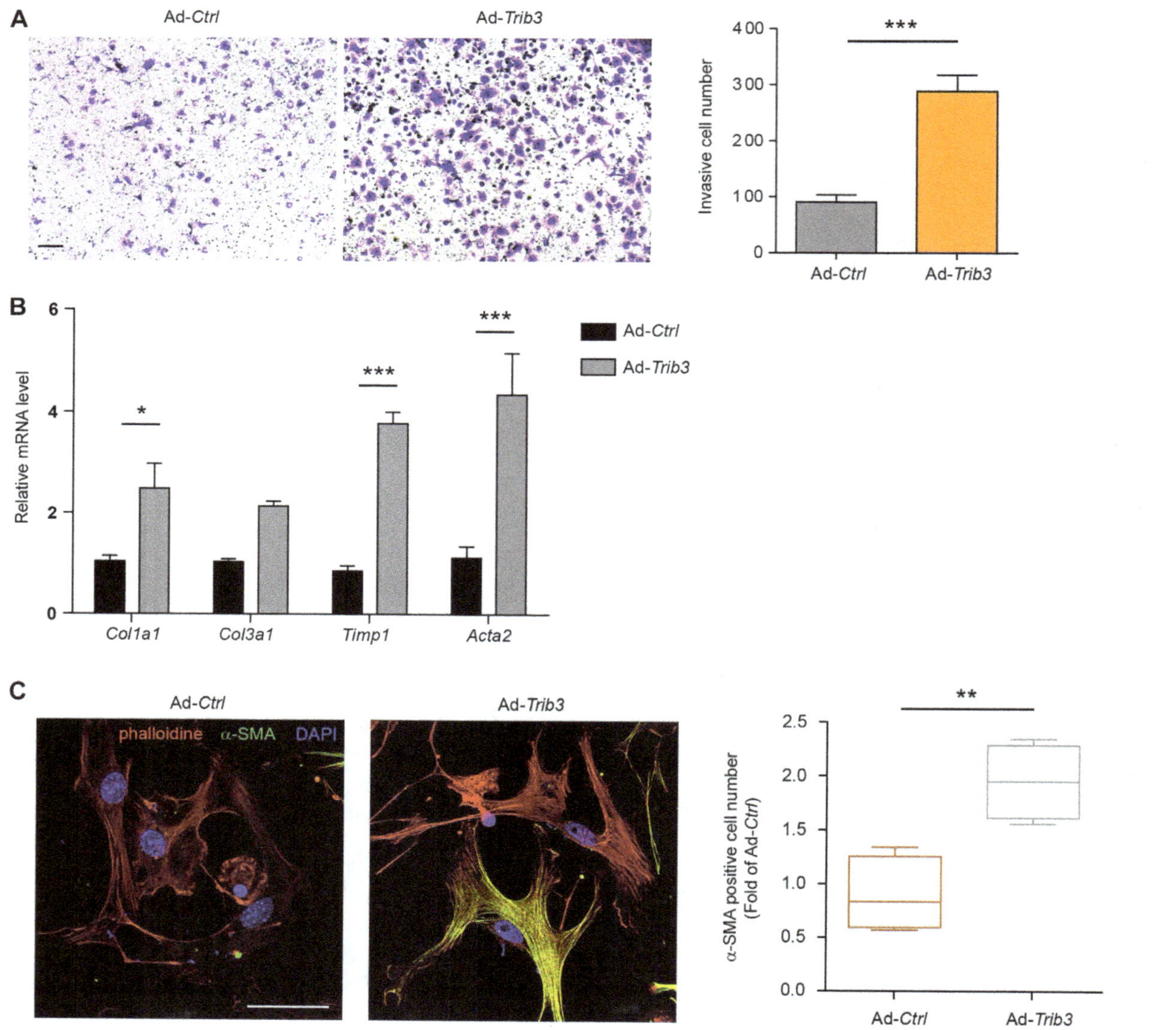

FIGURE 6 | Overexpression of TRIB3 activates lung fibroblasts. **(A)** Representative images and quantification of the invasion experiment results for mouse lung fibroblasts with or without TRIB3 overexpression. Scale bars, 100 μm. **(B)** mRNA expression of fibrosis genes in mouse lung fibroblasts with or without TRIB3 overexpression. **(C)** Representative images and quantification of α-SMA immunostaining in mouse lung fibroblasts with or without TRIB3 overexpression. Scale bars, 50 μm. Data are representative of 3 independent experiments. Data represent means ± SEM Statistical significance: *$p < 0.05$, **$p < 0.01$ or ***$p < 0.001$.

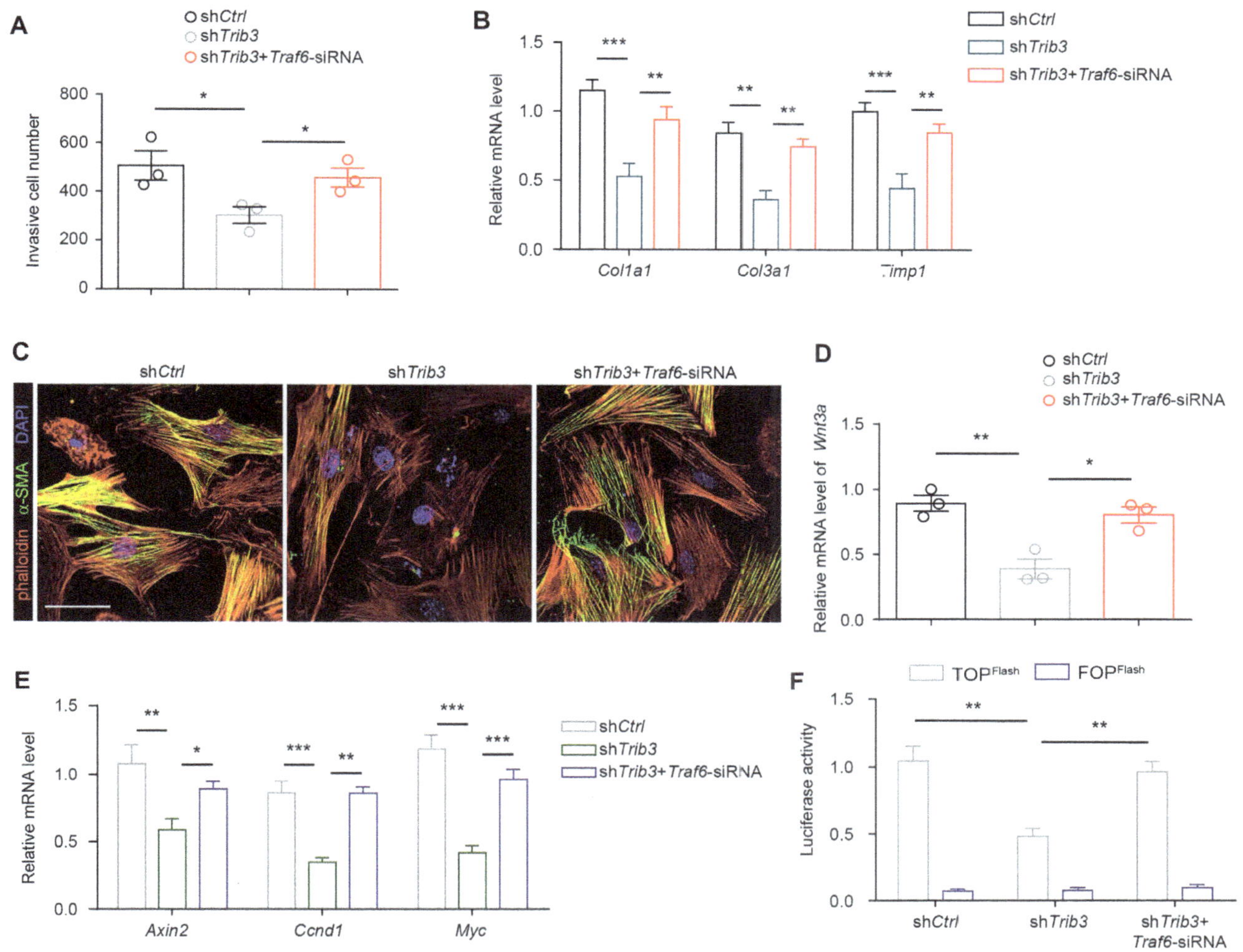

FIGURE 7 | TRIB3 activates lung fibroblasts by reducing TRAF6 expression. **(A)** Transwell assay for the evaluation of invasion of TRIB3-silenced PF lung fibroblasts with or without TRAF6 knockdown. **(B)** mRNA expression of fibrosis genes in TRIB3-silenced PF lung fibroblasts with or without TRAF6 knockdown. **(C)** Representative images of α-SMA immunostaining in TRIB3-silenced PF lung fibroblasts with or without TRAF6 knockdown. Scale bars, 50 μm. **(D)** mRNA expression of *Wnt3a* in TRIB3-silenced PF lung fibroblasts with or without TRAF6 knockdown. **(E)** mRNA expression of the β-catenin target genes in TRIB3-silenced PF lung fibroblasts with or without TRAF6 knockdown. **(F)** Wnt-reporter luciferase activity in TRIB3-silenced PF lung fibroblasts with or without TRAF6 knockdown. Data are representative of 3 independent experiments. Data represent means ± SEM Statistical significance: $^*p < 0.05$, $^{**}p < 0.01$ or $^{***}p < 0.001$.

decreased TRAF6 in PF lungs was associated with reduced pulmonary function (**Figure 1B**). The protein expression of TRAF6 was negatively correlated with the mRNA expression of *Acta2* (a marker of myofibroblasts) in fibrotic lungs (**Figure 1C**). These results prompted us to detect TRAF6 expression in lung fibroblasts, the effector cells in PF progression. Indeed, lower expression of TRAF6 was observed in lung fibroblasts from PF mice than in those from controls (**Figure 1D**). These findings demonstrate that TRAF6 in lung fibroblasts is negatively correlated with PF development.

To further confirm whether TRAF6 loss contributes to PF development *in vivo*, we instilled TRAF6-overexpressing lentivirus into lung tissue 10 days after BLM challenge. Overexpression of TRAF6 in lung tissue reduced BLM-induced PF changes, as revealed by the reduction in collagen deposition (**Figure 1E**), the improvement in lung function (**Figure 1F**), and the decreased hydroxyproline levels (an indicator of collagen content) in BLM mice (**Figure 1G**). Thus, TRAF6 may play an indispensable protective role in the progression of PF.

TRAF6 Overexpression Attenuates the Activation of Lung Fibroblasts From PF Mice

We next explored the functional relevance of TRAF6 in fibroblasts during PF progression. IHC staining showed that the expression of α-SMA was reduced in lung tissues from BLM-challenged mice under conditions of TRAF6 overexpression (**Figure 2A**), suggesting that TRAF6 overexpression suppressed fibroblast activation. To confirm

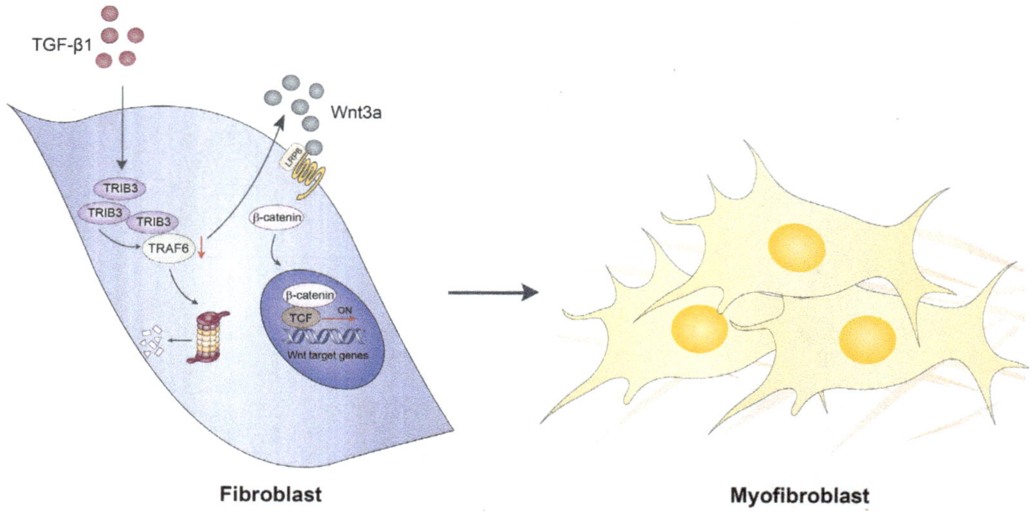

FIGURE 8 | Schematic diagram showing possible mechanisms by which TRAF6 involves in the development of pulmonary fibrosis.

this observation, primary mouse lung fibroblasts isolated from PF mice were transfected with a TRAF6-overexpressing adenovirus. PCR analysis revealed that the expression levels of several fibrosis-related genes and ECM proteins, including *Col1a1*, *Col3a1*, and *Timp1*, were reduced in fibroblasts overexpressing TRAF6 (**Figure 2B**). The matrigel invasion assay showed that the overexpression of TRAF6 decreased the invasive capacity of lung fibroblasts from PF mice (**Figure 2C**). In addition, the induction of TRAF6 overexpression in lung fibroblasts derived from PF mice decreased the percentages of α-SMA-positive cells (**Figure 2D**). Collectively, our data suggest that TRAF6 overexpression reverses the activation of myofibroblasts from PF mice and that TRAF6 deficiency during PF progression promotes the differentiation of lung fibroblasts into myofibroblasts.

TRAF6 Overexpression Decreases Wnt3a Expression

We explored how TRAF6 regulates the activation of lung fibroblasts. A previous study reported that TRAF6 overexpression in cardiac stem cells induced the downregulation of Wnt3a (Cao et al., 2015), which has been implicated in the pathogenesis of PF. We found that the overexpression of TRAF6 in lung fibroblasts from PF mice reduced the mRNA level of *Wnt3a* and that the depletion of TRAF6 in lung fibroblasts from control mice increased the mRNA level of *Wnt3a* (**Figures 3A,B**). TRAF6 depletion enhanced Wnt-reporter luciferase activity in PF lung fibroblasts (**Figure 3C**). In addition, western blot analysis demonstrated elevated expression of Wnt/β-catenin target genes in lung fibroblasts with TRAF6 depletion (**Figure 3D**). Moreover, the protein expression of TRAF6 was negatively correlated with the mRNA expression of *Wnt3a* in fibroblasts from PBS- and BLM-challenged mice (**Figure 3E**). The decreased expression of fibrosis-related genes caused by TRAF6 overexpression was reversed in lung fibroblasts treated with Wnt3a (**Figure 3F**). Furthermore, stimulation of lung fibroblasts with Wnt3a enhanced the invasive capacity that was suppressed by TRAF6 overexpression (**Figure 3G**). These data suggest that TRAF6 regulates fibroblast activation via Wnt3a.

TRIB3 Is Responsible for the Reduced Expression of TRAF6

We further investigated why TRAF6 expression is downregulated in fibroblasts during PF progression. PCR results showed that *Traf6* mRNA expression was comparable in lung fibroblasts from vehicle- and BLM-challenged mice (**Figure 4A**). We further analyzed TRAF6 gene expression in lung fibroblasts from IPF patients and healthy controls using a public microarray dataset (GSE129164). No difference in *TRAF6* mRNA expression was found between lung fibroblasts from IPF patients and healthy controls (**Figure 4B**). These data indicated that the decreased protein expression of TRAF6 in lung fibroblasts during PF progression might result from an alteration in its protein stability. Our group, along with others, has reported that TRIB3, a well-known stress sensor, is involved in regulating the stability of various proteins in the pathogenesis of chronic diseases (Lin et al., 2019; Yu J. M. et al., 2019; Liu S. et al., 2021). We then reasoned that TRIB3 might participate in regulating the altered protein expression of TRAF6. Indeed, an interaction between exogenous TRIB3 and TRAF6 was observed in HEK293T cells, and this was confirmed by the colocalization of TRIB3 and TRAF6 in primary mouse lung fibroblasts (**Figures 4C,D**). To map the interaction regions of TRAF6 and TRIB3, coIP assays were carried out using serial deletion mutants of either Myc-tagged TRAF6 or HA-tagged TRIB3. TRIB3 interacted with the ΔC domain but not with the ΔN domain of TRAF6 (**Supplementary Figure S1A**), and TRAF6 interacted with the KD and ΔN domains of TRIB3 (**Supplementary Figure S1B**). These data indicate that the ΔC domain of TRAF6 and the KD and ΔN domains of TRIB3 are required for the interaction between TRAF6 and TRIB3.

Overexpression of TRIB3 decreased the protein level of TRAF6, and depletion of TRIB3 increased the protein level of TRAF6 (**Figures 4E,F**). Moreover, the expression of TRAF6 was positively correlated with that of TRIB3 in lung fibroblasts from PBS- and BLM-challenged mice (**Figure 4G**). Indeed, the overexpression of TRIB3 reduced the half-life of TRAF6 (**Figure 4H**). Intracellular proteins are degraded by lysosomal autophagy pathways or the ubiquitin–proteasome system (UPS). We found that the UPS inhibitor MG132, but not the autophagy inhibitor 3-MA, reversed the TRIB3 overexpression-induced reduction in TRAF6 expression (**Figure 4I**). Furthermore, the overexpression and depletion of TRIB3 increased and blocked the ubiquitination of TRAF6, respectively (**Figures 4J,K**). These data indicate that the protein expression of TRAF6 can be regulated by TRIB3.

We then detected the expression of TRIB3 in lung fibroblasts during PF progression. TRIB3 exhibited markedly higher protein and mRNA expression levels in lung fibroblasts from PF mice than in those from control mice (**Figures 5A,B**). Based on the reanalysis of a published dataset (GSE129164), we found that stimulation of lung fibroblasts of IPF patients and normal controls with TGF-β1 (the principal profibrotic cytokines in lung fibrosis) increased *TRIB3* mRNA expression (**Figure 5C**). Another dataset also revealed higher *TRIB3* mRNA levels in human lung fibroblasts treated with TGF-β1 than in untreated cells (**Figure 5D**). Collectively, these data indicate that the enhanced expression of TRIB3 in lung fibroblasts results in a reduction in TRAF6 expression by promoting its ubiquitination and subsequent degradation.

TRAF6 Is Required for the Role of TRIB3 in Regulating Fibroblast Activation

Since the reduction in TRAF6 expression caused by TRIB3 contributes to the differentiation of fibroblasts to myofibroblasts, the above data prompted us to analyze the role of TRIB3 in regulating fibroblast activation. TRIB3 overexpression enhanced the invasive capacity of primary mouse lung fibroblasts (**Figure 6A**). Much higher levels of fibrosis-related genes were detected in TRIB3-overexpressing fibroblasts than in control fibroblasts (**Figure 6B**). Immunostaining analysis also indicated that TRIB3 overexpression in lung fibroblasts significantly increased the number of α-SMA-positive cells (**Figure 6C**), suggesting that TRIB3 induced the differentiation of fibroblasts into myofibroblasts. Consistently, we found that TRIB3 deficiency reversed the activation of myofibroblasts, as indicated by decreased invasive capacity, reduced expression of fibrosis-related genes, and fewer α-SMA-positive cells (**Figures 7A–C**). However, depletion of TRIB3 failed to inhibit the activation of TRAF6-silenced fibroblasts (**Figures 7A–C**). In addition, TRIB3 knockdown decreased the expression of *Wnt3a* and Wnt/β-catenin target genes in wild-type PF lung fibroblasts but not in fibroblasts with TRAF6 depletion (**Figures 7D,E**). Furthermore, TRIB3 depletion failed to reduce Wnt-reporter luciferase activity in lung fibroblasts with TRIB3 knockdown (**Figure 7F**). These results collectively demonstrate a TRIB3-TRAF6-Wnt3a signaling axis in regulating fibroblast activation.

DISCUSSION

TRAF6, a member of the TRAF family, plays a crucial role in immune signal transduction by acting as an adaptor protein downstream of multiple receptor families, including the interleukin-1 receptor (IL-1R) superfamily, the Toll-like receptor (TLR) family, and the TNFR superfamily. In recent years, TRAF6 has been extensively investigated in tumors, immunity, neurodegenerative diseases, ischemic stroke and osteoporosis (Li et al., 2017; Dou et al., 2018; Muto et al., 2022). Recent studies have also reported that TRAF6 is involved in the pathogenesis of NASH (Wang et al., 2020). They found that depletion of TRAF6 attenuated liver fibrosis in diet-induced NASH models, supporting a role for TRAF6 in promoting liver fibrosis. However, the role of TRAF6 in lung fibrosis remains unknown. In this study, we found that TRAF6 was downregulated in fibroblasts within the lung during the course of fibrotic processes. TRAF6 overexpression in fibroblasts from PF mice suppressed the activation of these cells. Furthermore, TRAF6 overexpression protected mice from BLM-induced lung fibrosis, with a decrease in the number of activated fibroblasts, also called myofibroblasts. Our data indicate that the downregulation of TRAF6 expression in fibroblasts contributes to PF progression by inducing the activation of those cells (**Figure 8**). This study selectively focused on the role of TRAF6 in fibroblasts. Given that TRAF6 is an intracellular protein widely expressed in epithelial cells, endothelial cells, and macrophages, future studies are needed to investigate the expression and role of TRAF6 in those cells during pulmonary fibrosis.

TRIB3, a stress sensor, is involved in the pathogenesis of various diseases, including obesity, diabetes, and tumors (Du et al., 2003; Oberkofler et al., 2010; Lin et al., 2019). Accumulating evidence has widely demonstrated that TRIB3 plays a vital role in organ fibrogenesis (Wang et al., 2014; Tomcik et al., 2016; Zhang et al., 2020). Our previous study, along with others, reported the key role of TRIB3 in promoting PF (Yu W. et al., 2019; Liu S. et al., 2021). We found that TRIB3 was substantially upregulated in alveolar macrophages (AMs) from patients with PF, inducing the profibrotic phenotype of AMs. Moreover, genetic knockout of TRIB3 specifically in AMs suppressed BLM-induced fibrotic changes in the lung. Another study found a central regulatory role of TRIB3 in fibroblast activation by stimulating canonical TGF-β1/Smad signaling in systemic sclerosis (Tomcik et al., 2016). Here, we found that elevated TRIB3 expression in fibroblasts from PF mice contributes to PF progression by enhancing the expression of Wnt3a, a crucial factor in the regulation of fibroblast activation (Li X. et al., 2020; Liu T. et al., 2021). Collectively, these data support that TRIB3 exerts profibrotic roles in different cell types during PF progression, demonstrating its potential value in the clinical treatment of PF.

As a member of the pseudokinase family, TRIB3 was found to regulate diverse processes in the progression of various diseases by interacting with functional proteins. For instance, the interaction of TRIB3 and the protein kinase GSK-3β interferes with the binding of GSK-3β to the E3 ligase UHRF1, thereby inhibiting the degradation of GSK-3β and leading to the profibrotic phenotype of Ams (Liu S. et al., 2021). TRIB3 interacted with MYC to suppress E3 ubiquitin ligase UBE3B-mediated MYC degradation, which induced the enhanced expression of MYC, causing the proliferation of lymphoma cells (Li K. et al., 2020). In the current study, the interaction of TRIB3 with TRAF6 in fibroblasts resulted in reduced TRAF6 expression. Intracellular proteins are degraded by the UPS or lysosomal autophagy pathway. We found that the UPS inhibitor MG132, but not the autophagy inhibitor 3-MA, reversed the TRIB3 overexpression-induced reduction in TRAF6 expression, indicating that the decrease in the protein level of TRAF6 caused by TRIB3 was related to its increased degradation through the UPS. This was consistent with previous studies showing that TRAF6 is degraded via the UPS (Li et al., 2014; Kim et al., 2017). Indeed, we observed increased ubiquitination and degradation of TRAF6 in TRIB3-overexpressing cells. We presumed that TRIB3, acting as a scaffolding protein, interacts with TRAF6 to recruit certain E3 ligases, thereby causing the ubiquitination and subsequent degradation of TRAF6. Obviously, further investigation of which kind of E3 ligase accounts for TRIB3 regulation of TRAF6 expression is warranted.

Increasing lines of evidence demonstrate that the aberrant activation of Wnt signaling is involved in the pathogenesis of PF (Morrisey, 2003; Skronska-Wasek et al., 2018). Attenuation of Wnt/β-catenin signaling can limit the development of fibrosis in mice. Wnt3a, the canonical ligand, is known to induce the activation of fibroblasts to myofibroblasts (Li X. et al., 2020). We found that depletion of TRAF6 in lung fibroblasts from control mice increased the expression of Wnt3a and Wnt/β-catenin target genes. A negative correlation was found between the expression of TRAF6 and Wnt3a in fibroblasts from PBS- and BLM-challenged mice. This was consistent with a prior study showing that TRAF6 overexpression induced the downregulation of Wnt3a in c-kit$^+$ cardiac stem cells. We also found that Wnt3a treatment reversed the suppressed activation of fibroblasts caused by TRAF6 overexpression. These results indicated that reduced expression of TRAF6 in lung fibroblasts induces the activation of fibroblasts by enhancing the expression of Wnt3a during PF progression. Thus, our work provides insight into the regulatory role of TRAF6 in Wnt3a expression in fibroblasts. Further investigation is necessary to determine the molecular mechanism by which TRAF6 controls Wnt3a expression.

Our findings revealed that the reduced expression of TRAF6 caused by TRIB3 overexpression in lung fibroblasts contributes to the progression of PF through upregulation of Wnt3a expression, which drives fibroblast differentiation into myofibroblasts. Accordingly, genetically enhancing TRAF6 expression or inhibiting the TRIB3-TRAF6 interaction may represent a novel therapeutic strategy for PF and other fibroproliferative lung diseases.

AUTHOR CONTRIBUTIONS

SL conceived the study. SL and JM designed the experiments. JM, QL, and MY performed the experiments. SL, QW, and YZ analyzed the data. BC and JY provided valuable suggestions and comments on the study design. JM and SL wrote and edited the manuscript.

REFERENCES

Cao, Q., Wang, Y., Huang, L., Wang, F., and Chen, S. (2015). TNF Receptor-Associated Factor 6 (TRAF6) Mediates the Angiotensin-Induced Non-canonical TGF-β Pathway Activation of C-Kit(+) Cardiac Stem Cells. *Am. J. Transl. Res.* 7 (11), 2233–43.

Cao, Z., Xiong, J., Takeuchi, M., Kurama, T., and Goeddel, D. V. (1996). TRAF6 Is a Signal Transducer for Interleukin-1. *Nature* 383 (6599), 443–446. doi:10.1038/383443a0

Dou, Y., Tian, X., Zhang, J., Wang, Z., and Chen, G. (2018). Roles of TRAF6 in Central Nervous System. *Curr. Neuropharmacol.* 16 (9), 1306–1313. doi:10.2174/1570159X16666180412094655

Du, K., Herzig, S., Kulkarni, R. N., and Montminy, M. (2003). TRB3: a Tribbles Homolog that Inhibits Akt/PKB Activation by Insulin in Liver. *Science* 300 (5625), 1574–1577. doi:10.1126/science.1079817

Frangogiannis, N. (2020). Transforming Growth Factor-β in Tissue Fibrosis. *J. Exp. Med.* 217 (3), e20190103. doi:10.1084/jem.20190103

George, P. M., Spagnolo, P., Kreuter, M., Altinisik, G., Bonifazi, M., Martinez, F. J., et al. (2020). Progressive Fibrosing Interstitial Lung Disease: Clinical Uncertainties, Consensus Recommendations, and Research Priorities. *Lancet Respir. Med.* 8 (9), 925–934. doi:10.1016/S2213-2600(20)30355-6

Hinz, B., and Lagares, D. (2020). Evasion of Apoptosis by Myofibroblasts: a Hallmark of Fibrotic Diseases. *Nat. Rev. Rheumatol.* 16 (1), 11–31. doi:10.1038/s41584-019-0324-5

Kim, E., Beon, J., Lee, S., Park, S. J., Ahn, H., Kim, M. G., et al. (2017). Inositol Polyphosphate Multikinase Promotes Toll-like Receptor-Induced Promotion of Tumor Necrosis Factor Receptor-Associated Factor 6 Protein Degradation. *Arthritis Rheumatol.* 66 (7), 1854–1863. doi:10.1002/art.38521

Li, T., Qin, J. J., Yang, X., Ji, Y. X., Guo, F., Cheng, W. L., et al. (2017). The Ubiquitin E3 Ligase TRAF6 Exacerbates Ischemic Stroke by Ubiquitinating and Activating Rac1. *J. Neurosci.* 37 (50), 12123–12140. doi:10.1523/JNEUROSCI.1751-17.2017

Li, X., Liu, X., Deng, R., Gao, S., Yu, H., Huang, K., et al. (2020). Nintedanib Inhibits Wnt3a-Induced Myofibroblast Activation by Suppressing the Src/β-Catenin Pathway. *Front. Pharmacol.* 11, 310. doi:10.3389/fphar.2020.00310

Lin, J., Zhang, W., Niu, L. T., Zhu, Y. M., Weng, X. Q., Sheng, Y., et al. (2019). TRIB3 Stabilizes High TWIST1 Expression to Promote Rapid APL Progression and ATRA Resistance. *Clin. Cancer Res.* 25 (20), 6228–6242. doi:10.1158/1078-0432.CCR-19-0510

Liu, G., Philp, A. M., Corte, T., Travis, M. A., Schilter, H., Hansbro, N. G., et al. (2021). Therapeutic Targets in Lung Tissue Remodelling and Fibrosis. *Pharmacol. Ther.* 225, 107839. doi:10.1016/j.pharmthera.2021.107839

Liu, S., Lv, X., Wei, X., Liu, C., Li, Q., Min, J., et al. (2021). TRIB3–GSK-3β Interaction Promotes Lung Fibrosis and Serves as a Potential Therapeutic Target. *Acta Pharm. Sin. B* 11 (10), 3105–3119. doi:10.1016/j.apsb.2021.06.017

Liu, S. S., Liu, C., Lv, X. X., Cui, B., Yan, J., Li, Y. X., et al. (2021). The Chemokine CCL1 Triggers an AMFR-SPRY1 Pathway that Promotes Differentiation of Lung Fibroblasts into Myofibroblasts and Drives Pulmonary Fibrosis. *Immunity* 54 (9), 2042–2048. doi:10.1016/j.immuni.2021.06.008

Liu, S. S., Lv, X. X., Liu, C., Qi, J., Li, Y. X., Wei, X. P., et al. (2019). Targeting Degradation of the Transcription Factor C/EBPβ Reduces Lung Fibrosis by

Restoring Activity of the Ubiquitin-Editing Enzyme A20 in Macrophages. *Immunity* 51 (3), 522–e7. e527. doi:10.1016/j.immuni.2019.06.014

Liu, T., Gonzalez De Los Santos, F., Hirsch, M., Wu, Z., and Phan, S. H. (2021). Noncanonical Wnt Signaling Promotes Myofibroblast Differentiation in Pulmonary Fibrosis. *Am. J. Respir. Cell Mol. Biol.* 65 (5), 489–499. doi:10.1165/rcmb.2020-0499OC

Lo Re, S., Lecocq, M., Uwambayinema, F., Yakoub, Y., Delos, M., Demoulin, J. B., et al. (2011). Platelet-derived Growth Factor-Producing CD4+ Foxp3+ Regulatory T Lymphocytes Promote Lung Fibrosis. *Am. J. Respir. Crit. Care Med.* 184 (11), 1270–1281. doi:10.1164/rccm.201103-0516OC

Morrisey, E. E. (2003). Wnt Signaling and Pulmonary Fibrosis. *Am. J. Pathol.* 162 (5), 1393–1397. doi:10.1016/S0002-9440(10)64271-X

Muto, T., Guillamot, M., Yeung, J., Fang, J., Bennett, J., Nadorp, B., et al. (2022). TRAF6 Functions as a Tumor Suppressor in Myeloid Malignancies by Directly Targeting MYC Oncogenic Activity. *Cell Stem Cell* 29 (2), 298–e9. doi:10.1016/j.stem.2021.12.007

Naito, A., Azuma, S., Tanaka, S., Miyazaki, T., Takaki, S., Takatsu, K., et al. (1999). Severe Osteopetrosis, Defective Interleukin-1 Signalling and Lymph Node Organogenesis in TRAF6-Deficient Mice. *Genes Cells* 4 (6), 353–362. doi:10.1046/j.1365-2443.1999.00265.x

Oberkofler, H., Pfeifenberger, A., Soyal, S., Felder, T., Hahne, P., Miller, K., et al. (2010). Aberrant Hepatic TRIB3 Gene Expression in Insulin-Resistant Obese Humans. *Diabetologia* 53 (9), 1971–1975. doi:10.1007/s00125-010-1772-2

Sgalla, G., Kulkarni, T., Antin-Ozerkis, D., Thannickal, V. J., and Richeldi, L. (2019). Update in Pulmonary Fibrosis 2018. *Am. J. Respir. Crit. Care Med.* 200 (3), 292–300. doi:10.1164/rccm.201903-0542UP

Skronska-Wasek, W., Gosens, R., Konigshoff, M., and Baarsma, H. A. (2018). WNT Receptor Signalling in Lung Physiology and Pathology. *Pharmacol. Ther.* 187, 150–166. doi:10.1016/j.pharmthera.2018.02.009

Tomcik, M., Palumbo-Zerr, K., Zerr, P., Sumova, B., Avouac, J., Dees, C., et al. (2016). Tribbles Homologue 3 Stimulates Canonical TGF-β Signalling to Regulate Fibroblast Activation and Tissue Fibrosis. *Ann. Rheum. Dis.* 75 (3), 609–616. doi:10.1136/annrheumdis-2014-206234

Walsh, M. C., Lee, J., and Choi, Y. (2015). Tumor Necrosis Factor Receptor-Associated Factor 6 (TRAF6) Regulation of Development, Function, and Homeostasis of the Immune System. *Immunol. Rev.* 266 (1), 72–92. doi:10.1111/imr.12302

Wang, W., Sun, A., Lv, W., Cheng, J., Lv, S., Liu, X., et al. (2014). TRB3, Up-Regulated in Kidneys of Rats with Type1 Diabetes, Mediates Extracellular Matrix Accumulation *In Vivo* and *In Vitro*. *Diabetes Res. Clin. Pract.* 106 (1), 101–109. doi:10.1016/j.diabres.2014.07.015

Wang, Y., Wen, H., Fu, J., Cai, L., Li, P. L., Zhao, C. L., et al. (2020). Hepatocyte TNF Receptor-Associated Factor 6 Aggravates Hepatic Inflammation and Fibrosis by Promoting Lysine 6-Linked Polyubiquitination of Apoptosis Signal-Regulating Kinase 1. *Hepatology* 71 (1), 93–111. doi:10.1002/hep.30822

Wu, H., and Arron, J. R. (2003). TRAF6, a Molecular Bridge Spanning Adaptive Immunity, Innate Immunity and Osteoimmunology. *Bioessays* 25 (11), 1096–1105. doi:10.1002/bies.10352

Yang, W. L., Wang, J., Chan, C. H., Lee, S. W., Campos, A. D., Lamothe, B., et al. (2009). The E3 Ligase TRAF6 Regulates Akt Ubiquitination and Activation. *Science* 325 (5944), 1134–1138. doi:10.1126/science.1175065

Yu, J. M., Sun, W., Wang, Z. H., Liang, X., Hua, F., Li, K., et al. (2019). TRIB3 Supports Breast Cancer Stemness by Suppressing FOXO1 Degradation and Enhancing SOX2 Transcription. *Nat. Commun.* 10 (1), 5720. doi:10.1038/s41467-019-13700-6

Yu, W., Song, X., and Liu, Y. (2019). TRB3 Regulates Pulmonary Interstitial Fibrosis through the MAPK Signaling Pathway. *Int. J. Clin. Exp. Pathol.* 12 (9), 3247–3257.

Zhang, J. L., Du, B. B., Zhang, D. H., Li, H., Kong, L. Y., Fan, G. J., et al. (2021). OTUB1 Alleviates NASH through Inhibition of the TRAF6-ASK1 Signaling Pathways. *Hepatology* 75, 1218–1234. doi:10.1002/hep.32179

Zhang, X. W., Zhou, J. C., Peng, D., Hua, F., Li, K., Yu, J. J., et al. (2020). Disrupting the TRIB3-SQSTM1 Interaction Reduces Liver Fibrosis by Restoring Autophagy and Suppressing Exosome-Mediated HSC Activation. *Autophagy* 16 (5), 782–796. doi:10.1080/15548627.2019.1635383

18

Identification of Hub Genes and Pathways Associated with Idiopathic Pulmonary Fibrosis *via* Bioinformatics Analysis

Hanxi Wan [1,2†], Xinwei Huang [2†], Peilin Cong [1,2], Mengfan He [1,2], Aiwen Chen [2], Tingmei Wu [1,2], Danqing Dai [1,2], Wanrong Li [1,2], Xiaofei Gao [1,2], Li Tian [1,2,3], Huazheng Liang [1,2] and Lize Xiong [1,2,3]**

[1]Department of Anesthesiology and Perioperative Medicine, School of Medcine, Shanghai Fourth People's Hospital, Tongji University, Shanghai, China, [2]Translational Research Institute of Brain and Brain-Like Intelligence, School of Medcine, Shanghai Fourth People's Hospital, Tongji University, Shanghai, China, [3]Clinical Research Center for Anesthesiology and Perioperative Medicine, Tongji University, Shanghai, China

***Correspondence:**
Lize Xiong
mzkxlz@126.com
Huazheng Liang
andyliang2018@126.com

†These authors have contributed equally to this work

Idiopathic pulmonary fibrosis (IPF) is a progressive disease whose etiology remains unknown. The purpose of this study was to explore hub genes and pathways related to IPF development and prognosis. Multiple gene expression datasets were downloaded from the Gene Expression Omnibus database. Weighted correlation network analysis (WGCNA) was performed and differentially expressed genes (DEGs) identified to investigate Hub modules and genes correlated with IPF. Gene Ontology (GO), Kyoto Encyclopedia of Genes and Genomes (KEGG) enrichment analysis, and protein-protein interaction (PPI) network analysis were performed on selected key genes. In the PPI network and cytoHubba plugin, 11 hub genes were identified, including ASPN, CDH2, COL1A1, COL1A2, COL3A1, COL14A1, CTSK, MMP1, MMP7, POSTN, and SPP1. Correlation between hub genes was displayed and validated. Expression levels of hub genes were verified using quantitative real-time PCR (qRT-PCR). Dysregulated expression of these genes and their crosstalk might impact the development of IPF through modulating IPF-related biological processes and signaling pathways. Among these genes, expression levels of COL1A1, COL3A1, CTSK, MMP1, MMP7, POSTN, and SPP1 were positively correlated with IPF prognosis. The present study provides further insights into individualized treatment and prognosis for IPF.

Keywords: idiopathic pulmonary fibrosiss, differentially expressed gene, hub genes, bioinformatics, WGCNA (weighted gene Co-expression network analyses), PPI

INTRODUCTION

Idiopathic pulmonary fibrosis (IPF), a chronic and progressive lung disease of unknown etiology (King et al., 2014; Martinez et al., 2017; Raghu et al., 2018), is characterized by diffuse alveolar inflammation and alveolar structural damage (Xu et al., 2016; Claude and Harold, 2018; David et al., 2019). The global annual incidence of IPF is 0.2–93.7 per 100,000 (Hutchinson et al., 2015) and the median survival time is only 2–3 years after diagnosis is confirmed (Tran and Suissa, 2018; Schäfer et al., 2020). Clinical biomarkers reliably reflecting the progression of IPF are small in number. In terms of treatment, medications recommended by current clinical guidelines - nintedanib and pirfenidone have a good therapeutic effect on IPF in general (Maher et al., 2019; Saito et al., 2019;

TABLE 1 | The main features of 7 selected datasets included in this analysis.

GEO datasets	Platform	Sample size		Publication years	Regions
		IPF	Normal		
GSE110147	GPL6244	22	11	2018	London
GSE53845	GPL6480	40	8	2014	South San Francisco
GSE24206	GPL570	11	6	2011	Durham
GSE32537	GPL6244	119	50	2013	Aurora
GSE68239	GPL1708	10	10	2017	Giessen
GSE10667	GPL153	23	15	2003	Bern
GSE70866	GPL17077	112	20	2018	Hannover

Behr et al., 2021), but not that effective for late stage IPF. Therefore, it is important to illuminate the pathogenesis of IPF and to explore potential biomarkers for early stage IPF in order to improve the therapeutic effect on IPF.

In recent years, the amount of biological data for research has dramatically increased with the development of transcriptomic analysis, providing new viewpoints for exploring the etiology, pathogenesis, and novel targets for clinical treatment (DePianto et al., 2015; Wang et al., 2017). Previous studies primarily tested individual genes in diseased conditions. However, genes with similar expression patterns are likely to be tightly co-regulated *in vivo* with closely related functions, expressed in the same signaling pathways or processes (Pei et al., 2017). Identifying these genes and their interactions will provide further understanding of biological pathways related to IPF.

In the present study, multiple bioinformatic methods were used to search for hub genes significantly correlated with the occurrence and prognosis of IPF. Their expression has also been validated using quantitative real-time PCR (qRT-PCR). This work will provide further insights into the underlying molecular mechanisms of IPF and potential molecular targets for developing novel interventional strategies.

MATERIALS AND METHODS

Acquisition of Microarray Data

In this study, seven gene array expression Series Matrix Files of IPF containing GSE110147, GSE53845, GSE24206, GSE32537, GSE68239, GSE10667, and GSE70866 were obtained from the Gene Expression Omnibus (GEO) repository (https://www.ncbi.nlm.nih.gov/geo/). The main features of these 7 datasets were shown in **Table 1**. These profiles consisted of gene expression matrices, probe sets, and clinical characteristics. Subsequent analyses were conducted on these datasets.

Removal of the Batch Effect

All of the raw data of GSE110147, GSE53845, GSE24206, GSE32537, and GSE68239 were merged and normalized into the training group using the RMA algorithm provided by the Limma package 3.40.6 of R, followed by removing the batch effect using R package SVA. The principal component analysis (PCA) was used to estimate whether the batch effect was removed. The validation group consisted of data from GSE10667 and GSE70866.

Identification of Significant Modules Using the Weighted Correlation Network Analysis

The WGCNA package was used to determine key genes significantly associated with IPF in the training and validation groups. The best soft threshold power was set to identify the module-trait relationship, module membership (MM), and gene significance (GS). In brief, a weighted adjacency matrix was first constructed based on the selected soft threshold power. Subsequently, the connectivity per gene was deduced through calculating connection strengths with other genes. After validating the module structure preservation using the module preservation R function, the gene expression profile of each module was summarized by the module eigengene on whom IPF traits were regressed in the Limma R package (Huang et al., 2020). The IPF-related module was selected with the highest coefficient square (r^2) and the p value <0.001.

TABLE 2 | Real-time PCR primers.

Gene		Primer
GAPDH	F	AGGTCGGTGTGAACGGATTTG
GAPDH	R	TGTAGACCATGTAGTTGAGGTCA
COL1A1	F	GCTCCTCTTAGGGGCCACT
COL1A1	R	CCACGTCTCACCATTGGGG
COL1A2	F	GTAACTTCGTGCCTAGCAACA
COL1A2	R	CCTTTGTCAGAATACTGAGCAGC
COL3A1	F	CCTGGCTCAAATGGCTCAC
COL3A1	R	CAGGACTGCCGTTATTCCCG
COL14A1	F	TTTGGCGGCTGCTTGTTTC
COL14A1	R	CGCTTTTGTTGCAGTGTTCTG
COL15A1	F	GCGGAGTCGGGTTTCAGAG
COL15A1	R	TACTTCGCCCGCAGAACAAA
MMP1	F	GGACAAGCAGTTCCAAAGGC
MMP1	R	GATGCTTAGGGTTGGGGTCT
MMP7	F	CTGCCACTGTCCCAGGAAG
MMP7	R	GGGAGAGTTTTCCAGTCATGG
CTSK	F	GAAGAAGACTCACCAGAAGCAG
CTSK	R	TCCAGGTTATGGGCAGAGATT
CDH2	F	AGCGCAGTCTTACCGAAGG
CDH2	R	TCGCTGCTTTCATACTGAACTTT
ASPN	F	AAGGAGTATGTGATGCTACTGCT
ASPN	R	ACATTGGCACCCAAATGGACA
POSTN	F	CCTGCCCTTATATGCTCTGCT
POSTN	R	AAACATGGTCAATAGGCATCACT
SPP1	F	AGCAAGAAACTCTTCCAAGCAA
SPP1	R	GTGAGATTCGTCAGATTCATCCG

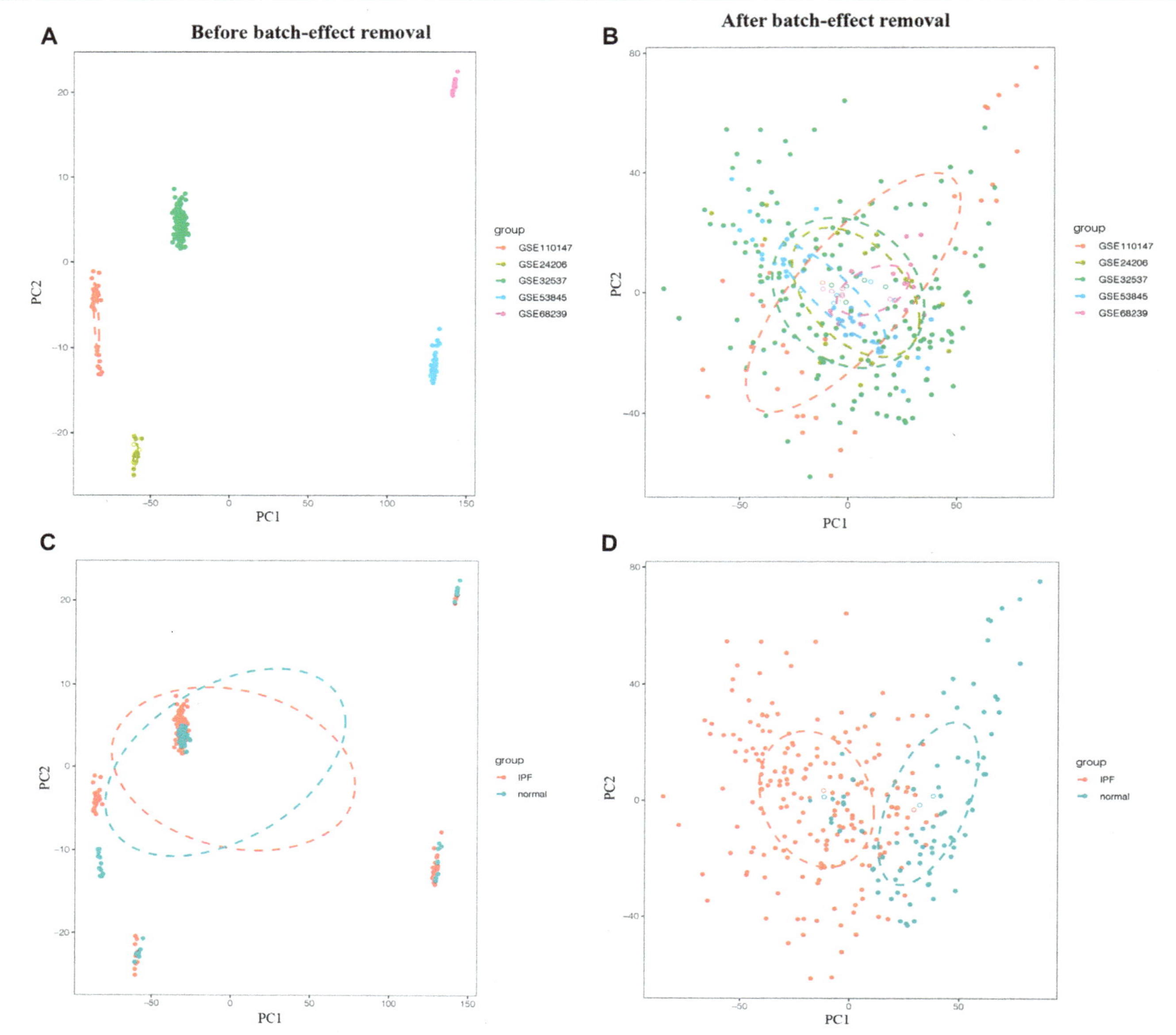

FIGURE 1 | Principal component analysis (PCA) of the training group. The points of the scatter plots represented the samples without **(A,C)** and with **(B,D)** the removal of batch effect based on the top two principal components (PC1 and PC2) of gene expression profiles. Samples from five different datasets were color coded **(A,B)**, and the colors represented the IPF group and the normal group, respectively **(C,D)**.

Identification of Differentially Expressed Genes

The Limma package 3.40.6 was used to compare DEGs between the normal group and the IPF group in the training group. The Benjamini-Hochberg's method was used to control the false discovery rate (FDR), and DEGs were selected through adopting the commonly used threshold of FDR p value <0.01 and |Log2 fold-change| > 1. The volcano plot of DEGs was generated by the ffplot2 package, and a heatmap of DEGs was produced using the pheatmap package in the R software.

Identification of Key Genes and Gene Set Enrichment Analysis

An online tool (http://bioinformatics.psb.ugent.be/webtools/Venn/) was employed to construct a Venn diagram to overlap the key genes in the significant modules and DEGs in the training group. The analyses of key genes of Gene Ontology (GO) and the Kyoto Encyclopedia of Genes and Genomes (KEGG) pathways were conducted using the GOplot, clusterProfiler, DOSE, colorspace, and the stringi packages in the R software.

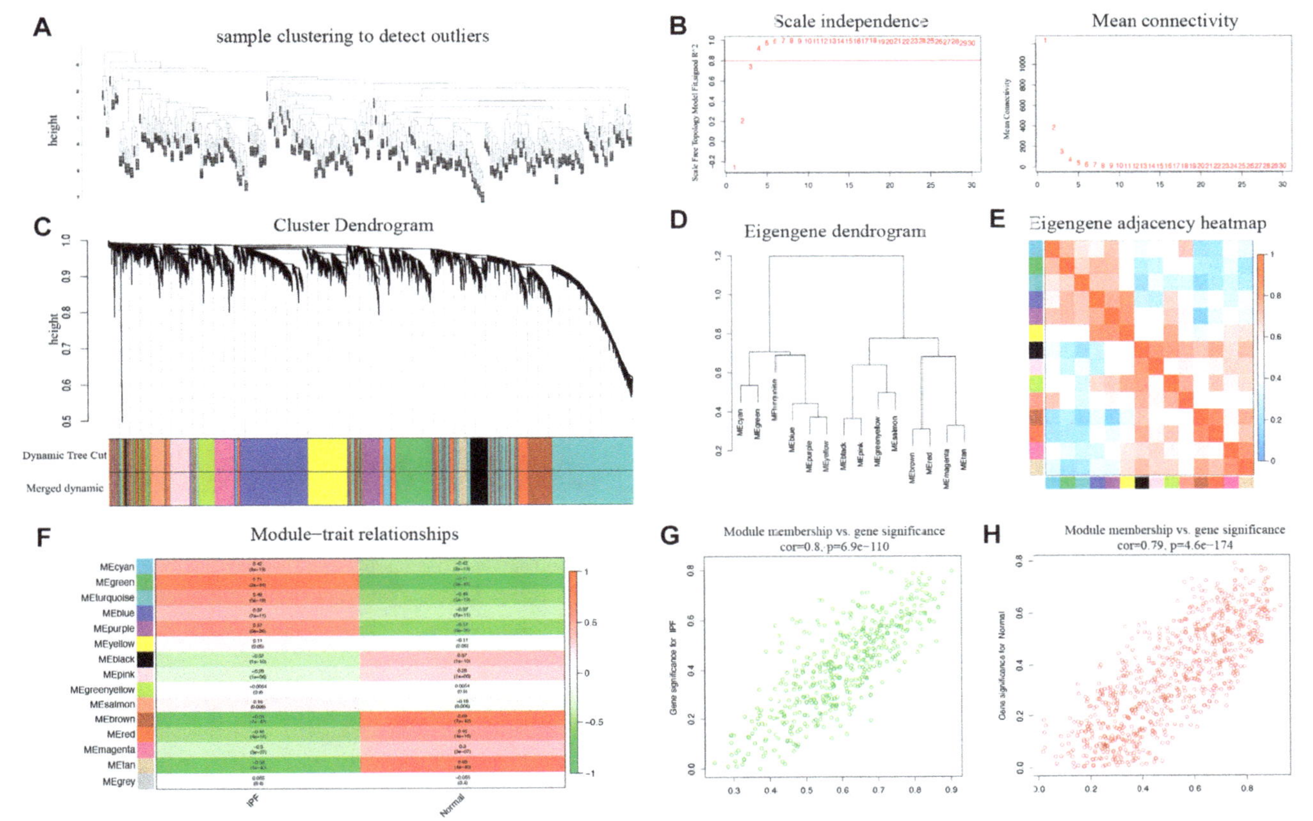

FIGURE 2 | Key modules identified by WGCNA in the training group. **(A)** Sample clustering to detect outliers. **(B)** Determination of soft-thresholding power. **(C)** Clustering dendrogram. Both of the original and the merged modules were presented. **(D)** Dendrogram of consensus module eigengenes obtained from WGCNA on the consensus correlation. **(E)** Dendrogram of merged module eigengenes obtained from WGCNA. **(F)** The module-trait relationships were evaluated by correlating module eigengenes with clinical traits. **(G)** Scatter plots of module eigengenes in the green modules. **(H)** Scatter plots of module eigengenes in the brown modules.

Protein-Protein Interaction Network Analysis

The Search Tool for the Retrieval of Interacting Genes (STRING, https://www. string-db. org/) was used to identify functional interactions between the products of the key genes in the training group. The PPI network was constructed using STRING by adopting the default threshold of a combined score >0.6. Then, the number of nodes of all the related proteins in the PPI network was counted using the R software and visualized using Cytoscape 3.8.2.

The Correlation Between Hub Genes

The ggcorrpolt and the ggthemes of the R package were used to determine the correlation between hub genes in the training and the validation groups, respectively. p value <0.01 was considered statistically significant.

Ethics Statement and Animal Treatment

In this study, 12 8 week-old male C57BL/6 mice weighing 20–25 g were obtained from Shanghai SLAC Laboratory Animal Ltd., China. Mice were bred at 22–24°C under a 12 h/12 h light/dark cycle and with free access to food and water. All procedures were implemented in conformity to the guidelines for animal care published by the United States' National Institutes of Health (NIH) for animal care (Guide for the Care and Use of Laboratory Animals, Department of Health and Human Services, NIH publication No. 86–23, revised 1985). All procedures were approved by Renji hospital, Shanghai Jiao Tong University School of Medicine, Shanghai, China (approval number: RJ-20170930). 5 mg/kg LPS was intraperitoneally injected for 5 consecutive days to 6 mice to induce pulmonary fibrosis as reported in our previous article (Wan et al., 2019). The other 6 mice served as control. The lung tissue of all mice was collected 30 days after LPS injection.

Hematoxylin and Eosin, Masson's Trichrome Staining and Immunohistochemistry

Lung tissue collected from both control and LPS injected mice was fixed in 4% paraformaldehyde solution for overnight, followed by dehydration in 70% ethanol and embedding in the paraffin wax. 5 μm thick sections were cut and subject to H&E

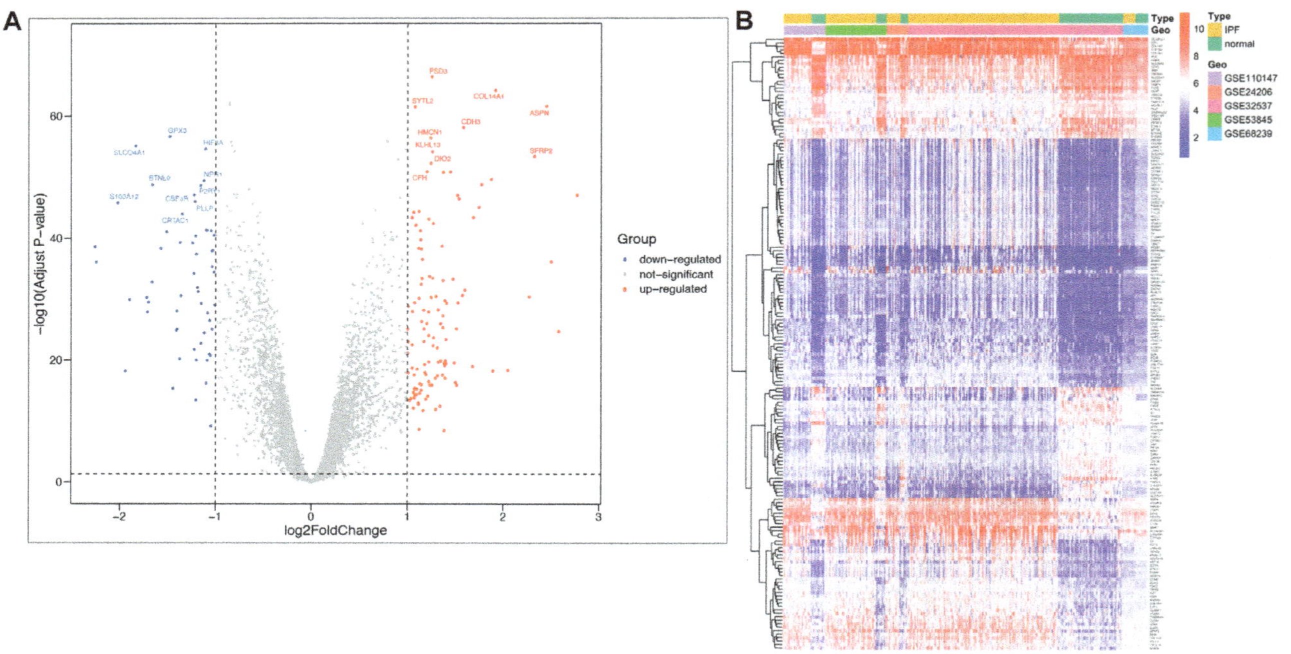

FIGURE 3 | Identification of DEGs in IPF and the enrichment of these genes in the training group. **(A)** Volcano plot of all DEGs. **(B)** Heatmap of all DEGs.

and Masson's trichrome staining, respectively, as previously described (Wan et al., 2019). Expression of α-SMA in the lung tissue was evaluated using immunohistochemical staining. Sample sections were deparaffinized and incubated with 5% goat serum containing 0.1% Triton X-100 at room temperature for 2 h, followed by sequential incubation in the primary (rabbit anti-α-SMA, 1:2000, CST, Cat No 19245) and secondary antibody solutions (goat anti-rabbit IgG, 1:1000, Jackson Immunoresearch Laboratory, Cat No 111-035-003) antibodies, each for 2 h. After 3 rinses with 1x PBS, the sections were incubated in a 3,3,-diaminobenzidine (DAB) reaction complex (Vector lab, Burlingame, CA, United States) until an optimal colour developed. At the end of the procedure, the sections were mounted and dehydrated before being coverslipped.

Quantitative Real-Time PCR and Statistical Analysis

Total RNA of the mouse lung tissue was isolated using Trizol (Thermofisher) according to the manufacturer's instructions. Primer Script RT reagent kit (Takara, Japan) was used to synthesize complementary DNA, and real-time PCR was run on a Quant Studio 1 real-time PCR system (Thermofisher, United States) using the TB Green Premix Ex Taq^{TM} kit (Takara, Japan). Glyceraldehyde-3-phosphate dehydrogenase (GAPDH) is stably expressed in the lung tissue during the process of pulmonary fibrosis. Therefore, it serves as a reliable endogenous control in the reverse transcription-polymerase chain reaction (Loitsch et al., 1999; Cruz-Bermúdez et al., 2019). The $2^{-\triangle\triangle Ct}$ method was employed to assess relative expression levels of genes of interest. All of the data were presented as mean ± standard error of mean (SEM) and analyzed using the GraphPad PRISM8 software (United States). Two-tailed Student's *t* test was used to compare between the two groups. $p < 0.001$ was considered statistically significant. Sequences of the primers could be found in **Table 2**.

Survival Analysis of Hub Genes

The Kaplan-Meier method (K-M method; product-limit method) is suitable for analysis with a small sample size. Survival analysis was performed using survfit R package in the R software. The difference in survival curves for IPF patients with different expression levels of hub genes was analyzed using the log-rank method provided by the survival package.

RESULTS

Removal of Batch Effects by Cross-Platform Normalization

To eliminate batch effects from different platforms and batches of datasets, the ComBat function of SVA package was used (Chen et al., 2020). Before the removal of batch effects, samples were clustered by batches based on the first two principal components (PC) of unnormalized expression values (**Figures 1A,C**). In contrast, the scatter plot of principal component analysis (PCA) based on normalized expression showed that batch processing effects from different platforms were eliminated (**Figures 1B,D**). These results confirmed that cross-platform standardization successfully eliminated batch effects.

TABLE 3 | DEGs in the training group.

DEGs	logFC	T	adj.*P*.Val	DEGs	logFC	T	adj.*P*.Val
MMP7	2.77203	17.63598	1.45E-45	TTC25	1.13038	8.34492	1.63E-14
MMP1	2.57792	11.49570	2.86E-24	SERPINB3	1.12534	6.17062	6.96E-09
CP	2.50036	14.67839	3.84E-35	COMP	1.12175	13.03885	1.84E-29
ASPN	2.45043	21.58471	2.65E-59	EPHA3	1.12035	16.91606	5.04E-43
SFRP2	2.32371	19.35112	1.18E-51	COL17A1	1.11795	15.28514	2.69E-37
KRT5	2.27018	13.10825	1.06E-29	CAPSL	1.11736	7.81414	4.85E-13
SPP1	2.04957	9.57238	3.87E-18	TEKT1	1.11608	7.72356	8.51E-13
COL14A1	1.91875	22.30443	1.38E-61	SLN	1.10315	9.63114	2.53E-18
PROM1	1.89389	9.54929	4.54E-18	ARMC4	1.09898	8.57409	3.58E-15
CD24	1.87693	18.33103	5.22E-48	C9orf135	1.09611	8.27343	2.58E-14
COL1A1	1.77486	18.10569	3.19E-47	CNTN3	1.08825	16.30609	7.36E-41
IL13RA2	1.74783	17.10082	1.11E-43	C10orf107	1.08106	8.24539	3.09E-14
COL3A1	1.69034	16.64818	4.49E-42	SYTL2	1.07978	21.56171	2.75E-59
SPAG6	1.68222	9.76954	9.58E-19	CCDC113	1.07764	8.61839	2.67E-15
POSTN	1.60165	13.40728	9.90E-31	FGF14	1.07645	12.83779	8.78E-29
CDH3	1.58629	20.63370	5.59E-56	DNAH11	1.07410	8.54680	4.30E-15
TDO2	1.57672	13.17209	6.44E-30	C6orf118	1.07219	8.08930	8.48E-14
THY1	1.54091	17.47384	5.18E-45	STK33	1.07050	9.32753	2.14E-17
SPATA18	1.53005	12.83180	9.10E-29	LTBP1	1.06576	16.87593	6.95E-43
SULF1	1.52483	17.62247	1.58E-45	SCGB3A1	1.06404	7.50102	3.34E-12
EFCAB1	1.51802	8.79445	8.24E-16	CLCA2	1.06387	8.38614	1.24E-14
WDR49	1.51485	11.61863	1.12E-24	CTSK	1.05448	12.43521	2.01E-27
ARMC3	1.50479	8.93218	3.24E-16	GPR87	1.05106	9.68485	1.74E-18
LRRIQ1	1.49233	9.94574	2.73E-19	CPA3	1.05092	10.85025	3.72E-22
CCDC80	1.47922	13.90511	1.87E-32	TRIM2	1.05023	16.64325	4.60E-42
FNDC1	1.45118	18.65814	3.50E-49	MDH1B	1.03320	8.05977	1.03E-13
MMP13	1.41253	12.81749	1.01E-28	RP1	1.02349	7.95282	2.03E-13
DSC3	1.40548	9.91334	3.42E-19	BCHE	1.01119	12.67214	3.19E-28
TMPRSS4	1.40534	11.10442	5.56E-23	FAM83D	1.01104	10.98620	1.34E-22
KRT15	1.39987	10.04997	1.28E-19	IGF1	1.00989	9.43908	9.76E-18
TSPAN1	1.39759	9.16860	6.38E-17	SERPINI2	1.00692	10.43532	7.83E-21
VSIG1	1.39411	9.79879	7.76E-19	NEK11	1.00509	11.60561	1.23E-24
SFRP4	1.39356	12.92391	4.51E-29	PTPRB	−1.00886	−12.73755	1.89E-28
SLC27A2	1.38762	9.93672	2.91E-19	GPR4	−1.01324	−15.86403	2.58E-39
MSMB	1.38711	6.09267	1.06E-08	CDH13	−1.01489	−14.21637	1.55E-33
LRRC17	1.37754	18.64756	3.67E-49	FAM107A	−1.02720	−15.18956	5.82E-37
FAP	1.37635	13.84266	3.06E-32	LRRC32	−1.03409	−14.46684	2.04E-34
VCAM1	1.37488	11.67872	7.09E-25	AFF3	−1.03498	−15.16171	7.31E-37
TMEM45A	1.37431	12.22798	1.00E-26	FPR1	−1.03536	−11.60303	1.25E-24
SPAG17	1.36994	9.32741	2.14E-17	PAPSS2	−1.04447	−16.05832	5.45E-40
HSPA4L	1.36353	15.37477	1.31E-37	ANKRD1	−1.04684	−6.38902	2.14E-09
CYP24A1	1.35190	10.04109	1.37E-19	PROK2	−1.05142	−10.31854	1.83E-20
SLITRK6	1.35026	11.86088	1.75E-25	PLA2G4F	−1.05968	−12.02025	5.07E-26
C20orf85	1.34465	7.61371	1.68E-12	HSD17B6	−1.06280	−10.37877	1.17E-20
WDR78	1.32791	9.98149	2.11E-19	CA4	−1.08075	−12.36029	3.54E-27
SLAMF7	1.32516	12.50422	1.19E-27	CACNA2D2	−1.08576	−10.07912	1.04E-19
GSTA1	1.31783	9.29345	2.71E-17	GRASP	−1.08796	−16.07649	4.82E-40
FANK1	1.31526	10.69559	1.15E-21	ACVRL1	−1.09478	−16.10034	4.06E-40
CLDN1	1.30119	13.12259	9.55E-30	FKBP5	−1.09614	−8.88744	4.39E-16
SCGB1A1	1.29900	7.41937	5.46E-12	HIF3A	−1.10235	−19.68359	8.92E-53
FAM81B	1.29639	9.15948	6.76E-17	SLC39A8	−1.11561	−11.43034	4.67E-24
RGS22	1.27438	11.18547	3.05E-23	NPR1	−1.11946	−18.27731	7.94E-48
LRRN1	1.27217	16.38499	3.81E-41	SMAD6	−1.14680	−12.80512	1.11E-28
MNS1	1.26945	10.80550	5.15E-22	CHI3L2	−1.14961	−10.91890	2.23E-22
CXCL14	1.26547	13.94959	1.33E-32	P2RY1	−1.15272	−18.05941	4.57E-47
KLHL13	1.26199	19.54838	2.33E-52	IL18R1	−1.17874	−13.34223	1.66E-30
C6	1.25902	8.78218	8.94E-16	SLCO2A1	−1.18823	−13.52812	3.82E-31
PSD3	1.25559	22.93054	1.21E-63	ID1	−1.19708	−15.01403	2.47E-36
PRSS12	1.24824	13.07355	1.39E-29	ZBTB16	−1.19762	−10.08938	9.64E-20
DIO2	1.24480	19.04587	1.42E-50	PGC	−1.20442	−7.95816	1.96E-13
HMCN1	1.24180	20.16614	2.28E-54	FASN	−1.20615	−15.82625	3.34E-39
CHST9	1.23465	8.79836	8.04E-16	PLLP	−1.21218	−17.35871	1.35E-44
DZIP3	1.23050	14.02285	7.40E-33	HHIP	−1.21951	−10.61885	2.03E-21
SPATA17	1.22401	9.99867	1.86E-19	CSF3R	−1.22052	−17.64669	1.36E-45

(Continued on following page)

TABLE 3 | *(Continued)* DEGs in the training group.

DEGs	logFC	T	adj.P.Val	DEGs	logFC	T	adj.P.Val
CXCL13	1.22326	8.97533	2.42E-16	INMT	−1.22178	−14.15692	2.48E-33
NELL2	1.22284	11.29983	1.27E-23	S100A9	−1.23775	−15.51469	4.21E-38
COL15A1	1.22278	16.57565	8.04E-42	CRTAC1	−1.34543	−16.80469	1.23E-42
SERPIND1	1.22108	12.41441	2.34E-27	IL18RAP	−1.35876	−13.16085	7.03E-30
DNAH9	1.21265	8.18456	4.61E-14	FMO5	−1.36614	−15.53888	3.46E-38
CFH	1.20440	18.66791	3.37E-49	AGER	−1.37110	−10.15923	5.84E-20
HHLA2	1.20322	11.86874	1.65E-25	ABCA3	−1.39859	−11.60612	1.22E-24
SOX2	1.19383	9.35110	1.82E-17	CLEC4E	−1.40101	−12.45507	1.74E-27
STOML3	1.19238	8.01573	1.36E-13	IL1RL1	−1.40643	−11.55651	1.78E-24
WDR63	1.18491	9.45155	8.98E-18	CPB2	−1.44059	-8.61043	2.81E-15
DNAH7	1.18030	9.86856	4.69E-19	GPX3	−1.47462	-20.23649	1.40E-54
CLIC6	1.17339	11.61737	1.13E-24	S100A8	−1.50688	−16.02132	7.36E-40
AMPD1	1.17332	11.00342	1.17E-22	MGAM	−1.56789	−15.28718	2.67E-37
SYNPO2	1.16962	12.49577	1.27E-27	BTNL9	−1.65868	−18.10805	3.19E-47
LRRC46	1.16388	7.35442	8.10E-12	PEBP4	−1.66297	−13.78816	4.80E-32
COL1A2	1.15626	14.78199	1.68E-35	PLA2G1B	−1.69918	−12.86725	7.02E-29
GEM	1.15200	13.93094	1.53E-32	MT1M	−1.70969	−12.41717	2.30E-27
MS4A2	1.14954	11.96580	7.75E-26	VIPR1	−1.71810	−13.07951	1.33E-29
CDH2	1.14648	15.24888	3.59E-37	SLCO4A1	−1.83259	−19.81841	3.06E-53
NEK10	1.14598	8.80644	7.61E-16	TMEM100	−1.89595	−12.98297	2.82E-29
ABCA13	1.14585	8.51578	5.27E-15	SLC6A4	−1.94099	-9.54127	4.80E-18
OGN	1.14330	13.67341	1.20E-31	S100A12	−2.02037	−17.30450	2.09E-44
CRISPLD1	1.13884	15.66068	1.29E-38	FCN3	−2.24401	−14.66999	4.09E-35
MXRA5	1.13572	16.05886	5.45E-40	IL1R2	−2.25735	−15.35214	1.57E-37
CASC1	1.13124	8.86592	5.08E-16				

Identification of IPF-Associated Weighted Correlation 26 Network Analysis Modules

A total of 287 samples and 6,263 genes retrieved from the training group were used for the co-expression network analysis (**Figure 2A**). An eigengene correlation coefficient square (r^2) of 0.8 and a soft threshold power of 3 were set to identify the module-trait relationship (**Figure 2B**). A hierarchical clustering tree was constructed following a dynamic hybrid cut (**Figure 2C**). The eigengene dendrogram and heatmap were used to quantify module similarity by eigengene correlation (**Figures 2D,E**). Among the 15 gene modules identified (**Figure 2F**), the green module (**Figure 2G**) showed a relatively higher positive correlation with the IPF group (cor = 0.71, $p < 0.001$), and the brown module (**Figure 2H**) exhibited significantly positive correlation with the IPF group (cor = −0.69, $p < 0.001$).

Idiopathic Pulmonary Fibrosis-Associated Key Genes and Their Functions

A total of 177 DEGs, including 121 up-regulated and 56 down-regulated genes, were identified in the training group (**Figures 3A,B, Table 3**). Among them, 72 genes were determined as key genes because they were shared by the green and brown modules (**Figure 4A** and **Table 4**). KEGG analysis revealed that the most notably enriched pathways were protein digestion and absorption and focal adhesion (**Figure 4B, Supplementary Table S1**). GO analysis showed that these genes were mainly involved in nine cellular components (**Figure 4D**), nine molecular functions (**Figure 4E**), and nine biological processes, including extracellular matrix organization (CCDC80, COL14A1, COL15A1, COL17A1, COL1A1, COL1A2, COL3A1, COMP, CTSK, FAP, MMP1, MMP7, POSTN, SFRP2, SPP1, SULF1, and VCAM1), extracellular structure organization (CCDC80, COL14A1, COL15A1, COL17A1, COL1A1, COL1A2, COL3A1, COMP, CTSK, FAP, MMP1, MMP7, POSTN, SFRP2, SPP1, SULF1, and VCAM1), response to TGF beta (ACVRL1, ASPN, CLDN1, COL1A1, COL1A2, COL3A1, ID1, LRRC32, LTBP1, MXRA5, POSTN, SMAD6), and others (**Figure 4C**), indicating that these genes could play important roles in the occurrence of IPF through influencing these biological processes and molecular functions.

Identification of Hub Genes

To explore hub genes, the PPI network analysis and cytoHubba plugin within cytoscape version 3.8.2 were performed based on the rank of the connection degree (number) of each gene. As shown in **Figures 5A,B,** nodes of 72 genes in the PPI network were identified according to the medium confidence ≥0.6. Finally, twelve hub genes were confirmed based on their node degrees within cytoHubba plugin (**Figure 5A**), including collagen alpha-1 chain (I) (COL1A1), collagen alpha-2 chain (I) (COL1A2), collagen alpha-1 (III) chain (COL3A1), collagen alpha-1 chain (XIV) (COL14A1), collagen alpha-1 chain (XV) (COL15A1), periostin (POSTN), secreted phosphoprotein 1 (SPP1), matrix metallopeptidase 1 (MMP1), matrix metallopeptidase 7 (MMP7), asporin (ASPN), cadherin 2 (CDH2), and cathepsin K (CTSK). In addition, correlation analysis showed a highly consistent positive correlation between 12 hub genes in both the training group (**Figures 5D,F**) and the validation group

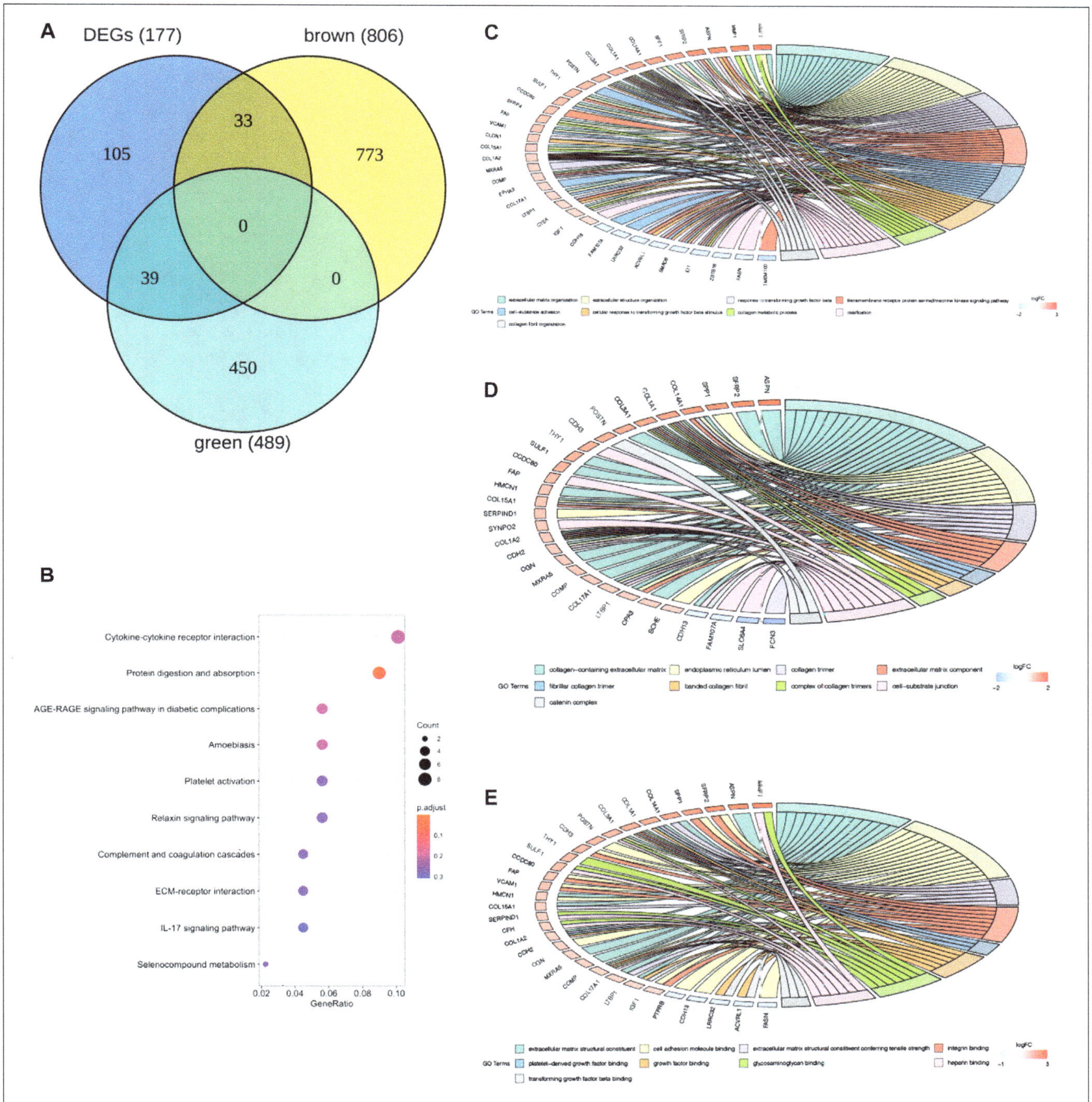

FIGURE 4 | GO and KEGG enrichment analysis of key genes in the training group. **(A)** The Venn diagram demonstrating key genes in the training group. **(B)** Kyoto encyclopedia of genes and genomes (KEGG) analysis of key genes **(E)**. Gene ontology (GO) analysis of key genes in the training group **(C–E)**, **(C)** BP: biological process, **(D)** CC: cellular component, **(E)** MF: molecular function.

(**Figures 5E,G**), such as COL1A2 and COL1A1, COL1A2 and COL3A1, COL1A2 and COL14A1, COL1A1 and COL3A1, COL1A1 and COL14A1, COL3A1 and COL14A1, SPP1 and MMP1, MMP1 and MMP7, POSTN and COL14A1, COL14A1 and COL15A1 ($0.17 < cor < 0.96$, $2.2E-16 < p < 0.039$), which further validated the results by PPI and cytoHubba plugin analysis (**Figure 5C**).

To further confirm the role of these 12 hub genes in IPF, another WGCNA for 6,252 genes obtained from GSE10667 of the training group was performed. It was found that the black

TABLE 4 | Key genes in the training group.

Key genes	logFC	adj.*P*.Val	module	*p*.GS.IPF	*p*.MMgreen	*p*.MMbrown
MMP7	2.77202754	1.45E-45	brown	5.30E-47	2.48E-21	2.87E-73
MMP1	2.57792316	2.86E-24	brown	5.09E-25	3.50E-15	7.98E-75
ASPN	2.45042861	2.65E-59	green	2.79E-61	6.46E-72	1.87E-19
SFRP2	2.32371277	1.18E-51	green	2.87E-53	7.07E-69	6.49E-40
SPP1	2.04957433	3.87E-18	brown	1.00E-18	1.07E-11	2.99E-69
COL14A1	1.91875456	1.38E-61	green	6.58E-64	1.08E-106	7.07E-38
COL1A1	1.77486012	3.19E-47	green	8.58E-49	1.23E-59	9.40E-31
IL13RA2	1.74782674	1.11E-43	green	4.06E-45	9.74E-37	4.43E-43
COL3A1	1.6903409	4.49E-42	green	1.82E-43	5.66E-63	2.63E-26
POSTN	1.6016506	9.90E-31	green	1.02E-31	2.69E-63	9.45E-26
CDH3	1.58629259	5.59E-56	brown	5.03E-58	1.08E-27	1.24E-83
THY1	1.54091349	5.18E-45	green	1.61E-46	2.66E-67	3.47E-27
SULF1	1.52483345	1.58E-45	green	4.55E-47	2.16E-71	3.70E-47
CCDC80	1.47922228	1.87E-32	green	1.65E-33	3.35E-65	4.08E-28
FNDC1	1.45118385	3.50E-49	green	6.98E-51	3.32E-61	1.85E-19
SFRP4	1.39356095	4.51E-29	green	5.09E-30	5.13E-56	2.73E-15
LRRC17	1.37753844	3.67E-49	green	7.23E-51	5.29E-76	2.11E-24
FAP	1.37635339	3.06E-32	green	2.68E-33	1.79E-44	2.49E-22
VCAM1	1.37488333	7.09E-25	green	1.11E-25	4.12E-37	3.64E-20
CLDN1	1.30119139	9.55E-30	brown	9.80E-31	2.17E-17	1.81E-60
CXCL14	1.26547198	1.33E-32	brown	1.06E-33	3.12E-30	2.76E-48
PSD3	1.25559334	1.21E-63	green	2.08E-66	3.62E-45	7.85E-42
DIO2	1.24479786	1.42E-50	green	2.21E-52	1.58E-63	2.59E-43
HMCN1	1.24179754	2.28E-54	green	1.77E-56	2.66E-69	5.68E-19
COL15A1	1.22278349	8.04E-42	green	2.65E-43	1.17E-78	1.18E-33
SERPIND1	1.22107917	2.34E-27	green	3.01E-28	1.52E-17	2.45E-24
CFH	1.20439698	3.37E-49	green	5.13E-51	9.50E-71	6.31E-29
SYNPO2	1.16962063	1.27E-27	green	1.53E-28	6.24E-68	4.75E-17
COL1A2	1.15626233	1.68E-35	green	9.57E-37	3.82E-65	7.11E-18
GEM	1.15200269	1.53E-32	green	1.17E-33	5.45E-56	2.55E-18
MS4A2	1.14954201	7.75E-26	green	1.07E-26	2.78E-44	2.17E-11
CDH2	1.14647827	3.59E-37	green	1.87E-38	2.24E-52	2.85E-27
OGN	1.14329874	1.20E-31	green	9.85E-33	2.86E-70	5.44E-14
MXRA5	1.13572189	5.45E-40	green	1.96E-41	2.90E-56	6.45E-27
COMP	1.12174857	1.84E-29	green	1.81E-30	2.67E-32	1.30E-24
EPHA3	1.12035363	5.04E-43	green	1.33E-44	1.15E-75	2.16E-18
COL17A1	1.11795013	2.69E-37	brown	1.35E-38	1.07E-22	3.90E-66
SLN	1.10315195	2.53E-18	green	6.10E-19	2.72E-34	1.93E-26
SYTL2	1.07977843	2.75E-59	green	1.13E-61	2.54E-64	3.95E-48
LTBP1	1.06576443	6.95E-43	green	1.76E-44	5.44E-93	4.58E-23
CTSK	1.05448468	2.01E-27	green	2.38E-28	4.70E-37	2.13E-33
CPA3	1.05091777	3.72E-22	green	6.51E-23	1.78E-38	1.02E-10
BCHE	1.01119209	3.19E-28	green	3.40E-29	1.02E-50	2.49E-11
FAM83D	1.01103826	1.34E-22	green	2.25E-23	5.23E-32	6.98E-24
IGF1	1.00988527	9.76E-18	green	2.41E-18	2.62E-51	1.22E-25
PTPRB	−1.0088593	1.89E-28	brown	1.99E-29	6.74E-12	1.22E-93
CDH13	−1.0148952	1.55E-33	brown	9.83E-35	9.31E-09	1.60E-64
FAM107A	−1.0272098	5.82E-37	brown	2.77E-38	1.90E-20	1.28E-60
LRRC32	−1.0340983	2.04E-34	brown	1.23E-35	1.19E-18	1.13E-45
AFF3	−1.0349871	7.31E-37	brown	3.54E-38	3.94E-25	2.76E-71
PAPSS2	−1.0444732	5.45E-40	brown	1.79E-41	5.89E-24	3.39E-92
CA4	−1.0807466	3.54E-27	brown	4.41E-28	6.60E-26	9.75E-78
GRASP	−1.0879563	4.82E-40	brown	1.61E-41	1.50E-23	6.02E-55
ACVRL1	−1.094783	4.06E-40	brown	1.33E-41	3.35E-23	1.21E-102
HIF3A	−1.1023551	8.92E-53	brown	8.22E-55	1.77E-27	4.71E-84
NPR1	−1.1194655	7.94E-48	brown	1.26E-49	4.32E-21	6.18E-96
SMAD6	−1.1468095	1.11E-28	brown	1.23E-29	6.60E-23	6.82E-85
P2RY1	−1.1527251	4.57E-47	brown	8.37E-49	2.79E-29	1.28E-64
SLCO2A1	−1.1882355	3.82E-31	brown	3.35E-32	7.44E-15	9.97E-90
ID1	−1.197083	2.47E-36	brown	1.40E-37	1.37E-30	4.03E-49
ZBTB16	−1.1976268	9.64E-20	brown	2.13E-20	8.96E-15	7.42E-30
FASN	−1.2061532	3.34E-39	brown	1.49E-40	6.58E-34	9.60E-35
PLLP	−1.2121833	1.35E-44	brown	3.42E-46	1.56E-36	2.59E-89
INMT	−1.2217822	2.48E-33	brown	1.85E-34	1.02E-13	1.67E-83

(Continued on following page)

TABLE 4 | *(Continued)* Key genes in the training group.

Key genes	logFC	adj.*P*.Val	module	*p*.GS.IPF	*p*.MMgreen	*p*.MMbrown
CRTAC1	−1.3454348	1.23E-42	brown	4.15E-44	4.62E-50	1.30E-54
FMO5	−1.3661473	3.46E-38	green	1.85E-39	3.11E-33	1.02E-42
GPX3	−1.4746242	1.40E-54	brown	1.26E-56	4.55E-26	1.03E-90
BTNL9	−1.6586875	3.19E-47	brown	8.05E-49	2.28E-29	1.37E-91
VIPR1	−1.7181029	1.33E-29	brown	1.52E-30	8.84E-25	8.16E-109
TMEM100	−1.8959563	2.82E-29	brown	3.41E-30	5.53E-22	8.15E-97
SLC6A4	−1.9409992	4.80E-18	brown	1.25E-18	3.81E-17	1.51E-82
FCN3	−2.2440192	4.09E-35	brown	3.23E-36	2.01E-31	1.07E-76

and greenyellow modules, containing 12 hub genes, out of the 14 gene modules identified (**Figure S1a**) showed strong association with IPF (black module: cor = -0.63, $p < 0.001$; greenyellow module: cor = 0.81, $p < 0.001$) (**Supplementary Figures S1B–D**). These hub genes were involved in many important IPF-related biological processes, such as extracellular matrix organization, response to TGF beta, collagen metabolic process, fibrillar collagen trimer, etc (**Supplementary Table S2**). These results suggested that the abovementioned hub genes play important roles in the occurrence of IPF.

Expression Validation of Hub Genes by Quantitative Real-Time -PCR

The clustering heatmap showed expression levels of hub genes in the training (**Figure 6A**) and the validation groups (**Figure 6B**). Expression levels of 12 hub genes showed consistent upregulation in both the training (**Figure 6C**) and the validation groups (**Figure 6D**). To further validate the results, qRT-PCR was conducted in the LPS-induced pulmonary fibrosis model. The modeling process was described in detail in our previous study (Wan et al., 2019). Firstly, mice were intraperitoneally injected with saline or LPS (5 mg/kg) for 5 consecutive days, and samples were collected on day 30 after LPS injection. H&E E/MASSON staining and α-SMA immunohistochemistry (**Figure 7A**) showed that the model of pulmonary fibrosis was successfully constructed. The lung tissue of 6 control and 6 LPS injected mice was collected. As shown in **Figure 7B**, expression levels of COL1A1, COL1A2, COL3A1, COL14A1, MMP1, MMP7, ASPN, CDH2, SPP1, POSTN, and CTSK were significantly increased in the lung tissue of LPS injected mice compared with that of control mice ($p < 0.001$), whereas the expression level of COL15A1 was undetectable in the lung tissue of either the control or LPS injected mice. These results demonstrated important roles COL1A1, COL1A2, COL3A1, COL14A1, MMP1, MMP7, ASPN, CDH2, SPP1, POSTN and CTSK play in IPF occurrence.

Survival Analysis of Hub Genes in the Validation Group

To explore the prognostic value of these 12 hub genes for IPF patients, overall survival analysis was performed using the GSE70866 dataset. It was found that IPF patients with high expression levels of COL1A1, CTSK, MMP1, MMP7, and SPP1 had poorer overall survival compared to those with low expression levels ($p < 0.05$). No significant correlation was found between expression levels of other hub genes and survival of IPF patients ($p > 0.05$, **Figure 8**).

DISCUSSION

Idiopathic pulmonary fibrosis (IPF) is an end-stage lung disease with a short survival time after diagnosis is confirmed (Liu et al., 2018). Therefore, it is vital to illuminate the underlying mechanism of IPF pathogenesis and to explore potential biomarkers for early diagnosis in order to improve the prognosis of IPF patients.

The present study used bioinformatic methods to screen IPF-related genes and tentatively tested their roles in the occurrence and prognosis of IPF based on the gene expression data of IPF patients in the GEO databases. Compared to other bioinformatics analyses, WGCNA is more valuable due to the comprehensive examination of links between co-expression modules and clinical traits with high reliability and biological significance (Wei et al., 2014; Kong et al., 2020; Lund et al., 2020). In the present study, 11 hub genes (COL1A2, COL1A1, COL3A1, SPP1, MMP1, POSTN, ASPN, CDH2, COL14A1, CTSK, MMP7) were found to be associated with the occurrence of IPF using WGCNA, differential gene expression analysis in the training datasets, PPI network analysis, and cytoHubba plugin analyses. Expression of these genes was validated in the GSE10667 dataset and in pulmonary fibrosis model mice using qRT-PCR. These results are consistent with those of previous studies in that COL1A1, COL1A2, COL3A1, COL14A1, POSTN, SPP1, MMP1, ASPN, MMP7, CDH2, and CTSK were up-regulated in a variety of samples from IPF patients and IPF-related mouse models, including blood, bronchoalveolar lavage, airway fibroblasts, and the lung tissue of human and mice, as well as involved in the occurrence of IPF (**Supplementary Table S3**) (Tzortzaki et al., 2003; Brule et al., 2005; Obermajer et al., 2006; Ivan et al., 2008; Naik et al., 2012; Vittal et al., 2013; Zhang et al., 2013; Hamai et al., 2016; Ghavami et al., 2018; Liu et al., 2018; Morimoto et al., 2018; Gao et al., 2019; Yu et al., 2020).

The collagen binding protein ASPN, a member of the family of leucine-rich repeat proteins, is produced by

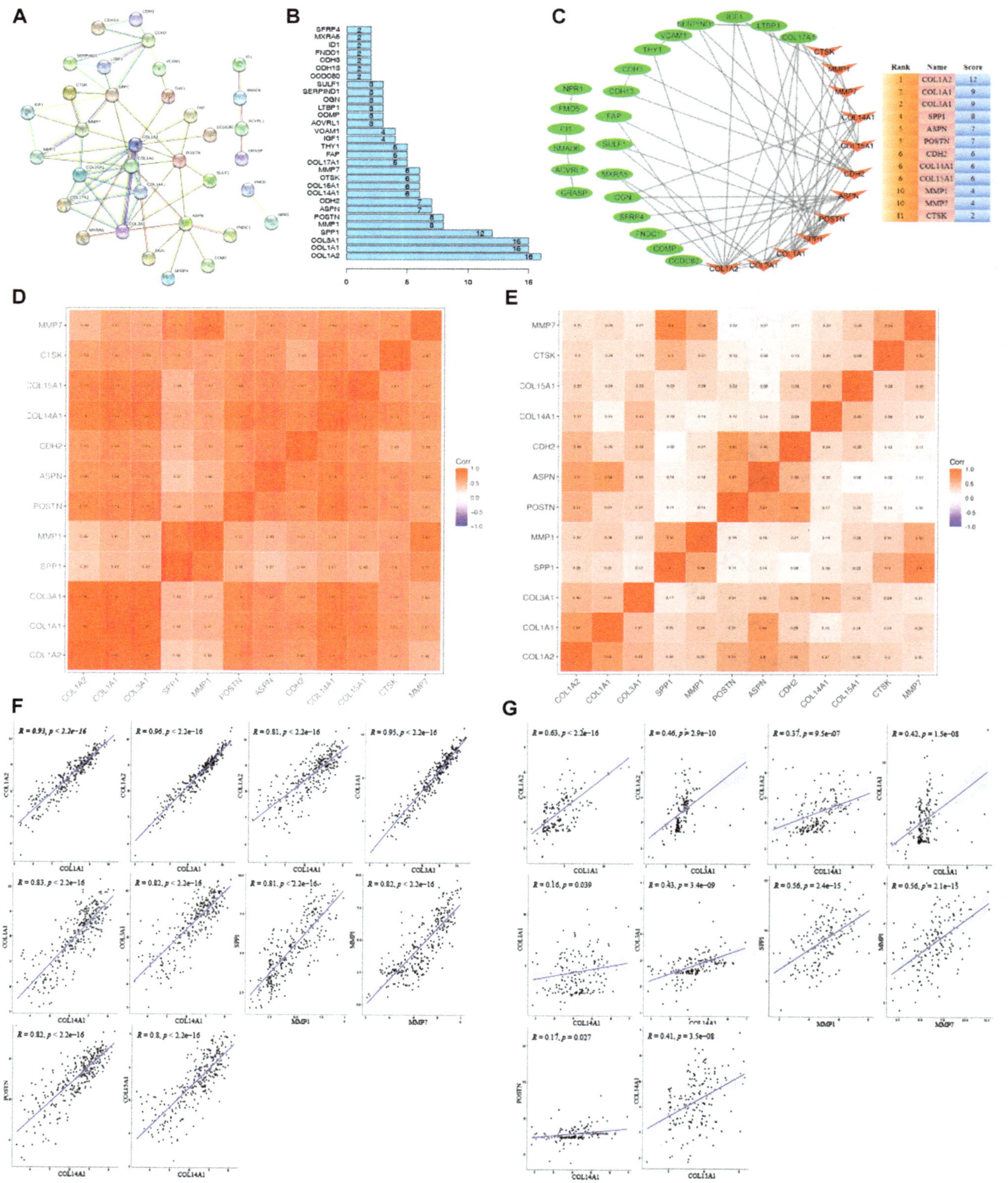

FIGURE 5 | Cluster analysis of the PPI network in the training group. **(A)** Protein-protein interaction (PPI) network for key genes. **(B)** Histogram of key genes. **(C)** The hub gene network analyzed by Cytosacpe. **(D)** Correlation between hub genes in the training group. **(E)** Correlation between hub genes in the validation group. **(F)** Display of correlations between ten groups of genes with a correlation coefficient >0.8 in the training group. **(G)** Display of correlations between ten groups of genes in the validation group.

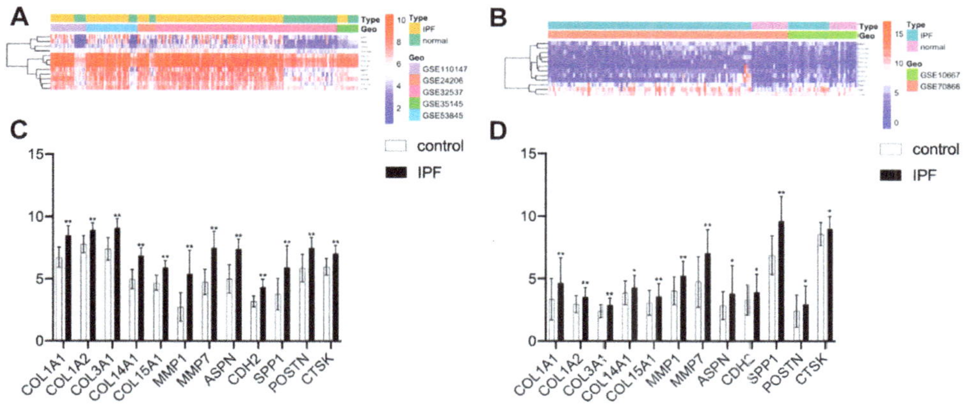

FIGURE 6 | Correlation analysis of hub genes. **(A)** Heatmap of the training group. **(B)** Heatmap of the validation group. **(C)** Expression levels of twelve hub genes (healthy control samples vs IPF samples) from the training group. **(D)** Expression levels of twelve hub genes from the validation group (*$p < 0.05$, **$p < 0.01$).

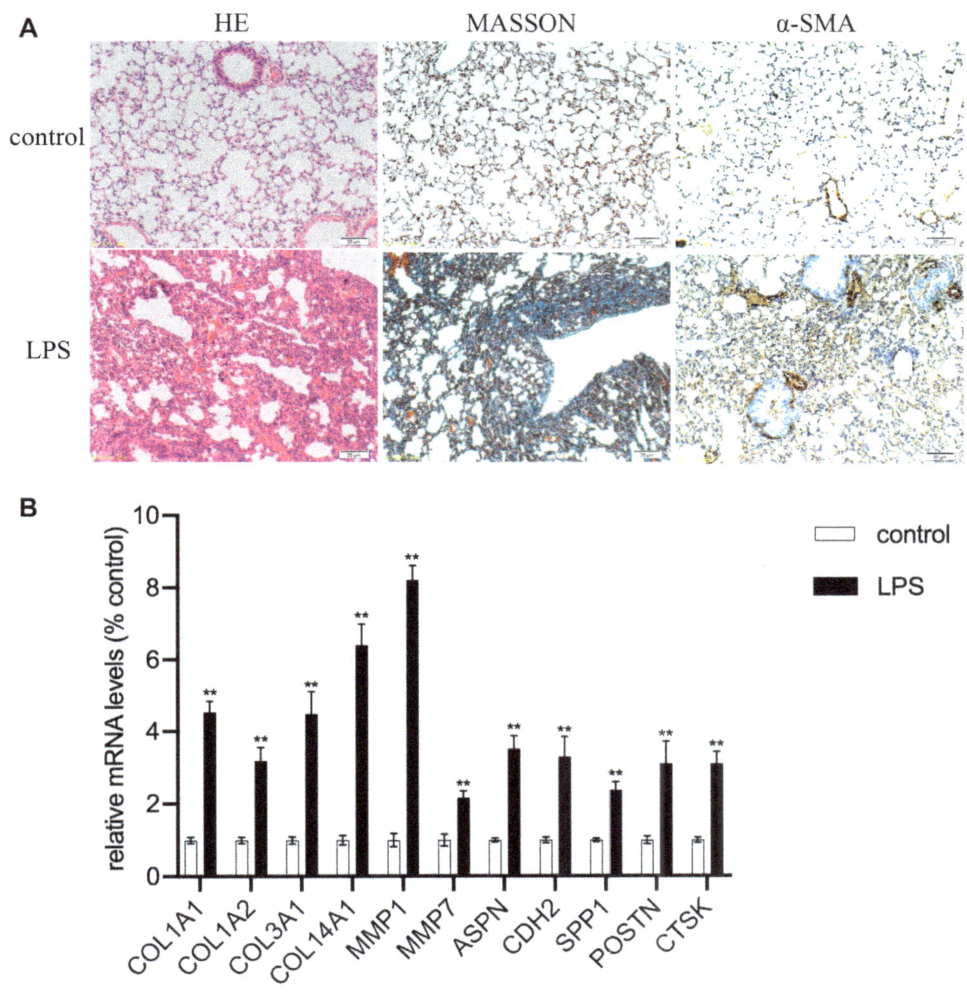

FIGURE 7 | Expression validation of hub genes. **(A)** The severity of pulmonary fibrosis was determined by hematoxylin-eosin (HE) staining, collagen deposition was assessed by Masson's trichrome staining, and α-SMA expression in the lung tissue was detected by immunohistochemistry (magnification, ×200). **(B)** Expression levels of COL1A1, COL1A2, COL3A1, COL14A1, MMP1, MMP7, ASPN, CDH2, SPP1, POSRN, CTSK mRNAs in lung tissue samples (**$p < 0.01$).

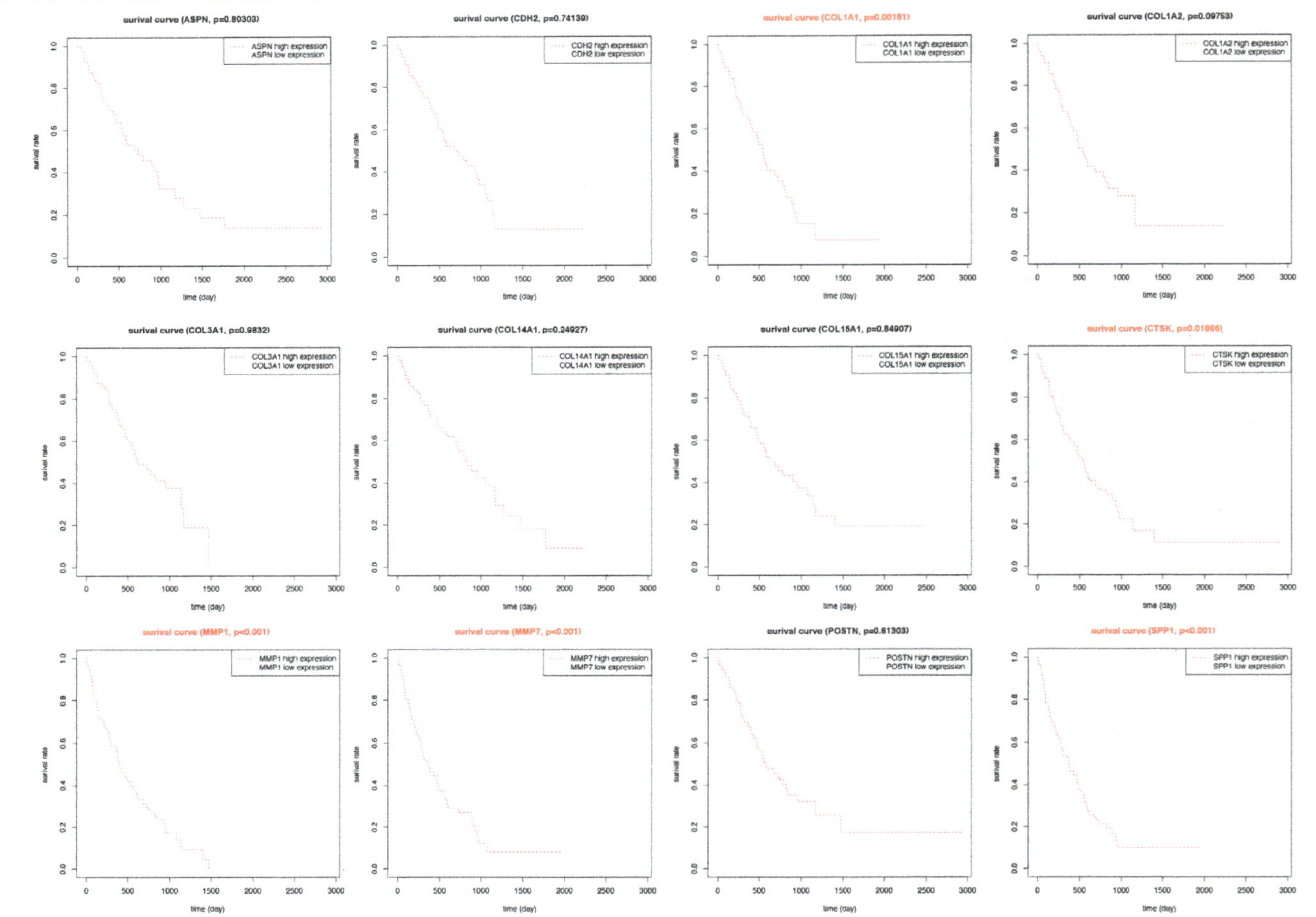

FIGURE 8 | Survival analysis for hub genes in the validation group. Kaplan-Meier plot depicting association of the expression level of twelve individual hub genes with patient survival.

fibroblasts (Nakajima et al., 2007). A previous study showed that the expression of ASPN was up-regulated in the IPF(+) soluble fractions (Åhrman et al., 2018). COL1A1, a functional gene that encodes the alpha 1 chain of type I collagen, is the main constituent of ECM component (Li et al., 2020) and participates in cell proliferation, infiltration, metastasis, and angiogenesis. Its expression is related to many types of tumors (Bi et al., 2017; Ma et al., 2019; Dong et al., 2020). It is known that type III collagen interacts with type I and type II collagen in fibril formation and is an essential regulator of fibril diameter. The increase in type I, III, XIV, XV collagen content will lead to the formation of fibrils. Like many fibrotic disorders, IPF is characterized by enhanced deposition and remodeling of ECM (Tjin et al., 2017). Matrix metalloproteinases (MMPs) are a family of calcium- and zinc-dependent endopeptidases (Visse and Nagase, 2003) whose function is to regulate abnormal epithelial response to injury, fibroblast proliferation, extracellular matrix accumulation, and aberrant tissue remodeling (Ivan et al., 2008). MMPs play a role in different pathological processes such as atherosclerosis (Wågsäter et al., 2011), arthritis (Huang et al., 2017), tumor invasion, and pulmonary fibrosis (Ivan et al., 2008). POSTN plays a notable role in ECM structure and organization and principally in collagen assembly. Secreted phosphoprotein 1 (SPP1), also known as osteopontin-like protein, is a multifunctional secretory acidic glycoprotein (Zhang et al., 2017). Earlier research displayed that POSTN can promote myofibroblast differentiation and type I collagen production, contributing to aberrant lung fibrosis. Serum levels of POSTN may predict the clinical progression of IPF (O'Dwyer and Moore, 2017; Morse et al., 2019; Alimperti and Andreadis, 2015). SPP1 can be secreted by various cells, such as osteoclasts, macrophages, epithelial cells, and endothelial cells. Prior studies reported that low-level local proliferation of macrophages that highly express SPP1 in the normal lung tissue was strikingly increased in IPF lungs, and macrophages that highly express SPP1 importantly contribute to lung fibrosis in IPF34. CDH2, a calcium-dependent cell adhesion protein and also a mesenchymal cell marker, preferentially mediates homotypic cell-cell adhesion by dimerization with a CDH2 chain from another cell (Alimperti and Andreadis, 2015). Previous study showed that CDH2 was involved in epithelial-mesenchymal transition (EMT) which contributes to pulmonary fibrosis (Gao et al., 2019). CTSK displays potent endoprotease activity against fibrinogen (Obermajer et al., 2006), and the expression level of CTSK was up-regulated in the silica induced pulmonary fibrosis model (Brule et al., 2005). These suggested that 11 hub genes identified in the present study play important roles in IPF occurrence.

To explore the prognostic value of these hub genes, survival analysis was performed. It was found that COL1A1, CTSK, MMP1, MMP7, and SPP1 could be potential biomarkers for poor prognosis of IPF patients because the survival rate of IPF patients with high expression levels of COL1A1, CTSK, MMP1, MMP7, and SPP1 was lower than that of those with low expression levels of the abovementioned genes. A number of studies have reported that type I (COL1A1) collagen and matrix metalloproteinases (MMP1 and MMP7) are fibrotic genes associated with the occurrence and prognosis of IPF (Ivan et al., 2008; Giménez et al., 2017; Adegunsoye et al., 2020; Liu et al., 2020; Xu et al., 2020; Mishra et al., 2021). However, further clinical investigation on these genes is warranted.

GO and KEGG pathway enrichment analyses revealed that COL1A1, COL1A2, COL3A1, COL14A1, POSTN, SPP1, MMP1, ASPN, MMP7, CDH2, and CTSK were involved in multiple biological processes related to extracellular matrix organization and collagen metabolism by protein digestion and absorption signaling pathways. In addition, correlation analysis, and PPI as well as cytoHubba plugin analyses showed a highly consistent positive correlation between hub genes in both the training group and the validation group. These results suggest that altered expression of these genes and their crosstalk might impact the development of IPF by modulating the above biological processes and signaling pathways.

The present study analyzed results of seven GEO datasets including 337 IPF samples and 120 control samples to identify possible biomarkers that facilitate elucidation of the underlying molecular mechanism of IPF using a variety of bioinformatics methods (WGCNA, different gene expression analysis, PPI, correlation analysis, etc.). These results were confirmed in 7 GEO datasets, indicating a high reliability and validity. They will shed light on the potential pathogenic mechanism of IPF and guide the development of more potent drugs for IPF.

CONCLUSION

In summary, results of the present study suggest that ASPN, CDH2, COL1A1, COL1A2, COL3A1, COL14A1, MMP1, POSTN, SPP1, MMP7, and CTSK are potential biomarkers of IPF. Altered expression of these genes and their cross-talk might impact the development of IPF by modulating IPF-related biological processes and signaling pathways. COL1A1, CTSK, MMP1, MMP7, and SPP1 are positively correlated with IPF prognosis. This study provides further insights into individualized treatment and prognosis for IPF.

AUTHOR CONTRIBUTIONS

HW and XH designed the experiments, prepared the manuscript and performed data analysis. PC, MH, AC, TW, DD, WL, LT and XG did the data curation. LX and HL oversaw the project and revised the manuscript.

REFERENCES

Adegunsoye, A., Alqalyoobi, S., Linderholm, A., Bowman, W. S., Lee, C. T., Pugashetti, J. V., et al. (2020). Circulating Plasma Biomarkers of Survival in Antifibrotic-Treated Patients with Idiopathic Pulmonary Fibrosis. *Chest* 158, 1526–1534. doi:10.1016/j.chest.2020.04.066

Åhrman, E., Hallgren, O., Malmström, L., Hedström, U., Malmström, A., Bjermer, L., et al. (2018). Quantitative Proteomic Characterization of the Lung Extracellular Matrix in Chronic Obstructive Pulmonary Disease and Idiopathic Pulmonary Fibrosis. *J. Proteomics* 189, 23–33. doi:10.1016/j.jprot.2018.02.027

Alimperti, S., and Andreadis, S. T. (2015). CDH2 and CDH11 Act as Regulators of Stem Cell Fate Decisions. *Stem Cel Res.* 14, 270–282. doi:10.1016/j.scr.2015.02.002

Behr, J., Nathan, S. D., Wuyts, W. A., Mogulkoc Bishop, N., Bouros, D. E., Antoniou, K., et al. (2021). Efficacy and Safety of Sildenafil Added to Pirfenidone in Patients with Advanced Idiopathic Pulmonary Fibrosis and Risk of Pulmonary Hypertension: a Double-Blind, Randomised, Placebo-Controlled, Phase 2b Trial. *Lancet Respir. Med.* 9, 85–95. doi:10.1016/s2213-2600(20)30356-8

Bi, S., Chai, L., Yuan, X., Cao, C., and Li, S. (2017). MicroRNA-98 Inhibits the Cell Proliferation of Human Hypertrophic Scar Fibroblasts via Targeting Col1A1. *Biol. Res.* 50, 22. doi:10.1186/s40659-017-0127-6

Brule, S., Misson, P., Buhling, F., Lison, D., and Huaux, F. (2005). Overexpression of Cathepsin K during Silica-Induced Lung Fibrosis and Control by TGF-Beta. *Respir. Res.* 6, 84. doi:10.1186/1465-9921-6-84

Chen, W., Zhang, S., Williams, J., Ju, B., Shaner, B., Easton, J., et al. (2020). A Comparison of Methods Accounting for Batch Effects in Differential Expression Analysis of UMI Count Based Single Cell RNA Sequencing. *Comput. Struct. Biotechnol. J.* 18, 861–873. doi:10.1016/j.csbj.2020.03.026

Claude, J., and Harold, A. (2018). Idiopathic Pulmonary Fibrosis: Cell Death and Inflammation Revisited. *Am. J. Respir. Cel Mol. Biol.* 59, 137–138. doi:10.1165/rcmb.2018-0083ED

Cruz-Bermúdez, A., Laza-Briviesca, R., Vicente-Blanco, R. J., García-Grande, A., Coronado, M. J., Laine-Menéndez, S., et al. (2019). Cancer-associated Fibroblasts Modify Lung Cancer Metabolism Involving ROS and TGF-β Signaling. *Free Radic. Biol. Med.* 130, 163–173. doi:10.1016/j.freeradbiomed.2018.10.450

DePianto, D. J., Chandriani, S., Abbas, A. R., Jia, G., N'Diaye, E. N., Caplazi, P., et al. (2015). Heterogeneous Gene Expression Signatures Correspond to Distinct Lung Pathologies and Biomarkers of Disease Severity in Idiopathic Pulmonary Fibrosis. *Thorax* 70, 48–56. doi:10.1136/thoraxjnl-2013-204596

Dong, X.-Z., Zhao, Z.-R., Hu, Y., Lu, Y.-P., Liu, P., and Zhang, L. (2020). LncRNA COL1A1-014 Is Involved in the Progression of Gastric Cancer via Regulating CXCL12-CXCR4 axis. *Gastric Cancer* 23, 260–272. doi:10.1007/s10120-019-01011-0

Gao, L., Jiang, D., Geng, J., Dong, R., and Dai, H. (2019). Hydrogen Inhalation Attenuated Bleomycin-induced Pulmonary Fibrosis by Inhibiting Transforming Growth Factor-β1 and Relevant Oxidative Stress and Epithelial-to-mesenchymal Transition. *Exp. Physiol.* 104, 1942–1951. doi:10.1113/ep088028

Ghavami, S., Yeganeh, B., Zeki, A. A., Shojaei, S., Kenyon, N. J., Ott, S., et al. (2018). Autophagy and the Unfolded Protein Response Promote Profibrotic Effects of TGF-B1 in Human Lung Fibroblasts. *Am. J. Physiology-Lung Cell Mol. Physiol.* 314, L493–L504. doi:10.1152/ajplung.00372.2017

Giménez, A., Duch, P., Puig, M., Gabasa, M., Xaubet, A., and Alcaraz, J. (2017). Dysregulated Collagen Homeostasis by Matrix Stiffening and TGF-B1 in Fibroblasts from Idiopathic Pulmonary Fibrosis Patients: Role of FAK/Akt. *Ijms* 18, 2431. doi:10.3390/ijms18112431

Hamai, K., Iwamoto, H., Ishikawa, N., Horimasu, Y., Masuda, T., Miyamoto, S., et al. (2016). Comparative Study of Circulating MMP-7, CCL18, KL-6, SP-A, and SP-D as Disease Markers of Idiopathic Pulmonary Fibrosis. *Dis. Markers* 2016, 4759040. doi:10.1155/2016/4759040

Huang, T.-L., Mu, N., Gu, J.-T., Shu, Z., Zhang, K., Zhao, J.-K., et al. (2017). DDR2-CYR61-MMP1 Signaling Pathway Promotes Bone Erosion in Rheumatoid Arthritis through Regulating Migration and Invasion of Fibroblast-like Synoviocytes. *J. Bone Miner Res.* 32, 407–418. doi:10.1002/jbmr.2993

Huang, X., Lv, D., Yang, X., Li, M., and Zhang, H. (2020). m6A RNA Methylation Regulators Could Contribute to the Occurrence of Chronic Obstructive Pulmonary Disease. *J. Cel. Mol. Med.* 24 (21), 12706–12715. doi:10.1111/jcmm.15848

Hutchinson, J., Fogarty, A., Hubbard, R., and McKeever, T. (2015). Global Incidence and Mortality of Idiopathic Pulmonary Fibrosis: a Systematic Review. *Eur. Respir. J.* 46, 795–806. doi:10.1183/09031936.00185114

Ivan, O., Thomas, J., and Kazuhisa, K. (2008). MMP1 and MMP7 as Potential Peripheral Blood Biomarkers in Idiopathic Pulmonary Fibrosis. *Plos Med.* 5, e93. doi:10.1371/journal.pmed.0050093

King, T. E., Jr., Bradford, W. Z., Castro-Bernardini, S., Fagan, E. A., Glaspole, I., Glassberg, M. K., et al. (2014). A Phase 3 Trial of Pirfenidone in Patients with Idiopathic Pulmonary Fibrosis. *N. Engl. J. Med.* 370, 2083–2092. doi:10.1056/nejmoa1402582

Kong, Y., Feng, Z. C., Zhang, Y. L., Liu, X. F., Ma, Y., and Zhao, Z. M. (2020). Identification of Immune-Related Genes Contributing to the Development of Glioblastoma Using Weighted Gene Co-expression Network Analysis. *Front. Immunol.* 11, 1281. doi:10.3389/fimmu.2020.01281

Li, H., Chang, H. M., Shi, Z., and Leung, P. C. K. (2020). The P38 Signaling Pathway Mediates the TGF-β1-induced Increase in Type I Collagen Deposition in Human Granulosa Cells. *FASEB j.* 34, 15591–15604. doi:10.1096/fj.202001377r

Liu, Y., Wang, Y., Lu, F., Wang, L., Miao, L., and Wang, X. (2020). BTB and CNC Homology 1 Inhibition Ameliorates Fibrosis and Inflammation via Blocking ERK Pathway in Pulmonary Fibrosis. *Exp. Lung Res.* 26, 1–11. doi:10.1080/01902148.2020.1849448

Liu, Y., Zhu, M., Geng, J., Ban, C., Zhang, S., Chen, W., et al. (2018). Incidence and Radiologic-pathological Features of Lung Cancer in Idiopathic Pulmonary Fibrosis. *Clin. Respir. J.* 12, 1700–1705. doi:10.1111/crj.12732

Loitsch, S. M., Kippenberger, S., Dauletbaev, N., Wagner, T. O., and Bargon, J. (1999). Reverse Transcription-Competitive Multiplex PCR Improves Quantification of mRNA in Clinical Samples-Application to the Low Abundance CFTR mRNA. *Clin. Chem.* 45 (5), 619–624. doi:10.1093/clinchem/45.5.619

Lund, J. B., Li, S., Baumbach, J., Christensen, K., Li, W., Mohammadnejad, A., et al. (2020). Weighted Gene Coregulation Network Analysis of Promoter DNA Methylation on All-Cause Mortality in Old-Aged Birth Cohorts Finds Modules of High-Risk Associated Biomarkers. *J. Gerontol. A. Biol. Sci. Med. Sci.* 75, 2249–2257. doi:10.1093/gerona/glaa066

Ma, H.-P., Chang, H.-L., Bamodu, O. A., Yadav, V. K., Huang, T.-Y., Wu, A. T. H., et al. (2019). Collagen 1A1 (COL1A1) Is a Reliable Biomarker and Putative Therapeutic Target for Hepatocellular Carcinogenesis and Metastasis. *Cancers* 11, 786. doi:10.3390/cancers11060786

Maher, T. M., Stowasser, S., Nishioka, Y., White, E. S., Cottin, V., Noth, I., et al. (2019). Biomarkers of Extracellular Matrix Turnover in Patients with Idiopathic Pulmonary Fibrosis Given Nintedanib (INMARK Study): a Randomised, Placebo-Controlled Study. *Lancet Respir. Med.* 7, 771–779. doi:10.1016/S2213-2600(19)30255-3

Martinez, F. J., Collard, H. R., Pardo, A., Raghu, G., Richeldi, L., Selman, M., et al. (2017). Idiopathic Pulmonary Fibrosis. *Nat. Rev. Dis. Primers* 3, 17074. doi:10.1038/nrdp.2017.74

Mishra, S., Shah, M. I., Udhaya Kumar, S., Thirumal Kumar, D., Gopalakrishnan, C., Al-Subaie, A. M., et al. (2021). Network Analysis of Transcriptomics Data for the Prediction and Prioritization of Membrane-Associated Biomarkers for Idiopathic Pulmonary Fibrosis (IPF) by Bioinformatics Approach. *Adv. Protein Chem. Struct. Biol.* 123, 241–273. doi:10.1016/bs.apcsb.2020.10.003

Morimoto, Y., Hirahara, K., Kiuchi, M., Wada, T., Ichikawa, T., Kanno, T., et al. (2018). Amphiregulin-Producing Pathogenic Memory T Helper 2 Cells Instruct Eosinophils to Secrete Osteopontin and Facilitate Airway Fibrosis. *Immunity* 49, 134–150. doi:10.1016/j.immuni.2018.04.023

Morse, C., Tabib, T., Sembrat, J., Buschur, K. L., Bittar, H. T., Valenzi, E., et al. (2019). Proliferating SPP1/MERTK-Expressing Macrophages in Idiopathic Pulmonary Fibrosis. *Eur. Respir. J.* 54, 1802441. doi:10.1183/13993003.02441-2018

Naik, P. K., Bozyk, P. D., Bentley, J. K., Popova, A. P., Birch, C. M., Wilke, C. A., et al. (2012). Periostin Promotes Fibrosis and Predicts Progression in Patients with Idiopathic Pulmonary Fibrosis. *Am. J. Physiology-Lung Cell Mol. Physiol.* 303, L1046–L1056. doi:10.1152/ajplung.00139.2012

Nakajima, M., Kizawa, H., Saitoh, M., Kou, I., Miyazono, K., and Ikegawa, S. (2007). Mechanisms for Asporin Function and Regulation in Articular Cartilage. *J. Biol. Chem.* 282, 32185–32192. doi:10.1074/jbc.m700522200

O'Dwyer, D. N., Ashley, S. L., Gurczynski, S. J., Xia, M., Wilke, C., Falkowski, N. R, et al. (2019). Lung Microbiota Contribute to Pulmonary Inflammation and Disease Progression in Pulmonary Fibrosis. *Am. J. Respir. Crit. Care Med.* 199, 1127–1138. doi:10.1164/rccm.201809-1650OC

O'Dwyer, D. N., and Moore, B. B. (2017). The Role of Periostin in Lung Fibrosis and Airway Remodeling. *Cell Mol Life Sci.* 74, 4305–4314. doi:10.1007/s00018-017-2649-z

Obermajer, N., Premzl, A., Zavašnik Bergant, T., Turk, B., and Kos, J. (2006). Carboxypeptidase Cathepsin X Mediates β2-integrin-dependent Adhesion of Differentiated U-937 Cells. *Exp. Cel Res.* 312, 2515–2527. doi:10.1016/j.yexcr.2006.04.019

Pei, G., Chen, L., and Zhang, W. (2017). WGCNA Application to Proteomic and Metabolomic Data Analysis. *Methods Enzymol.* 585, 135–158. doi:10.1016/bs.mie.2016.09.016

Raghu, G., Remy-Jardin, M., Myers, J. L., Richeldi, L., Ryerson, C. J., Lederer, D. J., et al. (2018). Diagnosis of Idiopathic Pulmonary Fibrosis. An Official ATS/ERS/JRS/ALAT Clinical Practice Guideline. *Am. J. Respir. Crit. Care Med.* 198, e44–e68. doi:10.1164/rccm.201807-1255st

Saito, S., Alkhatib, A., Kolls, J. K., Kondoh, Y., and Lasky, J. A. (2019). Pharmacotherapy and Adjunctive Treatment for Idiopathic Pulmonary Fibrosis (IPF). *J. Thorac. Dis.* 11, S1740–S1754. doi:10.21037/jtd.2019.04.62

Schäfer, S. C., Funke-Chambour, M., and Berezowska, S. (2020). Idiopathische Lungenfibrose - Epidemiologie, Ursachen und klinischer Verlauf. *Pathologe* 41, 46–51. doi:10.1007/s00292-019-00747-x

Tjin, G., White, E. S., Faiz, A., Sicard, D., Tschumperlin, D. J., Mahar, A., et al. (2017). Lysyl Oxidases Regulate Fibrillar Collagen Remodelling in Idiopathic Pulmonary Fibrosis. *Dis. Model. Mech.* 10, 1301–1312. doi:10.1242/dmm.030114

Tran, T., and Suissa, S. (2018). The Effect of Anti-acid Therapy on Survival in Idiopathic Pulmonary Fibrosis: a Methodological Review of Observational Studies. *Eur. Respir. J.* 51. doi:10.1183/13993003.00376-2018

Tzortzaki, E. G., Tischfield, J. A., Sahota, A., Siafakas, N. M., Gordon, M. K., and Gerecke, D. R. (2003). Expression of FACIT Collagens XII and XIV during Bleomycin-Induced Pulmonary Fibrosis in Mice. *Anat. Rec.* 275A, 1073–1080. doi:10.1002/ar.a.10120

Visse, R., and Nagase, H. (2003). Matrix Metalloproteinases and Tissue Inhibitors of Metalloproteinases. *Circ. Res.* 92, 827–839. doi:10.1161/01.res.0000070112.80711.3d

Vittal, R., Mickler, E. A., Fisher, A. J., Zhang, C., Rothhaar, K., Gu, H., et al. (2013). Type V Collagen Induced Tolerance Suppresses Collagen Deposition, TGF-Beta and Associated Transcripts in Pulmonary Fibrosis. *PLoS One* 8, e76451. doi:10.1371/journal.pone.0076451

Wågsäter, D., Zhu, C., Björkegren, J., Skogsberg, J., and Eriksson, P. (2011). MMP-2 and MMP-9 Are Prominent Matrix Metalloproteinases during Atherosclerosis Development in the Ldlr(-/-)Apob(100/100) Mouse. *Int. J. Mol. Med.* 28, 247–253. doi:10.3892/ijmm.2011.693

Wan, H., Xie, T., Xu, Q., Hu, X., Xing, S., Yang, H., et al. (2019). Thy-1 Depletion and Integrin β3 Upregulation-Mediated PI3K-Akt-mTOR Pathway Activation Inhibits Lung Fibroblast Autophagy in Lipopolysaccharide-Induced Pulmonary Fibrosis. *Lab. Invest.* 99 (11), 1636–1649. doi:10.1038/s41374-019-0281-2

Wang, Y., Yella, J., Chen, J., McCormack, F. X., Madala, S. K., and Jegga, A. G. (2017). Unsupervised Gene Expression Analyses Identify IPF-Severity Correlated Signatures, Associated Genes and Biomarkers. *BMC Pulm. Med.* 17, 133. doi:10.1186/s12890-017-0472-9

Wei, C., An-Lin, C., Marco, B., Chou, W. C., Cheng, A. L., and Brotto, M. (2014). Visual Gene-Network Analysis Reveals the Cancer Gene Co-expression in Human Endometrial Cancer. *BMC Genomics* 15, 300. doi:10.1186/1471-2164-15-300

Xu, Y., Mizuno, T., Sridharan, A., Du, Y., Guo, M., Tang, J., et al. (2016). Single-cell RNA Sequencing Identifies Diverse Roles of Epithelial Cells in Idiopathic Pulmonary Fibrosis. *JCI Insight* 1, e90558. doi:10.1172/jci.insight.90558

Xu, Z., Mo, L., Feng, X., Huang, M., and Li, L. (2020). Using Bioinformatics Approach Identifies Key Genes and Pathways in Idiopathic Pulmonary Fibrosis. *Medicine (Baltimore)* 99 (36), e22099. doi:10.1097/md.0000000000022099

Yu, D. H., Ruan, X. L., Huang, J. Y., Liu, X. P., Ma, H. L., Chen, C., et al. (2020). Analysis of the Interaction Network of Hub miRNAs-Hub Genes, Being Involved in Idiopathic Pulmonary Fibers and its Emerging Role in Non-small Cell Lung Cancer. *Front. Genet.* 11, 302. doi:10.3389/fgene.2020.00302

Zhang, X., Liu, H., Hock, T., Thannickal, V., and Sanders, Y. (2013). Histone Deacetylase Inhibition Downregulates Collagen 3A1 in Fibrotic Lung Fibroblasts. *Ijms* 14, 19605–19617. doi:10.3390/ijms141019605

Zhang, Y., Du, W., Chen, Z., and Xiang, C. (2017). Upregulation of PD-L1 by SPP1 Mediates Macrophage Polarization and Facilitates Immune Escape in Lung Adenocarcinoma. *Exp. Cel Res.* 359, 449–457. doi:10.1016/j.yexcr.2017.08.028

Permissions

All chapters in this book were first published by Frontiers; hereby published with permission under the Creative Commons Attribution License or equivalent. Every chapter published in this book has been scrutinized by our experts. Their significance has been extensively debated. The topics covered herein carry significant findings which will fuel the growth of the discipline. They may even be implemented as practical applications or may be referred to as a beginning point for another development.

The contributors of this book come from diverse backgrounds, making this book a truly international effort. This book will bring forth new frontiers with its revolutionizing research information and detailed analysis of the nascent developments around the world.

We would like to thank all the contributing authors for lending their expertise to make the book truly unique. They have played a crucial role in the development of this book. Without their invaluable contributions this book wouldn't have been possible. They have made vital efforts to compile up to date information on the varied aspects of this subject to make this book a valuable addition to the collection of many professionals and students.

This book was conceptualized with the vision of imparting up-to-date information and advanced data in this field. To ensure the same, a matchless editorial board was set up. Every individual on the board went through rigorous rounds of assessment to prove their worth. After which they invested a large part of their time researching and compiling the most relevant data for our readers.

The editorial board has been involved in producing this book since its inception. They have spent rigorous hours researching and exploring the diverse topics which have resulted in the successful publishing of this book. They have passed on their knowledge of decades through this book. To expedite this challenging task, the publisher supported the team at every step. A small team of assistant editors was also appointed to further simplify the editing procedure and attain best results for the readers.

Apart from the editorial board, the designing team has also invested a significant amount of their time in understanding the subject and creating the most relevant covers. They scrutinized every image to scout for the most suitable representation of the subject and create an appropriate cover for the book.

The publishing team has been an ardent support to the editorial, designing and production team. Their endless efforts to recruit the best for this project, has resulted in the accomplishment of this book. They are a veteran in the field of academics and their pool of knowledge is as vast as their experience in printing. Their expertise and guidance has proved useful at every step. Their uncompromising quality standards have made this book an exceptional effort. Their encouragement from time to time has been an inspiration for everyone.

The publisher and the editorial board hope that this book will prove to be a valuable piece of knowledge for researchers, students, practitioners and scholars across the globe.

List of Contributors

Jia He, Yue Du, Gaopeng Li, Peng Xiao, Xingzheng Sun, Wenjun Song, Lihua Lai, Meng Xia and Qingqing Wang
Institute of Immunology, Zhejiang University School of Medicine, Hangzhou, China
The Key Laboratory for Immunity and Inflammatory Diseases of Zhejiang Province, Hangzhou, China

Jianhua Zhang
Department of Medical Laboratory, School of Medicine, Shaoxing University, Shaoxing, China

Xiaohe Li, Rui Liu, Yunyao Cui, Jingjing Liang, Shimeng Li, Honggang Zhou and Cheng Yang
State Key Laboratory of Medicinal Chemical Biology, College of Pharmacy and Tianjin Key Laboratory of Molecular Drug Research, Nankai University, Tianjin, China
Tianjin Key Laboratory of Molecular Drug Research, Tianjin International Joint Academy of Biomedicine, Tianjin, China

Yang Miao and Zhun Bi
State Key Laboratory of Medicinal Chemical Biology, College of Pharmacy and Tianjin Key Laboratory of Molecular Drug Research, Nankai University, Tianjin, China

Liang Zhang and Xiaoping Li
Department of Thoracic Surgery, Tian Jin First Central Hospital, Tianjin, China

Pingping Bing, Wenhu Zhou and Songwen Tan
Academician Workstation, Changsha Medical University, Changsha, China

Cristina Estornut, María Amparo Bayarri and Nada Belhadj
Department of Pharmacology, Faculty of Medicine, University of Valencia, Valencia, Spain

Javier Milara
Department of Pharmacology, Faculty of Medicine, University of Valencia, Valencia, Spain
Pharmacy Unit, University General Hospital Consortium, Valencia, Spain
CIBERES, Health Institute Carlos III, Valencia, Spain

Julio Cortijo
Department of Pharmacology, Faculty of Medicine, University of Valencia, Valencia, Spain
Pharmacy Unit, University General Hospital Consortium, Valencia, Spain
CIBERES, Health Institute Carlos III, Valencia, Spain
Research and Teaching Unit, University General Hospital Consortium, Valencia, Spain

Hao Shen, Xuerong Yang, Yuanyuan He, Qi Li, Xiaoyan Shen and Yong Yang
Department of Pharmacy, Sichuan Academy of Medical Sciences and Sichuan Provincial People's Hospital, School of Medicine, University of Electronic Science and Technology of China, Chengdu, China
Personalized Drug Therapy Key Laboratory of Sichuan Province, School of Medicine, University of Electronic Science and Technology of China, Chengdu, China

Nu Zhang
Department of Pharmacy, People's Hospital of Fushun County, Fushun, China

Yuqing Liu
School of Basic Medicine and Clinical Pharmacy, China Pharmaceutical University, Nanjing, China

Yulian Zhu
Department of Pharmacy, Ziyang People's Hospital, Ziyang, China

Wan-Tong Zhang and Xu-Jie Wang
Xiyuan Hospital, China Academy of Chinese Medical Sciences, Beijing, China

Chun-Miao Xue, Lin Pan, Guo-Dong Hua and Bao-Chen Zhu
Dongzhimen Hospital, Beijing University of Chinese Medicine, Beijing, China

Xin-Yu Ji
Institute of Basic Research in Clinical Medicine, China Academy of Chinese Medical Sciences, Beijing, China

Wei-Liang Weng and Qiu-Yan Li
Xiyuan Hospital, China Academy of Chinese Medical Sciences, Beijing, China
National Clinical Research Center for Chinese Medicine Cardiology, Beijing, China

Menglin Zou, Xingxing Hu, Weishuai Zheng, Mingyang Zhang and Zhenshun Cheng
Department of Respiratory and Critical Care Medicine, Zhongnan Hospital of Wuhan University, Wuhan, China

Jingfeng Zou
Department of Respiratory and Critical Care Medicine, Jiangxi Provincial People's Hospital, Nanchang, China

Eric S. White
Boehringer Ingelheim Pharmaceuticals, Inc., Ridgefield, CT, United States

Matthew Thomas
Boehringer Ingelheim Pharma GmbH & Co. KG, Biberach, Germany

Susanne Stowasser
Boehringer Ingelheim International GmbH, Ingelheim am Rhein, Germany

Kay Tetzlaff
Boehringer Ingelheim International GmbH, Ingelheim am Rhein, Germany
Department of Sports Medicine, University of Tübingen, Tübingen, Germany

Laura Bergantini, Alessandro Mainardi, Miriana d'Alessandro, Paolo Cameli, David Bennett, Elena Bargagli and Piersante Sestini
Department of Medical Sciences, Surgery and Neurosciences, Respiratory Disease and Lung Transplant Unit, Respiratory Diseases and Transplant Unit, Siena University, Siena, Italy

Fei Jing, Jingbo Xue, Yuan Peng and Feng Xing
Institute of Liver Diseases, Shuguang Hospital Affiliated to Shanghai University of Traditional Chinese Medicine, Shanghai, China

Xi Chen and Kai Huang
Shanghai Key Laboratory of Traditional Chinese Clinical Medicine, Shanghai, China

Xudong Hu
School of Basic Medical Sciences, Shanghai University of Traditional Chinese Medicine, Shanghai, China

Chenghai Liu
Institute of Liver Diseases, Shuguang Hospital Affiliated to Shanghai University of Traditional Chinese Medicine, Shanghai, China
Shanghai Key Laboratory of Traditional Chinese Clinical Medicine, Shanghai, China
Key Laboratory of Liver and Kidney Diseases, Ministry of Education, Shanghai, China

Hongwei Han
Department of Biology, Georgia State University, Atlanta, GA, United States
Division of Pulmonary and Critical Care, Department of Medicine, Massachusetts General Hospital, Harvard Medical School, Boston, MA, United States

Guangda Peng and Zhi-Ren Liu
Department of Biology, Georgia State University, Atlanta, GA, United States

Maureen Meister and Xiangming Ji
Department of Nutrition, Georgia State University, Atlanta, GA, United States

Hongwei Yao
Division of Biology and Medicine, Department of Molecular Biology, Cell Biology and Biochemistry, Brown University, Providence, RI, United States

Jenny J. Yang
Department of Chemistry, Georgia State University, Atlanta, GA, United States

Ming-Hui Zou
Center for Molecular and Translational Medicine, Georgia State University, Atlanta, GA, United States

Yanzhen Yu, Xingzhi Liu and Zhongjuan Xu
School of Nano-Tech and Nano-Bionics, University of Science and Technology of China, Hefei, China
CAS Key Laboratory of Nano-Bio Interface, Suzhou Institute of Nano-Tech and Nano-Bionics, Chinese Academy of Sciences, Suzhou, China

Zhe Zhao, Yong Qiao and Guangli Suo
CAS Key Laboratory of Nano-Bio Interface, Suzhou Institute of Nano-Tech and Nano-Bionics, Chinese Academy of Sciences, Suzhou, China

Yuanshuai Zhou
Jiangsu Key Lab of Medical Optics, Suzhou Institute of Biomedical Engineering and Technology, Chinese Academy of Sciences, Suzhou, China

Hong Qiao
Department of Molecular Biosciences, the University of Texas at Austin, Austin, TX, United States

Junjie Zhong
Department of Neurosurgery, Fudan University Huashan Hospital, National Key Laboratory of Medical Neurobiology, Institutes of Brain Science, Shanghai Medical College, Fudan University, Shanghai, China

Jianwu Dai
State Key Laboratory of Molecular, Developmental Biology, Institute of Genetics and Developmental Biology, Chinese Academy of Sciences, Beijing, China

Zhen Li, Jing Geng, Bingbing Xie, Jiarui He, Yinan Hu, Huaping Dai and Chen Wang
Department of Pulmonary and Critical Care Medicine, Center of Respiratory Medicine, China-Japan Friendship Hospital; National Center for Respiratory Medicine; National Clinical Research Center for Respiratory Diseases; Institute of Respiratory Medicine, Chinese Academy of Medical Sciences, Peking Union Medical College, Beijing, China

Jing Wang
State Key Laboratory of Medical Molecular Biology, Department of Physiology, Institute of Basic Medical Sciences Chinese Academy of Medical Sciences, School of Basic Medicine Peking Union Medical College, Beijing, China

Liang Peng
Institute of Clinical Medical Sciences, China-Japan Friendship Hospital, Beijing, China

Xia Guo, Christudas Sunil and Guoqing Qian
Department of Cellular and Molecular Biology, The University of Texas Health Science Center at Tyler, The University of Texas at Tyler, Tyler, TX, United States

Yiliang Su, Li Shen, Fen Zhang, Xing Jiang, Xiaofeng Jin, Yuan Zhang, Yang Hu, Ying Zhou, Qiuhong Li and Huiping Li
Department of Respiratory and Critical Care Medicine, Shanghai Pulmonary Hospital, School of Medicine, Tongji University, Shanghai, China

Rosa Metella Refini, Valerio Alonzi, Carlo Magnoni and Paola Rottoli
Respiratory Diseases Unit, Department of Medicine, Surgery and Neurosciences, University of Siena, Siena, Italy

Jiali Min, Qiao Li, Suosi Liu, Qianrong Wang, Min Yin, Yan Zhang and Shanshan Liu
National Clinical Research Center for Metabolic Diseases, Key Laboratory of Diabetes Immunology, Ministry of Education, Department of Metabolism and Endocrinology, The Second Xiangya Hospital of Central South University, Changsha, China

Jun Yan
Beijing Institute of Brain Disorders, Capital Medical University, Beijing, China

Bing Cui
State Key Laboratory of Bioactive Substance and Function of Natural Medicines, Institute of Materia Medica, Chinese Academy of Medical Sciences and Peking Union Medical College, Beijing, China

Hanxi Wan, Peilin Cong, Tingmei Wu, Danqing Dai, Wanrong Li, Xiaofei Gao, Huazheng Liang and Mengfan He
Department of Anesthesiology and Perioperative Medicine, School of Medcine, Shanghai Fourth People's Hospital, Tongji University, Shanghai, China
Translational Research Institute of Brain and Brain-Like Intelligence, School of Medcine, Shanghai Fourth People's Hospital, Tongji University, Shanghai, China

Xinwei Huang and Aiwen Chen
Translational Research Institute of Brain and Brain-Like Intelligence, School of Medcine, Shanghai Fourth People's Hospital, Tongji University, Shanghai, China

Lize Xiong and Li Tian
Department of Anesthesiology and Perioperative Medicine, School of Medcine, Shanghai Fourth People's Hospital, Tongji University, Shanghai, China
Translational Research Institute of Brain and Brain-Like Intelligence, School of Medcine, Shanghai Fourth People's Hospital, Tongji University, Shanghai, China
Clinical Research Center for Anesthesiology and Perioperative Medicine, Tongji University, Shanghai, China

Index

www.ingramcontent.com/pod-product-compliance
Lightning Source LLC
LaVergne TN
LVHW061511220926
848485LV00017B/865
9781646475162